KU-031-034

VASCULAR TRAUMA

VASCULAR TRAUMA

SECOND EDITION

NORMAN M. RICH, M.D.
Leonard Heaton and David Packard Professor
Chairman, Department of Surgery, USUHS
Chief, Division of Vascular Surgery, Emeritus
F. Edward Herbert School of Medicine
Uniformed Services University of the Health Sciences
Bethesda, Maryland

KENNETH L. MATTOX, M.D.
Professor and Vice Chairman
Michael E. DeBakey Department of Surgery
Baylor College of Medicine
Chief of Staff and Chief of Surgery
Ben Taub General Hospital
Houston, Texas

ASHER HIRSHBERG, M.D.
Associate Professor
Michael E. DeBakey Department of Surgery
Baylor College of Medicine
Director of Vascular Surgery
Ben Taub General Hospital
Houston, Texas

ELSEVIER
SAUNDERS

ELSEVIER
SAUNDERS

The Curtis Center
Independence Square West
Philadelphia, Pennsylvania 19106

ISBN: 0-7216-4071-0

VASCULAR TRAUMA, SECOND EDITION
Copyright © 2004, Elsevier Science (USA). All rights reserved.

No part of this publication may be reproduced or transmitted in any form or by any means, electronic or mechanical, including photocopying, recording, or any information storage and retrieval system, without permission in writing from the publisher. Permissions may be sought directly from Elsevier's Health Sciences Rights Department in Philadelphia, PA, USA: phone: (+1) 215 238 7869, fax: (+1) 215 238 2239, e-mail: healthpermissions@elsevier.com. You may also complete your request on-line via the Elsevier Science homepage (http://www.elsevier.com), by selecting 'Customer Support' and then 'Obtaining Permissions'.

NOTICE

Surgery is an ever-changing field. Standard safety precautions must be followed, but as new research and clinical experience broaden our knowledge, changes in treatment and drug therapy may become necessary or appropriate. Readers are advised to check the most current product information provided by the manufacturer of each drug to be administered to verify the recommended dose, the method and duration of administration, and contraindications. It is the responsibility of the licensed prescriber, relying on experience and knowledge of the patient, to determine dosages and the best treatment for each individual patient. Neither the publisher nor the author assumes any liability for any injury and/or damage to persons or property arising from this publication.

The Publisher

Previous edition copyrighted 1978

International Standard Book Number: 0-7216-4071-0

Printed in the United States of America

Last digit is the print number: 9 8 7 6 5 4 3 2 1

To those who serve and have served our
country

—in the military, both at home and in
distant lands
—in our nation's trauma centers
—in the education of surgeons with an
interest in vascular disease
—in the development of new knowledge
—in safety net hospitals

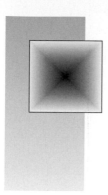

CONTRIBUTORS

JOHN T. ANDERSON, MD
Assistant Professor
Department of Surgery
Trauma Surgery and Surgical Critical Care
University of California, Davis
Sacramento, California

JUAN A. ASENSIO, MD
Associate Professor
Department of Surgery
University of Southern California Keck School of Medicine
Los Angeles, California

WALTER L. BIFFL, MD
Associate Professor
Department of Surgery
Brown Medical School
Chief, Division of Trauma and Surgical Critical Care
Rhode Island Hospital
Providence, Rhode Island

F. WILLIAM BLAISDELL, MD
Professor
Department of Surgery
University of California, Davis
Sacramento, California

KEVIN M. BRADLEY, MD
Assistant Professor
Department of Surgery
Temple University School of Medicine
Philadelphia, Pennsylvania

ROBERT F. BUCKMAN, MD
Professor
Department of Surgery
Drexel University College of Medicine
Trauma Program Director
Saint Mary Medical Center
Langhorne, Pennsylvania

JON M. BURCH, MD
Professor
Department of Surgery
University of Colorado Health Sciences Center
Denver, Colorado

NEAL S. CAYNE, MD
Assistant Professor
Department of Surgery
New York University School of Medicine
Director of Endovascular Surgery
New York University Medical Center
New York, New York

IRSHAD H. CHAUDRY, PhD
Professor, Departments of Surgery, Microbiology, Physiology, and Biophysics
Vice Chairmen, Department of Surgery
Director, Center for Surgical Research
The University of Alabama at Birmingham
Birmingham, Alabama

RAUL CIOMBRA, MD
Associate Professor
Department of Surgery
Division of Trauma, Surgical Critical Care and Burns
University of California, San Diego School of Medicine
San Diego, California

LORI D. CONKLIN, MD
Surgical Resident
Michael E. DeBakey Department of Surgery
Baylor College of Medicine
Houston, Texas

MICHAEL E. DeBAKEY, MD
Chancellor Emeritus
Distinguished Service Professor
Michael E. DeBakey Department of Surgery
Baylor College of Medicine
Houston, Texas

DEMETRIOS DEMETRIADES, MD, PhD
Professor
Department of Surgery
Division of Trauma and Critical Care
Keck School of Medicine University of Southern California
Los Angeles, California

JAMES W. DENNIS, MD
Professor
Department of Surgery
University of Florida Health Science Center
Chief, Division of Vascular Surgery
Shands Jacksonville Medical Center
Jacksonville, Florida

DAVID V. FELICIANO, MD
Professor
Department of Surgery
Emory University School of Medicine
Chief of Surgery
Grady Memorial Hospital
Atlanta, Georgia

ERIC R. FRYKBERG, MD
Professor
Department of Surgery
University of Florida College of Medicine
Chief, Division of General Surgery
Shands Jacksonville Medical Center
Jacksonville, Florida

PRISCILLA J. GARCIA, MD
Resident, Department of Anesthesia
Baylor College of Medicine
Houston, Texas

NICHOLAS J. GARGIULO, III, MD
Assistant Professor
Department of Surgery
The Albert Einstein College of Medicine
Chief of Endovascular Surgery
Jack D. Weiler Hospital
Bronx, New York

THOMAS S. GRANCHI, MD, MBA
Associate Professor
Michael E. DeBakey Department of Surgery
Baylor College of Medicine
Medical Director, Emergency Center
Ben Taub General Hospital
Houston, Texas

ASHER HIRSHBERG, MD
Associate Professor
Michael E. DeBakey Department of Surgery
Baylor College of Medicine
Director of Vascular Surgery
Ben Taub General Hospital
Houston, Texas

DAVID B. HOYT, MD
Professor and Interim Chairman
Department of Surgery
University of California, San Diego
Chief, Division of Trauma, Burns, and SICU
UCSD Medical Center
San Diego, California

RAO R. IVATURY, MD
Professor
Department of Surgery
Virginia Commonwealth University
Chief, Division of Trauma/Critical Care
VCU Medical Center
Richmond, Virginia

DORAID JARRAR, MD
Chief Resident
Department of General Surgery
The University of Alabama at Birmingham
Birmingham, Alabama

KAJ JOHANSEN, MD, PhD
Clinical Professor
Department of Surgery
University of Washington School of Medicine
Director, Peripheral Vascular Services
Swedisky Medical Center
Seattle, Washington

M. MARGARET KNUDSON, MD
Professor
Department of Surgery
University of California
Director, Injury Research Center
San Francisco General Hospital
San Francisco, California

ANNA M. LEDGERWOOD, MD
Professor
Department of Surgery
Wayne State University
Detroit, Michigan

SCOTT A. LeMAIRE, MD
Assistant Professor
Division of Cardiothoracic Surgery
Michael E. DeBakey Department of Surgery
Baylor College of Medicine
Houston, Texas

MICHAEL R. LePORE, MD
Medical Director of Peripheral Vascular Surgery
Sarasota Memorial Hospital
Sarasota, Florida

CHARLES E. LUCAS, MD
Professor
Department of Surgery
Wayne State University
Detroit, Michigan

KENNETH L. MATTOX, MD
Professor and Vice Chairman
Michael E. DeBakey Department of Surgery
Baylor College of Medicine
Chief of Staff and Chief of Surgery
Ben Taub General Hospital
Houston, Texas

SAMUEL R. MONEY, MD
Clinical Associate Professor
Department of Surgery
Tulane University
Head, Section of Vascular Surgery
Ochsner Clinic Foundation
New Orleans, Louisiana

ERNEST E. MOORE, MD
Vice Chairman and Professor
Department of Surgery
University of Colorado Health Sciences Center
Chief of Surgery and Trauma
Denver Health
Denver, Colorado

JAMES A. MURRAY, MD
Division of Trauma and Critical Care
Department of Surgery
Keck School of Medicine University of Southern California
Assistant Professor of Surgery
University of Southern California
Los Angeles, CA

TAKAO OHKI, MD, PhD
Associate Professor
Department of Surgery
Albert Einstein College of Medicine
Chief, Vascular and Endovascular Surgery
Montefiore Medical Center
Bronx, New York

ABHIJIT S. PATHAK, MD
Assistant Professor
Department of Surgery
Temple University School of Medicine
Director, Surgical Intensive Care Unit
Temple University Hospital
Philadelphia, Pennsylvania

DAVID C. RICE, MD, MB, BCH
Assistant Professor
Department of Thoracic and Cardiovascular Surgery
University of Texas M.D. Anderson Cancer Center
Houston, Texas

NORMAN M. RICH, MD
Leonard Heaton and David Packard Professor
Chairman, Department of Surgery, USUHS
Chief, Division of Vascular Surgery, Emeritus
F. Edward Herbert School of Medicine
Uniformed Services University of the Health Sciences
Bethesda, Maryland

AURELIO RODRIGUEZ, MD
Professor
Department of Surgery
Drexel University College of Medicine
Director, Division of Trauma Surgery
Allegheny General Hospital Shock Trauma Center
Pittsburgh, Pennsylvania

SALVATORE J.A. SCLAFANI, MD
Professor
Department of Radiology
State University of New York
Director, Department of Radiology
Kings County Hospital Center
Brooklyn, New York

BRADFORD G. SCOTT, MD
Assistant Professor
Michael E. DeBakey Department of Surgery
Baylor College of Medicine
Associate Trauma Medical Director
Ben Taub General Hospital
Houston, Texas

STEVEN R. SHACKFORD, MD
Stanley S. Fieber Professor and Chairman
Department of Surgery
University of Vermont College of Medicine
Surgeon-in-Chief
Fletcher Allen Health Care
Burlington, Vermont

MICHAEL J. SISE, MD
Clinical Professor
Department of Surgery
UCSD School of Medicine
Medical Director
Scripps Mercy Hospital
San Diego, California

ERNESTO SOLTERO, MD
Assistant Professor
Michael E. DeBakey Department of Surgery
Baylor College of Medicine
Chief of Cardiovascular Surgery
Michael E. DeBakey VA Medical Center
Houston, Texas

MICHAEL C. STONER, MD
Fellow
Division Vascular and Endovascular Surgery
Massachusetts General Hospital
Boston, Massachusetts

FRANK J. VEITH, MD
Professor and Vice Chairman
Department of Surgery
Albert Einstein College of Medicine
The William J. von Liebig Chair in Vascular Surgery
Montefiore Medical Center
Albert Einstein College of Medicine
Bronx, New York

MATTHEW J. WALL, Jr, MD
Professor
Michael E. DeBakey Department of Surgery
Baylor College of Medice
Deputy Chief of Surgery
Chief of Cardiothoracic Surgery
Ben Taub General Hospital
Houston, Texas

PING WANG, MD
Professor and Chief
Division of Surgical Research
Department of Surgery
North Shore-Long Island Jewish Medical Center
Manhasset, New York

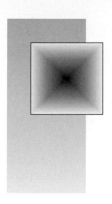

FOREWORD

Nearly 25 years have passed since the first edition of *Vascular Trauma* was published, edited by Norman Rich and myself. The first edition included experiences from both the Korean and Vietnam Conflicts. The Korean experiences demonstrated for the first time that arterial repair was imminently feasible in battle casualties without a serious hazard of infection. As cited by Hughes, a total of 304 arterial injuries underwent 269 repairs, with a 13% amputation rate as compared to the dismal 50% amputation rate following ligation in World War II. Our results in the U.S. Marine Corps were separately reported in the Annals of Surgery in 1955.

The Korean experience quickly led to widespread adoption of arterial repair, following which over 7500 such injuries were repaired in the Vietnam Conflict. These were entered into the Walter Reed Vascular Registry organized by Norman Rich; 1500 late results were then evaluated.

Arterial repair became possible primarily from the development of helicopter evacuation of wounded men. This coincided with the evolution of techniques of vascular repair, improved resuscitation, and antibiotics. Now, it is well established that the majority of arterial injuries can be effectively repaired if blood flow is restored within *6 to 7 hours* after injury. After *7 to 8 hours*, however, there is a rapid rise in the frequency of irreversible muscle necrosis, depending primarily upon extent of the associated soft tissue destruction with loss of collateral circulation.

Initially, it was feared that arterial repair would result in a prohibitive degree of wound infection, especially in Korea where the widespread use of cow manure for fertilizer resulted in gross contamination of virtually all injuries. Nonetheless, with adequate debridement, antibiotics and secondary closure, infection was rarely seen.

Several valuable developments have occurred since 1978 that make vascular repair even more feasible than before. These include the use of soft tissue pedicle flaps to cover arterial repair after radical debridement, the early detection of the vascular compartment syndrome by tissue pressure monitoring, and the recent development of endovascular techniques.

This book is of special importance because vascular injuries are uncommon in civilian trauma though increasing in frequency, primarily from automobile accidents and gunshot wounds. Civilian wounds fortunately often don't have the severe concomitant soft tissue destruction that often occurs with injury from high velocity missiles. Hence, extensive debridement and secondary closure are less often needed, but form the basis of the time-honored fact that the hazard of infection should virtually never prohibit arterial repair.

The rarity of arterial injuries makes continuing efforts with education, training, and referral to specialized vascular centers most important. Extremities are still lost because the gravity of early crucial symptoms of limb-threatening ischemia was missed. It has been known for over four decades that limb-threatening ischemia produces loss of peripheral nerve function within a few minutes after onset, manifested by numbness and paralysis in the affected extremity; but this crucial basic physiological fact is simply unknown to a surprisingly large number of personnel treating injured patients.

Another fact emphasizing the importance of experience is the fact that an acute vascular injury can be repaired with a success rate probably greater than 95% if treated with modern techniques within 6 to 7 hours after injury. If repair initially fails, however, prompt reoperation similarly has a success rate over 90%, for the cause of failure is usually thrombosis of an inadequate repair or thrombi incompletely removed at the first operation. Both of these preventable complications usually result from simple lack of experience.

These facts clearly show the importance of this book for all physicians and staff treating injured patients. Strong adherence to the basic principles described makes arterial repair achievable in the vast majority of patients. The authors are to be congratulated on their significant contributions.

Frank Spencer, MD

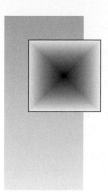

FOREWORD

Among traumatic injuries, those affecting the major vessels are of great importance, since they represent a serious threat to life and limb. These injuries assume special significance in light of the increasing number of trauma patients arriving at the hospital as a result of vehicular accidents, violent crimes, and other hazardous events.

Until relatively recently, therapy for vascular injuries was limited to lifesaving control of hemorrhage. Even during World War II, surgical repair of arterial injuries was rarely attempted. The pioneering developments in vascular surgery that evolved in the early 1950s and the successful surgical repair of vascular injuries in the Korean War provided the basis for effective surgical treatment of this form of trauma. Accordingly, in the care of patients with vascular trauma only, salvage of life is no longer acceptable; the goal is also rapid restoration of normal circulatory dynamics.

The authors, Norman Rich, Kenneth Mattox, and Asher Hirshberg, have had extensive and wide-ranging experience in the development of the most effective methods of treatment of vascular injuries, including civilian and military experience, especially during the Korean and Vietnam Wars. The authors have incorporated in this book a consideration of the entire subject of vascular injuries, including an interesting historical review of the topic; the relative frequency, and sites of their occurrence; and the clinical, anatomical, and surgical technical aspects of this subject. It will therefore be of immense value and usefulness to both civilian and military surgeons.

Micheal E. DeBakey, M.D.
Distinguished Service Professor
and Olga Keith Wiess Professor of Surgery
Michael E. DeBakey Department of Surgery
Director, DeBakey Heart Center
Chancellor Emeritus, Baylor College of Medicine
Houston, Texas

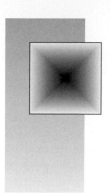

P R E F A C E

The first edition of this text was published in 1978 as a monograph written by Drs. Norman Rich and Frank Spencer. It was an extensive treatise on the pathophysiology, diagnosis, and management of traumatic injuries to blood vessels. It was and still is one of a kind. No other textbook on vascular trauma has been published before or since. The first edition was written in the aftermath of the Vietnam War, the first military conflict where modern principles of vascular surgery were applied to traumatic injuries of the blood vessels. Many of the lessons and concepts delineated in the first edition were based on the Vietnam Vascular Registry, an unprecedented effort, led by Dr. Rich, to systematically collect and analyze the vascular injuries in a large-scale military conflict. Yet with very few exceptions, most surgeons who performed vascular reconstructions in Vietnam did so only on a handful of patients.

In the 1980s, as surgeons began to encounter increasing numbers of major injuries to blood vessels in the civilian population, there was a surge of interest in vascular trauma and an exponential rise in the number of publications on the subject. Many of the advances in the field originated at urban trauma centers, and particularly at the Ben Taub General Hospital in Houston, where the modern concepts of cardiovascular surgery, pioneered by Drs. Michael E. DeBakey, Stanley Crawford, Arthur Beall and others at Baylor College of Medicine, were developed into new management strategies in vascular trauma by Dr. Kenneth L. Mattox and his team described in more than a hundred publications.

Ten years ago, Dr. Rich enlisted the assistance of Dr. Mattox in writing the second edition of *Vascular Trauma*. The objective was to combine the military and civilian experience into one cohesive text. However, the task rapidly proved to be a "mission impossible" as the rapid developments in the fields of trauma systems, care of the injured patient, damage control surgery, vascular imaging and endovascular intervention constantly outpaced the revision of the original text. This led to the addition of Dr. Asher Hirshberg to the editorial team. He represents a new generation of surgeons formally trained in both trauma and vascular surgery. The plan for the book has subsequently changed from a monograph to a multi-authored text containing cutting-edge concepts and information in vascular trauma. At the same time, we wished to keep some of the original exciting "flavor" from the first edition of *Vascular Trauma*, so expertly and lovingly compiled by Drs. Rich and Spencer.

Drs. Rich and Spencer assembled all their references at the end of the first edition, assuming that many of the references will be used in more than one chapter. Dr. Rich continued to collect key references during the next two decades, and his entire treasury of vascular trauma references, a unique and extremely valuable resource for any surgeon interested in the care of patients with injuries to blood vessels, is given at the end of this book. We have attempted to assure that all citations in each chapter are in this reference list, but because of the enormity of this project, it is inevitable that some might have been omitted. It is also inevitable that some vascular trauma references might have been missed by all three editors.

The editors are indebted to the numerous authors of this text, each one with a life-long commitment to the care of the injured. Ms. Mary Allen was the persistent force that brought the many aspects of this book together. In addition, we are grateful to the numerous individuals at Elsevier who contributed to the culmination of this endeavor.

Norman M. Rich, MD
Kenneth L. Mattox, MD
Asher Hirshberg, MD

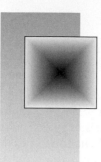

CONTENTS

GENERAL PRINCIPLES OF VASCULAR TRAUMA

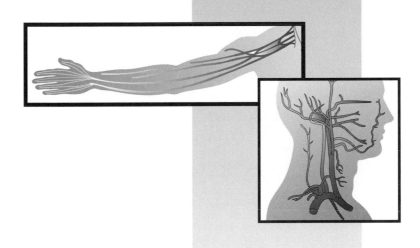

Historical and Military Aspects of Vascular Trauma (With Lifetime Reflections of Doctor Norman Rich)

NORMAN M. RICH

> *The advances in vascular surgery are typical of those in other fields of medicine and surgery. Each step is discovered and recorded only to be rediscovered by other individuals who failed to read and profit by the experience of others.*
> Carl W. Hughes (1961)

HISTORICAL OVERVIEW ON VASCULAR TRAUMA

Although the first crude arteriorrhaphy was performed about 243 years ago, only in the past 40 years has vascular surgery become widely practiced with the anticipation of consistently obtaining good results. By the turn of this century, extensive experimental work and some early clinical applications had occurred, employing most of the techniques of vascular surgery in use today. In retrospect, it is almost astonishing that it took nearly 50 years before the work of early pioneers such as Murphy, Goyanes, Carrel, Guthrie, and Lexer was widely accepted and applied in the treatment of vascular injuries. Since the days of Ambroise Paré in the mid-16th century, major advances in the surgery of trauma have occurred during the times of armed conflict, when it was necessary to treat large numbers of severely injured patients often under conditions far from ideal. This has been especially true with vascular injuries.

Although German surgeons accomplished a limited number of arterial repairs in the early part of World War I, it was not until the Korean Conflict in the early 1950s that ligation of major arteries was abandoned as the standard treatment for arterial trauma. The results of ligation of major arteries following trauma were clearly recorded in the classic manuscript by DeBakey and Simeone (1946), who found only 81 repairs in 2471 arterial injuries among U.S. troops in World War II. All but three of the arterial repairs were performed by lateral suture. Ligation was followed by gangrene and amputation in nearly one half of the cases. The pessimistic conclusion reached by many was expressed by Sir James Learmonth (1946), who said that there was little place for definitive arterial repair in the combat wound.

Between the end of World War II and the beginning of the Korean Conflict, advances in suture, noncrushing clamps, and arteriography were emerging. During the Korean Conflict continuing technology in polymerized material (plastic) added a new opportunity for vascular reconstruction.

The possibility of successfully repairing arterial injuries was established conclusively, stemming particularly from the works of Hughes, Howard, Jahnke, and Spencer. In 1958, Hughes emphasized the significance of this contribution in a review of the Korean experience, finding that the overall amputation rate was lowered to about 13%, compared to the approximately 49% amputation rate that followed ligation in World War II.

During the Vietnam hostilities, more than 600 young U.S. surgeons, representing most of the major surgical training programs in the United States, treated more than 7500 patients with vascular injuries. Rich and Hughes (1969) reported the preliminary statistics from the Vietnam Vascular Registry, established in 1966 at Walter Reed General Hospital to document and follow all servicemen who sustained vascular trauma in Vietnam. The interim Registry report, encompassing 1000 major acute arterial injuries, showed little change from the overall statistics presented in the preliminary report (Rich, 1970). Considering all major extremity arteries, the amputation rate remained near 13%. Although high-velocity missiles created more soft tissue destruction in injuries seen in Vietnam, the combination of a stable hospital environment and rapid evacuation of casualties, similar to that in Korea, made successful repair possible. Injuries of the popliteal artery remained an enigma, with an amputation rate remaining near 30%.

In the past 40 years, civilian experience with vascular trauma has developed rapidly under conditions much more favorable than those of warfare. As might be predicted, several series have reported results that are significantly better than those achieved with military casualties in Korea and Vietnam. Mattox (1989) published the epidemiology of the largest civilian experience in managing vascular trauma in the history of the world.

Control of Hemorrhage from the Time of Antiquity

The control of hemorrhage following injury has been of prime concern to humans since the beginning. Methods have included various animal and vegetable tissues, hot irons, boiling pitch, cold instruments, styptics, bandaging, and compression. These methods were described in a historical review by Schwartz in 1958. Ancient methods of hemostasis used by Egyptians about 1600 BC are described in the Ebers' papyrus, discovered by Ebers at Luxor in 1873 (Schwartz, 1958). Styptics prepared from mineral or vegetable matter were popular, including lead sulfate, antimony, and

copper sulfate. Several hundred years later, copper sulfate again became popular during the Middle Ages in Europe and was known as the hemostatic "button." In ancient India, compression, cold elevation, and hot oil were used to control hemorrhage, while the Chinese about 1000 BC used tight bandaging and styptics.

The writings of Celsus provide most of the knowledge of methods of hemostasis in the 1st and 2nd centuries AD, Celsus was the first to record an accurate account of the use of ligature for hemostasis in 25 AD. During the first three centuries AD, Galen, Heliodorus, Rufus of Ephesus, and Archigenes advocated ligation or compression of a bleeding vessel to control hemorrhage. The prevailing surgical practice when amputation was done for gangrene was to amputate at the line of demarcation to prevent hemorrhage. Archigenes, in the 1st century AD was apparently the first to advocate amputating above the line of demarcation for tumors and gangrene, using ligature of the artery to control hemorrhage.

Rufus of Ephesus (1st century AD) noted that an artery would continue to bleed when partly severed, but when completely severed, it would contract and stop bleeding within a short time. Galen, the leading physician of Rome in the 2nd century AD, advised placing a finger on the orifice of a bleeding superficial vessel for a period to initiate the formation of a thrombus and the cessation of bleeding. He noted, however, that if the vessel were deeper, it was important to determine whether the bleeding was coming from an artery or a vein. If a vein, pressure or a styptic usually sufficed, but ligation with linen was recommended for arterial injury. Herophilus, the Greek physician and anatomist of the 3rd century BC described the difference between veins and arterial as "veins were weak and thin-walled, containing only blood, whereas arteries were thick-walled, containing air 'pneuma' and blood."

Following the initial contributions of Celsus, Galen, and their contemporaries, the use of ligature was essentially forgotten for almost 1200 years. Throughout the Middle Ages, cautery was used almost exclusively to control hemorrhage. Jerome of Brunswick

(Hieronymus Brunschwig), an Alsatian Army surgeon, actually preceded Paré in describing the use of ligatures as the best way to stop hemorrhage (Schwartz, 1958). His recommendations were recorded in a textbook published in 1497 and provided a detailed account of the treatment of gunshot wounds. Ambroise Paré, with a wide experience in the surgery of trauma, especially on the battlefield, established firmly the use of ligature for control of hemorrhage from open blood vessels. In 1552, he startled the surgical world by amputating a leg above the line of demarcation, repeating the demonstration of Archigenes 1400 years earlier. The vessels were ligated with linen, leaving the ends long. Paré also developed the "bec de corbin," ancestor of the modern hemostat, to grasp the vessel before ligating it (Fig. 1–1). Previously, vessels had been grasped with hooks, tenaculums, or the assistant's fingers.

In the 17th century, Harvey's monumental contribution describing the circulation of the blood greatly aided the understanding of vascular injuries. Although Rufus of Ephesus apparently discussed arteriovenous communications in the 1st century AD, it was not until 1757 that William Hunter first described the arteriovenous fistula as a pathologic entity. The historical development of the treatment of arteriovenous fistulas and false aneurysms are discussed in Chapter 24. Also, similar review of false aneurysms is included. As early as the 2nd century AD, Antyllus described the physical findings and management by proximal

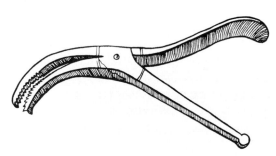

■ **FIGURE 1–1**
Artist's concept of the *bec de corbin*, developed by Paré and Scultetus in the mid-16th century. It was used to grasp the vessel before ligating it. (From Schwartz AM: Surgery 1958;44:604.) ■

and distal ligation. He was the first to document collateral circulation.

The development of the tourniquet was another advance that played an important role in the control of hemorrhage. Tight bandages had been applied since antiquity, but subsequent development of the tourniquet was slow. Finally, in 1674, a military surgeon named Morel introduced a stick into the bandage and twisted it until arterial flow stopped (Schwartz, 1958). The screw tourniquet came into use shortly thereafter. This method of temporary control of hemorrhage encouraged more frequent use of the ligature, which required time for its application. In 1873, Freidrich van Esmarch, a student of Langenbeck, introduced his elastic tourniquet bandage for first aid use on the battlefield. Previously, it was thought that such compression would injure vessels irreversibly. His discovery permitted surgeons to operate electively on extremities in a dry, bloodless field.

In addition to the control of hemorrhage at the time of injury, the second major area of concern for centuries was the prevention of secondary hemorrhage occurring days to weeks later. Because of its great frequency, styptics, compression, and pressure were used for several centuries after ligation of injured vessels became possible. Undoubtedly, the high rate of secondary hemorrhage after ligation was due to infection of the wound. Although John Hunter demonstrated the value of proximal ligation for control of a false aneurysm in 1757, failure to control secondary hemorrhage resulted in the use of ligature only for secondary bleeding from the amputation stump. Subsequently, Bell (1801) and Guthrie (1815) performed ligation both proximal and distal to the arterial wound with better results than those previously obtained.

Some of the first clear records of ligation of major arterial were written in the 19th century and are of particular interest. The first successful ligation of the common carotid artery for hemorrhage was performed in 1803 by Fleming but was not reported until 14 years later by Coley (1817), because Fleming died a short time after the operation was performed. A servant aboard the *HMS Tonnant* attempted suicide by slashing his throat.

When Fleming saw the patient, it appeared that he had exsanguinated. There was no pulse at the wrist and the pupils were dilated. It was possible to ligate two superior thyroid arteries and one internal jugular vein. A laceration of the outer and muscular layers of the carotid artery was noted, as well as a laceration of the trachea between the thyroid and cricoid cartilages. This allowed drainage from the wound to enter the trachea, provoking violent seizures of coughing. Although the patient seemed to be improving, approximately 1 week following the injury, Flemming recorded that "on the evening of the 17th, during a violent paroxysm of coughing, the artery burst, and my poor patient was, in an instant, deluged with blood!"

The dilemma of the surgeon is appreciated by the statement, "In this dreadful situation I concluded that there was but one step to take, with any prospect of success; mainly, to cutdown upon, and tie the carotid artery below the wound. I had never heard of such an operation being performed; but conceived that its effects might be less formidable, in this case, than in a person not reduced by hemorrhage."

The wound rapidly healed following ligation of the carotid artery and the patient recovered.

Ellis (1845) reported the astonishing experience of successful ligation of both carotid arteries in a 21-year-old patient who sustained a gunshot wound of the neck while he was setting a trap in the woods on October 21, 1844, near Grand Rapids, Michigan, when he was unfortunately mistaken for a bear by a companion. Approximately 1 week later, Ellis had to ligate the patient's left carotid artery because of a hemorrhage. An appreciation of the surgeon's problem can be gained by Ellis' description of the operation, "We placed him on a table, and with the assistance of Doctor Platt and a student, I ligatured the left carotid artery, below the omohyoideus muscle; an operation attended with a good deal of difficulty, owing to the swollen state of the parts, the necessity of keeping up pressure, the bad position of the parts owing to the necessity of keeping the mouth in a certain position to prevent his being strangulated by the blood, and the necessity of operating by candlelight."

There was recurrent hemorrhage on the 11th day after the accident and right carotid artery pressure helped control the blood loss. It was, therefore, necessary to ligate also the right carotid artery $4\frac{1}{2}$ days after the left carotid artery had been ligated. Ellis (1845) remarked, "For convenience, we had him in the sitting posture during the operation; when we tightened the ligature, no disagreeable effects followed; no fainting; no bad feeling about the head; and all the perceptible change was a slight paleness, a cessation of pulsation in both temporal arteries, and of the hemorrhage."

The patient recovered rapidly with good wound healing and returned to normal daily activity. There was no perceptible pulsation in either superficial temporal artery.

The importance of collateral circulation in preserving viability of the limb after ligation was well understood for centuries. The fact that time was necessary for establishment of this collateral circulation was recognized. Halsted (1912) reported cure of an iliofemoral aneurysm by application of an aluminum band to the proximal artery without seriously affecting the circulation or function of the lower extremity. The importance of asepsis had now been recognized, and the frequency of secondary hemorrhage and gangrene following ligation promptly decreased. Subsequently, Halsted (1914) demonstrated the roll of collateral circulation by gradually completely occluding the aorta and other large arteries in dogs by means of silver or aluminum bands, which were gradually tightened over a period of time.

EARLY DIRECT VASCULAR RECONSTRUCTION

About two centuries after Paré established the use of the ligature, the first direct repair of an injured artery was accomplished. This event, about 243 years ago, is credited as the first documented vascular repair. Hallowell (1762), acting on a suggestion by Lambert in

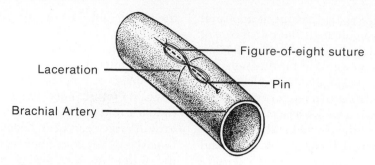

■ **FIGURE 1–2**

The first arterial repair performed by Hallowell, acting on a suggestion by Lambert in 1759. The technique, known as the farrier's (veterinarian's) stitch, was followed in repairing the brachial artery by placing a pin through the arterial walls and holding the edges in apposition with a suture in a figure-of-eight fashion about the pin. (From Lambert. Med Obser Inq 1762;30:360.) ■

1759, repaired a wound of the brachial artery by placing a pin through the arterial walls and holding the edges in apposition by applying a suture in a figure-of-eight fashion about the pin (Fig. 1–2). This technique (known as the Farrier stitch) had been used by veterinarians but had fallen into disrepute following unsuccessful experiments. Table 1–1 outlines early vascular techniques.

Unfortunately, others could not duplicate Hallowell's successful experience, almost surely because of the multiple problems of infection and lack of anesthesia. There was one report by Broca (1762) of a successful suture of a longitudinal incision in an artery. However, according to Shumacker (1969), an additional 127 years passed following the Hallowell-Lambert arterial repair before a second instance of arterial repair by lateral

TABLE 1–1
VASCULAR REPAIR PRIOR TO 1900

Technique	Year	Surgeon
Pin and thread	1759	Hallowell
Small ivory clamps	1881	Glück
Fine needles and silk	1889	Jassinowski
Continuous suture	1890	Burci
Invagination	1896	Murphy
Suture all layers	1899	Dörfler

Adapted from Guthrie GC: Blood Vessel Surgery and Its Application. New York: Longmans, Green, 1912.

suture of an artery in a man was reported by Postempski in 1886.

With the combined developments of anesthesia and asepsis, several reports of attempts to repair arteries appeared in the latter part of the 19th century. The work of Jassinowsky, who is credited in 1889 for experimentally proving that arterial wounds could be sutured with preservation of the lumen, was later judged by Murphy in 1897 as the best experimental work published at that time. In 1865, Henry Lee of London attempted repair of arterial lacerations with suture (Shumacker, 1969). Glück in 1883 reported 19 experiments with arterial suture, but all experiments failed because of bleeding from the holes made by suture needles. He also devised aluminum and ivory clamps to unite longitudinal incisions in a vessel, and it was recorded that the ivory clamps succeeded in one experiment on the femoral artery of a large dog. Von Horoch of Vienna reported six experiments, including one end-to-end union, in 1887, all of which thrombosed. In 1889, Bruci sutured six longitudinal arteriotomies in dogs; the procedure was successful in four. In 1890 Muscatello successfully sutured a partial transection of the abdominal aorta in a dog. In 1894 Heidenhain closed by catgut suture, a 1-cm opening in the axillary artery made accidentally while removing the adherent carcinomatous glands. The patient recovered without any circulatory disturbance. In 1883, Israel, in a discussion of a paper by Glück, described closing a laceration in the common iliac artery created during an operation for perityphlitic abscess. The closure was accomplished by five silk sutures. However, Murphy (1897) did not believe it could be possible from his personal observations to have success in this type of arterial repair. In 1896, Sabanyeff successfully closed small openings in the femoral artery with sutures.

The classic studies of John B. Murphy (1897) of Chicago contributed greatly to the development of arterial repair and culminated in the first successful end-to-end anastomosis of an artery in 1896. Previously, Murphy had carefully reviewed earlier clinical and experimental studies of arterial repair and had evaluated different techniques extensively in laboratory studies. Murphy attempted to determine experimentally how much artery could be removed and still allow an anastomosis. He found 1 inch of calf's carotid artery could be removed and the ends still approximated by invagination suture technique because of the elasticity of the artery. He concluded that arterial repair could be done with safety when no more than three fourths of an inch of an a artery had been removed, except in certain locations such as the popliteal fossa or the axillary space where the limb could be moved to relieve tension on the repair. He also concluded that when more than one half of the artery was destroyed, it was better to perform and end-to-end anastomosis by invagination rather than to attempt repair of the laceration. This repair was done by introducing sutures into the proximal artery, including only the two outer coats, and using three sutures to invaginate the proximal artery into the distal one, reinforcing the closure with an interrupted suture (Fig. 1–3).

In 1896 Murphy was unable to find a similar recorded case involving the suture of an artery after complete division, and he consequently reported his experience (1897) in one patient and then and carried out a number of experiments to determine the feasibility of his procedure. Murphy's patient was a 19-year-old male shot twice, with one bullet entering the femoral triangle. The patient was admitted to Cook County Hospital in Chicago on September 19, 1896, approximately 2 hours after wounding. There was no hemorrhage or

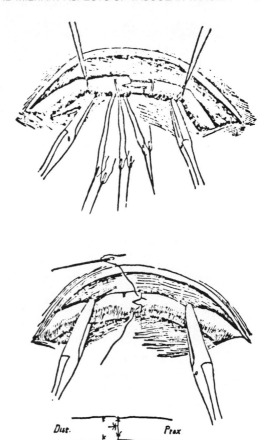

■ **FIGURE 1–3**
The first successful clinical end-to-end anastomosis of an artery was performed in 1896. Sutures were placed in the proximal artery, including only the few outer costs, and three sutures were used to invaginate the proximal artery into the distal one; the closure was reinforced with an interrupted suture. (From Murphy JB: Exp Clin Res Med Rec 1897;51:73-104.) ■

increased pulsation noted at the time. Murphy first saw the patient 15 days later, October 4, 1896, and found a large bruit surrounding the site of the injury. Distal pulses were barely perceptible. Two days later, when demonstrating this patient to students, a thrill was also detected. An operative repair was decided. Because of the historical significance, the operation report is quoted:

Operation, October 7, 1896. An incision five inches long was made from Poupart's ligament along the course of the femoral artery. The artery was readily exposed about one inch above Poupart's ligament; it was separated from its sheath and a provisional ligature thrown about it but not tied. A careful dissection was then made down along the wall of the vessel to the pulsating clot. The artery was exposed to one inch below the point and a ligature thrown around it but not tied; a careful dissection was made upward to the point of the clot. The artery was then closed above and below with gentle compression clamps and was elevated, at which time there was a profuse hemorrhage from an opening in the vein. A cavity, about the size of a filbert, was found posterior to the artery communicating with its caliber, the aneurysmal pocket. A small aneurysmal sac about the same size was found on the anterior surface of the artery over the point of perforation. The hemorrhage from the vein was very profuse and was controlled by digital compression. It was found that one-eighth of an inch of the arterial wall on the outer side of the opening remained, and on the inner side of the perforation only a band of one-sixteenth of an inch of adventitia was intact. The bullet had passed through the center of the artery, carried away all of its wall except the strands described above, and passed downward and backward making a large hole in the vein in its posterior and external side just above the junction of the vena profunda. Great difficulty was experienced in controlling the hemorrhage from the vein. After dissecting the vein above and below the point of laceration and placing a temporary ligature on the vena profunda, the hemorrhage was controlled so that the vein was greatly diminished in size, but when the clamps were removed it dilated about one-third the normal diameter or one-third the diameter of the vein above and below. There was no bleeding from the vein when the clamps were removed. Our attention was then turned to the artery. Two inches of it had been exposed and freed from all surroundings. The opening in the artery was three-eighths of an inch in length; one-half inch was resected and the proximal was invaginated into the distal for one-third of an inch with four double needle threads which penetrated all of the walls of the artery. The adventitia was peeled off the invaginated portion for a distance of one-third of an inch: a row of sutures was placed around the edge of the overlapping distal end, the sutures penetrating only the medial of the proximal portion; the adventitia was then brought over the end of the union and sutured. The clamps were removed. Not a drop of blood escaped at the line of suture. Pulsation was immediately restored in the artery below the line of approximation and it could be felt feebly in the posterior tibial and dorsalis pedis pulses. The sheath and connective tissue around the artery were then approximated at the position of the suture with catgut, so as to support the wall of the artery. The whole cavity was washed out with a five percent solution of carbolic acid and the edges of the wound were accurately approximated with silk worm-gut sutures. No drainage. The time of the operation was approximately two and one-half hours, most of the time being consumed in suturing the vein. The artery was easily secured and sutured, and the hemorrhage from it readily controlled. The patient was placed in bed with the leg elevated and wrapped in cotton.

The anatomic location of the injuries, the gross pathology involved and the repair for Murphy's historically successful arterial anastomosis are shown in Figure 1–4. Murphy mentioned that a pulsation could be felt in the dorsalis pedis artery 4 days following the operation. The patient had no edema and no disturbance of his circulation during the reported 3 months of observation.

Subsequently, Murphy (1897) reviewed the results of ligature of large arteries before the turn of the century. He found that the abdominal aorta had been ligated 10 times with only one patient surviving for 10 days. Lidell

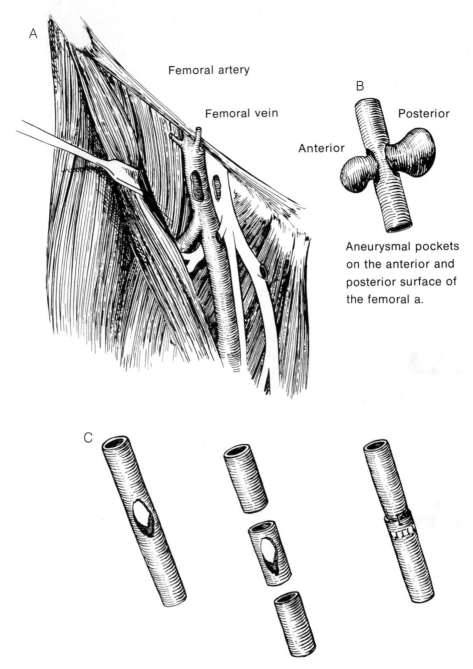

A

Femoral artery

Femoral vein

B

Anterior

Posterior

Aneurysmal pockets
on the anterior and
posterior surface of
the femoral a.

C

■ FIGURE 1-4
The first successful end-to-end arterial anastomosis in man by Murphy in 1896. *A*, The anatomic location of the injury. *B*, The close pathology involved. *C*, Degree of destruction, portion resected and appearance after invagination of femoral artery. See text for details including venous repair. (From Murphy JB: Med Rec 1897;51:73-104.) ■

reported only 16 recoveries after ligation of the common iliac artery 68 times, a mortality of 77%. Balance and Edmunds reported a 40% mortality following ligation of a femoral artery aneurysm in 31 patients. Billroth reported secondary hemorrhage from 50% of large arteries ligated in continuity. Wyeth collected 106 cases of carotid artery aneurysms treated by proximal ligation, with a mortality rate of 35%.

In 1897 Murphy summarized techniques he considered necessary for arterial suture. They bear a close resemblance to principles generally followed today:

1. Complete asepsis
2. Exposure of the vessel with as little injury as possible
3. Temporary suppression of the blood current
4. Control of the vessel while applying the suture
5. Accurate approximation of the walls
6. Perfect hemostasis by pressure after the clamps are taken off
7. Toilet of the wound

Murphy also reported that Billroth, Schede, Braun, Schmidt, and others had successfully sutured wounds in veins. He personally had used five silk sutures to close an opening three eighths of an inch in the common jugular vein. Several significant accomplishments occurred in vascular surgery within the next few years. Matas (1903) described his technique with endoaneurysmorrhaphy for aneurysm, a technique that remained the standard technique for aneurysms for more than 40 years. In 1906 Carrel and Guthrie performed classic experimental studies over a period with many significant results. These included direct suture repair of arteries, vein transplantation, and transplantation of blood vessels, organs, and limbs (Fig. 1–5).

In 1912 Guthrie independently published his continuing work on vascular surgery. Following Murphy's successful case in 1896, the next successful repair of an arterial defect came 10 years later when Goyanes used a vein graft to bridge an arterial defect in 1906. Working in Madrid, Goyanes excised a popliteal artery aneurysm and used the accompanying popliteal vein to restore continuity (Fig. 1–6).

He used the suture technique, developed by Carrel and Guthrie, of triangulation of the arterial orifice with three sutures, followed by continuous suture between each of the three areas.

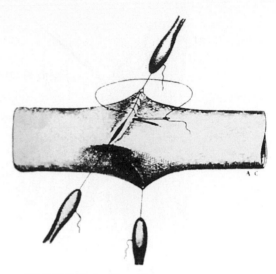

■ **FIGURE 1–5**
The triangulation method of suturing vessels. Initially conceived in 1902 by Carrel, this method was used by Carrel and Guthrie in their monumental contributions in the direct suture repair of arteries, vein transplants, and transplantation of blood vessels and organs. (Courtesy the New York Academy of Medicine Library.) ■

A year later in Germany, Lexer (1907) first used the saphenous vein as an arterial substitute to restore continuity after excision of an aneurysm of the axillary artery. In his 1969 review, Shumacker commented that within the first few years of this century, the triangulation stitch of Carrel (1902), the quadrangulation method of Frouin (1908), and the Mourin modification (1914) (Fig. 1–7) had developed.

By 1910 Stich reported more than 100 cases of arterial reconstruction by lateral suture. His review also included 46 repairs by end-to-end anastomosis or by insertion of a vein graft (Nolan, 1968). It is curious with this promising start that more than 30 years had elapsed before vascular surgery was widely employed. A high failure rate, usually by thrombosis, attended early attempts at repair, and few surgeons were convinced that repair of an artery was worthwhile. Matas (1913) stated that vascular injuries, particularly arteriovenous aneurysms, had become a conspicuous feature of modern military surgery, and he felt that this class of injury must command the closest attention of the modern military surgeon:

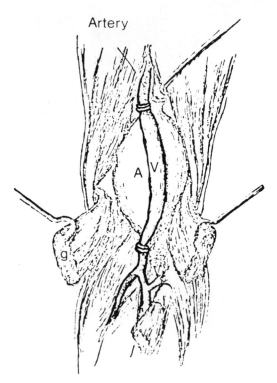

Artery

■ **FIGURE 1–6**
The first successful repair of an arterial defect utilizing a vein graft. Using the triangulation technique of Carrel with endothelial coaptation, a segment of the adjacent popliteal vein was used to repair the popliteal artery. (From Goyanes DJ: El Siglo Med 1906;53:546,561.) ■

A most timely and valuable contribution to the surgery of blood vessels resulted from wounds in war. . . . Unusual opportunities for the observation of vascular wounds inflicted with modern military weapons . . . based on material fresh from the field of action, and

fully confirmed the belief that this last war, waged in closed proximity to well equipped surgical centers, would also offer an unusual opportunity for the study of the most advanced methods of treating injuries of blood vessels.

MILITARY VASCULAR TRAUMA EXPERIENCE

Balkin Wars

In 1913 Soubbotitch (Fig. 1–8) described the experience of Serbian military surgeons during the Serbo-Turkish and Serbo-Bulgarian Wars. Seventy-seven false aneurysms and arteriovenous fistulas were treated. There were 45 ligations, but 32 vessels were repaired, including 19 arteriorrhaphies, 13 venorrhaphies, and 15 end-to-end anastomoses (11 arteries and 4 veins). It is impressive that infection and secondary hemorrhage were avoided. Matas (1913), in discussing Soubbotitch's report, emphasized that a notable feature was the suture (circular and lateral repair) of blood vessels and the fact that it had been used more frequently in the Balkan Conflict than in previous wars. He also noted that judging by Soubbotitch's statistics, the success obtained by surgeons in the Serbian Army Hospital in Belgrade far surpassed that obtained by other military surgeons in previous wars, with the exception perhaps of the remarkably favorable results in the Japanese Reserve Hospital reported by Kikuzi during the Russo-Japanese War (1904/1905). It is ironic that

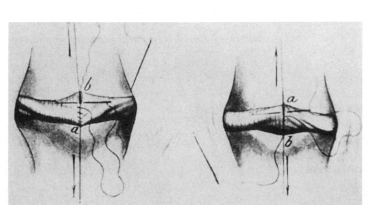

■ **FIGURE 1–7**
The original triangulation stitch of Carrel in 1902 was modified to a quadrangulation method by Frouin in 1908. Another modification, as shown here, was that of Mourin in 1914. (From Moure P. Les Greffes Artérielles, 1914.) ■

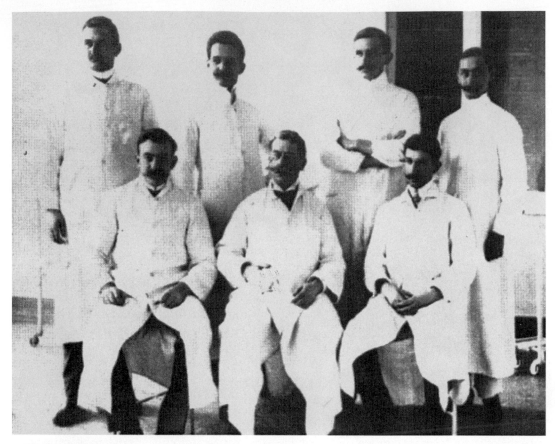

■ FIGURE 1–8
Dr. V. Soubbotitch (front-row center), Lt Col., Serbian Army Reserves, is flanked by members of his staff at the Belgrade State Hospital (circa 1912-1913). The reference provides additional details regarding the Matas–Soubbotitch connection. (From Rich NM, Clagett GP, Salander JM, Piščević S: Surgery 1983;93:17-19.) ■

the vascular experience continued in the Balkans, in the early 1990s. Additional information regarding Soubbotitch came directly from Geza De Takats (Fig. 1–9) who was in Belgrade early in World War II. Table 1–2 identifies the Soubbotitch experience.

World War I Experience

During the early part of World War I, with the new techniques of vascular surgery well established, the German surgeons attempted repair of acutely injured arteries and were successful in more than 100 cases (Nolan, 1968). During the first 9 months of World War I, low-velocity missiles caused arterial trauma of a

TABLE 1–2
TREATMENT OF TRAUMATIC ANEURYSMS FROM THE SERBO-TURKISH AND SERBO-BULGARIAN WARS

	Ligation	Partial Suture	Circular Suture
Arteries	41	8	11
Veins	4	9	4

Modified from Soubbotitch V: Lancet 1913;2:720-721.

MILITARY SURGICAL HERITAGE
DEPARTMENT OF SURGERY, USUHS
Geza de Takats 1892 - 1985

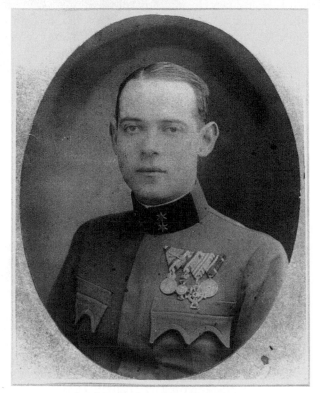

1st. LT, MC Austro-Hungarian Army
At Funeral of Emperor Franz Joseph 1916
A Dedicated Friend of Military Surgeons
Consultant, Great Lakes Naval Hospital, 1946 - 1954

■ **FIGURE 1-9**
An internationally acclaimed pioneer in vascular surgery Geza De Takats is among the early contributors to our military surgical heritage. (From Rich NM: Am J Surg 1993;166:91-96.) ■

limited extent. In 1915, however, the widespread use of high explosives (the high explosive artillery shells replaced the Shrapnel shell in use since British action in Surinam in 1904) and high-velocity bullets, combined with mass casualties and slow evacuation of the wounded, made arterial repair impractical.

Bernheim (1920), who had performed vascular research in a Hunterian Laboratory, performed the first vascular repair using saphenous vein in the United States at Johns Hopkins University and went to France with the specific intent of repairing arterial injuries. Despite extensive prior experience and equipment, however, he concluded that attempts at vascular repair were unwise (1920). He wrote

Opportunities for carrying out the more modern procedures for repair or reconstruction of damaged blood vessels were conspicuous by their absence during the recent military activities. . . . Not that blood vessels were immune from injury; not that gaping arteries and veins and vicariously united vessels did not cry out for relief by fine suture or anastomosis. They did, most eloquently, and in great numbers, but he would have been a foolhardy man who would have essayed sutures of arterial or venous trunks in the presence of such infections as were the rule in practically all of the battle wounded.

The great frequency of infection with secondary hemorrhage virtually precluded arterial repair. In addition, there were inadequate statistics about the frequency of gangrene following ligation, and initial reports subsequently proved to be unduly optimistic. Poole (1927), in the Medical Department History of World War I, remarked that if gangrene was a danger following arterial ligation, primary suture should be performed and the patient watched very carefully.

Despite the discouragement of managing acute arterial injuries in World War I, fairly frequent repair of false aneurysms and arteriovenous fistulas was carried out by many surgeons. These cases were treated after the acute period of injury, when collateral circulation had developed with the passage of time and ensured viability of extremities. Matas (1921) recorded that most of these repairs consisted of arteriorrhaphy by lateral or circular suture, with excision of the sac or endoaneurysmorrhaphy.

Makins (1919), who served in World War I as a British surgeon, recommended ligating the concomitant vein when it was necessary to ligate a major artery. He thought that this reduced the frequency of gangrene. This hypothesis was debated for more than 20 years before it was finally abandoned.

Goodman (1918), in describing his experience at the number 1 (Presbyterian U.S.A.) General Hospital in France during World War I, reported a successful closure with continuous silk suture of 5-mm longitudinal openings in both the popliteal artery and the popliteal vein in one patient with a shell fragment. However, the patient was followed for only 9 days before being transferred to the Base Hospital. Goodman reported, "An attempt to obtain further information covering the case is now underway and will be embodied in a subsequent report."

If there was any further follow-up information obtained or reported, it became obscured in the available literature. At least this military surgeon recognized the importance of obtaining long-term follow-up information to thoroughly evaluate his method of managing vascular trauma.

In 1987, Shumacker identified that Weglowski was a neglected pioneer in vascular surgery. Weglowski served first in a Russian Military Hospital and later as Surgeon General of the Polish Army. Based on his experience with more than 600 patients, he summarized his recommendations in 1919 that all arterial injuries and post-traumatic aneurysms, including those of the aorta, carotid, iliac, and subclavian arteries, and the arteries of the extremities, should be repaired by vascular suture either immediately after the injury or after 1 month for pulsating hematomas. In 1924 Weglowski presented the results of 193 personal vascular repairs including 46 by lateral sutures, 12 by end-to-end anastomosis and 56 using venous grafts. Ligation was required in the remaining 79 patients because of infection and the risk of postoperative bleeding. His results were surprisingly good. In 1994, Nunn wrote in detail about Ernst Jeger, who he called a "forgotten pioneer in cardiovascular surgery." Jeger's work was recorded only in the German language. Jeger described his research in a book, *Die Chirgurie der Blutgefasse und des Herzens* in 1913. He was drafted as a physician for the German Army in 1914 and died tragically in a Russian prison camp in 1915. Jeger did report his operative experience with 10 soldiers with vascular injuries. He had success in seven patients using lateral suture or end-to-end anastomosis. Based on his successful experience, he recommended increased use of vascular repair in war injuries.

World War II Experience

Experiences with vascular surgery in World War II are well recorded in the classic review of DeBakey and Simeone (1946), analyzing 2471 arterial injuries. Almost all were treated by ligation, with a subsequent amputation rate near 49%. Only 81 repairs were attempted, 78 by lateral suture and 3 by end-to-end anastomosis, with an amputation rate of approximately 35%. The use of vein grafts was even more disappointing: They were attempted in 40 patients, with an amputation rate of nearly 58%. Early patency of a venous graft in the arterial system was demonstrated angiographically. DeBakey (Fig. 1–10) has had the opportunity to contribute to the development and progress in vascular surgery over more than 50 years, from 1946 to 1996.

The controversial question of ligation of the concomitant vein remained, although few observers were convinced that the procedure enhanced circulation. The varying opinions were summarized by Linton in 1949.

A refreshing exception to the dismal World War II experience in regard to ligation and gangrene was the case operated on by Doctor Allen M. Boyden: an acute arteriovenous fistula of the femoral vessels repaired shortly after D-Day in Normandy. The following comments are taken from his field notes about 26

years later Boyden (personal communication, 1970) and emphasize the value of adequate records, even in military combat:

High explosive wound left groin, 14 June 1944, at 2200 hours. Acute arteriovenous aneurysm femoral artery
Preoperative blood pressure 140/70; pulse 104
Operation: 16 June 1944, nitrous oxide and oxygen
Operation: 1910 to 22 hours
One unit blood transfused during the operation

Continued

MILITARY SURGICAL HERITAGE
Department of Surgery, USUHS
Michael E. DeBakey, MD

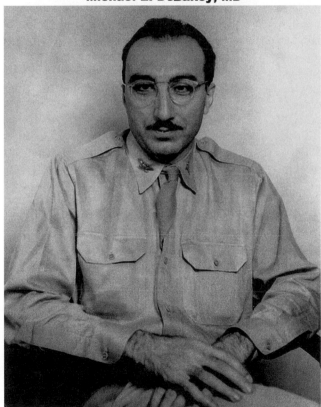

Colonel, MC, AUS   Third AMEDD Surgical Consultant 1946
Consultant Department of Surgery USUHS, 1977-
Visiting Board Department of Surgery USUHS, 1978-
Advisor, USU Surgical Associates, 1980-   President 1990
Michael E. Debakey International Military Surgeon's Award

■ **FIGURE 1–10**
Doctor DeBakey is recognized for his numerous and valuable contributions to surgery, in general, and specifically to military vascular surgery. The Michael DeBakey International Military Surgeons Award is presented at the Uniformed Services University Surgical Associates Day each spring at the Uniformed Services University of the Health Sciences, Bethesda, Maryland. (From Rich NM: Am J Surg 1993;166:91-96.) ■

*Arteriovenous aneurysms isolated near
    junction with profunda femoris artery*
Considerable hemorrhage
*Openings in both artery and vein were sutured
    with fine silk*
*Postoperative blood pressure 120/68; pulse
    118*
*Circulation of the extremity remained intact
    until evacuation*

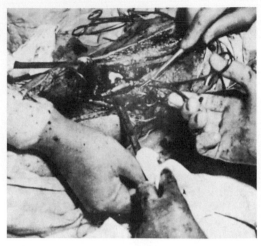

■ **FIGURE 1–11**
Completed unsutured vein graft of the popliteal
artery which was complicated by a severe
compound fracture of the tibia. This was
representative of 40 cases utilizing the double-
tube graft technique in World War II as
advocated by Blakemore, Lord and Stefko in
1942. (From DeBakey ME, Simeone FA: Ann
Surg 1946;123:534-579.) ■

As this case demonstrated Boyden's interest in vascular surgery, the Consulting Surgeon
for the First Army presented him with one half
of the latter's supply of vascular instruments
and material. This supply consisted of two sets
of Blakemore tubes, two bulldog forceps, and
a 2-mL ampule of heparin!

The conclusion that ligation was the treatment of choice for injured arteries was
summarized by DeBakey and Simeone in 1946,
"It is clear that no procedure other than ligation is applicable to the majority of vascular
injuries which come under the military surgeons' observation. It is not a procedure of
choice. It is a procedure of stern necessity, for
the basic purpose of controlling hemorrhage,
as well as because of the location, type, size
and character of most battle injuries of the
arteries."

In retrospect it should be remembered that
the average time lag between wounding and
surgical treatment was more than 10 hours in
World War II, virtually precluding successful
arterial repair in most patients. Of historical
interest is the nonsuture method of arterial
repair used during World War II (Figs. 1–11
and 1–12).

Although considerable time and effort
were expended following World War II in an
attempt to provide additional long-term
follow-up information, the results of this
effort are not generally available. Individual
follow-up has been possible in a random way
for some patients, such is the case of an acute
femoral arteriovenous fistula that was repaired
shortly after D-Day in Normandy on June 16,
1944 (Boyden, 1970). This was an unusual case
because it involved the successful repair of
both the common femoral artery and the

common femoral vein in a combat zone at a
time when ligation of vascular injuries was the
accepted principle. Unfortunately, when it was
possible more than 26 years later to obtain
follow-up data on this patient, it was learned
that hemorrhage occurred in the left inguinal
wound after the patient was evacuated to a
General Hospital in England. Ligation of both
the common femoral artery and the common
femoral vein was required. Additional follow-
up was not possible because the patient died
of tuberculosis approximately 16 months
after receiving the wound. Shumacker (1946,
1947a, 1947b, 1948a, 1948b) (Fig. 1–13)
(Table 1–3) made many valuable contributions to vascular surgery with the U.S. Army,
as did Rob (Fig. 1–14) with the British Army.

Experiences During the Korean Conflict

The successful repair of arterial injuries in the
Korean Conflict, in pleasant contrast to the
experiences of World War I and World War

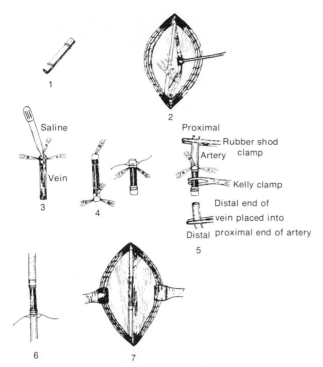

■ FIGURE 1-12
The various steps of a nonsuture method of bridging arterial defects designed during World War II (1) The Vitallium tube with its two ridges (sometimes grooves). (2) The exposed femoral artery and vein retracted and clamps placed on a branch. (3) The removed segment of vein is irrigated with saline solution. (4) The vein has been pushed through the inside of the Vitallium tube, and the two ends everted over the ends of the tube held in place with one or two ligatures of fine silk. (5) Distal end of the segment of vein is placed into the proximal end of the artery and held there by two ligatures of fine silk. (6) The snug ligature near the end of the Vitallium tube is tied to provide apposition of the artery and vein. (7) The completed operation, showing the bridging of a 2-cm gap in the femoral artery. (From Blakemore AH, Lord JW, Stefko PL: Surgery 1942;12:488-508.) ■

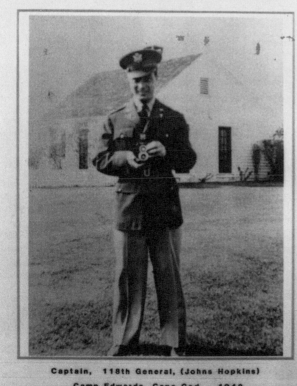

MILITARY SURGICAL HERITAGE
DEPARTMENT OF SURGERY, USUHS
Harris B Shumacker, Jr.

Captain, 118th General, (Johns Hopkins)
Camp Edwards, Cape Cod   1942
Professor of Surgery, USUHS
1 July 1981 –

■ FIGURE 1-13
Doctor Harris Shumacker made many valuable contributions in World War II to the early development of military vascular surgery. Subsequently, he received appropriate recognition by being named the first, and only, distinguished professor in the Department of Surgery at the Uniformed Services University of the Health Sciences, Bethesda, Maryland. (From Rich NM: Am J Surg 1993;166:91-96.) ■

TABLE 1–3
CASES IN WHICH ARTERY WAS REPAIRED BY END-TO-END SUTURE*

Case No.	Age of Patient (yr)	Duration of Lesion (mo)	Type of Lesion	Location of Lesion	Preoperative Symptoms	Length of Artery Excised (mm)	Period of Follow-ups (mo)	Result
1	20	5.7	Saccular aneurysm	Brachial distal third	0	1.5	2	Excellent
2	35	7.5	Saccular aneurysm	Brachial distal third	0	1.5-2	2	Excellent
3	27	8	Saccular aneurysm	Brachial proximal third	0	1.5-2	3.5	Excellent
4	28	8.5	Saccular aneurysm	Brachial middle third	0	1.5	2	Excellent
5	23	5.5	Saccular, aneurysm	Axillary distal third	+	2-2.5	2	Excellent
6	19	6	Saccular aneurysm	Brachial middle third	0	1.5	2	Excellent
7	24	6	Saccular aneurysm	Brachial distal third	0	2	1	Segment thrombosed Good circulation
8	21	3	Saccular aneurysm	Brachial distal third	0	2	5	Probably thrombosed and recannulized
9	29	3	Arteriovenous saccular aneurysm	Axillary distal third	0	2	4	Excellent
10	29	3	Arteriovenous	Femoral and profunda arteries Femoral veins	0	3-femoral 2-profunda	2.5	Excellent

*Anastomosis between proximal end of profunda and distal segment of femoral artery.
From Shumacker HB Jr: Problems of maintaining continuity of artery in surgery of aneurysms and arteriovenous fistulae. Notes on developmental and clinical application of methods of arterial suture. Ann Surg 127:207-230, 1948.

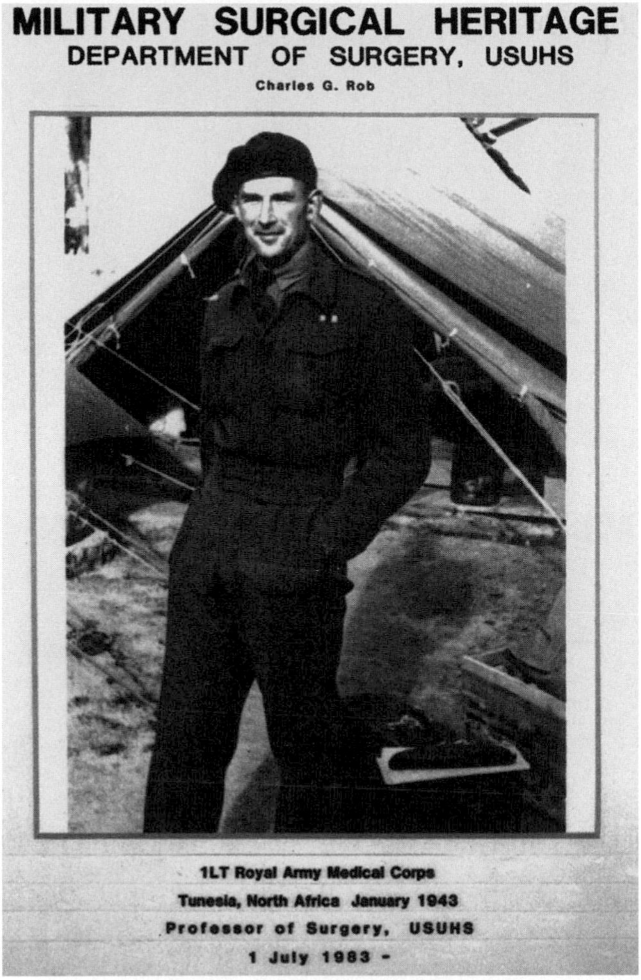

MILITARY SURGICAL HERITAGE
DEPARTMENT OF SURGERY, USUHS
Charles G. Rob

1LT Royal Army Medical Corps
Tunesia, North Africa January 1943
Professor of Surgery, USUHS
1 July 1983 -

■ **FIGURE 1–14**
Doctor Charles Rob has had a distinguished career, both in the United Kingdom and in the United States; he has been recognized for his international contributions in vascular surgery. Dr. Rob continues to serve as professor and senior advisor at the Uniformed Services University of the Health Sciences, Bethesda, Maryland. (From Rich NM: Am J Surg 1993;166:91-96.) ■

II, was due to several factors. There had been substantial progress in the techniques of vascular surgery, accompanied by improvements in anesthesia, angiography, blood transfusion, and antibiotics. Perhaps of the greatest importance was rapid evacuation of wounded men often by helicopter, permitting their transport from time of wounding to surgical care often within 1 to 2 hours (Fig. 1–15). In addition, a thorough understanding of the importance of dèbridement, delayed primary closure, and antibiotics greatly decreased the hazards of infection.

Initially in the Korean Conflict, attempts at arterial repair were disappointing. During one report of experiences at a surgical hospital for 8 months between September 1951 and April 1952, only 11 of 40 attempted arterial repairs were thought to be successful (Hughes, 1959). Only 6 of 29 end-to-end anastomoses were considered initially successful, and all 6 venous grafts failed. In another report from a similar period, only 4 of 18 attempted repairs were considered successful. Warren (1952) emphasized that an aggressive approach was needed, with the establishment of a research team headed by a surgeon experienced in vascular grafting. Surgical research teams were established in the Army, and there was improvement in results of vascular repairs in 1952. Significant reports were published by Jahnke and Seeley (1953), Hughes (1955, 1958), and Inui, Shannon, and Howard (1955). Hughes (Fig. 1–16) continued his

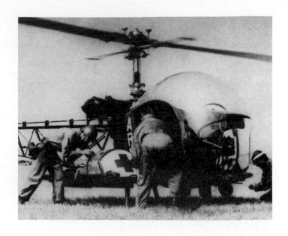

■ **FIGURE 1–15**
Helicopter evacuation of the wounded during the Korean Conflict helped reduce the lag time between injury and definitive surgical care. Continued improvement in Vietnam in helicopter evacuation of the wounded allowed some patients with vascular trauma to reach a definitive surgical center within 15 to 30 minutes. (US Army photograph.) ■

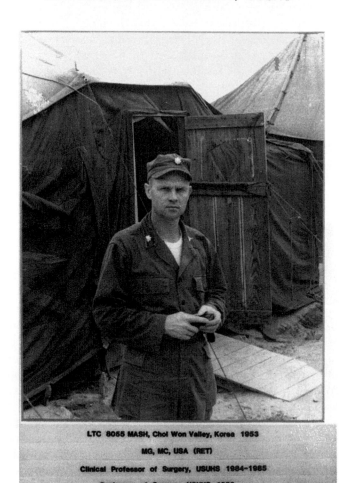

MILITARY SURGICAL HERITAGE
DEPARTMENT OF SURGERY, USUHS

LTC 8055 MASH, Chol Won Valley, Korea 1953

MG, MC, USA (RET)

Clinical Professor of Surgery, USUHS 1984–1985

Professor of Surgery, USUHS 1986 –

■ **FIGURE 1–16**
Doctor Carl Hughes had a distinguished military career providing valuable contribution during the Korean Conflict and, subsequently, during the Vietnam War. He continues to serve as professor at the Uniformed Services University of the Health Sciences, Bethesda, Maryland. (From Rich NM. Am J Surg 1993;166:91-96.) ■

efforts in vascular surgery rising to the rank of Major General. He continues at the Uniformed Services University of the Health Sciences, a Distinguished Professor of Surgery. Howard reflected in 1998 on his clinical and research experiences during the Korean Conflict. Similar work in the Navy was done with the U.S. Marines during 1952 and 1953 by Spencer and Grewe (1955). These surgeons worked in specialized research groups under fairly stabilized conditions, considering that they were in a combat zone (Fig. 1–17). Spencer reflected on his experiences during the Korean Conflict during his Presidential Address to the American Surgical Association in 1998.

Brigadier General Sam Seeley, who was Chief of the Department of Surgery at Walter Reed Army Hospital in 1950, had the foresight to establish Walter Reed Army Hospital as a vascular surgery center, and this made it possible for patients with vascular injuries to be returned there for later study (Fig. 1–18). In a total experience with 304 arterial injuries, 269 were repaired and 35 ligated (Hughes, 1958). The overall amputation rate was 13%, a marked contrast to that of about 49% in World War II. Because the amputation rate is only one method of determining ultimate

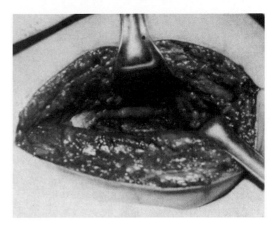

■ **FIGURE 1–18**
An autogenous greater saphenous vein graft was utilized in 1952 at Walter Reed General Hospital to repair a traumatized proximal popliteal artery. Each anastomosis is an everting type with intima-to-intima held by everting mattress sutures. (Rich NM, Hughes CW. Bull Am Coll Surg 1972;57:35.) ■

success or failure in arterial repair, it is important to emphasize that Jahnke (1958) revealed that in addition to the lowered rate of limb loss, limbs functioned normally when arterial repair was successful. The arteriovenous fistula experience is expanded on in Chapter 24.

Experience in Vietnam

In Vietnam the time lag between injury and treatment was reduced even further by the almost routine evacuation by helicopter, combined with the widespread availability of surgeons experienced in vascular surgery. In one study of 750 patients with missile wounds in Vietnam, 95% of the patients reached the hospital by helicopter (Rich, 1968) (Fig. 1–18). This prompt evacuation, however, similarly created an adverse effect on the overall results, for patients with severe injuries from high-velocity missiles survived only long enough to reach the hospital. During initial care, they expired. These patients would never have reached the hospital alive in previous military conflicts.

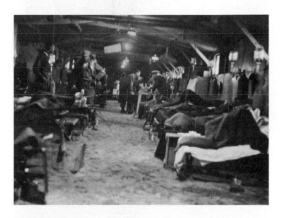

■ **FIGURE 1–17**
Postoperative ward in a *mobile* army surgical hospital (MASH) shows some of the conditions at the time of the Korean Conflict when it was demonstrated that arterial repair could be successful, even under battlefield conditions. (Hughes CW. Milit Med 1959;124:30-46.) ■

In the initial Vietnam studies, between October 1, 1965, and June 30, 1966, there were 177 known vascular injuries in U.S. casualties, excluding those with traumatic amputation (Heaton and colleagues, 1966). One hundred sixteen operations were performed on 106 patients with 108 injuries (Table 1–4). These results included the personal experience of one of us (N.M.R.) at the Second Surgical Hospital. The results reported included a short-term follow-up of approximately 7 to 10 days in Vietnam. In Vietnam, amputations were required for only 9 of the 108 vascular injuries, a rate of about 8%. Subsequently, more detailed analysis from the Vietnam Vascular Registry (Rich and Hughes, 1969; Rich, 1970) found the amputation rate of approximately 13%, identical to that of the Korean Conflict. Almost all amputations were performed within the first month after wounding.

The Vietnam Vascular Registry (Figs. 1–19 and 1–20) was established at Walter Reed General Hospital in 1966 to document and analyze all vascular injuries treated in Army Hospitals in Vietnam. A preliminary report

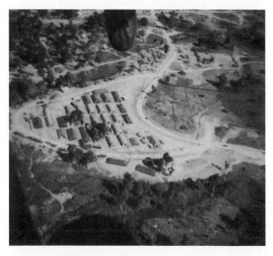

■ **FIGURE 1-19**
During the war in Vietnam, most patients were rapidly treated in fixed installations. An early example is the 2nd Surgical Hospital at An Khe in January, 1966. Ninety-five per cent of the wounded reached a hospital by helicopter. (Rich NM, Georgiade NG. Plastic and Maxillo-facial Trauma Symposium. CV Mosby, St Louis, 1969.) ■

(Rich and Hughes, 1969) involved the complete follow-up of 500 patients who sustained 718 vascular injuries (Table 1–5). Although vascular repairs on Vietnamese and allied military personnel were not included, the Registry effort was soon expanded to include all U.S. service personnel, rather than limiting the effort to soldiers.

Fisher (1967) collected 154 acute arterial injuries in Vietnam covering the 1965 to 1966 period. There were 108 arterial injuries with significant information for the initial review from Army hospitals. In 1967, Chandler and Knapp reported results in managing acute vascular injuries in the U.S. Navy hospitals in Vietnam. These patients were not included in the initial Vietnam Vascular Registry report, but after 1967, an attempt was made to include all military personnel sustaining vascular trauma in Vietnam. This included active-duty members of the U.S. Armed Forces treated at approximately 25 Army hospitals, six Navy hospitals, and one Air Force hospital.

As with any registry, success of the Vietnam Vascular Registry has depended on the cooperation of hundreds of individuals within the military and civilian communities. In the initial report from the Registry, the names of 20 surgeons who had done more than five vascular repairs were included (Rich and Hughes, 1969). In the first edition of *Vascular Trauma,* the names of many more who contributed to the Vietnam Vascular Registry are included (Rich and Spencer, 1978).

We would be remiss if we did not gain something positive from an experience with as many negative aspects as the U.S. involvement in Southeast Asia between 1965 and 1972. The Vietnam Vascular Registry provides a unique opportunity for long-term follow-up of thousands of young men with vascular repairs. The challenge remains and the potential is great. Additional historical details regarding the Registry activities are included in the first edition of *Vascular Trauma.* Unfortunately, the majority in the United States did not want to hear the word *Vietnam* for nearly 25 years. Only recently has the value of the Vietnam Vascular Registry been appreciated appropriately and it is hoped that the efforts can be completed.

TABLE 1–4
EARLY EXPERIENCE WITH VASCULAR SURGERY IN VIETNAM 108 ARTERIAL INJURIES AT ARMY HOSPITALS*

Artery	No. of Injuries	Type of Repair					Total Repairs	Results		
		Anastomosis	Vein Graft	Lateral Repair	Thrombectomy	Pros Graft		Pulse Present	Pulse Absent	Am
									No. Amputation	
Common carotid	7	1	3	3	0	0	7	7	0	0
Axillary	9	3	4	2	0	0	9	8	1	0
Brachial	33	15	11	9	1	0	36	29	3	1
Innominate	1	1	0	0	0	0	1	1	0	0
Subclavian	1	0	0	1	0	0	1	1	0	0
External iliac	4	2	1	0	0	1	4	4	0	0
Common femoral	7	3	4	1	0	0	8	7	0	0
Superficial femoral	30	21	3	6	0	0	30	26	1	3
Popliteal	16	7	7	5	1	0	20	10	1	5
TOTAL	108	53	33	27	2	1	116	93	6	9

*Including 2nd Surg, 3rd Surg, 85th Evac, 91st Evac, 3rd Field 8th Field Hospitals.
Modified from Heaton LD, Hughes CW, Rosegay H, et al: Military surgical practices of the United States Army in Vietnam. In Current Problems in Surgery. Chicago Year Book Medical Publishers, 1966.

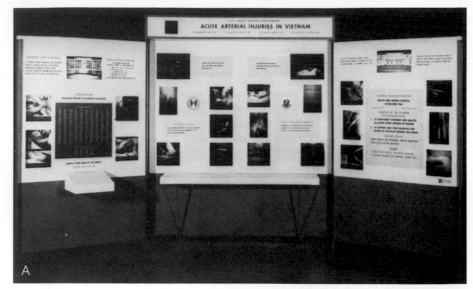

■ **FIGURE 1–20**

A, This exhibit representing the management of acute arterial trauma in Vietnam was presented from material in the Vietnam Registry to the Clinical Congress of the American College of Surgeons in Chicago in 1970. At least 110 surgeons who had previously performed arterial repairs in Vietnam visited the exhibit. *B,* Identification card sent to armed forces personnel who were wounded in Vietnam. This card was issued in an attempt to identify participation in the Registry and with the hope that additional long-term follow-up information will be generated. (*A,* From A.F.I.P. photograph; *B,* From Walter Reed General Hospital.) ■

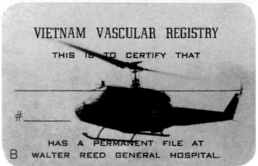

TABLE 1–5

MANAGEMENT OF ARTERIAL TRAUMAIN VIETNAM CASUALTIES PRELIMINARY REPORT FROM THE VIETNAM VASCULAR REGISTRY*

Artery	End-to-End Anastomosis	Vein Graft	Lateral Suture	Prosthetic Graft	Thrombectomy	Ligation
Common carotid	2	6 (2)	3		(2)	1
Internal carotid			2			1
Subclavian	1					
Axillary	6 (3)	12 (3)	2 (3)	(1)	(3)	(1)
Brachial	57 (8)	32 (10)	2 (1)		1 (9)	1 (2)
Aorta			3 (1)			
Renal						1
Iliac	1	1		1 (1)	(1)	(1)
Common femoral	4 (2)	11 (1)	4 (1)	1 (2)	(2)	(4)
Superficial femoral	63 (5)	37 (14)	7 (7)	(4)	2 (6)	(4)
Popliteal	31 (5)	28 (13)	6 (4)		(10)	2 (4)
TOTAL	165 (23)	127 (43)	29 (17)	2 (8)	3 (33)	6 (16)

*Numbers in parenthesis represent additional procedures performed after the initial repair in Vietnam and repair of major arterial injuries not initially treated in Vietnam.

Modified from Rich NM, Hughes CE: Vietnam vascular registry: a preliminary report. Surgery 65:218-226, 1969.

TABLE 1-6

LOCATION OF EXTREMITY VENOUS INJURIES IN VIETNAM (1965-1969), ISRAEL (1973), LEBANON (1969-1982), AND CROATIA (1991-1992)

Vein	Vietnam (%) ($n = 361$)	Israel (%) ($n = 26$)	Lebanon (%) ($n = 348$)	Croatia (%) ($n = 41$)
Subclavian	1	8	3	—
Axillary	6		3	10
Brachial	15	31	—	20
Iliac	3	—	10	12
Femoral	43	35	51	39
Popliteal	32	27	32	20

From Leppäniemi A, Rich NM, Browner BD (eds): Techniques in Orthopaedics, vol 10, pp 265-271, 1995, Philadelphia, JB. Lippincott.

Military Armed Conflicts Following Vietnam

From Beruit (1982) to Grenada (1983), Panama (1989), the Gulf War (1991), Somalia (1992), as well as recent experiences in Croatia, Rwanda, and Haiti (and even the 2001/2002 War against Terrorism), no United States military surgeons have had more than an antidotal vascular case or two to manage. The data from Vietnam remain pertinent and valuable today! Leppäniemi (1995) makes comparisons between Vietnam and recent wars in Israel (1973), Lebanon (1969 to 1982) and Croatia (1992) (Table 1–6). Roostar (1995) adds the Soviet experience in Afghanistan in the early 1980s (Table 1–7). There are military sources such as Croatia and Serbia; however, these are generally limited in coverage considering the large numbers of casualties. The following report is outlined because of the information contained. Luetic and colleagues, at the "Doctor Ozren Novosel" Clinical Hospital at the University of Zagreb, has documented experience in the management of military vascular injuries in Croatia. He presented a single center experience in the recent conflict, documenting results from April through December 1991. Luetic and colleagues (1993) managed 1020 casualties with 76 patients sustaining 120 vascular injuries. This is a relatively high 7.5% of the casualties with vascular trauma. Also, patients averaging

TABLE 1-7

LOCATION OF INJURIES IN THE AFGHANISTAN WAR

Location	Artery	Vein	Artery and Vein	Total
Carotid	3	—	1	4
Subclavian	10	2	3	15
Axillary	6	—	1	7
Brachial	39	—	6	45
Radial	7	—	1	8
Iliac	5	—	2	7
Femoral	45	9	22	76
Popliteal	19	2	1	22
Tibial	22	—	—	22
TOTAL	156	13	37	206

Modified from Roostar L: Treatment plan used for vascular injuries in the Afghanistan war. Cardiovasc Surg 3:42-45, 1995.

1.58 vascular injuries is a very high percent of multiple injuries. It is particularly pertinent to note that the casualties were transported after initial treatment in forward surgical facilities, reaching the university hospital within 3 to 18 hours, with a mean time of 7 hours. The most common injuries were to the popliteal artery (12.5%) and the brachial veins (10%). There was a relatively high incidence of concomitant fractures, occurring in 90.4% of the cases. They routinely employed external fixation of the concomitant fractures. They used venous interposition grafts in 45 arterial injuries and 20 venous injuries. Prostheses were used in only three arterial injuries. They did have a relatively high incidence of arteriovenous fistulas and pseudoaneurysms, with the former occurring in seven patients and the latter in six patients (9.8%) with one patient having injury to the popliteal artery and five having injuries to the superficial femoral artery. Sepsis, deep venous thrombosis, and extensive myonecrosis contributed to the required amputations, with three patients not receiving definitive surgical repair until 12 hours after injury. All patients requiring amputations had concomitant injury to bone, nerve, soft tissue, veins, and arteries. There was a mortality rate of 3.9%, with three patients dying.

CIVILIAN VASCULAR INJURIES

Several differences exist between civilian and military vascular injuries. First, military injuries are characteristically in young persons without arterial disease. They frequently result from high-velocity missiles with extensive soft tissue destruction, often with injuries of multiple organ systems and in circumstances in which surgical treatment is less than ideal. Civilian injuries, however, are usually from wounds associated with minimal soft tissue destruction. Prompt treatment and excellent hospital facilities are usually available. Although young civilians are commonly injured, there is also a significant percentage of older patients who often have preexisting arterial disease. In addition, there are frequent injuries from blunt trauma, such as automobile or industrial accidents, and fractures of long bones. Finally, an increasing number of vascular injuries are being seen as a complication of diagnostic procedures involving cannulation of peripheral arteries, as in angiography or cardiac catheterization.

> *Currently accepted principles regarding management of acute vascular injuries is largely based on military experience.*
> Theodore Drapanas (1970)

The frequency of arterial injuries in civilian life has increased greatly in the past decade. This is due to more automobile accidents, the appalling increase in gunshot and stab wounds, and the increasing use of therapeutic and diagnostic techniques involving the cannulation of major arteries. As recently as 1950, most general surgeons had little experience or confidence in techniques of arterial repair. The experiences in the Korean Conflict, combined with the widespread teaching of techniques of vascular surgery in surgical residencies, resulted in a great increase in frequency of arterial repair between 1950 and 1960.

One of the first large series of civilian arterial trauma was reported by Morris, Creech, and DeBakey in 1957. They described a series of 136 patients with acute arterial injuries treated over 7 years at Baylor University–affiliated hospitals in Houston (Fig. 1–21). Sixty-

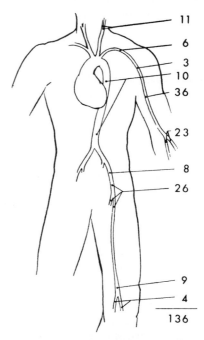

■ **FIGURE 1-21**
Anatomic locations of arterial injuries in the civilian experience in Houston. In addition to the fact that nearly one half of the injuries involved the brachial and femoral arteries, exactly 50% of the injuries also involved arteries supplying the upper extremity. (From Morris GC Jr, Creech O Jr, DeBakey ME: Am J Surg 1957;93:565-567.) ■

TABLE 1–8

THE CIVILIAN EXPERIENCE IN ATLANTA COMPARING TWO CONSECUTIVE 5-YEAR PERIODS SHOWS THE INCREASE IN INCIDENCE OF INJURY AND THE MARKED IMPROVEMENT OF SUCCESSFUL REPAIR FROM 36 PERCENT TO 90 PERCENT. THERE WAS ALSO AN ASSOCIATED REDUCTION IN THE MORTALITY RATE BY ONE-THIRD AND AMPUTATION RATE BY ONE HALF

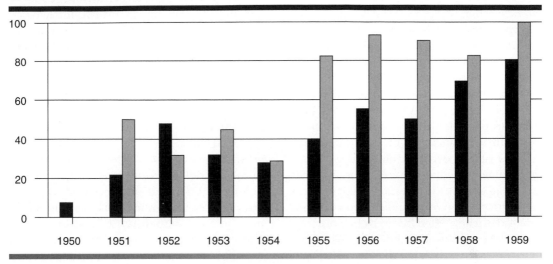

■ Percentage of cases treated by repair
▣ Percentage of repairs successful (restoration of distal pulses)
From Ferguson IA, Byrd WM, McAfee DK: Experiences in the management of arterial injuries. Ann Surg 153:980-986, 1961.

eight injuries, one half of the group, involved the upper extremities, and forty-seven injuries (about 35%) involved the lower extremities. There were injuries of either the abdominal or the thoracic aorta and 11 of the carotid artery. One hundred twenty of the patients, 88%, were male, and most of the injuries were caused by acts of violence. Primary arterial repair was possible in a high percentage of these patients.

In 1961, Ferguson, Byrd, and McAfee, reported from Grady Memorial Hospital in Atlanta, 200 arterial injuries treated over 10 years. The superficial femoral artery was injured most often, 39 patients, or nearly 20% of the total group. However, 54 of the 200 patients had injuries of minor arteries such as the radial or ulnar arteries. The proportion of patients treated by arterial repair increased from less than 10% in 1950 to more than 80% in 1959. In the latter part of the study, ligation was done only for injuries of minor arteries, such as the radial or ulnar, or certain visceral arteries. The mortality rate was reduced by one third and the amputation rate

by one half when two consecutive 5-year periods were compared. The rate of success of arterial repair improved from 36% to 90% (Table 1–8). As in Houston, most resulted from acts of violence (Table 1–9). Automobile, industrial, and domestic accidents accounted for most of the remaining injuries.

TABLE 1–9

TYPE OF ACUTE ARTERIAL INJURIES IN CIVILIAN PRACTICE, HOUSTON, PRIOR TO 31 JULY 1956

	No.	No.
Transection	71	52.2
Laceration	56	41.2
Contusion	6	4.4
Spasm	3	2.2
TOTAL	136	100.0

Modified from Morris GC Jr, Creech O Jr, DeBakey ME: Acute arterial injuries in civilian practice. Am J Surg 93:565-572, 1957.

In 1963, Smith, Foran, and Gaspar described experiences with 59 patients with 61 vascular injuries in Detroit, including both acute and chronic arterial injuries (Table 1–10). They properly emphasized that a careful distinction must be made between results with acute and chronic lesions. Collateral circulation has usually developed when a chronic lesion is treated and the problem of soft tissue is not present. Acts of violence, gunshot and stab wounds, caused 18 injuries, 44% of the penetrating lesions (Table 1–11). Their patients included ten industrial injuries and eight iatrogenic injuries resulting either from surgical operations or from diagnostic procedures. These eight included three injuries of the external iliac artery during inguinal herniorrhaphy, three arterial injuries following diagnostic arterial catheterization, one injury of the internal iliac artery during removal of a herniated intravertebral disc, and one arteriovenous fistula developing after a mass suture ligature of the renal pedicle during nephrectomy.

In 1964, Patman, Poulos, and Shires described experiences with 256 patients, with a total of 271 arterial injuries, treated at the Parkland Memorial Hospital in Dallas over 12 years starting in July 1949. As in other U.S. series, most resulted from acts of violence, and only a few resulted from industrial or automobile accidents. Multiple arterial injuries occurred in 6% of the group. Although chronic lesions from trauma were included, it was noteworthy that these were few: only 6 arteriovenous fistulas and 12 false aneurysms among the entire group of 256 patients.

A somewhat different group of cases was reported from Europe by Vollmar in 1968. In an analysis of 85,000 injured patients treated in the Heidelberg University Surgery Clinic between 1953 and 1966, there were only 172 arterial lesions, an incidence of 0.3%. In marked contrast to the U.S. experience, only 1% of the injuries were due to gunshot wounds. Most patients were injured in industrial accidents (Table 1–12). Approximately

TABLE 1–10
CIVILIAN ARTERIAL TRAUMA IN DETROIT, 61 ARTERIAL INJURIES

Type of Trauma	Laceration	28 Early Lesions		Spasm
		Transection	Thrombosis	
Penetrating injuries	10	6	2	—
Nonpenetrating injuries	2	2	4	2
TOTAL	12	8	6	2

Modified from Smith RF, Szilagyi DE, Pfeifer JR: Arterial trauma. Arch Surg 86:825-835, 1963.

TABLE 1–11
ETIOLOGIC FACTORS CAUSING 61 ARTERIAL INJURIES, 59 PATIENTS IN CIVILIAN SERIES IN DETROIT

42 Penetrating Injuries	%	19 Nonpenetrating Injuries	%
Gunshot 13	21.3	Industrial 11	18.0
Industrial 10	16.4	Auto 4	6.6
Iatrogenic 8	13.1	Athletic 2	3.3
Household 6	9.8	Household 2	3.3
Stab 5	8.2		

Modified from Smith RF, Szilagyi DE, Pfeifer JR: Arterial trauma. Arch Surg 86:825-835, 1963.

TABLE 1-12
TYPE OF ACCIDENT RESPONSIBLE FOR 169 PATIENTS WITH ARTERIAL INJURIES, HEIDELBERG UNIVERSITY SURGICAL CLINIC 1953-1966

Etiology	No.	%
Industrial accident	59	35
Domestic accident	44	26
Suicide	32	19
Traffic	24	14
Iatrogenic	10	6
TOTAL	169	100

Modified from Vollmar J: In Hiertonn T, Rybeck B (eds): Traumatic arterial lesions. Stockholm: Försvarets Forskningsanstalt, 1968.

TABLE 1-13
NATURE OF 197 ARTERIAL LESIONS IN 168 PATIENTS, HEIDELBERG UNIVERSITY, SURGICAL CLINIC

	Type	No.	%	
Sharp penetrating	Cut	95	48	}
	Stab	19	10	} 59
	Shot	3	1	}
Blunt	Closed	22	11	}
	Open	58	30	} 41

Modified from Vollmar J: In Hiertonn T, Rybeck B (eds): Traumatic arterial lesions. Stockholm: Försvarets Forskningsanstalt, 1968.

one fourth resulted from simple domestic accidents. Twelve resulted from automobile accidents. It was significant in this group that 41% of the total resulted from blunt trauma (Table 1–13).

In 1968, Saletta and Freeark described experiences with 57 patients with partially severed major peripheral arteries treated in Chicago (Table 1–14). Most of the injuries resulted from physical violence from gunshot wounds

TABLE 1-14
LOCATION AND CAUSE OF INJURY IN 57 PATIENTS WITH PARTIALLY SEVERED ARTERIES

Location and Artery	No.	Etiology				
		Gunshot	Knife	Glass	Blunt	Other
Head and neck						
Temporal	3			1	2	
Internal carotid	2	2				
External carotid	2	1	1			
Vertebral	1		1			
Lingual	1		1			
Upper extremity						
Axillary	6	2	3	1		
Brachial	5	1	4			
Innominate	1	1				
Subclavian	1		1			
Lower extremity						
Femoral	15	11	3			1 (needle)
Common femoral	6	3	1	1		1 (needle)
Popliteal	6	6				
External iliac	4	3	1			
Deep femoral	2	1	1			
Anterior tibial	1			1		
Posterior tibial	1					1 (tin can)
Tibioperoneal	1	1				

Modified from Saletta JD, Freeark RJ: The partially severed artery. Arch Surg 97:198-205, 1968.

or knives. Also, in 1968 Dillard, Nelson, and Norman described the treatment of 85 arterial injuries in St. Louis over 8 years beginning in 1958 (Table 1–15). Eighty-one percent of the injuries involved an extremity. Penetrating injuries from knives or glass caused 35 of the injuries, 31 resulted from gunshot wounds, and 19 were caused by blunt trauma or crushing injuries (Table 1–16).

Two large series are those of Drapanas and colleagues (1970) from New Orleans, which included 226 arterial injuries, and the cumulative report by Perry, Thal, and Shires from Dallas (1971), which included 508 arterial injuries. At Charity Hospital in New Orleans, 226 patients with arterial injuries were treated between 1942 and 1969 (Drapanas and colleagues, 1970) (Fig. 1–22). Of 226 patients, 173 had major arterial injuries and 53 had minor injuries. The most frequently injured arteries were the brachial (39 injuries) and the superficial femoral (31 injuries). There was an unusually large number (23) of aortic injuries involving the thoracic or abdominal aorta.

In 1971, Perry Thal, and Shires reported additional series of 259 arterial injuries from Dallas. About 55% of these were associated with gunshot wounds (Table 1–17). Combined with the 1964 report (Patman, Poulos, and Shires), there were a total of 508 injuries (Table 1–18). These included 442 injuries of

TABLE 1–15
DISTRIBUTION OF ARTERIAL INJURIES, ST. LOUIS, MISSOURI, 1958-1966

Artery	No.	%
Axillary artery	6	7.1
Brachial artery	26	30.6
Subclavian artery	4	4.7
Thoracic aorta	8	9.4
Abdominal aorta and branches	8	9.4
Iliac artery	2	2.3
Common femoral artery	7	8.2
Superficial femoral artery	14	16.5
Popliteal artery	10	11.8
TOTAL	85	100.0

Modified from Dillard BM, Nelson DL, Norman HG Jr: Review of 85 major traumatic arterial injuries. Surgery 63:391-395, 1968.

TABLE 1–16
ETIOLOGY AND ANATOMIC DISTRIBUTION OF 85 ARTERIAL INJURIES, ST. LOUIS, MISSOURI, 1958-1966

A. Knife or glass penetrating injuries	
Upper extremities	15
Thoracic aorta	3
Abdominal aorta and branches	5
Lower extremities	12
TOTAL	35 (41.2%)

B. Penetrating gunshot injuries	
Upper extremities	13
Thoracic aorta	2
Abdominal aorta and branches	2
Lower extremities	14
TOTAL	31 (36.5%)

C. Blunt trauma or crush injuries	
Upper extremities	8
Thoracic aorta	3
Abdominal aorta and branches	3
Lower extremities	5
TOTAL	19 (22.3%)

Modified from Dillard BM, Nelson DL, Norman HG Jr: Review of 85 major traumatic arterial injuries. Surgery 63:391-395, 1968.

arteries in the extremities, representing 87% of the total. There were also 42 cervical arterial injuries and 24 visceral arterial injuries. Moore and colleagues in 1971 reported 250 vascular injuries treated in Galveston, 45% of which occurred in the extremities (Table 1–19). In this series, 40% of the cases involved either the chest, the abdomen, or the head and neck, a percentage higher than that in other reports. The injuries resulted from either gunshot or stab wounds in 60% of the group (Table 1–20). Thirteen percent resulted from blunt trauma, and iatrogenic injuries were responsible for ten percent. Among the 25 iatrogenic injuries, there were 16 acute arterial thromboses resulting from a total of more than 3000 cardiovascular radiographic procedures, a frequency of less than 1% (Table 1–21).

Smith, Elliot, and Hageman (1974) reported a survey of 268 patients in Detroit with 285 penetrating wounds of the limbs and neck. There were 127 peripheral arterial injuries identified. Kelly and Eiseman (1975)

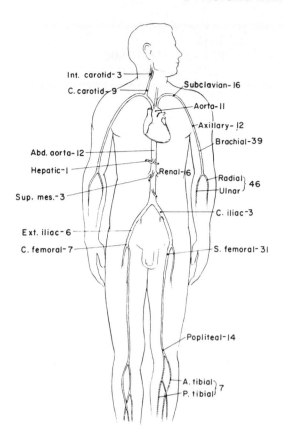

Int. carotid-3
C. carotid-9
Subclavian-16
Aorta-11
Axillary-12
Brachial-39
Abd. aorta-12
Hepatic-1
Renal-6
Radial }
Ulnar } 46
Sup. mes.-3
C. iliac-3
Ext. iliac-6
C. femoral-7
S. femoral-31
Popliteal-14
A. tibial }
P. tibial } 7

■ **FIGURE 1–22**
Distribution of 226 acute civilian arterial injuries covering a 30-year period in New Orleans starting in 1942. Eighty percent of the injuries involve arteries to the extremities. (From Drapanas T, Hewitt RL, Weichert RF 3rd, Smith AD: Surg 1970;172:351-360.) ■

reported 43% of 143 patients in Denver with vascular injuries sustained gunshot wounds. The brachial artery was injured most often, 37 times. Hardy and colleagues (1975) in Jackson recorded 192 arterial injuries from firearms (155 gunshot and 37 shotgun), 91 stab wounds and lacerations, 48 injuries from blunt trauma, and 20 iatrogenic injuries. The series included 36 aortic injuries. However, approximately two thirds involved extremity vessels. Cheek and colleagues (1975) reviewed 200 operative cases of major vascular injuries in Memphis, which included 155 arterial injuries. Bole and colleagues (1976) reported 126 arterial injuries in 122 patients in New York City from 1968 to 1973.

Reynolds, McDowell, and Diethelm (1979) documented results in managing 191 consecutive patients treated for arterial injuries during an 8-year period at the University of Alabama Medical Center starting in 1970. Most of their patients sustained penetrating wounds, either gunshot or shotgun; however, there were also 46 patients, or 24%, who had blunt trauma associated with their arterial injuries. Barros D'Sa and colleagues (1980) from the Queen's University Hospital at Belfast reviewed their experience with missile-induced vascular trauma over $7\frac{1}{2}$ years of serious hostilities involving the civilian population of northern Ireland. They documented the results in managing 113 patients with 191 vascular injuries treated at the Royal Victoria Hospital. It is particularly important to note that treatment commenced within 1 hour in 87% of the patients. Etiology of the

TABLE 1–17
CAUSE AND TYPE OF INJURY, CIVILIAN ARTERIAL TRAUMA, DALLAS, TEXAS

Cause	No.	%	Arterial Injury	No.	%
Gunshot wound	143	55.2	Laceration	133	51.4
Edged instruments	93	35.5	Transection	99	38.2
Blunt trauma	24	9.3	Puncture	18	6.9
TOTAL	259	100.0	Contusion	7	2.7
			Spasm	2	0.8
			TOTAL	259	100.0

Modified from Perry MO, Thal ER, Shires GT: Management of arterial injuries. Ann Surg 173:403-408, 1971.

TABLE 1–18

DISTRIBUTION OF CIVILIAN ARTERIAL INJURIES, DALLAS, TEXAS, 508 ARTERIAL INJURIES

Extremity (89.0%)		Cervical (8.3%)		Visceral (4.7%)	
Aorta	26	Common carotid	24	Celiac	2
Innominate	1	Internal carotid	8	Splenic	2
Subclavian	23	External carotid	6	Superior mesenteric	7
Axillary	38	Vertebral	4	Renal	9
Brachial	78	TOTAL	42	Hepatic	4
Radial	58			TOTAL	24
Ulnar	39				
Common iliac	20				
External iliac	11				
Hypogastric	7				
Common femoral	11				
Superficial femoral	93				
Profunda femoral	8				
Popliteal	17				
Tibial	12				
TOTAL	442				

Modified from Perry MO, Thal ER, Shires GT: Management of arterial injuries. Ann Surg 173:403-408, 1971.

TABLE 1–19

LOCATION OF VASCULAR TRAUMA IN 250 CIVILIAN INJURIES, GALVESTON, TEXAS, 1960-1970

Location	%
Head and neck	10
Thoracic outlet	16
Chest	15
Abdomen	14
Extremities	45
TOTAL	100

Modified from Moore CH, Wolma FJ, Brown RW, Derrick JR: Vascular trauma. A review of 250 cases. Am J Surg 122:576-578, 1971.

TABLE 1–20

LOCATION OF VASCULAR TRAUMA IN 250 CIVILIAN INJURIES, GALVESTON, TEXAS, 1960-1970

Type	%
Gunshot	39.0
Stab	25.0
Blunt	13.0
Iatragenic	10.0
Other	13.0
TOTAL	100.0

Modified from Moore CH, Wolma FJ, Brown RW, Derrick JR: Vascular trauma. A review of 250 cases. Am J Surg 122:576-578, 1971.

TABLE 1–21

25 CASES OF IATROGENIC VASCULAR INJURIES, GALVESTON, TEXAS, 1960-1970

Procedure	Injury	Treatment	No.
Central venous catheterization	Thrombosis	Thrombectomy	16
Lumbar laminectomy	Arteriovenous fistula	Repair of fistula	3
Osteotomy of hip	Arteriovenous fistula	Repair of fistula	1
Renal hemodialysis arteriovenous shunts	False aneurysm	Resection of aneurysm	2
Pelvic irradiation	Femoral artery rupture	Aortofemoral bypass	1
Fracture of humerus closed reduction	Volkmann's ischemia	Open reduction; free artery and fasciotomy	1
Subclavian catheterization	Arteriovenous fistula	Repair of fistula	1
TOTAL			25

Modified from Moore CH, Wolma FJ, Brown RW, Derrick JR: Vascular trauma. A review of 250 cases. Am J Surg 122:576-578, 1971.

injuries is outlined in Table 1–22. A special group of 38 patients had "knee capping" contributed to most of the popliteal vascular injuries.

Koivunen (1982) documented the experience in managing vascular trauma in a rural population in Missouri. During a 10-year period, they identified 89 cases of vascular trauma. Recognizing that the considerable delay in abdominal vasculature accounted for 33.7% of the injuries. Multiple injuries were common, with 1057 patients having two or more concurrent vascular injuries. There were three patients who had four or more separate vascular injuries. The increasing inci-

TABLE 1–22

INCIDENCE OF VASCULAR INJURIES RELATED TO TYPE

Wounding Missile	Patient	
	No.	%
Bullet		
Low velocity	48	42.5
High velocity	28	24.8
Uncertain velocity	22	19.5
Fragments from explosions	15	13.2
TOTAL	113	

From Barros D, Sa AA, Hassard TH, Livingston RH, et al: Missile-induced vascular trauma. Injury 12:13-30, 1980.

dence of vascular trauma in urban centers is emphasized by the marked increase from an average of 27 patients per year in the early 1960s to nearly a tenfold increase to the current average of 213 patients per year. These data can be compared and contrasted to other civilian and military experience, as noted in Table 1–23.

Feliciano and colleagues (1984) reported a 1-year experience with 456 vascular and cardiac injuries among 312 patients during 1982 at the Ben Taub Hospital in Houston. More than 87% of the injuries were penetrating, as identified in Table 1–24. Specifically, there were 408 vascular injuries and 48 cardiac injuries. Thirty-four percent of the patients had two or more vascular or cardiac injuries. The majority were penetrating, with more than 87% secondary to gunshot wounds, stab wounds, or shotgun wounds. The largest number of injuries occurred in the extremities, 39.9%, with the brachial artery being the most common arterial injury. There was a relatively large number of abdominal vascular injuries, accounting for 31.9% of the total. The most common venous injury occurred in the internal jugular vein in 26 patients.

Mattox and colleagues (1989) detailed a unique epidemiologic evolutionary profile from the civilian trauma registry at Baylor College of Medicine in Houston. During a 30-year period from 1958 to 1987, where consistent evaluation and treatment philosophy

TABLE 1–23

LOCATION OF REPORTED VASCULAR INJURIES IN MAJOR WARS

	Neck	Chest	Abdomen	Upper Extremity	Lower Extremity	Total
Makins (WWI[4])	176	—	11	367	648	1202
DeBakey (WWII[2])	34	—	49	871	1517	2471
Hughes (Korea[3])	14	—	7	109	304	304
Rich (Vietnam[7])	76	4	354	416	840	1377
TOTAL	300	4	421	1763	3179	5667

LOCATION OF CARDIOVASCULAR INJURIES IN CIVILIAN EPIDEMIOLOGIC VASCULAR TRAUMA REPORTS

Author	City	Year	Neck	Chest	Abdomen	Upper Extremities	Lower Extremities	Total
Morris[19]	Houston	1957	16	5	13	62	39	136
Ferguson[13]	Atlanta	1961	15	1	32	93	56	200
Smith[23]	Detroit	1962	3	2	8	25	21	57
Treiman[24]	Los Angeles	1966	14	10	56	67	86	233
Dilard[10]	St. Louis	1968	4	8	10	32	31	85
Drapanas[11]	New Orleans	1970	28	11	31	97	59	226
Perry[21]	Dallas	1971	65	14	75	213	141	508
Moore[16]	Galveston	1971	45	57	35	56	37	250
Cheek[9]	Memphis	1975	46	10	88	30	60	200
Kelly[15]	Denver	1975	14	—	62	52	47	175
Hardy[16]	Jackson	1975	39	41	66	98	116	360
Bole[8]	New York	1976	8	12	31	25	50	126
Sirinek[22]	San Antonio	1983	17	35	218	—	—	270
TOTAL			315	206	725	850	763	2859

From Mattox KL, Feliciano DV, Burch J, et al: Five thousand seven hundred sixty cardiovascular injuries in 4459 patients. Epidemiologic evolution, 1958 to 1987. Ann Surg 209:698-707, 1989.

TABLE 1–24

MECHANISMS OF INJURY; ALL VASCULAR AND CARDIAC INJURIES

Mechanism	No.	
Gunshot wound	166 (53.2%)	
Stab wound	88 (28.2%)	87.2%
Shotgun wound	18 (5.8%)	
Laceration	17 (5.4%)	
Iatrogenic	14 (4.5%)	
Blunt	9 (2.9%)	
TOTAL	312 (100%)	

From Feliciano DV, Bitando CG, Mattox KL, et al: Civilian trauma in the 1980s. A 1-year experience with 456 vascular and cardiac injuries. Ann Surg 199:717-724, 1984.

existed, they treated 5760 cardiovascular injuries in 4459 patients. Eighty-six percent of the patients were male, with an average age of 30 years. Penetrating trauma accounted for more than 90.0% of the injuries, with 51.1% resulting from gunshot wounds, 31.1% from stab wounds, and 6.8% from shotgun wounds (Table 1–25). The remaining injuries were iatrogenic or secondary to blunt trauma. Table 1–26 outlines the specific cardiovascular injuries by etiology and grouped by body region. Of particular interest and note, and in marked contrast with military experience and many previous civilian series, truncal injuries, including the neck, accounted for 66% of all injuries treated. The lower extremities, including the groin, accounted for only 19% of the injuries, specifically, injuries to the six patients. In the decade of the 1980s, there was marked increase in the number of

TABLE 1–25
ETIOLOGY OF PATIENT CARDIOVASCULAR INJURIES PER 5-YEAR TIME INTERVAL

Etiology	1958-1963	1964-1968	1969-1973	1974-1978	1979-1983	1984-1988	Total
Gunshot wound	42	236	436	501	625	456	2296
Stab/laceration	64	110	161	229	362	463	1389
Blunt trauma	1	17	58	90	62	76	304
Shotgun wound	1	15	45	55	61	37	214
Iatrogenic	1	1	0	0	4	25	31
Other/unknowns	54	20	111	25	3	12	225
TOTAL	163	399	811	900	1117	1069	4459

From Mattox KL, Feliciano DV, Burch J, et al: Five thousand seven hundred sixty cardiovascular injuries in 4459 patients: Epidemiologic evolution 1958 to 1987. Ann Surg 209:698-707, 1989.

manuscripts devoted to the management of civilian vascular trauma culminated by the extensive review of Mattox and colleagues.

During the 1990s, there continued to be a significant number of reports of the management of civilian arterial injuries. Oller and colleagues (1992) established a State Trauma Registry that had an early report of 1148 vascular injuries suffered by 978 patients in North Carolina over 39 months (October 1987 to January 1991) (Table 1–27). Whether human made or natural, there will continue to be trauma patients with associated vascular injuries. Internationally Kurtoglu and colleagues (1991) described treating 115 peripheral arterial injuries in Istanbul (Table 1–28). There will be additional details throughout the text emphasizing the recent experience of the past decade. The following, however, identifies areas of historical significance related to specific considerations involving vascular injuries.

HISTORICAL NOTES ON 20th CENTURY PROGRESS WITH VENOUS INJURIES

It could be recorded in history that outstanding contributions based on experience of managing Vietnam casualties by American military surgeons did as much to stimulate and direct interest and success

in repair of venous injuries as was established during the Korean Conflict with repair of arterial injuries. Vietnam Vascular Registry, Rich (1977)

Several excellent historic reviews of the development of venous trauma have been published (Haimovici, 1963; Shumacker, 1969; Rob, 1972). Two earlier outstanding references are Guthrie (1912) and Murphy (1897). As early as 1816, Travers supposedly closed a small wound in a femoral vein. In 1830, Guthrie reported more precisely that he closed a laceration of the internal jugular vein by placing a tenaculum through the cut edges, after which he tied a suture around the tenaculum to constitute a lateral ligature. In 1878, Agnew used lateral sutures to close venous wounds. Only a year earlier, Eck had performed the first vascular anastomosis by suturing the portal vein to the inferior vena cava. Schede in 1882 in Germany is generally given credit for performing the first successful lateral suture repair of a laceration in a vein in clinical practice, and he advocated repair of wounds of the femoral vein in man.

In the late 19th century, other surgeons who with apparent success sutured wounds of veins include Billroth, Braun of Koenigsberg, and Schmidt. In his experimental laboratory, Hirsch in 1881 successfully repaired divided veins in dogs. When Dörfler in 1889 outlined his method of arterial repair, he recommended the same technique for repairing

TABLE 1–26

SPECIFIC CARDIOVASCULAR INJURIES BY ETIOLOGY AND GROUPED BY BODY REGION

	Gunshot wound	Stab wound/ laceration	Blunt trauma	Shotgun wound	Iateogenic	Unknown/ Other	Total
Carotid artery	115	45	6	14	—	10	190
Jugular vein	116	154	4	9	—	13	296
Vertebral artery	18	13	3	3	—	2	40
Subclavian vessel	91	50	8	6	—	13	168
Heart	220	261	32	3	5	8	539
Coronary artery	3	10	—	—	3	1	14
Ascending aorta	15	12	3	3	—	—	33
Innominate artery	20	8	7	2	2	—	39
Pulmonary artery	43	25	7	3	—	1	79
Desc thorac aorta	25	5	59	—	—	—	89
Aortic arch	13	7	1	1	—	—	22
Thorac vena cava	34	15	4	1	—	1	55
Innominate vein	25	15	2	—	—	—	42
Pulmonary vein	29	5	4	1	—	1	40
Azygous vein	13	2	—	1	—	—	16
Thoracic duct	3	8	—	1	—	—	12
Int mammary artery	18	71	3	—	—	6	98
Intercostal artery	25	54	—	—	—	2	81
Abdominal aorta	180	40	5	17	2	5	249
Inf vena cava	353	100	44	21	—	17	535
Mesentric artrey	136	45	14	7	—	14	216
Portal venous	116	44	22	3	—	4	189
Iliac artery	172	30	11	11	2	6	232
Iliac vein	224	32	9	11	1	12	289
Renal vessel	86	33	32	4	—	8	163
Epigastric artery	3	14	—	3	—	1	52
Hepatic veins	36	6	8	1	—	1	21
Axillary vessel	85	40	3	6	1	8	143
Brachial artery	184	163	14	38	10	37	446
Radial/ulnar art	38	169	1	10	2	41	261
Cephalic/basilic vein	4	3	—	1	1	—	0
Femoral artery	316	58	14	70	5	37	500
Femoral vein	184	34	7	36	—	19	280
Popliteal artery	88	3	36	18	—	11	156
Popliteal vein	45	5	9	14	—	9	68
Tibial artery	31	8	11	9	—	9	68
Tibial vein	4	1	—	1	—	1	7
Saphenous vein	12	—	1	1	—	1	15
TOTAL	3134	1543	385	341	56	293	5760

From Mattox KL, Feliciano DV, Burch J, et al: Five thousand seven hundred sixty cardiovascular injuries in 4459 patients: Epidemiologic evolution 1958 to 1987. Ann Surg 209(6):698-707, 1989.

veins. Haimovici (1963) described Dörfler's method, "The essential features of this method consisted of the use of fine, round needles and fine silk and his suture was continuous, embracing all of the coats of the vessel. From his experience, although limited to 16 cases, he concluded that aseptic silk thread in the lumen of the vessel does not necessarily lead to thrombosis and, therefore, the penetration of the intima was not contraindicated."

TABLE 1–27
VASCULAR INJURIES IN A RURAL STATE: A REVIEW OF 978 PATIENTS FROM A STATE TRAUMA REGISTRY

Vessels Injured by Region	No. (%)
Head carotid and neck	133 (9.9)
Common	12
Internal	17
External	9
Unspecified	10
Jugular internal	22
Other vessels of neck	63
Thorax	166 (12.4)
Aorta	58
Innominate/subclavian A & V	37
Pulmonary vessels	14
Intercostals, mammary, superior vena cava, other, unspecified	57
Abdomen/pelvis	211 (15.7)
Aorta	16
Interior vena cava	38
Celiac and mesenteric artery	40
Porta and splenic vessel	19
Renal vessel	23
Iliac vessels	45
Ovarian, other, unspecified	30
Upper extremity	361 (26.9)
Axillary vessels	17
Brachial vessels	93
Radial artery	79
Ulnar artery	81
Digital	69
Other, unspecified	22
Lower extremity	271 (20.2)
Common femoral artery	16
Superficial femoral artery	54
Femoral vessel	25
Popliteal artery	38
Popliteal vein	12
Popliteal vessels	14
Tibital vessels	63
Plantar, other, unspecified	49

From Oller DW, Rutledge R, Clancy T, et al: Vascular injuries in a rural state: a review of 978 patients from a state trauma registry. J Trauma 32:740-746, 1992.

TABLE 1–28
ETIOLOGIC FACTORS MANAGEMENT OF VASCULAR INJURIES OF THE EXTREMITIES (115 CASES)

Etiologic Factors	Number of Cases	%
Penetrating trauma	50	43
Stab wounds	25	21
Traffic accidents	22	19
Gunshot injury	9	8
Industrial accidents	5	5
Failing from heights	2	2
Iatragenic	2	2

From Kurtoğlu M, Ertekin C, Bulut T, et al: Management of vascular injuries of the extremities: 115 cases, Int Angiol 10:95-99, 1991.

In 1889, Kümmel performed the first clinical end-to-end anastomosis of a femoral vein. In 1901, Clermont successfully reunited the ends of a divided vena cava with a continuous fine silk suture. A month later, the lumen of the vena cava was found to be smooth and unobstructed at the site of the anastomosis. Jensen in 1903 was successful in four of seven operations in anastomosing transected veins, using a continuous suture technique.

In World War I the clinical use of lateral suture repair of venous lacerations was reported by Goodman (1918). He reported experiences with five patients with vascular injuries in whom a lateral suture repair of venous lacerations was done in four, involving two popliteal and two superficial femoral veins. The defects ranged from 5 to 20 mm in length. The results are unknown because there was no follow-up evaluation.

The importance of venous repair was minimized by the proposal of Makins in 1917, which was that the concomitant vein should be ligated when an arterial injury was treated by ligation. The results reported by Makins to support this hypothesis were later found to have no statistical significance (Table 1–29). The influence persisted even until World War II. Data from World War II showed no benefit from ligation of the concomitant vein, however (DeBakey and Simeone, 1946). During the Korean Conflict, repair of injuries of major veins was again undertaken in selected patients (Hughes, 1959). This was expanded in Vietnam (Rich, 1970 to 1995).

One of the most bizarre recommendations in the history of vascular surgery is the mid-19th century recommendation that ligation of the concomitant uninjured artery should be done when a venous injury was treated by

TABLE 1–29

A COMPARISON OF THE RESULTS OF LIGATIONS OF THE ARTERY ALONE WITH THOSE OF SIMULTANEOUS LIGATIONS OF ARTERY AND VEIN

Artery	Artery Alone				Artery and Vein			
	No. of Cases	Good Result	Gangrene	Percent Gangrene*	No. of Cases	Good Result	Gangrene	Percent Gangrene*
Subclavian	4	3	1	25.0	1	1	—	0.0
Axillary	6	5	1	16.6	4	4	—	0.0
Brachial	13	10	3	23.0	1	1	—	0.0
Femoral	32	24	8	25.0	32	25	7	21.0
Popliteal	24	14	10	41.6	28	22	6	21.4
Tibial	4	4	—	0.0	1	1	—	0.0
Carotid	18	12	6	3.3	4	3	1	25.0
TOTAL	101	72	29	28.0	71	57	14	19.7

*All the percentages were added to the table by the author, except the total percentages, which appear in Makins' original table. Modified from Montgomery ML: Arch Surg 1932;24:1016-1027.

ligation (Rich and Rob, 1996). Apparently this astonishing recommendation was first made by Gensoul in 1883, who feared the hazards of venous engorgement if the vein alone was ligated. Other surgeons (Dupuytren, 1839; Chassaignac, 1855; Langenbeck, 1861; Pilcher, 1886) made similar recommendations, although these were intended primarily to minimize hemorrhage with venous injuries (Simeone, Grillo, and Rundle, 1951).

Moreover, during the Korean Conflict, there was a renewal of interest in repair of the involved vein during the elective repair of arteriovenous fistulas that usually was performed several months after the initial injury. Traditionally such fistulas were treated by ligation of both the artery and the vein. The technique of repair gradually evolved to include repair of the artery and often repair of the concomitant vein. Successful results in such patients generated some enthusiasm for repair of acute venous injuries (Hughes, 1958):

> . . . noted 63 percent major vein injuries accompanying major artery injuries. A number of other vein injuries were treated in which there was no arterial involvement. Most of these veins were treated by ligation, but in some, ligations resulted in various

> degrees of venous stasis. On rare occasion, massive venous stasis resulted in amputation of the extremity. To eliminate this complication two investigators . . . [sic] Hughes and Spencer independently . . . began the repair of major veins. They reported 20 major veins repaired, all by lateral suture except one which was repaired by direct anastomosis. Some of these are known to have thrombosed later without complications. No embolic complications resulted.

A review concerned primarily with the management of venous injuries in civilian practice was published by Gaspar and Treiman in 1960; it described injuries of 52 major veins in 51 patients. Venous reconstruction when performed was usually by lateral suture.

During the Vietnam Conflict, with the interest and experience resulting from the necessity of treating thousands of vascular injuries, there was a significant effort to perform venous repairs in the last 5 years of the conflict (from 1968 to 1972). In a symposium on venous surgery in the lower extremities at Walter Reed Army Institute of Research, the combined experiences of both civilian and military surgeons were summarized (Swan and colleagues, 1975). *Venous Trauma,* by Hobson, Rich, and Wright (1983), reviews civilian and military experience with venous injuries.

Venous injuries are unimportant to many surgeons, so the true frequency is not documented accurately. This is particularly true in the case of combined arterial and venous injuries. Analysis of the Vietnam experience found numerous cases in which venous trauma was not documented in the records. The first major interest in the frequency of venous injuries in military trauma was during the Korean Conflict. In analysis of 180 acute vascular injuries (Table 1–30), Hughes (1954) found nearly as many injuries in major veins (71) as there were in major arteries (79). Similarly, in civilian practice, the frequency of venous trauma was documented only occa-

sionally, most reports describing only arterial trauma until 1980. There are numerous large series of arterial injuries reported that give no details regarding venous trauma and this continues through 1996. The report by Gaspar and Treiman (1960) is one of the first to have a detailed analysis of venous injuries alone. In a group of 228 patients with vascular injuries at the Los Angeles County General Hospital over a period of 10 years, about 22% (51 patients) had venous injuries. The superficial femoral vein was most commonly injured (nine times). The inferior vena cava and the internal jugular vein were each injured eight times, and the brachial veins seven. In 1966 40 patients were added to the original series in a supplementary report by Treiman. The frequency of venous injury in the different locations is shown in Table 1–31. Mullins, Lucas, and Ledgerwood (1980) published a large series of civilian venous injuries from Detroit.

In the preliminary Vietnam Vascular Registry report, approximately one fourth of the patients had venous trauma (Table 1–32) (Rich and Hughes, 1969). There were only 28 injuries of isolated veins, and most of the venous injuries were combined with arterial trauma. The increased incidence of venous trauma when associated with arterial trauma was emphasized in an interim Registry report, which documented concomitant venous injuries in 37.7% of cases with acute major arterial trauma (Table 1–33) (Rich, 1970).

TABLE 1–30
INCIDENCE OF ACUTE VASCULAR TRAUMA IN KOREAN CASUALTIES

Vessel	No.	%
Major arteries	79	43.9
Major veins	71	39.4
Minor arteries	30	16.7
TOTAL	180	100.0

Modified from Hughes CW: Acute vascular trauma in Korean casualties: analysis of 180 cases. Surg Gynecol Obstet 99:91-100, 1954.

TABLE 1–31
INCIDENCE OF VENOUS INJURIES

Vein	No. 1948-1958	No. 1958-1963	Total 1948-1963	%
Axillary brachial	8	5	13	14.1
Innominate subclavian	3	5	8	8.7
Superior vena cava	1	0	1	1.1
Inferior vena cava	8	4	12	13.0
Iliac	7	4	11	12.0
Femoral	11	6	17	18.5
Other	14	16	30	32.6
TOTAL	52	40	92	100.0

Modified from Treiman RL, Doty D, Gaspar MR: Acute vascular trauma a fifteen year study. Am Surg 111:469-473, 1966.

TABLE 1–32
INCIDENCE OF VENOUS TRAUMA; PRELIMINARY VIETNAM VASCULAR REGISTRY REPORT (500 PATIENTS)

Total vascular injuries	718	
Venous injuries	194	(27.0%)
Isolation	28	(14.4%)
Combined	166	(85.6%)

Modified from Rich NM, Hughes CW: Vietnam vascular registry: a preliminary report. Surgery 65:218-226, 1969.

TABLE 1–33
CONCOMITANT VENOUS TRAUMA ASSOCIATED WITH ACUTE ARTERIAL TRAUMA

Cases	1000	
Venous injuries	377	(37.7%)

Modified from Rich NM, Baugh JH, Hughes CW: Acute arterial injuries in Vietnam: 1000 cases. J Trauma 1970;10:359-369.

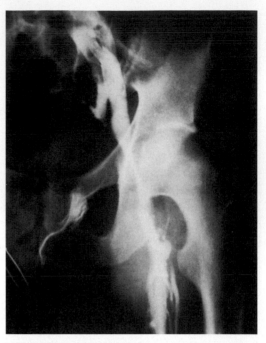

■ **FIGURE 1–23**
Clinical success is demonstrated angiographically by the patent compilation vein graft used to repair an injured common femoral vein. (Courtesy Dr. William G. Sullivan.) ■

Combat situations provide fertile opportunities for young surgeons to learn by managing many similar injuries in a short period under similar circumstances and this has been emphasized repeatedly. Over an 8-year period in Vietnam (from 1965 to 1972), this opportunity was provided for approximately 600 young U.S. surgeons. The consensus developed toward an increased emphasis for repair of major lower extremity veins that were injured with a particular emphasis for repair of the popliteal vein. Valid statistical data are still badly needed to determine the best method of venous repair, especially when end-to-end venous anastomosis or vein grafts are required. Only by such long-term evaluation can the reliability of different types of venous reconstruction be determined. Figure 1–23 demonstrates patency of a compilation graft of autogenous greater saphenous vein used successfully to repair a defect in the left common femoral vein. Although this repair was successful in the immediate postoperative period, it is also important to know whether long-term patency can be anticipated. The second important area in which long-term data are needed is the frequency of significant venous insufficiency following ligation. Because venous insufficiency may not develop for several years, often after repeated episodes of phlebitis induced by stasis from the original vein ligation, long periods of observation are necessary. Another consideration is the possibility of delayed venous reconstruction in some patients with chronic venous insufficiency following ligation. In such patients, serial venography may be useful. This is shown in a report by Rich and Sullivan (1972) of a patient with recanalization of an autogenous vein graft in the popliteal vein (Figs. 1–24 and 1–25). Early recanalization can be seen in Figure 1–26. Additional phlebograms area needed in the extended follow-up, and some findings have been encouraging, such as the long-term patency $3\frac{1}{2}$ years after lateral suture repair (Fig. 1–27).

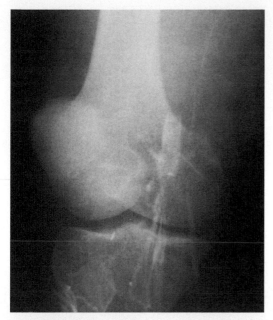

■ **FIGURE 1–24**
This venogram was performed 72 hours postoperatively at the 12th Evacuation Hospital in the Republic of Vietnam. It revealed thrombosis of the autogenous cephalic vein graft placed in the right popliteal vein. (From Rich NM, Sullivan WG: J Trauma 1972;12:919-920.) ■

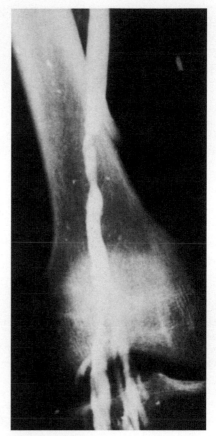

■ **FIGURE 1–25**
An additional venogram was performed at Walter Reed General Hospital approximately $4^{1}/_{2}$ months following a venogram performed in Vietnam (see Fig. 1–24). Note recanalization of the 3-cm cephalic vein graft in the right popliteal vein. (From Rich NM, Sullivan WG: J Trauma 1972;12:919-920.) ■

The importance of repair of the popliteal vein when associated with injuries of the popliteal artery is discussed in further detail in Chapter 18. Recently, additional experience has been accumulated regarding the use of adjunctive measures. Schramek and Hashmonai (1974) and Schramek and colleagues (1975) in Israel have used a branch of the profunda femoris artery to reconstruct a distal arteriovenous fistula with an autogenous vein graft for repair of the femoral in three patients (Fig. 1–28).

A study from the Vietnam Vascular Registry (Rich and colleagues, 1976) evaluates the management and long-term follow-up of 110 patients with isolated popliteal venous trauma. Nearly an equal number were repaired and ligated. Thrombophlebitis and pulmonary embolism were not significant complications in this series. The only pulmonary embolus occurred after ligation of an injured popliteal vein. However, there was a significant increase in edema in the involved extremity following ligation of the popliteal vein (Table 1–34). Rich (1977) also provided a 10-year follow-up of 51 Vietnam casualties who had lower extremity venous injuries repaired using autogenous interposition venous grafts. Only one patient (2%) developed thrombophlebitis in the postoperative period and this was transitory in nature (Table 1–35).

Although repair rather than ligation of arterial injuries has been widely and enthusiastically accepted for the past 40 years, the same approach has not developed for venous

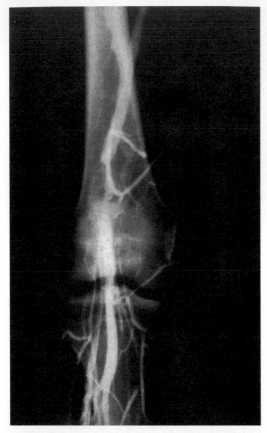

■ FIGURE 1–26
The venogram shows minimal recanalization of a segment of the left greater saphenous vein, which was used to repair the right popliteal vein 2$\frac{1}{2}$ months earlier in Vietnam. Also note some of the remaining collateral venous development. Interestingly, the patient had no distal edema. (From Rich NM, Hobson RW: *In* Swan KE, et al. [eds]: Venous Surgery in the Lower Extremity. St. Louis: Warren H. Green Publishers, Inc., 1975.) ■

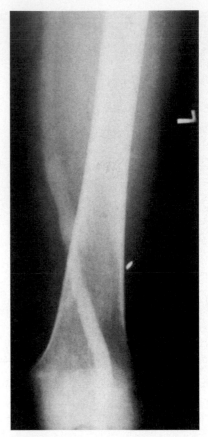

■ FIGURE 1–27
Venogram demonstrating patency of the popliteal vein at its junction with the superficial femoral vein. Note the metallic fragments that caused the injury. The vein was repaired by lateral suture 3$\frac{1}{2}$ years earlier in Vietnam. Repair of concomitant venous injuries is advocated as one of the methods that will help lower the relatively high amputation rate associated with popliteal artery trauma. (From Rich NM, Jarstfer BS, Geer TM: J Cardiovasc Surg 1974;15:340-351.) ■

injuries (Fig. 1–29). In many instances, these have been simply treated by ligation. There are several reasons for this paucity of interest in repair. First, many veins can be ligated and little or no disability follows. Even when very large veins are ligated, the extremity may not be threatened, although months or years later venous insufficiency may appear. Second, the effectiveness of repair of many venous injuries is uncertain. With the low pressure in the venous system, thrombosis is much more common than it is after repair of arterial

injuries. Acquisition of data to show the effectiveness of repair is particularly difficult because there is no simple method for patency of a venous reconstruction; with arterial repair, simple palpation of a peripheral pulse is usually adequate.

The degree of disability from chronic venous insufficiency is not recognized by many, because it may become evident only months or years after injury. A clinical example of disability including venous stasis, edema, skin pigmentation, and ulceration following

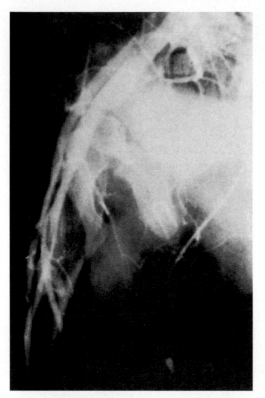

■ FIGURE 1–28

Operative photograph showing the H-type arteriovenous fistula, which measures approximately 1 cm in length and 8 mm in diameter *(arrow)*, constructed approximately 2 to 3 cm distal to the suture line of the vein graft *(between two vascular forceps)* in the femoral vein of the canine model. Patency of the autogenous vein graft in the venous system was enhanced by the adjuvant distal arteriovenous fistula. (From Rich NM, Levin PM, Hutton JE Jr: *In* Swan KE, et al. Venous Surgery in the Lower Extremity. St. Louis: Warren H. Green Publishers, Inc., 1975.) ■

TABLE 1–34
INCIDENCE OF EDEMA FOLLOWING LIGATION AND REPAIR OF INJURED POPLITEAL VEINS

Management	No.	With Edema	%
Ligation	57	29	50.9
Repair	53	7	13.2

Modified from Rich NM, Hobson RW, Collins GJ Jr, Anderson CA: The effect of acute popliteal venous interruption. Ann Surg 183:365–368, 1976.

TABLE 1–35
COMPLICATIONS OF VENOUS REPAIR USING AUTOGENOUS VENOUS GRAFTS

Complication	No.	%
Thrombophlebitis	1	2.0
Pulmonary embolism	0	0.0
Amputation	0	0.0
Death	0	0.0

Edema	No.	%
None	34	66.6
Early	11	21.6
Residual	6	11.8
TOTAL	51	100.0

From Rich NM, Collins GJ, Andersen CA, McDonald PT: Autogenous venous interposition grafts in repair of major venous injuries. J Trauma 17:512-520, 1977.

ligation of the superficial femoral and greater saphenous veins is shown in Figure 1–30. Because of the uncertainty of the importance and the effectiveness of repair of venous injuries, an analysis and a preliminary report from the Vietnam Vascular Registry were prepared in 1970; this report encouraged the repair of major veins in the lower extremities (Rich, 1970). Although data thus far are meager and the effectiveness of some types of venous reconstruction is yet unproved, certain clinical guidelines are now well established.

Venous trauma remains a continuing challenge with controversy regarding appropriate management. Selective references (1980-1996) emphasize experience from an expanding literature. Ironically, John B. Murphy emphasized in 1987 in Chicago that injured veins, like injured arteries, should be repaired. Including all medium and large-caliber veins in a general description might add to the existing confusion. There is a considerable difference in injury to the inferior or superior vena cava compared and contrasted to the axillary or superficial femoral veins, with the latter two being duplicated more frequently. Additional controversial exchanges have centered on the management of injured veins by ligation or repair particularly in larger caliber

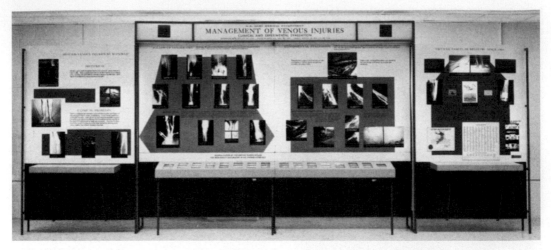

■ FIGURE 1–29

This exhibit, entitled "Management of Venous Injuries: Clinical and Experimental Evaluation," has been used to stimulate an increased interest in the repair of venous injuries. Although repair of arterial injuries has been accepted during the past 20 years, all too often the repair of venous injuries has been treated with minimal interest and even disdain. (A.F.I.P. photograph.) ■

lower extremity veins. It has been widely recognized that most patients can tolerate ligation of injured veins, although the contest has been in identifying the challenge to determine which patients will not tolerate the ligation of medium and larger veins, again, particularly in the lower extremities. General agreement emphasizes that the patient's overall condition must be considered primarily, and the requirement to save a patient's life when multiple injuries are present may necessitate ligation of injured veins. Prevention of long-term disability, particularly from lower extremity swelling, on the other hand, should be considered and this is what has emphasized the importance to place a priority on the repair of major lower extremity veins when possible.

Venous repair may be important in at least three circumstances. First, when popliteal injuries, repair of the vein may be necessary to prevent loss of the leg despite successful arterial reconstruction. This observation was first made during the Korean Conflict and has been confirmed repeatedly since that time (Hobson and Rich, 1995; Rich, 1995). A major factor in this decision is the anatomy of the popliteal space, where an injury often critically impedes venous return from the lower extremity. Second, venous repair may be nec-

essary in the presence of massive soft tissue injury in the extremities, where the widespread loss of soft tissue interrupts venous return to a crucial degree. Third, repair should be routinely considered with large veins, especially when the damage is proximal to the profunda femoris, to prevent chronic venous insufficiency. This includes the common femoral, and the external and common iliac veins.

For a long time, a natural concern with repair of venous injuries was the fear of producing venous thrombosis and pulmonary embolization. Though an apparently likely hazard, this dangerous sequence has been surprisingly absent. Conceivably, small emboli may not be recognized clinically, but the absence of clinically detectable pulmonary emboli has been uniformly documented in both the Vietnam Vascular Registry and in civilian reports (1980 to 1995).

There have been an increasing number of reports from the civilian community in the United States and from a variety of locations around the world since the documented experience from U.S. surgeons in Vietnam. Confirming and conflicting military and civilian experiences have been reported. Civilian reports have identified that ligation of injured veins, including those in the lower extremi-

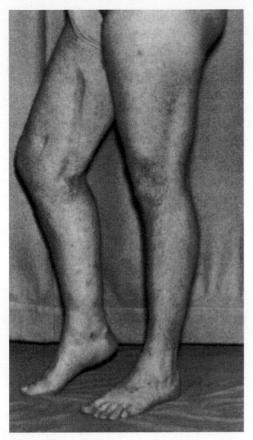

■ FIGURE 1-30
Chronic venous insufficiency has been seen in the Registry with increasing frequency in patients who had lower extremity venous ligation in Vietnam. In addition to edema, other changes similar to the postphlebitic syndrome have been evident, including venous stasis changes in the skin and even some superficial ulcerations. Some of these changes are present in the right lower extremity of this patient, who had ligation of his superficial femoral vein. (Walter Reed General Hospital 1969. Vietnam Vascular Registry #225, NMR.) ■

ties, did not result in significant morbidity. Recognizing that civilian and military wounds are considerably different, this should not be a surprise. Civilian wounds had in general less soft tissue destruction, less interruption of lymphatics, and less interruption of venous collaterals with fewer associated fractures with wounds resulting more often from knives or low-velocity handguns in contrast to the more massive military wounds, which lead to increas-

ing morbidity with ligation of major caliber veins, particularly in the lower extremities. Ideally, determination of patients in jeopardy for complications would be desired. Noninvasive examinations, ambulatory venous pressures, and phlebography can all be of assistance. These studies are, however, often impractical. Also, it is important to emphasize the inconsistency in venous anatomy. It would be helpful to know the anatomy before making claims regarding success or failure of management whether by ligation or repair. In summation, it is important to emphasize the difference in wounds in civilian and military experiences around the world recognizing that many civilian wounds have become more military in nature in recent years. This latter fact emphasizes the validity of continuing to analyze the military experiences. Long-term follow-up remains a major requirement. Nevertheless, it is becoming increasingly obvious that there are patients who suffer life-long disability from ligation of medium and larger caliber lower extremity veins. Many studies have evaluated the pathophysiology of acute interruption of major caliber veins. Correlation with clinical experiences and long-term follow-up are part of the remaining challenge.

SPECIAL HISTORIC OBSERVATIONS

Site of Injury

The specific site of arterial injury is important. All of the cited series, except that of Mattox in 1989, emphasize the predominance of extremity arterial injuries. On the other hand, arterial injuries in the thorax or abdomen may be more difficult to diagnose or may present additional problems in management. There has been a relatively high mortality rate associated with arterial injuries at the base of the neck as a result of uncontrollable hemorrhage and cerebral ischemia. In 1964, Pate and Wilson described experiences with 21 patients with arterial injuries at the base of the neck treated at the City of Memphis Hospital over a 12 year period. As would be expected, there was a significant percentage of permanent crippling neurologic injuries. The interesting observation was made that 93% of the patients who were stabbed were injured on the left side, suggesting that most of the assailants were right handed.

Until the past 20 years, little had been published about intra-abdominal vascular injuries, perhaps because most victims died of exsanguinating hemorrhage. In 1968, Perdue and Smith reported a group of 90 patients with 126 separate injuries treated in Atlanta over a period of 10 years beginning in 1956. Most injuries resulted from low-velocity bullet wounds. Five were injured with a shotgun and fourteen were stab wounds. Mattox's epidemiologic study reported in 1989 emphasized the increasing number of truncal vascular injuries from civilian vascular experience in contrast to the military vascular experience where extremity arteries are involved predominantly.

Iatrogenic Injury

Of historical interest is the fact that one of the first hospital-incurred vascular injuries (iatrogenic injuries) was described approximately 100 years ago. Murphy (1897) reported that Heidenhain used a catgut suture to close a 1-cm laceration of the axillary artery, accidentally injured during removal of adherent carcinomatous glands on May 28, 1894. The patient made a good recovery with no disturbance of the circulation in the extremity.

Several reports have described arterial injuries complicating the removal of a herniated nucleus pulposus; usually the injury involves the common iliac artery. One of the first detailed reports of this complication was made by Seeley (1954). The injury resulted from the anatomic location of the iliac vessels on the anterior surface of the lumbar vertebrae, especially at the intervertebral spaces between the fourth and fifth lumbar vertebrae and between the fifth lumbar and first sacral ribs. In addition to the anatomic susceptibility to injury, the use of a pituitary rongeur for removal of the intervertebral discs was found to predispose to this type of injury (Fig. 1–31).

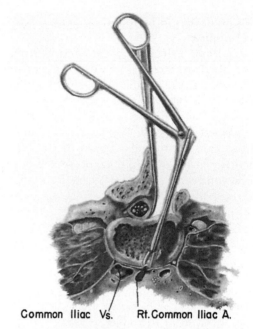

Common Iliac Vs.   Rt. Common Iliac A.

■ **FIGURE 1–31**
Manner in which the common iliac artery can be injured while using an angled pituitary rongeur at the intervertebral space between L4 and L5 during removal of a herniated nucleus pulposus. (From Seeley SF, Hughes CW, Jahnke EJ Jr: Surgery 1954;35:421-429.) ■

At least eight such cases have been seen at Walter Reed General Hospital over a period of 25 years, including the report by Jarstfer and Rich (1976). Salander and colleagues (1984) expanded the Walter Reed Army Medical Center report to six patients operated on from 1949 to 1982 for vascular injury following lumbar disc surgery. All six patients had common iliac artery injuries.

Arteriovenous fistulas have occurred at numerous sites after ligation in continuity of an artery and a vein, such as a renal artery and vein following nephrectomy, the splenic artery and vein following splenectomy, or the superior thyroid artery and vein following thyroid lobectomy. Pritchard and colleagues (1977) reported an interesting case of traumatic popliteal arteriovenous fistula following meniscectomy treated at the Mayo Clinic. Jimenez and colleagues (1988) presented an interesting case of a popliteal artery and venous aneurysm as a complication of arthroscopic meniscectomy. There was an associated arteriovenous fistula. It was emphasized that this is a rare finding following open surgical techniques.

In 1968, Dillard, Nelson, and Norman described an arterial injury developing from a Kirschner wire placed through the popliteal artery while applying skeletal traction for a femoral fracture. Saletta and Freeark (1972) described injury of the profunda femoris artery caused by a drill point during an orthopedic procedure. Injuries of the femoral artery and vein have occurred during inguinal herniorrhaphy, especially during attempts to control hemorrhage with deep, blindly inserted sutures. A series of 11 iatrogenic injuries were reported by Lord and colleagues in 1958 (Table 1–36). Although retrograde dissection of an iliac artery and the aorta have been uncommon, Kay, Dykstra, and Tsuji (1966) have emphasized this catastrophic complication of cannulation and perfusion of the common femoral artery in open heart surgery. Aust, Bredenberg, and Murray (1981) reported five cases of arterial complications associated with total hip replacement. All five injuries resulted from intraoperative injury.

Kozloff and colleagues (1980) presented a report of eight patients seen over 18 months who had significant iliofemoral arterial comprise secondary to cannulation for cardiopulmonary bypass or intra-aortic balloon pumping. Perler and colleagues (1983) documented an incidence of vascular complications of 8.8 percent utilizing the intra-aortic balloon pump in 794 patients at the Massachusetts General Hospital in Boston. Eighty-seven major vascular complications occurred in 70 patients. Specifically, 36 patients had a limb ischemia and arterial trauma occurred in 20. No limbs were lost. Todd and colleagues (1983) identified vascular complications related to percutaneous intra-aortic balloon pump inserted in 112 patients (Table 1–37). While six patients had reversal of ischemic signs following removal of the device, nine patients required exploration of the femoral artery for thrombectomy, femoral laceration repair, or false aneurysm repair.

Vascular injuries following angiographic procedures have increased in number with the rapid development of precise techniques of angiography. The actual incidence of these injuries has decreased somewhat with the availability of skilled vascular radiologists, specifically trained for angiography, but the increasing utilization of such diagnostic techniques has resulted in an overall increase in the number of cases seen. Complications include hemorrhage, hematoma formation, false aneurysm, arteriovenous fistula, subintimal dissection (with and without thrombus), distal embolization of thrombi material, and breakage of a guidewire or catheter.

In 1971, Bolasny and Killen reviewed the frequency and management of arterial injuries following angiography at Vanderbilt University over a period of $2\frac{1}{2}$ years, starting in January 1968. Almost 4000 angiographic procedures were performed, following which there were 33 vascular injuries requiring surgical intervention (0.8%) (Table 1–38). Twenty-six of thirty-three complications were thrombosis at the site of catheterization. Sixteen involved the femoral artery, three the axillary, and five the brachial. In three instances, there was extensive dissection of the intima in association with thrombosis (Fig. 1–32).

Two patients developed arteriovenous fistulas and one had a distal embolus from the puncture site in the femoral artery. Almost none of the arterial injuries resulted simply from the needle puncture, in only one case did the injury occur from uncomplicated passage of a single arterial catheter. Most injuries occurred when manipulation of the catheter was "difficult" or multiple catheters were inserted. Complications were more common with arteries with atherosclerotic plaques. Spasm alone did not cause serious problems in any patient. Among numerous other recent papers describing complications associated with angiographic procedures is the 1973 report by Brener and Couch from Boston. They reported a thrombosis rate of 13% in using the brachial route for angiocardiographic catheterization (Table 1–39). Their overall complication rate was 6% when the femoral route was used, and 28% when the brachial route was used.

Rich, Hobson, and Fedde (1974) described the Walter Reed Hospital experience with hospital-incurred vascular trauma. This was updated by Youkey and colleagues in 1983

TABLE 1–36
MAJOR VASCULAR INJURY DURING ELECTIVE OPERATIVE PROCEDURES

Case	Age	Sex	Date	Operation	Artery Injured	Management	Pulses	Results
Injuries to the axillary carotid and subclavian arteries								
1	42 yr	F	1949	Radical mastectomy	Axillary	End-to-end anastomosis	Yes	Recovery
3	37 yr	F	1956	Z-plasty contracture of axilla	Axillary	End-to-end anastomosis	Yes	Recovery
4	22 mo	F	1955	Emergency tracheostomy	Common carotid	Ligation	No	Died 2 days later from aspiration, pneumonia
5	66 yr	M	1956	Radical neck dissection	Common carotid	Ligation and preservation of carotid bifurcation	In both internal and external branches	Recovery
7	64 yr	M	1953	Radical neck dissection	Subclavian	Ligation	No	Recovery
Injuries to the iliac and femoral arteries								
2	37 yr	F	1955	Posthysterectomy bleeding	Common iliac	Ligation at aortic bifurcation end-to-side, left-to-right common iliac artery	Yes	Recovery
6	48 yr	F	1951	Anterior resection	Common iliac	Ligation	No	2-yr postoperative, good
10	21 yr	F	1955	Varicose vein ligation	Common femoral	Delayed bypass vein graft	Yes	Recovery
11	29 yr	M	1949	Right inguinal hernia	Common femoral	End-to-end anastomosis	Yes	Recovery

Modified from Lord JW Jr, Stone PW, Cloutier WA, Breidenbach L: Major blood vessel injury during electric surgery. Arch Surg 77:282-288, 1958.

TABLE 1-37
INCIDENCE OF VASCULAR COMPLICATIONS

	No. (%) of Complications	
	Total Group (N = 102)	Survivors Until Balloon Removal (N = 67)
Total no. of clinically evident vascular complications	**15 (14.7)**	**15 (22.4)**
Limb ischemia responding to balloon removal	6 (5.9)	6 (8.9)
Limb ischemia requiring thrombectomy	6 (5.9)	6 (8.9)
Hemorrhage requiring operation	3 (2.9)	3 (4.5)

From Todd GJ, Bregman D, Voorhees AB, Reemtsma K: Vascular complications associated with percutaneous intra-acute balloon pumping. Arch Surg 118:963-964, 1983.

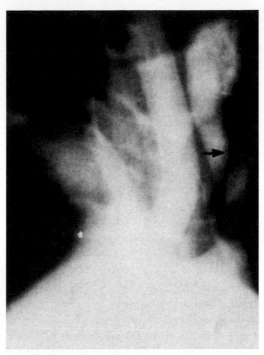

■ **FIGURE 1-32**
Arch aortogram in a patient with angiographic dissection of the subclavian artery shows an intimal dissection caused by transfemoral selective arteriography. View is of the origin of the arch vessels. Arrow indicates intimal "septum" in the first portion of the left subclavian artery. (From Bolasny BL, Killen DA: Ann Surg 1971;174:962-964.) ■

TABLE 1-38
ARTERIAL INJURY RESULTING FROM 3934 ANGIOGRAPHIC PROCEDURES: 0.8% INCIDENCE, VANDERBILT UNIVERSITY MEDICAL CENTER, 1 JANUARY, 1968 – 1 JULY 1977

Complications	Cases	%
Thrombosis at site of entry	26	78.8
Femoral 18		
Axillary 3		
Brachial 5		
Intimal dissection with occlusion	3	9.1
Arteriovenous fistula	2	6.1
Embolus from puncture site	1	3.0
Perforation with hemorrhage	1	3.0
TOTAL	33	100.0

Modified from Bolasny BL, Killen DA: Surgical management of arterial injuries secondary to angiography. Ann Surg 174:962-964, 1971.

TABLE 1-39
INCIDENCE OF ANGIOGRAPHIC CATHETER COMPLICATIONS

Complications	Femoral (223 Patients)	Brachial (96 Patients)
Thrombosis	2 (1%)	12 (13%)
Stenosis	—	14 (15%)
Embolus	7 (3%)	—
False aneurysm	4 (2%)	—
TOTAL	13 (6%)	26 (28%)

Modified from Brener BJ, Couch MP: Surgical arterial complications of left heart catheterization and their management. Am J Surg 125:521-526, 1973.

noting many similarities. Natali and Ben-hemori (1979) reviewed an interesting group of 125 cases of iatrogenic vascular injuries excluding angiographic injuries from Paris. Included were three cases in which there was inadvertent arterial stripping during a vein stripping operation.

Alpert and colleagues (1980) presented five patients who sustained limb ischemia in neonates after umbilical artery catheterization. Gangrene developed in three patients and two patients died from primary illness, with the third patient surviving after leg amputation. In the remaining two infants who had advanced ischemia, there was a favorable response to catheter removal and heparinization.

Cronenwett, Walsh, and Garrett (1988) identified an unusual case of multiple tibial artery pseudoaneurysms that appeared 4 years after balloon catheter embolectomy. They reviewed the literature and found 46 cases of balloon catheter injuries reported, including arterial disruption (29), intimal rupture (12), or catheter malfunction (5). The injuries resulted in hemorrhage (13), arteriovenous fistula (12), pseudoaneurysm (4), thrombosis (3), dissection (5), accelerated atherosclerosis (4), and catheter fragment embolism (5). Only 41% of these complications were recognized during the initial operation.

Gurri and Johnson (1980) reviewed operative management of 42 patients who sustained brachial arterial injury following cardiac catheterization at the University of North Carolina at Chapel Hill.

Adar, Bass, and Walden (1982) reviewed a University Hospital experience with iatrogenic vascular complications. They emphasized that a concerted effort to study these injuries can lead to a decrease in incidence.

Orcutt and colleagues (1985) reviewed 46 patients who were treated for iatrogenic vascular injuries at the University of Texas Health Science Center in San Antonio during a 6-year period ending in December 1982. Diagnostic procedures led to 24 injuries and therapeutic procedures were responsible for 22 vascular injuries.

Flanigan and colleagues (1983) documented a 32-month period involving iatro-genic pediatric vascular injuries in 79 extremities in 76 children in Chicago. They emphasized that iatrogenic pediatric vascular injuries are common and can result in significant limb growth impairment.

Historic Observations on Mechanism of Injury

FRACTURES

Although an arterial injury can occur with almost any type of fracture or dislocation, it is surprising that such an injury does not occur more often. The usual injury is confusion with spasm and subsequent thrombosis, rather than laceration or transection (Collins and Jacobs, 1961; Makins, Howard, and Green, 1966). Such injuries commonly have been overlooked in the past, confusing the signs of acute arterial insufficiency with soft tissue trauma, hemorrhage, and "arterial spasm." The availability of angiography has greatly facilitated the management of such problems; the question of arterial injury in a patient with a fracture can be resolved simply by performing an angiogram. Fractures of the midshaft of the femur may lacerate the superficial femoral artery (Kirkup, 1963), whereas fractures of the distal tibia and fibula may lacerate the posterior and anterior tibial arteries (Miller, 1957). Pelvic fractures have traumatized the iliac arteries, whereas medial angulation of the radial fragments of a fracture of the neck of the humerus may lacerate the axillary or brachial artery (Hughes, 1958).

POSTERIOR DISLOCATION OF THE KNEE

Dislocation of the knee has frequently been associated with injury of the popliteal artery, often leading to amputation. In one series of 22 dislocated knees, the popliteal artery was injured in 13 patients, an incidence of nearly 60% (Kennedy, 1959). Similarly, Hoover, reporting from the Mayo Clinic in 1961, found 9 popliteal artery occlusions associated with 14 knee dislocations. Less commonly, dislocation of the elbow has injured the brachial or radial arteries. Anterior dislocation of the shoulder has injured the axillary artery (McKenzie and Sinclair, 1958). Trauma to the axillary artery may be compounded by trauma to the subscapular and humeral circumflex branches; this may make the injury more serious by destroying important collateral pathways for arterial flow to the upper extremity. Fractures or the clavicle may injury the subclavian artery, the subclavian vein and the brachial plexus.

BLUNT INJURY IN PRESENCE OF OTHER VASCULAR PATHOLOGY

The types of blunt trauma that may in unusual instances injure an artery are almost endless. Gibson (1962) described injury from direct blunt force. Instances of intimal dissection, prolapse, and eventual thrombosis were reported by Elliott in 1956 and Moore in 1958. Ngu and Konstam (1965) reported the case of a woman who developed traumatic dissection of the abdominal aorta following blunt trauma from a surfboard.

USE OF CRUTCHES

Lesions of the axillary artery have resulted from long-term use of crutches (Rob and Standeven, 1956). In 1973, Abbott and Darling added eight cases of axillary artery aneurysm secondary to crutch trauma from the Massachusetts General Hospital between 1965 and 1971 to a review of the English literature that contained only 11 cases of arterial thrombosis and 2 cases of arterial aneurysms. Ettien (1980) reported the case of a crutch-induced aneurysm of the axillary artery, which resulted in distal embolism.

ATHLETIC INJURIES

In baseball players, effort thrombosis of the subclavian artery and vein has been described. In addition, the syndrome has developed in the index finger of the catching hand, where the major force of the baseball is received. Although signs of ischemia may become marked, amputations have not been necessary. In baseball pitchers, thrombosis of the axillary artery has developed apparently as a result of the motion of the throwing arm from a position of exaggerated hyperabduction through a wide downward arc with great force. The two possibilities of injury are a tear of the intima from repeated stretching or twisting and compression from hypertrophy of the pectoralis minor tendon, causing repetitive trauma to the artery (Whelan and Baugh, 1967). The importance of complete angiography in these unusual instances of arterial trauma has recently been emphasized. Aneurysms of the ulnar artery in the wrist or palm, which without angiographic investigation would have gone undetected, have been found to be responsible for distal emboli.

VASCULAR INJURY IN CHILDREN

Meagher and colleagues (1979) performed a retrospective evaluation of vascular trauma in infants and children in Houston. They identified 53 cases of blunt and penetrating vascular injuries in pediatric patients. The brachial artery, superficial femoral artery, and inferior vena cava were the vessels most often involved. There were 41 major arterial and 32 major venous injuries.

Richardson and colleagues (1981) reviewed the management of arterial injuries in 29 children treated at the University of Louisville. Blunt trauma was responsible for 11 injuries, gunshot wounds for 9, penetrating injuries by sharp objects for 5 injuries, and angiographic-related injury occurred in the remaining 4. The femoral artery was most often injured.

RADIATION

The extent of arterial trauma secondary to radiation therapy is not completely understood. However, it is generally believed that only smaller vessels are usually affected. Frequent observations have been made that there seems to be an increase in the friable nature of the vena cava during a retroperitoneal node dissection following radiation for pelvic carcinoma.

VIBRATORY TOOLS

Chronic use of vibratory tools such as an air hammer has caused thrombosis of the distal arteries (Barker and Hines, 1944; De Takats, 1959).

Historic Classification of Vascular Injury

The types of arterial injury that can occur can be conveniently divided into five groups, as follows: lacerations, transections, contusions, spasm, and arteriovenous fistulas (Fig. 1–33). In almost every series reported, laceration or transection accounts for 85% to 90% of the total injuries seen.

A laceration varies from a simple puncture wound to almost complete transection of the arterial wall. Transection varies from simple division of the artery to actual loss of substance from a high velocity bullet, often with injury of the ends of the divided artery. Contusion ranges from a trivial hematoma in the adventitia to diffuse fragmentation and hematomas throughout the arterial wall. In the most severe form, there is fracture of the intima, subsequent prolapse into the lumen and eventual thrombosis. Spasm is a definite entity that can occur in the absence of any organic injury, but it is extremely rare. It can be demonstrated simply in the laboratory by repetitively stretching an artery. This initiates a sustained contraction of "spasm" of the concentric bands of smooth muscle in the media of the arterial wall. When it occurs, it is important to appreciate that spasm is a mechanical myogenic response and not a neurogenic response that is typically see in smaller arterial tributaries under the influence of the sympathetic nervous system. Arteriovenous fistulas classically occur with a fortuitous injury of concomitant artery and

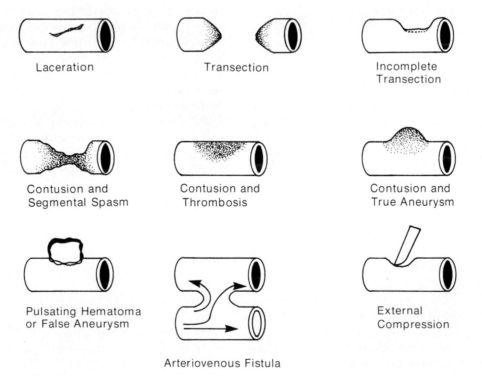

Laceration   Transection   Incomplete Transection

Contusion and Segmental Spasm   Contusion and Thrombosis   Contusion and True Aneurysm

Pulsating Hematoma or False Aneurysm   External Compression

Arteriovenous Fistula

■ **FIGURE 1–33**
Common types of arterial trauma. Lacerations and transections account for the vast majority of arterial injuries. Transections may be associated with avulsions with missing segments of artery. External compression can be caused by displaced bone from comminuted fractures. ■

vein, but the overall frequency of their occurrence is small. False aneurysms evolve from lacerations of an artery temporarily sealed by blood clot. Eventually the thrombosis liquefies and the lesion begins to expand. Often only after the appearance of an expanding lesion is the presence of an arterial injury first recognized.

HISTORY OF BALLISTICS AND VASCULAR INJURY

Primary damage and wounding results from direct crushing of tissue in front of the moving missile and from stretching and tearing in a wide range around the missile path. The stretching results from the formation of a large temporary cavity behind the missile which leaves a region of extravasated blood on collapse. The cavity formation is explosive in character and a comparison is drawn between a shot into tissue and an underwater explosion.
Harvey (1947)

Primary damage and wounding results from direct crushing of tissue in front of the moving missile and from stretching and tearing in a wide range around the missile path. The stretching results from the formation of a large temporary cavity behind the missile, which leaves a region of extravasated blood on collapse. The cavity formation is explosive in character and a comparison is drawn between a shot into tissue and an underwater explosion (Harvey, 1947).

Experimental effort has been expended by a small number of individuals in an attempt to better understand the wounding power of missiles, particularly during the last 50 years. This knowledge is of paramount importance before one can gain a full appreciation of the various etiologies of arterial trauma and the resultant degree of damage. As stated in the aforementioned quote, the temporary cavitational affect of a missile has an extremely important adverse effect on tissues, including

arteries. This can be demonstrated best experimentally. The effort is warranted in view of an alarming increase in the number of gunshot wounds, including those involving arterial trauma, even in civilian experience. The mechanical disruption of arteries by high-velocity missiles has presented additional problems in arterial repair. Controversy regarding the extent of arterial trauma and the significance of this trauma to the eventual success of the arterial repair stimulated additional experimental work based on clinical impressions from both the Korean and Vietnam experiences. Many misconceptions regarding wound ballistics have been corrected through experimental research. Even a lower velocity missile creates a temporary cavity, as shown in Figure 1–34. Nevertheless, the wounding power of high-velocity missiles, in comparison to that of lower velocity missiles, is greatly accentuated by the additional energy in the larger temporary cavity. Within microseconds after impact, the missile transfers energy to the tissues struck. Herget (1956) emphasized that high internal pressures and shockwaves as high as 100 atmospheres (1500 pounds per square inch) exist in the temporary cavity as the tissue along the

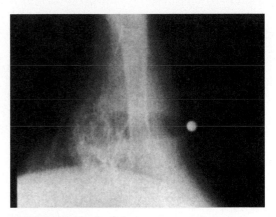

■ **FIGURE 1–34**
A 16-grain sphere traveling at 1000 feet per second through the suspended hindlimb of a canine model demonstrates that there is even a small temporary cavity formed in muscle by a low velocity missile. (From Amato JJ, Billy LJ, Lawson NS, Rich NM: High velocity missile injury. An experimental study of the retentive forces of tissue. Am J Surg 1974;127:454-459.) ■

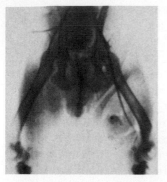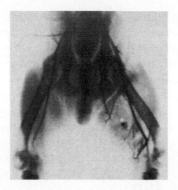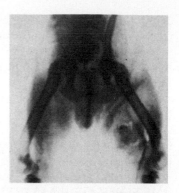

■ **FIGURE 1–35**

These angiograms of a canine model, started 10 minutes after missile wounding (the entrance wound is marked), show the marked increase in arterial flow in the injured leg on the dog's left side, compared to the contralateral side, as judged by the rapid transit of contrast media. Note in *C* the earlier venous filling. (From Rybeck B: Acta Chir Scand Suppl 1974;450:1.) ■

wound tract expands after the high-velocity missile passes through it.

Under the auspices of the International Commission of the Red Cross, a series of meetings have been held by many interested nations to discuss the possibility of prohibition of certain weapons used in warfare (Rich, 1975). Included in the weapons systems that have been criticized are those that fire high-velocity bullets. In 1974 in Sweden, Rybeck conducted an interesting series of five experiments to determine the hemodynamic effects if energy absorption following missile wounding. Among their results is a graphic demonstration of the increased arterial flow in the injured limb compared to that in the opposite uninjured limb (Fig. 1–35).

Experimental vascular trauma continues to challenge the interested investigator. Some might say this is only a problem for military medicine. However, with the increasing number of gunshot wounds in our cities, including those caused by high-velocity missiles, this information also has practical value in our civilian community. Despite the international prohibition at the turn of the century, the "dum-dum" bullet is again being used. It is no longer used on the battlefield; however, numerous law enforcement agencies in the United States have reinstituted or are considering reinstitution of its use. Yet very little is understood regarding either the experimental or the clinical aspects of the wounding power of this missile.

Additional international symposia on wound ballistics has been conducted. The interested reader is referred to the 1988 and 1996 supplements from the *Journal of Trauma,* where additional detailed studies are reported from numerous investigators around the world. Additional material from individuals investigators is available from the Sixth International Symposium in Wound Ballistics held in November 1988 in Chongqing, Peoples Republic of China and in St. Petersburg, Russia in September 2 through 7, 1994.

With the rapidly expanding increase in the management of civilian vascular trauma, it is equally important that long-term follow-up be obtained to evaluate the true success of various acceptable procedures and to develop new techniques that will help continue to improve the results of managing patients with vascular trauma.

HISTORICAL REFLECTIONS AND PROJECTIONS

We should not rest content with the work of our predecessors, or assume that it has proved everything conclusively, on the contrary it should serve only as a stimulus to further investigation. Ambroise Paré (sixteenth century)

This quote from the translated review by Billroth (1931) on studies on the nature and treatment of gunshot wounds emphasizes the historical development and current status of vascular surgery. Although some might say that all the principles of vascular surgery are established and accepted by the vast majority of surgeons, we must not lose sight of the need for continued analysis of results and continued investigation to solve the problems that remain.

As a prime example, the "ideal conduit" still has not been discovered, appreciating the pioneering work of Voohrees reported first in 1952. A substitute for both the arterial and the venous system is greatly needed. A conduit of varied size in diameter and length that would be an acceptable biologic substitute will always be needed in the repair of traumatized arteries and veins. Although some might argue that the ravages of atherosclerosis can be greatly helped by drug therapy and other conservative medical regimens in the future, the increasing incidence of injured arteries and veins in civil life (urban violence) and on the battlefield accentuates the importance of the need for a substitute vascular conduit. Many materials have been investigated, both clinically and under laboratory conditions. At Walter Reed Army Institute of Research, an assortment of grafts and prostheses have been used in the venous system without universal success. The problem remains more significant in the repair of injured veins than of injured arteries. Considering that the Nobel Prize in Medicine was awarded to Carrel in 1912 based in part on his contributions to vascular surgery, including the reconstruction of arteries and veins, this might be an additional stimulus to the serious investigator in search of the "ideal conduit."

The first vascular surgery procedures were described in patients with vascular trauma. For almost two centuries, the treatment of vascular conditions was basically a very early history of the evaluation and treatment of injured vessels. The observations in the patients with injured arteries and veins led to innumerable concepts and laboratory experiments that made significant contributions to the field of surgery. It was the concomitant availability of angiography, antibiotics, plastics, vascular instruments developed through metallurgy, and synthetic monofilament suture that allowed the explosion of vascular surgery development during the 1950s and 1960s. Ironically, the principles established in treatment of wounded arteries and veins were immediately available and adaptable to the receptive new vascular surgeons eager to develop new imaginative horizons. Concomitant with this new composite technology and surgical vision, three major campaigns allowed for the field testing of many of the emerging concepts and instrumentation. Ironically, the types of lessons learned in Korea and Vietnam became adaptable to the third major warfare in the urban hospitals of America. There was a paradigm shift from the military vascular injury where over 90% were in the extremities to the civilian vascular trauma arena where over 60% were in the trunk. It is also ironic that this epidemic continued through the writing of the second edition of this book. It is further ironic that during the military conflicts in Grenada (1983), Panama (1989), and the Persian Gulf (1991) and Somalia (1992), as well as "peace keeping" in Haiti (1994 to 1996) and Bosnia (1996 to 1999), that no single surgeon handled more than two or three vascular injuries.

Continuing technology, at the time of the writing of the second edition of this book, innumerable controversies, and advancements are dynamically evolving. These include the areas of imaging, noninvasive evaluation, use of the intravascular technology, changing roles of the surgeon and interventional radiologists, improvements in substitute conduits and suture material, and changing adjuncts in autotransfusion and extracorporeal bypass and various shunts. There are also changes in hospital and specialty credentialing and recognition, as well as an explosion of specialty organizations with interests in vascular surgery and in trauma. The areas of infection and thrombosis continue to plague the vascular surgical investigator. In the interim between the writing of the first two editions of this book, the viral infections of hepatitis B and C, human immunodeficiency virus, and others create challenges, paranoia, and ethical issues for the patient and the clinician alike.

Finally, the issue of training, role models, and the practice of vascular trauma has considerable problems in the arena of managed care, health maintenance organizations, trauma center development, and specialty drift. The push for increased numbers of primary care physicians and primary surgeons will increase to the detriment to not only the vascular surgery specialists, but individuals who choose to enter the field of trauma care. Furthermore, the current regulatory and medical/legal climate and the perceptions of potential litigation involving the patient with a vascular injury may cause the patient who literally needs the care of an advanced specialist the most to not be able to find one during their moment of greatest need.

A major factor in this remaining problem in vascular surgery has been the obvious paucity of long-term follow-up studies of vascular repairs. The importance of long-term follow-up of patients with vascular injuries cannot be overemphasized. This would be true of both patients who have had successful repair and those in whom repair failed or was not possible. In the former group, periodic evaluation of the function of the repair should be carried out. There is early documentation of the value of providing details of vascular cases with appropriate follow-up information. Although arterial aneurysms previously had been treated by proximal ligation, excision, or the Matas repair from within the sac, Pringle (1913) developed a modification of the method used by Carrel and Guthrie in excising an aneurysm of the popliteal artery and reestablishing continuity with an autogenous saphenous vein graft. Both the resected popliteal aneurysm and the vein graft specimen were obtained years later postmortem, and the findings are shown in Figure 1–36.

Goodman (1918), in describing his experience at the number 1 (Presbyterian U.S.A.) General Hospital in France during World War I, reported a successful closure with continuous silk suture of 5-mm longitudinal openings in both the popliteal artery and vein in one patient with a shall fragment. However, the patient was followed only 9 days before being transferred to the Base Hospital. Goodman reported that "an attempt to obtain further

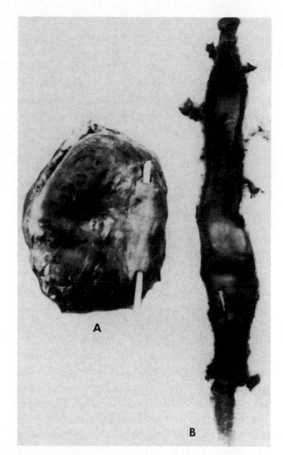

■ **FIGURE 1–36**
The value of adequate documentation and follow-up of vascular cases was demonstrated early by Pringle. *A,* An excised popliteal aneurysm is shown, and *B,* the vein specimen obtained years later at postmortem. Pringle reported his work in 1913, when he modified the method of Carrel and Guthrie in excising an aneurysm of the popliteal artery by reestablishing continuity with an autogenous saphenous vein graft. (Photograph obtained from and used with permission of the Royal College of Surgeons of Edinburgh.) ■

information covering the case is now underway and will be embodied in a subsequent report."

If there was any further follow-up information obtained or reported, it became obscured in the available literature. At least this military surgeon recognized the importance of obtaining long-term follow-up information to thoroughly evaluate his method of managing vascular trauma.

In the classic report by DeBakey and Simeone (1946) from the U.S. experience in World War II, early patency of venous graft in the arterial system was demonstrated angiographically (Fig. 1–37). Although considerable time and effort were expended following World War II in an attempt to provide additional long-term follow-up information, the results of this effort are not generally available. Individual follow-up has been possible in a random way for some patients, such as in the case of an acute, femoral arteriovenous fistula, mentioned earlier, which was repaired shortly after D-Day in Normandy on June 16, 1944 (Boyden, personal communication, 1970). Rob (1985) had a 10-year follow-up of a patient from World War II (Fig. 1–38).

The importance of a well-documented past medical history covering previous vascular trauma was emphasized in the long-term follow-up of a 50-year-old former United States Army Officer who entered the Peripheral Vascular Surgery Clinic at Walter Reed General Hospital for evaluation to rule out cerebrovascular ischemia. The patient had complained of several episodes of visual disturbance and weakness of his left hand during the past year. The patient knew that he had a ligation of "some of the arteries in his neck" during World War II. An angiogram of the aortic arch and its major branches was obtained to determine the amount of arterial flow to the brain. The study demonstrated no identifiable right common carotid artery or its branches, and there was no late retrograde filling of the right internal carotid artery. A copy of part of his old military medical records was finally obtained and it was revealed that he had sustained a fragment wound on the right side of the neck on January 19, 1945, on Saipan when an ammunition dump exploded. Although only dèbridement was necessary at first, approximately 6 months later ligation of the right common internal and external carotid arteries was necessary. In subsequent follow-up through the Vascular Clinic, the patient had no significant problems. Jackson, Brengman, and Rich (1997) have added the latest long-term delayed vascular injury from Walter Reed Hospital. The patient was a World War II casualty who developed a false aneurysm of the brachial arterial branch about 50 years after injury (Fig. 1–39).

Murray (1952) stated approximately 45 years ago that the fate of venous grafts in the arterial system had been under considerable

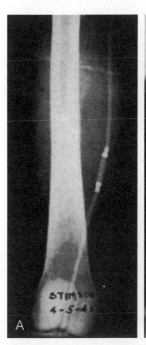
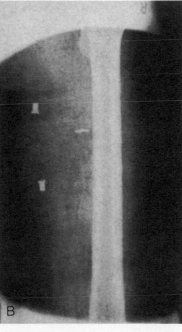

■ **FIGURE 1–37**

A, This arteriogram was performed there and one-half weeks after a nonsuture anastomosis of the superficial femoral artery. There is patency of the anastomosis and no evidence of undue ballooning of the vein segment. The operation was performed at the 8th Evacuation Hospital during World War II. *B,* This roentgenogram of a successful nonsuture anastomosis of the superficial femoral artery shows the extent of the defect bridged by the position of the Vitallium tubes. (From DeBakey ME, Simeone FA: Ann Surg 1946;123:534-579.) ■

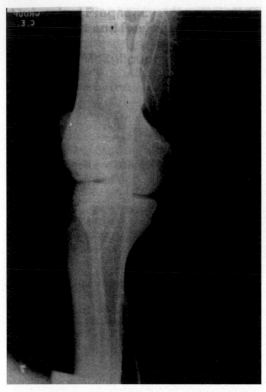

■ **FIGURE 1–38**
This follow-up angiogram was obtained by
Professor Charles G. Rob at St. Mary's Hospital
in London in 1954, which was 10 years after
successful repair of a popliteal arteriovenous
fistula during World War II. Although patency
was maintained, aneurysmal dilation occurred
at the site where a portion of the sac had been
included in the repair. This was replaced with a
vein graph. (From Rob CG: JR Army Med
Corps 1986;132:11-15.) ■

discussion. However, he felt that the saphenous grafts would continue to function
without complications for a long period of
time. He reported that he had removed a
venous graft that had functioned in the
carotid artery of a dog for nine years. Although
the graft was slightly larger than the adjacent
artery and there was some arteriosclerotic
change in one area, it continued to function
well. There are some reports of good results
with aneurysmal formation in utilizing an
adjacent vein, such as the femoral vein next
to the common femoral artery as documented
by Murray (1952), but the greater saphenous

vein still appears to be the best arterial substitute, particularly for major arteries of the
extremities.

The outstanding documentation of the U.S.
experience during the Korean Conflict by
Hughes, Jahnke, Spencer, and others has provided an opportunity for long-term follow-up.
Figure 1–40 is an angiogram of a patient followed up after 19 years with a patent interposition greater saphenous vein in the
proximal right superficial femoral artery.
The establishment of a Vascular Registry and
Blood Flow Laboratory at Walter Reed General
Hospital in 1966 provided an opportunity for
long-term follow-up of former combat casualties who sustained vascular injuries. In the
early efforts of the Vietnam Vascular Registry,
the problems of obtaining long-term follow-
up of patients who had vascular injuries in
Vietnam were illustrated by an attempt to
follow those listed in Fisher's report (1967)
of 108 vascular injuries. After intensive investigation at the time of organization of statistics for the preliminary report for the Vietnam
Vascular Registry, it was possible to find only
60 of his patients whose postoperative period
and convalescence could be completely evaluated. This represents slightly more than 50%
of the patients of the original study. In subsequent years, however, the long-term follow-
up percentage continued to improve.

What is the long-term fate of the autogenous greater saphenous vein used as an interposed segmental graft in the arterial system?
Most surgeons continue to believe that the
long-term patency is excellent. However, few
recognize the development of aneurysmal
changes in these grafts. The long-term follow-
up effort in the Vietnam Vascular Registry has
continued to demonstrate an increasing
number of patients with these changes. The
true significance and the actual percentage
of these changes remain unknown. This does,
however, emphasize the great need for continued long-term follow-up studies. This complication of fusiform aneurysmal dilation of
an autogenous greater saphenous interposition segment used for repair of an injured
artery was first brought to our attention by
Carrasquilla and Weaver (1972) when they
reported on the follow-up of a 22-year-old
Marine who had originally been wounded and

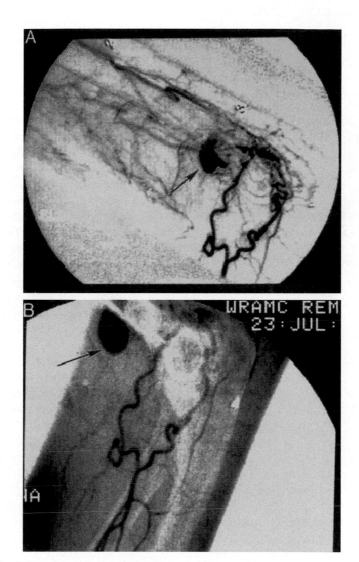

■ **FIGURE 1-39**
Angiogram demonstrates a false aneurysm of a branch of the brachial artery diagnosed 49 years after the original injury in World War II. Successful treatment was carried out at Walter Reed Army Medical Center. (From Jackson MR, Brengman ML, Rich NM: J Trauma 1997;43:159-616.) ■

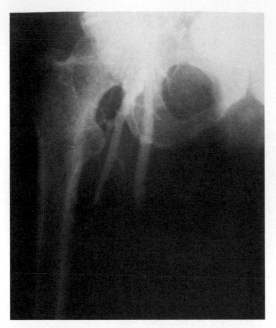

■ **FIGURE 1–40**
This long-term follow-up femoral angiogram
demonstrates patency of an interposition
autogenous greater saphenous vein used to
repair the proximal right superficial femoral
artery. The follow-up period extended from
1953 until the patient was evaluated at Walter
Reed General Hospital in 1972 (19 years). This
is one of the longest known follow-ups and
represents the continued effort to provide this
type of data for former combat casualties from
the Korean Conflict. (From Rich WR: General
Hospital, 1978.) ■

treated in Vietnam. Figure 1–41 demonstrates
the findings. With the accumulation of
approximately 250 follow-up angiograms of
Vietnam casualties, with the range in time from
months to years, the number of recognized
aneurysmal dilation of these venous interposition grafts is in the range of 6%.

It is often not practical or economically feasible to routinely obtain follow-up angiograms,
particularly in asymptomatic patients. The
long-term follow-up through the Vietnam Vascular Registry relies to a great extent on the
noninvasive approach through the Blood
Flow Laboratory. Figure 1–42 demonstrates
this type of follow-up, using the measurement
of wrist pressures and obtaining tracings with
the Doppler ultrasound method. Unfortunately, aneurysmal changes in venous grafts
in the arterial system cannot be detected in

this manner. B-mode ultrasonography has
been tested to augment this information;
however, data remain fragmentary and unsatisfactory. Color-flow duplex offers good eval-
uations of many arteries and veins, although
the equipment is expensive (Fig. 1–43).

The continuing challenge that remains in
the management of patients with vascular
injuries is exemplified by the questions and
problems involving the search for the "ideal
conduit" for segmental replacement of injured
arteries and veins. There are also many other
aspects of the management of injured patients
with vascular injuries that could be expanded.
The management of concomitant fractures
associated with vascular injuries, the use of
fasciotomy, the use of fasciotomy in extremities with vascular injuries, and other associated considerations are among these factors.
Moreover, there are a multitude of professional challenges that exist in unusual situations involving vascular trauma. The following
is cited as an example. Kapp, Gielchinsky,
and Jelsma (1973) stated that they could
find only four cases of intravascular metallic
fragment embolization to the cerebral circulation. To their surgical review they added the
report of two patients who were treated by the
24th Evacuation Hospital in the Republic of
South Vietnam. Because of the unusual
problem, some details of one of these cases
follow:

*A 19-year-old American soldier received a
fragment wound of the right side of the neck
from a grenade explosion, associated with
immediate onset of weakness of the left side
of his body. An exploration of his neck was
carried out and showed no evidence of
vascular trauma. Three days after
wounding, the patient was transferred to the
24th Evacuation Hospital where he showed
slight improvement in his left-sided
weakness.*

Roentgenograms of the skull showed a
small, jagged, metallic fragment, and an arteriogram revealed that the fragment was lodged
at the origin of the middle cerebral artery,
completely occluding the middle cerebral
artery and projecting into the carotid artery
(Fig. 1–44).

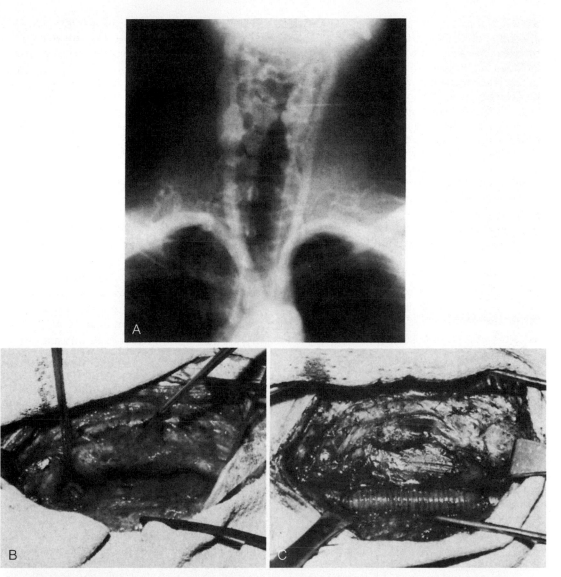

■ **FIGURE 1–41**
A, Fusiform aneurysmal dilation of an autogenous greater saphenous vein segment used as an interposition graft in the right common carotid artery of a Vietnam casualty is demonstrated angiographically. *B,* The operative photograph demonstrates the dilated segment of saphenous vein. *C,* Arterial reconstruction was completed with a Dacron prosthesis. (From Carrasquilla C, Weaver AW: Aneurysm of the saphenous graft to the common carotid artery. Vasc Surg 1972;6:66-68.) ■

It was also thought that there was thrombus formation around the fragment. Six days following injury, the right internal carotid artery, the anterior cerebral artery and the middle cerebral artery were exposed through a right front temporal craniotomy. After applying temporary vascular clamps, the fragment was removed without difficulty through a longitudinal arteriotomy in the internal carotid artery. A thrombus was also extracted from the middle cerebral artery. An arteriorrhaphy was performed, with some initial spasm at the repair site. In the postoperative period the patient's neurologic status improved. An arteriogram performed on the 25th postoperative day revealed that the carotid artery was patent and without stenosis or aneurysmal formation (Fig. 1–45). The middle cerebral artery was thrombosed at its origin, but its branches filled readily via

■ **FIGURE 1-42**

The long-term follow-up through the Vietnam Vascular Registry includes the recording of wrist pressures and Doppler ultrasonicgraphic tracings. The two tracings at the top show the comparison of the right side and the abnormal left side, where occlusion of the repair of the left brachial artery with a saphenous vein graft had occurred in 1969. The two lower tracings show the change after reconstruction of the left brachial artery with a new segment autogenous greater saphenous vein. There is considerable improvement in the wrist pressure and Doppler tracing on the left. (From NM. Walter Reed General Hospital, 1978.) ■

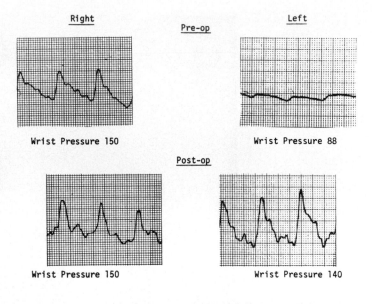

Right

Left

Pre-op

Wrist Pressure 150   Wrist Pressure 88

Post-op

Wrist Pressure 150   Wrist Pressure 140

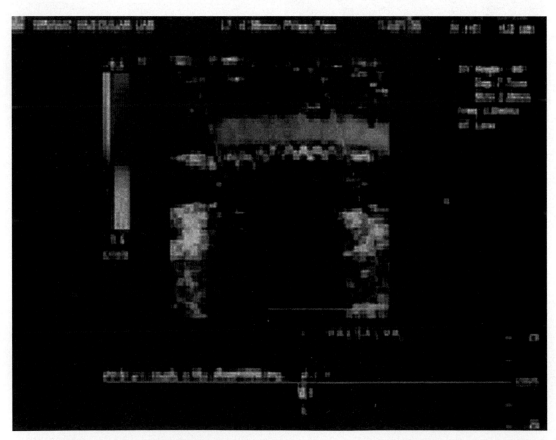

■ **FIGURE 1-43**

Color-flow duplex sonogram of axillary vein valve transfer 1 year postoperatively. No venous reflux is found when the patient performs a Valsalva maneuver, indicating that the valve remains competent. (From Goff JM, Gillespie DL, Rich NM: J Trauma 1998;44:209-211.) ■

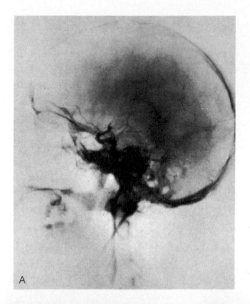

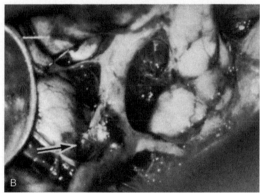

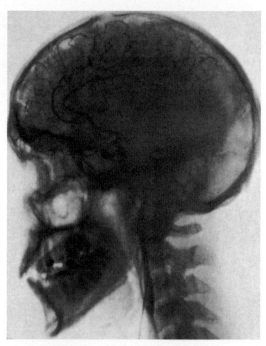

■ **FIGURE 1–45**
This angiogram performed 25 days after removal of the intra-arterial metallic fragment shown in Figure 1–44 *A* and *B* demonstrates patency of the carotid artery, a patent anterior cerebral artery that is larger than normal, and thrombosis of the origin of the middle cerebral artery. (From Kapp JP, Gielchinsky I, Jelssma R: J Trauma 1973;13:256-261.) ■

■ **FIGURE 1–44**
A, Reports of migration of intravascular metallic fragments have been rare. This right carotid angiogram demonstrates an intra-arterial metal fragment at the intracranial bifurcation of the carotid explosion. *B,* This operative photograph taken at the 24th Evacuation Hospital in Vietnam shows an intra-arterial fragment with extreme thinning of the wall of the artery overlying the fragment at the origin of the middle cerebral artery. (From Kapp JP, Gielchinsky I, Jelssma R: J Trauma 1973;13:256-261.) ■

collateral channels with a large patent right anterior cerebral artery.

The authors outlined the possible problems that might occur when a metallic fragment lodges in a cerebral vessel:

1. Neurologic defect secondary to arterial occlusion and infarction

2. Proximal and distal propagation of thrombus, which could extend the infarcted area

3. Erosion with hemorrhage

4. Infection, arteritis, and then abscess formation or meningitis

5. Infection with mycotic aneurysm formation and probable subsequent rupture

They emphasized that one of their main concerns was the possibility of erosion through the small, thin-walled artery caused by pulsatile motion of the fragment. They also stressed the importance of maintaining a high index of suspicion in patients with neurologic symptoms who have wounds of the neck and chest.

International exchange of information is important in the treatment of patients with vascular trauma. In some parts of the world,

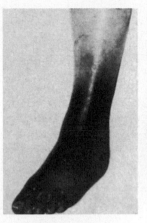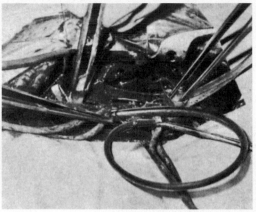

■ **FIGURE 1–46**
Temporary intraluminal arterial shunts have been used in Munich, Germany, to reduce the ischemic time, to diminish thrombosis in the peripheral venous system, and to allow repair of concomitant lacerated veins for major arterial repair. This use of the temporary intraluminal arterial shunt in the management of acute arterial injuries is somewhat unique in that it was not documented in the United States during the same period between 1965 and 1970. (From Mack D, Scherer H, Maurer P: Mschr Unfallheilk 1973;76:217-224.) ■

specific vascular trauma, such as avulsion of the femoral vessels by a bull's horn in the bullring in Mexico or in Spain, may be unique to a certain region or country. Nevertheless, the common goal of all surgeons to provide the best medical care possible creates a desirable situation for exchange of data and experience among surgeons in all parts of the world who have an interest in the management of vascular injuries. Language difficulties can often be overcome through personal exchange and translation of scientific articles. An example of this is the personal exchange that took place with Doctor Peter Mauer in Munich in 1973. Mack, Scherer, and Maurer (1973) described the treatment of 154 patients with vascular injuries in Munich between January 1965 and December 1971. They found that 80% of 129 of their patients had suffered additional trauma, including fractures, trauma to the head, and rupture abdominal organs. Also, 60% of their patients had vascular injuries in association with concomitant fractures. They found angiography to be of great value in diagnosing the vascular injury. One relatively unique aspect of their management, in contrast to the management of arterial injuries in the United States during the same time, was reestablishing arterial flow by temporary intraluminal shunts (Fig. 1–46). They felt that

this reduced ischemic time, diminished thrombosis in the peripheral venous system, and allowed repair of lacerated veins before arterial repair was instituted. They were successful in restoring circulation in 75.8% of their patients; 12.6% showed remaining symptoms secondary to complications associated with vascular injuries, and their amputation rate was 4.2%. Barros D'Sa (1990) champions intraluminal shunts in northern Ireland.

In the United States, Weinstein and Golding (1975) used temporary external Silastic arterial and venous shunts in replanting a traumatically amputated upper extremity in a 10-year-old boy who was involved in an automobile accident (Fig. 1–47). The level of the incomplete traumatic amputation was at the upper third of the arm, with only a posterior skin bridge intact. These authors emphasized that early arterial perfusion decreased the total anoxic time. The challenge persists with unusual and complex injuries such as this, and the varied and unique additions to the surgeon's armamentarium that might assist in obtaining satisfactory results should be known and understood.

The following quote by Carleton Mathewson, Jr., (Fig. 1–48) in the discussion of the paper by Morris, Creech, and DeBakey (1957) is most apropos:

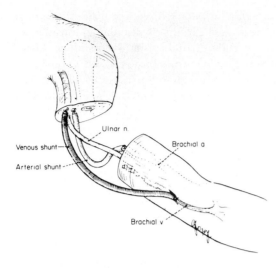

■ **FIGURE 1–47**
This diagrammatic drawing demonstrates the use of temporary external Silastic arterial an venous shunts during replantation of a traumatically amputated upper extremity in a 10-year-old boy involved in an automobile accident. The shunts, which were 20 cm long and 2.5 mm in internal diameter, reduced the anoxic time during replantation of the upper extremity. (From Weinstein MH, Golding AL: J Trauma 1975;15:912-915.) ■

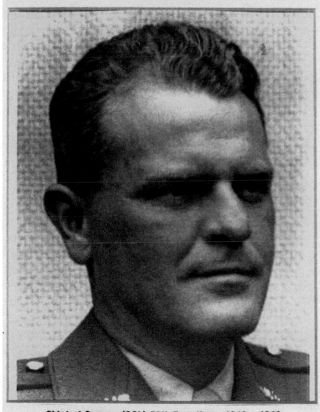

■ **FIGURE 1–48**
Doctor Carleton Mathewson (1902-1989) as professor of surgery at Stanford, and subsequently at the University of California, provided leadership in establishing residency programs in surgery in the military following World War II. He served on the Visiting Board at the Uniformed Services University of the Health Sciences, (Bethesda, Maryland) with other senior surgeons identified in this manuscript. ■

Unfortunately in many quarters these lessons so well emphasized during the stress of world conflict have been neglected in the complacency of civilian life. It is important, therefore, that we re-emphasize the seriousness of vascular injury and, where possible, stress the favorable circumstances that present themselves in civilian life with the successful primary repair of injured vessels.

Endovascular procedures offer a new and alternative consideration to the more traditional suture repair of injured arteries and veins in the 1990s. Parodi (1990) in Buenos Aires championed this approach. In collaboration with Marin and Veith in New York City (1994) endovascular approaches have been used for primary repairs of arteriovenous fistulas and false aneurysms in most cases (Fig. 1–49). Durability and ultimate success await needed follow-up.

Exciting challenges remain. From the microbiology research, we know of a connection between P-55 receptor site alterations and complications of vascular manipulation to include thrombosis and possible stenosis. Nevertheless, while basic research continues so does daily examples of man's inhumanity to man resulting in vascular trauma now in regional conflicts and in urban violence.

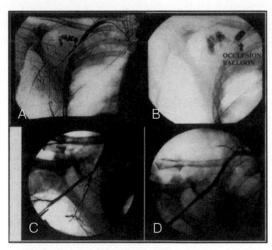

■ **FIGURE 1–49**
Angiographic images of a patient who sustained a gunshot wound to the right chest. *A,* Prograde arteriogram showing subclavian artery and active bleeding in the region. *B,* Image after proximal balloon occlusion, which stopped the bleeding. *C,* Retrograde brachial arteriogram showing extent of injury. *D,* Completion arteriogram after successful repair. (From Patel AV, Marin MD, Veith FJ, et al. J Endovasc Surg 1996;3:382-388.) ■

REFERENCES

Abbott WM, Darling RC: Axillary artery aneurysms secondary to crutch trauma. Am J Surg 1973; 125:515-520.

Adar R, Bass A, Walden R: Five years' experience in general and vascular surgery in a university hospital. Ann Surg 1982;196:725-729.

Agnew D II: The Principles and Practice of Surgery. Philadelphia, JB Lippincott Co, 1978.

Alpert J, O'Donnell JA, Parsonnet V, et al: Clinically recognized limb ischemia in the neonate after umbilical artery catheterization. Am J Surg 1980;140:413-418.

Aust JC, Bredenberg CE, Murray DG: Mechanisms of arterial injuries associated with total hip replacement. Arch Surg 1981;116:345-349.

Barker NW, Hines EA Jr: Arterial occlusion in the hands and fingers associated with repeated occupational trauma. Proc Staff Meet Mayo Clin 1944;19:345-349.

Barros D'Sa AAB, Hassard TH, Livingston RH, Irwin JW: Missile-induced vascular trauma. Injury 1980;12:13-30.

Bell J: Principles of surgery. Discourse 1801;9:4.

Bernheim BM: Blood vessel surgery in the war. Surg Gynecol Obstet 1920;30:564-567.

Billroth T: Historical studies on the nature and treatment of gunshot wounds from the 15th century to the present time. Yale J Biol Med 1931;4:16-36.

Bolasny BL, Killen DA: Surgical management of arterial injuries secondary to angiography. Ann Surg 1971;174:962-964.

Bole PV, Purdy RT, Munda RT, et al: Civilian arterial injuries. Ann Surg 1976;183:13-23.

Boyden AM: Personal communication, 1970.

Brener BJ, Couch N: Peripheral arterial complications of left heart catheterization and their management. Am J Surg 1973;125:521-526.

Carrasquilla C, Weaver AW: Aneurysm of the saphenous graft to the common carotid artery. Vasc Surg 1972;6:66-68.

Carrel A: La technique opératories des anastomoses vasculaires et la transplantation des viscéres. Lyon Medical 1902;98:859.

Carrel A, Guthrie CC: Uniterminal and biterminal venous transplantations. Surg Gynecol Obstet 1906;2:266-286.

Chandler JG, Knapp RW: Early definitive treatment of vascular injuries in the Vietnam conflict. JAMA 1967;202:960-966.

Cheek RC, Pope JC, Smith HF, et al: Diagnosis and management of major vascular injuries: A review of 200 operative cases. Am Surg 1975;41:755-760.

Clermont G: Suture laterale et circulaire des veines. Presse Med 1901;1:229.

Coley RW. Case of rupture of the carotid artery and wound of several of its branches successfully treated by tying off the common trunk of the carotid itself. Med Chir J (Lond) 1817;3:2.

Collins HA, Jacobs JK: Acute arterial injuries due to blunt trauma. J Bone Joint Surg 1961;43-A:193-197.

Cronenwett JL, Walsh DB, Garrett HE: Tibial artery pseudoaneurysms: delayed complication of balloon catheter embolectomy. J Vasc Surg 1988;8:483-488.

DeBakey ME, Simeone FA: Battle injuries of the arteries in World War II: An analysis of 2,471 cases. Ann Surg 1946;123:534-579.

De Takats G: Vascular Surgery. Philadelphia, WB Saunders, 1959.

Dillard BM, Nelson DL, Norman HG: Review of 85 major traumatic arterial injuries. Surgery 1968;63:391-395.

Dörfler J: Uber arteriennaht. Beitr Klin Chir 1889;25:781.

Drapanas T, Hewitt RL, Weichert RF III, Smith AD: Civilian vascular injuries: A critical appraisal of three decades of management. Ann Surg 1970;172:351-360.

Eck NV: K. voprosu o perevyazkie vorotnois veni. Predvaritelnoye soobshtshjenye (Ligature of the portal vein). Voen Med J 2001;130:1-2.

Elliot JA: Acute arterial occlusion: an unusual cause. Surgery 1956;39:825-827.

Ellis J: Case of gunshot wound, attended with secondary hemorrhage in which both carotid arteries were tied at an interval of four and a half days. N Y J Med 1845;5:187.

Ettien JT: Crutch-induced aneurysms of the axillary artery. Am Surg 1980;46:267-269.

Feliciano DV, Bitondo CG, Mattox KL, et al: Civilian trauma in 1980s: A one-year experience with 456 vascular and cardiac injuries. Ann Surg 1984;199:717-724.

Ferguson IA, Byrd WM, McAfee DK: Experiences in the management of arterial injuries. Ann Surg 1961;153:980-986.

Fisher GW: Acute arterial injuries treated by the United States Army Medical Service in Vietnam, 1965-1966. J Trauma 1967;7:844-855.

Flanigan DP, Keifer TJ, Schuler JJ, et al: Experience with iatrogenic pediatric vascular injuries: Incidence, etiology, management, and results. Ann Surg 1983;198:430-442.

Gaspar MR, Treiman RL: The management of injuries to major veins. Am J Surg 1960;100:171-175.

Gensoul: Note sur les Bless és reçus á l'Hôtel Dieu de Lyon, pendant les troubles de 1831. Gaz Méd Paris 1883;297.

Gibson JMC: Rupture of axillary artery. J Bone Joint Surg 1962;44B:114-115.

Glück T: Uber zwei fälle von aortenaneurysmen nebst bemerkungen uber die naht der blutgefässe. Arch Klin Chir 1883;28:548.

Goodman C: Suture of blood vessel from projectiles of war. Surg Gynecol Obstet 1918;27:528.

Goyanes J: Neuvos trabajos de chirurgial vascular: substitucion plastica de las the arterias por las venas, o arterio-plastia venosa, aplicado, como neuvo metodo, al traitamiento de los aneurismas. El Siglo Med 1906;53:546-561.

Gurri JA, Johnson G Jr: Management of brachial artery occlusion after cardiac catheterization. Am Surg 1980;46:233-235.

Guthrie GJ: Disease and injuries of arteries. 1830.

Haimovici H: History of arterial grafting. J Cardiac Surg 1963;4:152-174.

Hallowell. Extract of a letter from Mr. Lambert, surgeon at Newcastle upon Tyne, to Dr. Hunter, giving an account of new method of treating an aneurysm. Med Obser Inq 1762;30:360.

Halsted WS: The effect of ligation of the common iliac artery on the circulation and function of lower extremity. Report of a cure of iliofemoral aneurysm by their application of an aluminum band to the vessel. Bull Johns Hopkins Hosp 1912;23:191-220.

Hardy JD, Raju S, Neely WA, Berry DW: Aortic and other arterial injuries. Ann Surg 1975;181:640-653.

Heaton LD, Hughes CW, Rosegay H, et al: Military surgical practices of the United States Army in

Vietnam. In Current Problems in Surgery. Chicago, Year Book Medical Publishers, 1966.

Herget CH: Wound ballistics. In Bowers WB (ed): Surgery of Trauma. Philadelphia, JB Lippincott Co, 1956.

Hobson RW II, Rich NM: Traumatismes veineux des membres inférieurs. In Kieffer E (ed): Traumatismes Artériels. Paris, AERCV, 1995.

Hobson RW II, Rich NM, Wright CB: Venous Trauma: Pathophysiology, Diagnosis and Surgical Management. Mt. Kisco, NY, Futura Publishing, 1983.

Hoover NW: Injuries of the popliteal artery associated with fractures and dislocations. Surg Clin North Am 1961;41:1099-1112.

Hughes CW: Acute vascular trauma in Korean War casualties: An analysis of 180 cases. Surg Gynec Obstet 1954;99:91-100.

Hughes CW: The primary repair of wounds of major arteries: An analysis of experience in Korea in 1953. Ann Surg 1955;141:297-303.

Hughes CW: Arterial repair during the Korean War. Ann Surg 1958;147:555-561.

Hughes CW: Vascular surgery in the armed forces. Milit Med 1959;124:30-46.

Hunter W: The history of an aneurysm of the aorta, with some remarks on aneurysms in general. Med Obs Soc Phys Lond 1757;1:323.

Inui FK, Shannon J, Howard JM: Arterial injuries in the Korean conflict: Experiences with 111 consecutive injuries. Surgery 1955;37:850-857.

Jackson MR, Brengman ML, Rich NM: Delayed presentation of 50 years after a World War 2 vascular injury with intraoperative localization by duplex ultrasound of a traumatic false aneurysm. J Trauma 1997;43:159-161.

Jahnke EJ Jr: Late structural and functional results of arterial injuries primarily repaired. Surgery 1958;43:175-183.

Jahnke EJ Jr, Seeley SF: Acute vascular injuries in the Korean War: An analysis of 77 consecutive cases. Ann Surg 1953;138:158-177.

Jarstfer BS, Rich NM: The challenge of arteriovenous fistula formation following disk surgery: A collective review. J Trauma 1976;16:726-733.

Jassinowsky A: Die arteriennhat: Eine experimentelle studie. Inaug Diss Dorpat 1889.

Jensen: Ueber circulare gefassutur. Arch Klin Chir 1903;69:938-998.

Jimenez F, Utrilla A, Cuesta C, et al: Popliteal artery and venous aneurysm as a complication of arthroscopic meniscectomy. J Trauma 1988;28:1404-1405.

Kapp JP, Gielchinsky I, Jelsma R: Metallic fragment embolization to the cerebral circulation. J Trauma 1973;13:256-261.

Kay JK, Dykstra PC, Tsuji HK: Retrograde ilioaortic dissection. A complication of common femoral artery perfusion during open-heart surgery. Am J Surgery 1966;111:464-468.

Kelly GL, Eiseman B: Civilian vascular injuries. J Trauma 1975;15:507-514.

Kennedy JC: Complete dislocations of the knee. J Bone Joint Surg 1959;41:878.

Kozloff L, Rich NM, Brott WH, et al: Vascular trauma secondary to diagnostic and therapeutic procedures: Cardiopulmonary bypass and intra-aortic balloon assist. Am J Surg 1980;140:302-305.

Kümmel: Über circuläre naht der gefässe. Munch Med Wschr 1899;46:1398.

Kirkup JR: Major arterial injury complicating fracture of the femoral shaft. J Bone Joint Surg 1963;45:337-343.

Kurtoglu M, Ertekin C, Bulut T, et al: Management of vascular injuries of the extremities. One hundred and fifteen cases. Int Angiol 1991;10:95.

Langenbeck B: Beitrage zur chirurgischen pathologie der venen. Arch Klin Chir 1861;1:1.

Learmonth J: Vascular injuries in war. Royal Soc Med 1946;39:488.

Lexer E: Die ideale operation des arteriellen und des arteriell-venosen aneurysma. Arch Klin Chir 1907;83:459-477.

Linton R: Injuries to major arteries and their treatment. N Y J Med 1949;49:2039.

Lord JW, Stone P, Clouthier W, Breidenbach L: Major blood vessel injury during elective surgery. Arch Surg 1958;77:282.

Luetic V, Sosa T, Tonkovic I, et al: Military vascular injuries in Croatia. Cardiovasc Surg 1993;1:3-6.

Makins G: Gunshot injuries to the blood vessels. Bristol, England, John Wright and Sons, 1919.

Makins G, Howard JM, Green R: Arterial injuries complicating fractures and dislocations: The necessity for a more aggressive approach. Surgery 1966;59:203-209.

Matas R: An operation for radical cure of aneurysm based on arteriography. Ann Surg 1903;37:161-196.

Matas R: Military Surgery of the Vascular System. Philadelphia, WB Saunders, 1921.

Mattox KL: Approaches to trauma involving the major vessels of the thorax. Surg Clin North Am 1989;69:77-92.

Mattox KL, Feliciano DV, Burch J, et al: Five thousand seven hundred sixty cardiovascular injuries in 4459 patients: epidemiologic evolution 1958 to 1987. Ann Surg 1989;209:698-707.

McKenzie A, Sinclair A: Axillary artery occlusion complicating shoulder dislocation: a report of two cases. Ann Surg 1958;148:139-144.

Meagher DJ, Defore W, Mattox KL, Harberg F: Vascular trauma in infants and children. J Trauma 1979;19:532-536.

Miller D: Gangrene from arterial injuries associated with fractures and dislocations of the leg in the young and in adults with normal circulation. Am J Surg 1957;93:367-375.

Moore T: Acute arterial obstruction due to the traumatic circumferential intimal fracture. Ann Surg 1958;148:111-114.

Moore C, Wolma F, Brown R, Derrick J: Vascular trauma: A review of 250 cases. Am J Surg 1971;122:576-578.

Morris GC Jr, Creech O Jr, DeBakey ME: Acute arterial injuries in civilian practice. Am J Surg 1957;93:565-572.

Mullins R, Lucas C, Ledgerwood A: The natural history following venous ligation for civilian injuries. J Trauma 1980;20:737-743.

Murphy J: Resection of arteries and veins injured in continuity end-to-end suture. Exp Clin Res Med Rec 1897;51:73-104.

Murray G: Surgical repair of injuries to main arteries. Am J Surg 1952;83:480.

Natali J, Benhemori AC: Iatrogenic vascular injuries. J Cardiovasc Surg 1979;20:169-176.

Ngu V, Konstam PG: Traumatic dissecting aneurysm of the abdominal aorta. Br J Surg 1965;52:981-982.

Nolan B: Vascular injuries. J Royal Coll Surg 1968;13:72.

Oller D, Rutledge R, Clancey T, et al: Vascular injuries in a rural state: A review of 978 patients from a state trauma registry. J Trauma 1992;32:740-746.

Orcutt M, Levine B, Gaskill H III, Sirinek K: Iatrogenic vascular injury: A reducible problem. Arch Surg 1985;120:384-385.

Pate J, Wilson H: Arterial injuries of the base of the neck. Arch Surg 1964;89:1106-1110.

Patman R, Poulos E, Shires G: The management of civilian arterial injuries. Surg Gynecol Obstet 1964;118:725-738.

Perdue GJ, Smith RI: Intra-abdominal vascular injury. Surgery 1968;64:562-568.

Perler B, McCabe C, Abbott WM, Buckley MJ: Vascular complications of intra-aortic balloon counterpulsation. Arch Surg 1983;118:957-962.

Perry MO, Thal E, Shires G: Management of arterial injuries. Ann Surg 1971;173:403-408.

Postempski P: La sutura dei vasi sanguigni. Arch Soc Ital Chir Roma 1886;3:391.

Pritchard D, Maloney J, Barnhorst DA, Spittel JJ: Traumatic popliteal arteriovenous fistulas. Arch Surg 1977;112:849-852.

Reynolds R, McDowell H, Diethelm A: The surgical treatment of arterial injuries in the civilian population. Am Surg 1979;189:700-708.

Rich NM: Vietnam missile wounds evaluated in 750 patients. Milit Med 1968;133:9-22.

Rich NM: Vascular trauma in Vietnam. J Cardiovasc Surg 1970;11:368-377.

Rich NM: Venous injuries. In Sabiston DJ (ed): Textbook of Surgery. Philadelphia, WB Saunders, 1995.

Rich NM, Hobson RW II, Collins GJ Jr, Anderson CA: The effect of acute popliteal venous interruption. Ann Surg 1976;183:365-368.

Rich NM, Hobson RW II, Fedde C: Vascular trauma secondary to diagnostic and therapeutic procedures. Am J Surg 1974;128:715-721.

Rich NM, Hughes CW: Vietnam Vascular Registry: A preliminary report. Surgery 1969;65:218-226.

Rich NM, Spencer FC: Vascular Trauma. Philadelphia, WB Saunders, 1978.

Rich NM, Sullivan W: Clinical recanalization of an autogenous vein graft in the popliteal vein. J Trauma 1972;12:919-920.

Richardson JD, Fallat M, Nagaraj H, et al: Arterial injuries in children. Arch Surg 1981;116:685-690.

Rob CG: A history of arterial surgery. Arch Surg 1972;105:821-823.

Rob CG, Standeven A: Closed traumatic lesions of the axillary and brachial arteries. Lancet 1956;1:597-599.

Rybeck B: Missile wounding and hemodynamic effects of energy absorption. Acta Chir Scand 1974;450:1.

Salander J, Youkey J, Rich NM, et al: Vascular injury related to lumbar disk surgery. J Trauma 1984;24:628-631.

Saletta J, Freeark R: The partially severed artery. Arch Surg 1968;97:198-205.

Saletta J, Freeark R: Injuries to the profunda femoris artery. J Trauma 1972;12:778.

Schede M: Zur frage von der jodoformvergiftung. Zentralb Chir Beil 1882;9:33-38.

Schramek A, Hashmonai M: Distal arteriovenous fistula for the prevention of occlusion of venous interposition grafts to veins. J Cardiovasc Surg 1974;15:392-395.

Schramek A, Hashmonai M, Farbstein J, Adler O: Reconstructive surgery in major vein injuries in the extremities. J Trauma 1975;15:816-822.

Schwartz A: The historical development of methods of hemostasis. Surgery 1958;44:604.

Seeley S: Vascular surgery at Walter Reed Army Hospital. US Armed Forces Med J 1954;8.

Shumacker HB Jr: Incisions in surgery of aneurysm: With special reference to explorations in the antecubital and popliteal fossae. Ann Surg 1946;124:586-598.

Shumacker HB Jr: Surgical cure of innominate aneurysm; report of a case with comments on applicability of surgical measures. Surgery 1947a;22:729-739.

Shumacker HB Jr: Resection of the clavicle with particular reference to the use of bone chips in the periosteal bed. Surg Gynecol Obstet 1947b;84:245-248.

Shumacker HB Jr: Problem of maintaining the continuity of artery in surgery of aneurysms and arteriovenous fistulae; notes on the development and clinical application of methods of arterial suture. Ann Surg 1948a;127:207-230.

Shumacker HB Jr: Operative exposure of the blood vessels in the superior anterior mediastinum. Am Surg 1948b;127:464-475.

Shumacker HB Jr: Arterial suture techniques and grafts: Past, present and future. Surgery 1969;66:419-433.

Simeone F, Grillo H, Rundle F: On the question of ligation of the concomitant vein when a major artery is interrupted. Surgery 1951;29:932-951.

Smith R, Elliot J, Hageman J: Acute penetrating arterial injuries of the neck and limbs. Arch Surg 1974;109:198-205.

Smith L, Foran R, Gaspar MR: Acute arterial injuries of the upper extremity. Am J Surg 1963;106:144-151.

Soubbotitch V: Military experiences of traumatic aneurysms. Lancet 1913;2:720-721.

Spencer FC, Grewe R: The management of acute arterial injuries in battle casualties. Ann Surg 1955;141:304-313.

Stich R: Ueber gefaess und organ transplantationen mittelst gefaessnaht. Ergeon Chir Orth 1910;1:1.

Swan KG, Hobson RW II, Reynolds D, et al: Venous surgery in the lower extremities. In Swan KG, Hobson R, Reynolds D, et al (eds): St Louis, Warren H Green Publishers, 1975.

Todd G, Bregman D, Voorhees A, Reemtsma K: Vascular complications associated with percutaneous intra-aortic balloon pumping. Arch Surg 1983;118:963-964.

Vollmar J: Surgical experience with 197 traumatic arterial lesions (1953-66). In Hiertonn T, Rybeck B (eds): Traumatic Arterial Lesions. Stockholm, Försvarets Forskningsanstalt, 1968.

Warren R: Report to the Surgeon General. Washington, DC, Department of the Army, 1952.

Weinstein M, Golding A: Temporary external shunt bypass in the traumatically amputated upper extremity. J Trauma 1975;15:912-915.

Whelan TJ, Baugh JH: Non-Atherosclerotic Arterial Lesions and Their Management. Current Problems in Surgery. Chicago, Year Book Medical Publishers, 1967.

Youkey J, Clagett GP, Rich NM, et al: Vascular trauma secondary to diagnostic and therapeutic procedures: 1974 through 1982. Am J Surg 1983;146:788-791.

Ischemia and Reperfusion Injury

IRSHAD H. CHAUDRY
PING WANG
DORAID JARRAR

INTRODUCTION

The original Greek words *ischein* and *haima* mean to hold and blood. In the modern medical field, this means the lack of circulation or perfusion. In this chapter, the pathophysiology of ischemia and the clinical implications for the clinician are outlined. Specific attention is devoted to ischemia caused by vascular injury, as well as the potential therapeutic options under those conditions (Bickwell and colleagues, 1989; Burch and colleagues, 1990; Bickell and colleagues, 1994; de Guzman and colleagues, 1999). Vascular injury is present in approximately 20% of all trauma admissions to a tertiary care center. Besides obvious vascular trauma with the threat of immediate exsanguination, vascular compromise with subtle changes in perfusion and subsequent ischemia is an important issue in the secondary survey of the traumatized host. A thorough physical examination of the patient is, therefore, mandatory to identify vascular compromise and possible ischemia of the dependent organ or system.

With the evolution of multicellular organisms, the development of the cardiovascular system was essential, because the exchange of nutrients and oxygen is limited by diffusion and, therefore, is feasible only for single-cell organisms. In an adult human, thousands of miles of vessels of various size, shape, and capacity provide the body with oxygen and nutrients. This complex system also is responsible for the clearance of waste products and serves as the transport medium for hormones to reach their target sites. With the dependence of virtually all organs on aerobic metabolism, a stasis or even a reduction of blood flow will inevitably result in tissue damage or death, unless the collateral blood flow is sufficient to meet the metabolic demands of the affected organ bed.

The terms *ischemia* and *hypoxia* have been used indiscriminately. In view of this, differentiation between these two terms is important. In this chapter, *ischemia* refers to a total lack of oxygen, whereas *hypoxia* refers to decreased oxygen availability. Furthermore, whereas *ischemia,* that is, stasis of blood flow, inevitably leads to hypoxia of the dependent organ or organ system, *hypoxia* can occur in the presence of normal blood flow. Moreover, it appears that the detrimental effects of ischemia are not only due to the lack of oxygen, but also to the role of blood both to preserve tissue homeostasis and to deliver oxygen.

Clinical decision making is highly dependent on whether the ischemic event occurred acutely or has evolved over a prolonged time. If there has been a slow onset of decreased blood flow, leading ultimately to ischemia, collateral blood supply may have developed. However, in the case of traumatic vascular injury to an extremity, revascularization must be accomplished within 6 hours, because warm ischemia time for striated muscle results in irreversible damage after 6 to 8 hours.

With the re-establishment of blood flow to a previous ischemic organ or limb, reperfusion is initiated, that is, ischemia-reperfusion (I/R). This event also marks the onset of reperfusion injury, a complex event that involves many cellular and hormonal components including oxygen radicals, neutrophils, and complement activation. Reperfusion of an ischemic vascular bed not only produces local injury but also could produce distant organ injury.

The clinical hallmarks of ischemia are the five *P*s: pain, pulselessness, paresthesia, pallor, and paralysis. In the event of acute ischemia, pain and pulselessness are the leading clinical symptoms. Nevertheless, it should be kept in mind that in the multi-injured or unconscious patients, the clinical diagnosis may be difficult, and an appropriate vascular examination including Doppler flow ultrasound is mandated if vascular injury or compromise is suspected. If vascular trauma is present, the therapeutic goal should be restoration of function to the preinjury level (Burch and colleagues, 1990; Bickell and colleagues, 1994). In case of extremity trauma, warm ischemia time should not exceed 6 hours to ensure complete recovery of the extremity.

ISCHEMIA-REPERFUSION INJURY

Ischemia caused by conditions such as hemorrhagic shock, vascular trauma, and cardiac arrest, followed by reperfusion of the tissues with oxygenated blood, can compromise microvascular and cellular integrity (Massberg and Messmer, 1998; Ikeda and colleagues, 2000; Lefer, 1999; Lefer, 1994). The pathophysiologic mechanisms causing the so-called I/R injury are quite complex and involve a variety of cell populations including endothelial cells, leukocytes, hormones, up-regulation of cell surface proteins, and activation of the complement system. Part of the I/R injury is attributable to the phenomenon of slow reflow or no reflow, which is characterized by reduced blood flow despite the restoration of adequate perfusion pressure (Menger and colleagues, 1992). Although this phenomenon is still poorly understood, apparently, leukocytes, at least partially, mediate postischemic microvascular compromise (Schlag and colleagues, 2001; Kadambi and Skalak, 2000; Menger and colleagues, 1997; Waxman, 1996; Nolte and colleagues, 1991; Lehr and colleagues, 1991). Leukocyte adhesion to the endothelium is significantly enhanced following I/R injury, which is mediated by several adhesion molecules on the surface of leukocytes and/or endothelial cells such as immunoglobulin-like receptors (intercellular adhesion molecule-1 [ICAM-1], platelet endothelial cell adhesion molecule-1 [PECAM-1], vascular cell adhesion molecule-1 [VCAM-1]), integrins (CD11/CD18), and selectins (E-, P-, L-selectin) (Nolte and colleagues, 1994; Thorlacius and colleagues, 1998; Jaeschke, 1998; Weiser and colleagues, 1996; Farhood and colleagues, 1995). The endothelium now has been recognized not just to be a lining of the vascular conduit, but also to play a key role in the multistep process of leukocyte accumulation and emigration (Ikeda and colleagues, 2000). Moreover, soluble mediators, which are released after reperfusion, such as proinflammatory cytokines (tumor necrosis factor-α [TNF-α], interleukins, platelet-activating factor [PAF]), and leukotrienes, contribute to postischemic endothelial edema formation and perfusion dysfunction (Lefer, 1999; Jarrar and colleagues, 1999; Wang and colleagues, 1995; Jarras and colleagues, 2001; Linden, 2001). Moreover, radicals generated during reperfusion with oxygen-rich blood are factors that cause membrane damage and microvascular dysfunction.

The depletion of energy-rich phosphates such as adenosine triphosphate (ATP) diminishes the ability of the endothelial cell to maintain a transmembrane gradient of cations and anions as during normal homeostasis and leads to cell swelling and impairs cell integrity, causing extravasation of macromolecules, the so-called *leakage* (Wang and colleagues, 1999; Chaudry, 1983; Chaudry, 1990; Wang and colleagues, 1995; Wang and colleagues, 1994; Clemens and colleagues, 1985; Chaudry, 1989). The bioavailability of nitric oxide (NO) under those conditions is also markedly reduced (Ikeda and colleagues, 2000; Kim and Hwan, 2001; Hierholzer and colleagues, 2001; Uhlmann and colleagues, 2000; Traber, 2000). NO plays an important role in maintaining vascular tone and has antiadhesive properties (Wang and colleagues, 1995; Carden and Granger, 2000; Zhou and colleagues, 1997, Wang and colleagues, 1995; Wang and colleagues, 1994). With the advances in molecular biology techniques and knowledge, it has been shown that the proinflammatory milieu and generation of oxygen radicals trigger the activation of intracellular signaling pathways, leading to translocation of nuclear transcription factors and induction of stress genes and *de novo* protein synthesis (Okubo and colleagues, 2000; McDonald and colleagues, 2001; Jarrar and colleagues, 2000; Massberg and colleagues).

The key role of leukocytes in the manifestation of I/R injury has been documented using anti-adhesion molecule strategies, for example, monoclonal antibodies or antineutrophil serum. Through polymorphonuclear (PMN) leukocytes accumulation and leukocyte-capillary plugging, reperfusion is further impaired, enhancing the vicious cycle of no-reflow under those conditions (Massberg and Messmer, 1998; Lefer, 1999; Schlag and colleagues, 2001; Yamaguchi and colleagues, 1999).

The gut has been proposed as the motor for initiating multiorgan dysfunction following trauma and I/R. Although endotoxin and bacteria translocation may play a role in inducing cell and organ dysfunction following I/R, mediators that are released to the portal blood or lymph can activate neutrophils and Kupffer cells to release proinflammatory mediators, causing organ dysfunction. Characterization of the role of gut-derived mediators and/or factors during I/R will provide further insight into the mechanism responsible for cell and organ dysfunction following I/R.

ROLE OF ENDOTHELIAL CELLS FOLLOWING ISCHEMIA-REPERFUSION

Unstressed endothelial cells express a distinct set of genes that produce a nonthrombogenic lining of the blood vessels (Linden, 2001; Boyle and colleagues, 1999). This minimizes interaction between the endothelial lining and circulating blood cells and platelets. Moreover, during homeostasis, antithrombotic and procoagulatory mechanisms are balanced. This includes the production of thrombomodulin and vasoactive molecules such as NO and prostacyclin, which promote vasodilation and inhibition of smooth muscle cell contraction (Boyle and colleagues, 1999; Massberg and colleagues, 1999; Lefer and Lefer, 1993). Following I/R, genes favoring an inflammatory milieu are preferentially induced. This leads to the increased production of E-selectin, ICAM, VCAM, and interleukin-8 (IL-8), which promote leukocyte rolling, aggregation, subsequent adhesion and trans-endothelial cell migration (Massberg and Messmer, 1998; Schlag and colleagues, 2001; Massberg and colleagues, 1999; Boyle and colleagues, 1999). Moreover, the production of the vasoactive molecule NO by constitutive NO synthetase (NOS) is diminished, whereas superoxide production is increased. Experimental data have shown that following I/R, endothelium-dependent vasodilation in arterioles is reduced because NO is not available in sufficient quantities to serve as a second messenger in response to endogenous vasodilators such as acetylcholine (Farhood and colleagues, 1995; Lefer and Leafer, 1993). Arteriolar smooth muscle cell responsiveness, however, is maintained under those conditions. At a molecular level, studies have shown that the transcription factor NF-κB plays a key in the phenotypic changes of the endothelial cell lining toward an inflammatory phenotype. NF-κB is activated by oxidative stress, and upon degradation of its inhibitory molecule IκBα, NF-κB is translocated to the nucleus where it

binds to specific deoxyribonucleic acid (DNA) binding sequences, commonly the promotor region of inflammatory proteins and adhesion molecules, thereby increasing their rate of gene transcription. This includes E-selectin, VCAM, ICAM, IL-8, TNF-α, and the interleukins. Moreover, PAF receptor, tissue factor, and plasminogen activator are regulated by NF-κB and are induced following I/R, leading to microthrombosis, reduced blood flow, and leukocyte activation (McDonald and colleagues, 2001).

LEUKOCYTE-ENDOTHELIAL CELL INTERACTION FOLLOWING ISCHEMIA-REPERFUSION

Leukocyte trafficking through the microcirculation of tissues is essential for immune surveillance of tissues and early detection of pathologic conditions. Leukocyte recruitment is tightly regulated not only by the neutrophils, but also by the endothelial cell and adjacent tissue cells such as monocytes and mast cells. Several distinct steps regulate the recruitment of leukocytes into the extravascular space following inflammatory stimuli as observed after I/R (Fig. 2–1). The first step in this process is the rolling of leukocytes along the microvascular endothelium. Under normal flow conditions, leukocytes travel along an axial stream, whereas rolling allows contact of the blood cells with the endothelium. P-selectin, an adhesion glycoprotein, primarily regulates this process. In the second step, which is mediated via the expression of CD11/CD18, a member of the β_2-integrins, on the surface of leukocytes and ICAM-1, a member of the immunoglobulin superfamily, on the apical site of endothelial cells, the rolling leukocyte adheres firmly to the endothelium (Massberg and colleagues, 1998; Becker and colleagues, 1994; Menger and colleagues, 1994; Menger and colleagues, 1997; Pickelmann and colleagues, 1998; Steinbauer and colleagues, 1998; Kaeffer and colleagues, 1997). Finally, transendothelial migration occurs, requiring PECAM-1. The primary target sites for the aforementioned process

Proinflammatory milieu: E-selectin, P-selectin, IL-6, IL-8   Oxidative stress   Procoagulant

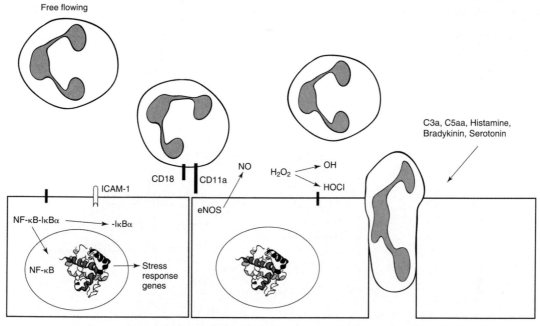

■ **FIGURE 2–1**
This figure shows the leukocyte-endothelium cell interactions following ischemia-reperfusion. Under normal conditions, the cellular components of the blood are separated from the endothelium by a rim of plasma. Following adverse circulatory conditions such as ischemia-reperfusion, the leukocyte gets in proximity to the endothelial wall by rolling along the wall. Up-regulation of adhesion molecules such as intercellular adhesion molecule-1 on the endothelial surface and the CD11/CD18 complex on polymorphonuclear (PMN) leukocytes then promotes sticking of the leukocytes to the venules. Subsequently, transendothelial migration of PMN is enhanced by tissue mast cells and the release of inflammatory meditators. Together with activation of platelets, this leads to the no-reflow phenomenon in postcapillary venules following ischemia-reperfusion. ■

are the postcapillary venules. This multistep process is markedly enhanced by local oxidative stress. Although initially the endothelium via xanthine oxidase serves as a production site of superoxide and hydrogen peroxide, the adherent leukocyte then amplifies this event and accounts for the substantially greater amount of radicals produced. Reperfusion and reintroduction of molecular oxygen add significantly to oxidative stress in the postcapillary venules. Furthermore, this results in an imbalance in the production of NO and superoxide, accounting for microvascular dysfunction and the no-reflow phenomenon. The lack of sufficient NO by the endothelial NOS leads to the unavailability of NO to serve as a second messenger and to effectively scavenge superoxide. Studies by Massberg and Messmer (1998) have demonstrated that

leukocyte-endothelial cell interaction precedes capillary perfusion failure and is the primary step responsible for the pathophysiologic sequelae following I/R (Fig. 2–2).

ROLE OF PLATELETS AND COMPLEMENT SYSTEM

Other than PMN cells and the endothelium, other blood components such as the anuclear platelets play an important role in I/R injury. Platelets are a source of oxygen radicals, release inflammatory mediators including thromboxane A_2, leukotrienes, serotonin, and platelet factor-4. Recruitment of platelets early following I/R to the postischemic vasculature leads to luminal narrowing and local

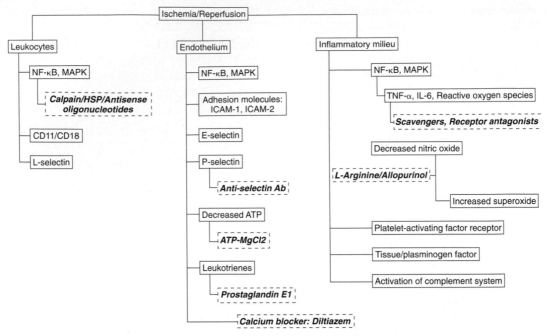

■ **FIGURE 2–2**
This schema shows the pathophysiologic changes occurring following ischemia-reperfusion and possible therapeutic interventions. Activation of intracellular stress signaling pathways are the key event on a molecular level. The inflammatory milieu then results in a vicious cycle on the level of the microcirculation. The potential therapeutic strategies are highlighted in dashed boxes. ■

thrombosis. Concomitantly, fibrinogen is deposited at the endothelium, which displays a procoagulant phenotype under those conditions (Massberg and colleagues, 1997; Massberg and colleagues, 1999). This is dependent on the expression of ICAM-1.

DIVERGENT EFFECTS OF NITRIC OXIDE AND SUPEROXIDE FOLLOWING ISCHEMIA-REPERFUSION

NO plays a critical role in I/R injury. As mentioned earlier in this chapter, this is partially due to the role of NO to scavenge superoxide, which is produced by xanthine oxidase. The substrate of xanthine oxidase, hypoxanthine, accumulates as the ATP stores are depleted. The imbalance between reduced availability of NO and the enhanced production of toxic radicals increases leukocyte

accumulation and impairs microvascular perfusion. The role of xanthine oxidase as a contributor to I/R injury has been demonstrated using inhibitors of this enzyme such as allopurinol. Experimental data support the notion that xanthine oxidase-derived oxidants act as a chemoattractant that regulates leukocyte trafficking in the microvasculature. The studies of Suzuki and colleagues (1991) have shown that exposure of postcapillary venules to oxidative stress increases leukocyte accumulation. The precise contribution of NO to I/R injury, however, is complicated because depending on the enzymatic source, NO may have beneficial or deleterious effects on tissue perfusion. Both constitutive and inducible forms of the enzyme NOS account for the production of NO. Constitutive Ca^{2+}-dependent production by constitutive NOS (cNOS) (endothelial and neuronal NOS) is present before the injury and is thought to be beneficial. The Ca^{2+}-independent, inducible isoform (inducible NOS [iNOS], NOS-2) accounts for the detrimental effects of NO, including the production of peroxynitrite. Insight into the complicated role of NOS following I/R has been gained using mice with targeted disruption of the iNOS (NOS-2) isoform (Kozlov and colleagues, 2001). Deficiency in iNOS-derived NO resulted in a significant reduction of skeletal muscle necrosis following hind-limb ischemia and reperfusion. Moreover, L-arginine supplementation during I/R prevents microvascular perfusion dysfunction by providing substrate for cNOS and maintaining tissue NO levels while concomitantly decreasing superoxide production (Ikeda and colleagues, 2000; Uhlmann and colleagues, 2000; Traber, 2000; Carden and Granger, 2000; Suzuki and colleagues, 1991; Rahat and colleagues, 2001). These findings not only underscore the significance of NO in maintaining microvascular integrity and perfusion under normal and pathologic conditions but also imply that L-arginine may be a useful therapeutic agent under those conditions.

CONFOUNDING COMORBIDITIES FOLLOWING ISCHEMIA-REPERFUSION

Although most trauma patients are in the younger population with no prior medical history, the consequences of I/R injury secondary to vascular trauma and/or compromise require special attention in comorbid patients. Comorbidities such as diabetes mellitus, hypertension, and hypercholesterolemia are all associated with arteriosclerotic disease and preexisting microvascular compromise (Huk and colleagues, 2000; Tailor and Granger, 2000; Hoshida and colleagues, 2000; Salas and colleagues, 1999; Bouchard and Lamontagne, 1998; Panes and colleagues, 1996). It is very conceivable and proven experimentally using animal strains expressing the aforementioned diseases that these confounding factors further aggravate I/R injury following vascular trauma and successful revascularization. This should be kept in mind when taking care of elderly patients, because the window for successful therapeutic interventions is even narrower under those conditions.

SYSTEMIC LEVELS OF INFLAMMATORY MEDIATORS AND REMOTE ORGAN INJURY

Following ischemia and reperfusion, local production and release of inflammatory mediators such cytokines, oxygen radicals, and vasoactive peptides are markedly enhanced. As discussed earlier in this chapter, this local inflammatory milieu contributes to PMN and platelet adhesion and ultimately to the no-reflow phenomenon. However, following I/R, this is not contained to the affected organ or organ system and leads to significant increased levels of mediator in the systemic circulation. For example, even simple laparotomy increased TNF-α messenger ribonucleic acid (mRNA) production in lung tissues, which was even further enhanced after remote, that is, intestinal, I/R. Circulating levels of xanthine oxidase are markedly elevated following I/R and accounted for activation of Kupffer cells and elevated liver enzyme release following hind-limb ischemia. Moreover, similar results were obtained by the administration of exogenous xanthine oxidase. From experimental and clinical data, it appears that the lungs are the most susceptible organ to low-flow conditions including ischemic events. The acute respiratory distress syndrome (ARDS) is a threaded event following adverse circulatory conditions, with a high mortality once fully developed. Apparently, once the initial I/R insult has been severe enough to lead to the systemic inflammatory response syndrome, circulating neutrophils are activated, leading to leukocyte-endothelial cell interaction in multiple vascular beds. The radiologic hallmark of ARDS, bilateral infiltrates, are caused by leukocyte influx, interstitial edema, and alveolar wall thickening. The development of respiratory insufficiency usually begins within 24 to 72 hours after the initiating ischemic event. As outlined earlier, the risk of developing ARDS corresponds to the length of the ischemic time and is markedly increased in the elderly comorbid patient.

SIGNIFICANCE OF ISCHEMIC PRECONDITIONING

Preconditioning refers to the phenomenon in which the exposure of cells, tissues, or organ systems to brief periods of ischemia protects them from the deleterious effects of subsequent prolonged ischemia. Although preconditioning, for obvious reasons, is not available in the acute setting of vascular trauma and because of the need for subsequent immediate revascularization, it should be discussed because important insights into the mechanism of I/R injury have been gained from this phenomenon. Preconditioning blunts the impairment of endothelium-dependent relaxation to acetylcholine, capillary plugging, leukocyte adhesion, and the no-reflow phenomenon usually observed following I/R. Among other mechanisms, a distinct set of genes the family of heat shock proteins (HSPs) confers protection against adverse circulatory events. HSPs maintain cellular survivability by preserving metabolic and structural integrity of cells. Recent data suggest that via the adenosine A_1 receptor and activation of protein kinase C, as well as tyrosine kinases, HSP27 is phosphorylated, thereby conferring protection against a subsequent lethal insult (Davies and Hagen, 1993; Speechly-Dick and colleagues, 1995). Summarizing ongoing efforts, it appears that selective induction of the HSPs might become a therapeutic modality.

MODIFYING FACTORS DETERMINING ISCHEMIA-REPERFUSION INJURY

Several factors modify the consequences, that is, the extent of tissue injury following I/R. Ambient temperature is well known to modulate the extent of necrosis. These lessons are learned from transplantation of solid organs, a classic example of I/R injury. Decreasing the temperature of the storage solution to 4°C can accomplish later reestablishment of the venous and arterial blood flow with complete return of organ func-

tion. In the case of extremity trauma with complete amputation, the recommendations are that the severed limb be stored in ice water until the patient is transported to an appropriate center with expertise in vascular surgery.

TREATMENT OF ISCHEMIA-REPERFUSION INJURY: ROLE OF PHARMACOLOGIC ADJUNCTS

A key event during ischemia is the decrease in the cellular levels of energy-rich phosphates, such as ATP. In view of this, studies have used the approach of administrating $ATP-MgCl_2$ after I/R, and such studies have shown that endothelial cell function can be restored following adverse circulatory conditions (Wang and colleagues, 1999; Wang and colleagues, 1995; Dana and colleagues, 2000; Gaudio and colleagues, 1982; Chaudry and colleagues, 1983; Ohkawa and colleagues, 1983; Chaudry and colleagues, 1984). Moreover, monoclonal antibodies against adhesion molecules such as CD11/CD18 or the P-selectin family have also been beneficial in preventing I/R injury (Ohkawa and colleagues, 1984).

Improvement of blood flow using rheologic agents such as dextran are also effective in improving capillary reflow following I/R (Sharar and colleagues, 1991; Schott and colleagues, 1998). Administration of prostaglandin E_1 following I/R normalized NO and superoxide release and thus improved microvascular blood flow with reduced adherence of leukocytes (Berglund and colleagues, 1981).

Although all the aforementioned agents have been shown to reduce I/R injury in experimental models, they have not been used clinically to improve outcome in patients following vascular trauma and subsequent ischemic events. Only the intraoperative administration of heparin following vascular extremity injury has been shown to significantly improve the rate of limb salvage (Forrest and colleagues, 1991; Melton and colleagues, 1997; Wang and colleagues, 1990; Rana and colleagues, 1992; Wang and colleagues, 1993; Wang and colleagues, 1994; Zellweger, 1995).

SUMMARY

This chapter has covered pathophysiology of ischemia and reperfusion injury, including the consequences of re-establishment of blood flow following a variable period of cessation of perfusion with oxygenated blood (Wang and colleagues, 1996; Wall and colleagues, 1996). Apparently, I/R injury is due not only to the lack of oxygen as seen during ischemia, but also to the absence of whole blood with its scavenging properties. Generally speaking, I/R injury is the most common cause of death in the Western Hemisphere because of the prevalence of arteriosclerotic disease including the coronary arteries (Shin and colleagues, 2000; Beebe and colleagues, 1996; Brengman and colleagues, 2000; Eifert and colleagues, 2000). The key pathophysiologic events following I/R have been investigated in depth. In this regard, the leukocyte-endothelial cell interactions appear to be a key element, which results in the phenomenon of no reflow following adverse circulatory conditions, secondary to enhanced PMN leukocyte recruitment to the postcapillary venules. Using intravital microscopy, it has been shown that an orderly sequence of events takes place including leukocyte rolling, sticking, and adherence, followed by transendothelial migration. These processes are modified by the inflammatory milieu generated following I/R injury. Reactive oxygen species, proinflammatory cytokines, superoxide, and other paracrine messengers all intensify the leukocyte-endothelial cell interaction, leading to microvascular perfusion failure. Paradoxically, most of the damage occurs during the reperfusion period and to a lesser extent during the actual ischemic time.

The probably most significant independent factor determining injury following vascular injury and subsequent ischemia of an organ or limb is time until re-establishment of blood flow. Modifying factors, however, include ambient temperature and preexisting comorbidities. Although a variety of therapeutic agents have been effectively used in experimental studies, this has not yet been translated into an accepted modality in clinical practice. Of note, the decrease in hematocrit during vascular injury caused by blood loss has beneficial effects on the rheology of the microvasculature but does mandate immediate blood transfusion.

With the use of molecular biology tools, the changes on the cellular mRNA and protein level have also been characterized following I/R. A distinct set of stress response genes and signaling pathways appear activated, leading to a change in the phenotype of leukocytes and endothelial cells. This propagates the local inflammatory milieu, resulting in the upregulation of adhesion molecules and the no reflow following ischemia and reperfusion. With the advances in our understanding of the molecular mechanisms of I/R injury, selective modulation of the aforementioned phenotypic changes in leukocytes and endothelial cells should be forthcoming.

REFERENCES

Barker JE, Knight KR, Romeo R, et al: Targeted disruption of the nitric oxide synthase 2 gene protects against ischemia/reperfusion injury to skeletal muscle. J Pathol 2001;194:10-115.

Becker M, Menger MD, Lehr HA: Heparin-released superoxide dismutase inhibits postischemic leukocyte adhesion to venular endothelium. Am J Physiol 1994;267:H925-H930.

Beebe HG, Bergan JJ, Bergqvist D, et al: Classification and grading of chronic venous disease in the lower limbs. A consensus statement. Eur J Vasc Endovasc Surg, 1996;12:487-492.

Berglund B, Swanbeck G, Hedin H: Low molecular weight dextran therapy for digital ischemia due to collagen vascular disease. Dermatologica 1981;163:353-357.

Bickell WH, Shaftan GW, Mattox KL: Intravenous fluid administration and uncontrolled hemorrhage. J Trauma 1989;29:409.

Bickell WH, Wall MJ Jr, Pepe PE, et al: Immediate versus delayed fluid resuscitation for hypotensive patients with penetrating torso injuries. N Engl Med 1994;331:1105-1109.

Bouchard JF, Lamontagne D: Protection afforded by preconditioning to the diabetic heart against ischemic injury. Cardiovasc Res 1998;37:82-90.

Boyle EM Jr, Canty TG Jr, Morgan EN, et al: Treating myocardial ischemia-reperfusion injury by targeting endothelial cell transcription. Ann Thorac Surg 1999;68:1949-1953.

Brengman ML, O'Donnell SD, Mullenix P, et al: The fate of a patent carotid artery contralateral to an occlusion. Ann Vasc Surg 2000;14:77-81.

Burch JM, Richardson RJ, Martin RR, Mattox KL: Penetrating iliac vascular injuries: recent experience with 233 consecutive patients. J Trauma 1990;30:1450-1459.

Carden DL, Granger DN: Pathophysiology of ischemia-reperfusion injury. J Pathol 2000;190:255-266.

Chaudry IH: Cellular mechanisms in shock and ischemia and their correction. Am J Physiol 1983;245:R117-R134.

Chaudry IH: ATP-MgCl$_2$ and liver blood flow following shock and ischemia. Prog Clin Biol Res 1989;299:19-31.

Chaudry IH: The use of ATP following shock and ischemia. Ann N Y Acad Sci 1990;603:130-141.

Chaudry IH, Ohkawa M, Clemens MG: Improved mitochondrial function following ischemia and reflow by ATP-MgCl$_2$. Am J Physiol 1984;246:R799-R804.

Chaudry IH, Ohkawa M, Clemens MG, Baue AE: Alterations in electron transport and cellular metabolism with shock and trauma. Prog Clin Biol Res 1983;111:67-88.

Clemens MG, McDonah PF, Chaudry IH, Baue AE: Hepatic microcirculatory failure after ischemia and reperfusion: Improvement with ATP-MgCl$_2$ treatment. Am J Physiol 1985;248:H804-H811.

Dana A, Skarli M, Papakrivopoulou J, Yellon DM: Adenosine A(1) receptor induced delayed preconditioning in rabbits: Induction of p38 mitogen-activated protein kinase activation and Hsp27 phosphorylation via a tyrosine kinase— and protein kinase C-dependent mechanism. Circ Res 2000;86:989-997.

Davies MG, Hagen PO: The vascular endothelium. A new horizon. Ann Surg 1993;218:593-609.

de Guzman E, Shankar MN, Mattox KL: Limited volume resuscitation in penetrating thoracoabdominal trauma. AACN Clin Issues 1999;10:61-68.

Eifert S, Villavicencio JL, Kao TC, et al: Prevalence of deep venous anomalies in congenital vascular malformations of venous predominance. J Vasc Surg 2000;31:462-471.

Farhood A, McGuire GM, Manning AM, et al: Intercellular adhesion molecule 1 (ICAM-1) expression and its role in neutrophil-induced ischemia-reperfusion injury in rat liver. J Leukoc Biol 1995;57:368-374.

Forrest CR, Pang CY, Zhong AG, Kreidstein ML: Efficacy of intravenous infusion of prostacyclin (PG12) or prostaglandin E$_1$ (PGE$_1$) in augmentation of skin flap blood flow and viability in the pig. Prostaglandins 1991;41:537-558.

Gaudio KM, Taylor MR, Chaudry IH, et al: Accelerated recovery of single nephron function by the postischemic infusion of ATP-MgCl$_2$. Kidney Int 1982;22:13-20.

Geller DA, Chia SH, Takahashi Y, et al: Protective role of the L-arginine-nitric oxide synthase pathway on preservation injury after rat liver transplantation. J Parenter Enter Nutr 2001;25:142-147.

Hierholzer C, Harbrecht BG, Billiar TR, Tweardy DJ: Hypoxia-inducible factor-1 activation and cyclo-oxygenase-2 induction are early reperfusion-independent inflammatory events in hemorrhagic shock. Arch Orthop Trauma Surg 2001;121:219-222.

Hoshida S, Yamashita N, Otsu K, et al: Cholesterol feeding exacerbates myocardial injury in Zucker diabetic fatty rats. Am J Physiol Heart Circ Physiol 2000;278:H256-H262.

Huk I, Brovkovych V, Nanobashvili J, et al: Prostaglandin E$_1$ reduces ischemia/reperfusion injury by normalizing nitric oxide and superoxide release. Shock 2000;14:234-242.

Ikeda Y, Young LH, Scalia R, Lefer AM: Cardioprotective effects of citrulline in ischemia/reperfusion injury via a non-nitric oxide-mediated mechanism. Methods Find Exp Clin Pharmacol 2000;22:563-571.

Jaeschke H: Mechanisms of reperfusion injury after warm ischemia of the liver. J Hepatobiliary Pancreat Surg 1998;5:402-408.

Jarrar D, Chaudry IH, Wang P: Organ dysfunction following hemorrhage and sepsis: Mechanisms and therapeutic approaches [Review]. Int J Mol Med 1999;4:575-583.

Jarrar D, Wang P, Chaudry IH: Hepatocellular dysfunction: Basic considerations. In Holzheimer RG, Mannick JA (eds): Surgical Treatment: Evidence-Based and Problem-Oriented. Munich, Germany, Zuckschwerdt Verglad, 2001:763-767.

Jarrar D, Wang P, Song GY, et al: Inhibition of tyrosine kinase signaling after trauma-hemorrhage: A novel approach for improving organ function and decreasing susceptibility to subsequent sepsis. Ann Surg 2000;231:399-407.

Kadambi A, Shalak TC: Role of leukocytes and tissue-derived oxidants in short-term skeletal muscle ischemia-reperfusion injury. Am J Physiol Heart Circ Physiol 2000;278:H435-H443.

Kaeffer N, Richard V, Thuillez C: Delayed coronary endothelial protection 24 hours after preconditioning: Role of free radicals. Circulation 1997;96:2311-2316.

Kim H, Hwan KK: Role of nitric oxide and mucus in ischemia/reperfusion-induced gastric mucosal injury in rats. Pharmacology 2001;62:200-207.

Kozlov AV, Sobhian B, Duvigneau C, et al: Organ specific formation of nitrosyl complexes under intestinal ischemia/reperfusion in rats involves NOS-independent mechanism(s). Shock 2001; 15:366-371.

Lefer AM: Endotoxin, cytokines, and nitric oxide in shock. Shock 1994;1:79-80.

Lefer AM: Role of the beta2-integrins and immunoglobulin superfamily members in myocardial ischemia-reperfusion. Ann Thorac Surg 1999;68:1920-1923.

Lefer AM, Lefer DJ: Pharmacology of the endothelium in ischemia-reperfusion and circulatory shock. Ann Rev Pharmacol Toxicol 1993;33:71-90.

Lehr HA, Guhlman A, Nolte D, et al: Leukotrienes as mediators in ischemic-reperfusion injury in a microcirculation model in the hamster. J Clin Invest 1991;87:2036-2041.

Linden J: Molecular approach to adenosine receptors: Receptor-mediated mechanisms of tissue protection. Ann Rev Pharmacol Toxicol 2001; 41:775-787.

Massberg S, Enders G, Matos FC, et al: Fibrinogen deposition at the postischemic vessel wall promotes platelet adhesion during ischemia-reperfusion in vivo. Blood 1999;94:3829-3838.

Massberg S, Messmer K: The nature of ischemia/ reperfusion injury. Transplant Proc 1998;30: 4217-4223.

Massberg S, Sausbier M, Klatt P, et al: Increased adhesion and aggregation of platelets lacking cyclic guanosine 3',5'-monophosphate kinase I. J Exp Med 1999;189:1255-1264.

McDonald MC, Mota-Filipe H, Paul A, et al: Calpain inhibitor I reduces the activation of nuclear factor-kappaB and organ injury/ dysfunction in hemorrhagic shock. FASEB J 2001;15:171-186.

Melton SM, Croce MA, Patton JH Jr, et al: Popliteal artery trauma. Systemic anticoagulation and intraoperative thrombolysis improves limb salvage. Ann Surg 1997;225:518-527.

Menger MD, Kerger H, Geisweid A, et al: Leukocyte-endothelium interaction in the microvasculature of postischemic striated muscle. Adv Exp Med Biol 1994;361:541-545.

Menger MD, Pelikan S, Steiner D, Messmer K: Microvascular ischemia-reperfusion injury in striated muscle: significance of reflow paradox. Am J Physiol 1992;263:H1901-H1906.

Menger MD, Rucker M, Vollmar B: Capillary dysfunction in striated muscle ischemia/ reperfusion: on the mechanisms of capillary no-reflow. Shock 1997;8:2-7.

Menger MD, Volmmar B: In vivo analysis of microvascular reperfusion injury in striated muscle and skin. Microsurgery 1994;15:383-389.

Nolte D, Hecht R, Schmid P, et al: Role of Mac-1 and ICAM-1 in ischemia-reperfusion injury in a microcirculation model of BALB/C mice. Am J Physiol 1994;267:H1320-H1328.

Nolte D, Lehr HA, Messmer K: Adenosine inhibits postischemic leukocyte-endothelium interaction in postcapillary venules of the hamster. Am J Physiol 1991;261:H651-H655.

Ohkawa M, Chaudry IH, Clemens MG, Baue AE: ATP-MgCl$_2$ produces sustained improvement in hepatic mitochondrial function and blood flow after hepatic ischemia. J Surg Res 1984;37:226-234.

Ohkawa M, Clemens MG, Chaudry IH: Studies on the mechanism of beneficial effects of ATP-MgCl$_2$ following hepatic ischemia. Am J Physiol 1983; 244:R695-R702.

Okubo S, Bernardo NL, Elliott GT, et al: Tyrosine kinase signaling in action potential shortening and expression of HSP72 in late preconditioning. Am J Physiol Heart Circ Physiol 2000;279: H2269-H2276.

Panes J, Kurose I, Rodriguez-Vaca D, et al: Diabetes exacerbates inflammatory responses to ischemia-reperfusion. Circulation 1996;93:161-167.

Pickelmann S, Nolte D, Leiderer R, et al: Attenuation of postischemic reperfusion injury in striated skin muscle by diaspirin-cross-linked Hb. Am J Physiol 1998;275:H361-H368.

Rahat MA, Lahat N, Smollar J, et al: Divergent effects of ischemia/reperfusion and nitric oxide donor on TNF-alpha mRNA accumulation in rat organs. Shock 2001;15:312-317.

Rana MW, Singh G, Wang P, et al: Protective effects of preheparinization on the microvasculature during and after hemorrhagic shock. J Trauma 1992;32:420-426.

Salas A, Panes J, Rosenbloom CL, et al: Differential effects of a nitric oxide donor on reperfusion-induced microvascular dysfunction in diabetic and non-diabetic rats. Diabetologia 1999;42:1350-1358.

Schlag MG, Harris KA, Potter RF: Role of leukocyte accumulation and oxygen radicals in ischemia-reperfusion-induced injury in skeletal muscle. Am J Physiol Heart Circ Physiol 2001; 280:H1716-H1721.

Schott U, Lindbom LO, Sjostrand U: Hemodynamic effects of colloid concentration in experimental hemorrhage: A comparison of Ringer's acetate, 3% dextran-60, and 6% dextran-70. Crit Care Med 1998;16:346-352.

Sharar SR, Winn RK, Murry CE, et al: A CD18 monoclonal antibody increases the incidence and severity of subcutaneous abscess formation after high-dose *Staphylococcus aureus* injection in rabbits. Surgery 1991;110:213-220.

Shin DD, Wall MJ Jr, Mattox KL: Combined penetrating injury of the innominate artery, left common carotid artery, trachea, and esophagus. J Trauma 2000;49:780-783.

Speechly-Dick ME, Grover GJ, Yellon DM: Does ischemic preconditioning in the human involve protein kinase C and the ATP-dependent K+ channel? Studies of contractile function after simulated ischemia in an atrial *in vitro* model. Circ Res 1995;77:1030-1035.

Steinbauer M, Harris AG, Leiderer R, et al: Impact of dextran on microvascular disturbances and tissue injury following ischemia/reperfusion in striated muscle. Shock 1998;9:345-351.

Tailor A, Granger DN: Role of adhesion molecules in vascular regulation and damage. Curr Hypertens Rep 2000;2:78-83.

Thorlacius H, Vollmar B, Westermann S, et al: Effects of local cooling on microvascular hemodynamics and leukocyte adhesion in the striated muscle of hamsters. J Trauma 1998;45:715-719.

Traber DL: Nitric oxide synthase and tissue injury. Shock 2000;14:243-244.

Uhlmann D, Uhlmann S, Spiegel HU: Endothelin/nitric oxide balance influences hepatic ischemia-reperfusion injury. J Cardiovasc Pharmacol 2000;36:S212-S214.

Wall MJ Jr, Granchi T, Liscum K, Mattox KL: Penetrating thoracic vascular injuries. Surg Clin North Am 1996;76:749-761.

Wang P, Ba ZF, Chaudry IH: Endothelial cell dysfunction occurs after hemorrhage in nonheparinized but not in preheparinized models. J Surg Res 1993;54:499-506.

Wang P, Ba ZF, Chaudry IH: Chemically modified heparin improves hepatocellular function, cardiac output, and microcirculation after trauma-hemorrhage and resuscitation. Surgery 1994;116:169-175.

Wang P, Ba ZF, Chaudry IH: Nitric oxide. To block or enhance its production during sepsis? Arch Surg 1994;129:1137-1142.

Wang P, Ba ZF, Chaudry IH: ATP-MgCl$_2$ restores depressed endothelial cell function after hemorrhagic shock and resuscitation. Am J Physiol 1995;268:H1390-H1396.

Wang P, Ba ZF, Chaudry IH: Endothelium-dependent relaxation is depressed at the macro- and microcirculatory levels during sepsis. Am J Physiol 1995;269:R988-R994.

Wang P, Ba ZF, Reich SS, et al: Effects of nonanticoagulant heparin on cardiovascular and hepatocellular function after hemorrhagic shock. Am J Physiol 1996;270:HI294-HI302.

Wang P, Ba ZF, Stepp KJ, Chaudry IH: Pentoxifyline attenuates the depressed endothelial cell function and vascular muscle contractility following trauma and hemorrhagic shock. J Trauma 1995;39:121-126.

Wang P, Singh G, Rana MW, et al: Preheparinization improves organ function after hemorrhage and resuscitation. Am J Physiol 1990;259:R645-R650.

Wang P, Tait SM, Ba ZF, Chaudry IH: ATP-MgCl$_2$ administration normalizes macrophage cAMP and beta-adrenergic receptors after hemorrhage and resuscitation. Am J Physiol 1994;267:G52-G58.

Waxman K: Shock: ischemia, reperfusion, and inflammation. New Horiz 1996;4:153-160.

Weiser MR, Gibbs SA, Valeri CR, et al: Anti-selectin therapy modifies skeletal muscle ischemia and reperfusion injury. Shock 1996;5:402-407.

Yamaguchi Y, Matsumura F, Liang J, et al: Neutrophil elastase and oxygen radicals enhance monocyte chemoattractant protein-expression after ischemia/reperfusion in rat liver. Transplantation 1999;68:1459-1468.

Zellweger R, Ayala A, Zhu XL, et al: A novel nonanticoagulant heparin improves splenocyte and peritoneal macrophage immune function after trauma-hemorrhage and resuscitation. J Surg Res 1995;59:211-218.

Zhou M, Wang P, Chaudry IH: Endothelial nitric oxide synthase is downregulated during hyperdynamic sepsis. Biochim Biophys Acta 1997;1335:182-190.

Minimal Vascular Injuries

JAMES W. DENNIS

Arterial injuries come in various shapes and sizes. Regardless of the etiology, complete transections, occlusions, bleeding lacerations, and large pseudoaneurysms almost universally require immediate surgical intervention or the patient faces the loss of life or limb. These types of arterial injuries make up the vast majority (80% to 90%) of cases (Hardy and colleagues, 1975). Since the earliest times, surgeons have recognized that the type of injury can have a profound effect on the ultimate outcome. A special class of injuries has been recognized over the past 15 years that can be called "minimal injuries." This small select group appears to have a unique natural history and must be considered in this light. By understanding this natural history, management plans for patients presenting with certain types of injuries can be formulated so that they ensure proper and safe treatment in the acute setting.

DEFINITION

Minimal injuries are generally defined as identifiable damage to a blood vessel, usually by arteriography or ultrasound, with no clinical signs of that injury. By definition, hard signs of vascular trauma including pulse

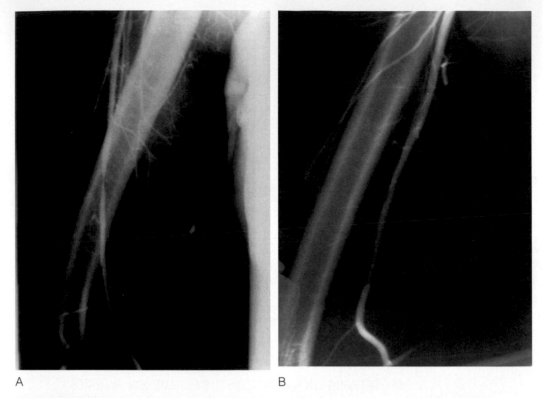

A   B

■ FIGURE 3–1

A, Short segmental narrowing and intimal irregularity after a gunshot wound to the right brachial artery. *B,* Complete resolution of injury 6 weeks later. (From Dennis JW, Frykberg ER, Crump JM, et al: New perspectives on the management of penetrating trauma in proximity to major limb arteries. J Vasc Surg 1990;11:84-93.) ■

deficit, active hemorrhage, expanding hematoma, distal ischemia, and bruit or thrill are absent. Soft signs such as a history of bleeding, stable hematoma, associated nerve deficit, or unexplained hypotension may or may not be present and have no direct relationship to these injuries. Minimal injuries will also regularly demonstrate prograde flow of contrast on arteriography or flow on ultrasound. In addition, no gross, uncontained extravasation of blood or contrast is seen outside the normal lumen of the vessel involved.

Studies have identified four basic types of minimal injuries, of which two dominate. The first major type is focal segmental narrowing or constriction that is characteristically smooth in nature with tapering at both ends (Figs. 3–1*A* and 3–2*A*). Arteries can demonstrate this abnormality secondary to external compression, intramural hematoma (contusion), or

reactive spasm. Spasm is due to the myogenic response of blood vessels to the blast effect of penetrating missiles or direct effects of blunt forces. Blood flow can be demonstrated throughout this narrowed segment, which can vary in length from just a few millimeters to several centimeters.

The second predominant type of minimal injury is that of the intimal flap or irregularity (Fig. 3–3*A*). This is usually seen as a luminal surface abnormality in which the intimal layer has a raised portion extending into the lumen. Flaps may be lifted in either a proximal or a distal orientation. It may also appear as a focal, roughened area of the luminal surface. In both forms, flow is present within the lumen and there is no extravasation outside of it.

Small pseudoaneurysms and arteriovenous (AV) fistulas make up the other two smaller categories of minimal injuries.

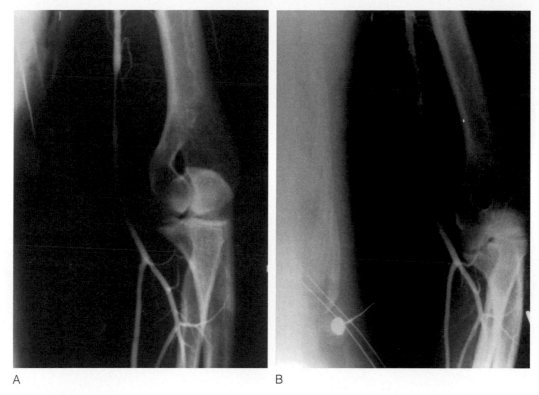

A   B

■ **FIGURE 3–2**
A, Long smooth area of narrowing of the left brachial artery after a gunshot wound. *B,* Complete resolution after 1 week. (From Dennis JW, Frykberg ER, Crump JM, et al: New perspectives on the management of penetrating trauma in proximity to major limb arteries. J Vasc Surg 1990; 11:84-93.) ■

Pseudoaneurysms are formed when there is an incomplete laceration of an artery with the resultant hemorrhage contained by the surrounding tissue (Fig. 3–4*A*). These lesions are easily seen by arteriography or ultrasound and will appear as contained extravasation of contrast or blood outside the normal arterial lumen. AV fistulas develop when an arterial laceration and simultaneous laceration or tear occurs in the adjacent vein causing flow to enter into the low-pressure venous channel. This is also clearly identified by arteriography or ultrasound as a direct passage of contrast or blood from an artery into a vein without passing through a capillary system.

In each of these minimal injuries, distal pulses usually remain intact. In patients with a pseudoaneurysm or AV fistula, an audible bruit or thrill may be present on physical examination, indicating the need for further

evaluation to determine the nature and extent of these injuries.

HISTORY OF THE MANAGEMENT OF MINIMAL INJURIES

Early information concerning vascular trauma was the result of military experience in World Wars I and II (DeBakey and Simeone, 1946). Direct vascular repair of injuries was not performed on a widespread basis, however, until the 1950s in both the Korean conflict and civilian settings (Hughes, 1958; Ferguson, Byrd, and McAfee, 1961). The decision to operate was initially based on physical examination alone, as there was no other available or reliable means to diagnose vascular injuries.

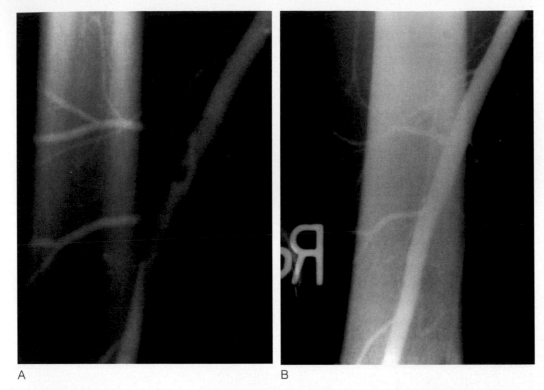

A   B

■ FIGURE 3–3

A, Intimal irregularity or flap in the superficial femoral artery after a through-and-through gunshot wound of the right thigh. *B,* Complete resolution of the injury after 1 week. (From Dennis JW, Frykberg ER, Crump JM, et al: New perspectives on the management of penetrating trauma in proximity to major limb arteries. J Vasc Surg 1990;11:84-93.) ■

Penetrating wounds in proximity to major arteries began to be routinely explored to determine the presence or absence of a vascular injury. This policy continued into the 1970s when arteriography began to be widely used to evaluate patients for vascular trauma and avoid unnecessary surgery.

Multiple studies were published in the late 1970s and early 1980s that showed arteriography to be as accurate as surgical exploration for detecting any type of vascular injury following penetrating trauma to the extremities (Synder and colleagues, 1978; Sirinek and colleagues, 1981). These studies consistently showed a more than 95% chance of having a significant arterial injury when hard signs were present on physical examination. In addition, there was a 10% to 20% risk of an arteriographic abnormality found even in the face of normal physical examination results (Table 3–1). This new use of arteriography first demonstrated the presence of these minimal arterial injuries that had not been seen before

its use. Because no data existed about their clinical significance, surgeons erred on the side of operating on any abnormalities found. This approach was based on the fear of missing an injury that needed repair even in the absence of any clinical findings. Universal recommendations resulting from these series were to either surgically explore or obtain an arteriogram on every patient with penetrating trauma to the extremities. If any abnormalities were seen on arteriography, they required immediate exploration and repair if needed.

DEFINING THE NATURAL HISTORY OF MINIMAL INJURIES

The first evidence that minimal vascular injuries might have the potential to

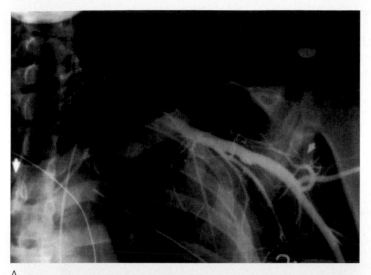

A

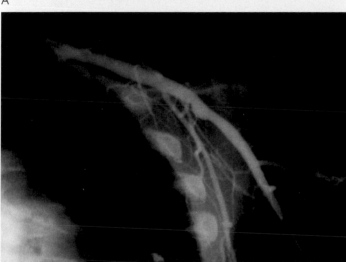

B

■ **FIGURE 3–4**
A, Small pseudoaneurysm of the left distal axillary artery after a gunshot wound to the shoulder. B, Pseudoaneurysm 10 months later—essentially unchanged with possibly slight improvement. (From Dennis JW, Frykberg ER, Crump JM, et al: New perspectives on the management of penetrating trauma in proximity to major limb arteries. J Vasc Surg 1990;11:84-93.) ■

TABLE 3–1
MECHANISM OF PENETRATING PROXIMITY EXTREMITY TRAUMA AND ULTIMATE OUTCOME

Injury	Total (No.)	No. Arterial Injuries	No. Requiring Surgery (%)
Gunshot	247	24 (9.7)	2 (0.8)*
Stab	54	5 (9.3)	2 (3.7)
Shotgun	17	3 (17.6)	2 (11.8)*
Total	318	32 (10.0)	6 (1.8)

*One operated on immediately.
From Dennis JW, Frykberg ER, Crump JM, et al: New perspectives on the management of penetrating trauma in proximity to major limb arteries. J Vasc Surg 1990;11:84-93.

TABLE 3–2

RESULTS OF NONOPERATIVE OBSERVATION OF 29 CLINICALLY OCCULT ARTERIAL INJURIES ACCORDING TO MORPHOLOGY

		Repeat Arteriogram (No.)				Clinical Follow-up (No.)	
	Total No.	RES	IMP	UNC	WOR	UNC	WOR
Narrowing	12	7	0	1	0	4	0
Intimal flap	12	6	2	0	1*	2	1*
Pseudoaneurysm	5	2	1	0	2*	0	0
Total	29	15	3	1	3	6	1

*Underwent surgical repair.
IMP, improved; RES, resolved; UNC, unchanged; WOR, worsened.
From Dennis JW, Frykberg ER, Crump JM, et al: New perspectives on the management of penetrating trauma in proximity to major limb arteries. J Vasc Surg 1990;11:84-93.

spontaneously heal was work done by Glover in 1986. He induced intimal tears in rat arteries and harvested them for up to 1 year later. All vessels remained patent and the endothelial injury was consistently healed by 8 weeks with no long-term sequelae (Glover, 1986). Clinical studies suggesting this might hold true in humans began to appear soon (Stain and colleagues, 1989; Kestenberg, 1990). These scientific studies began to look at the natural history of this unique class of injuries. The first prospective series on penetrating extremity injuries was performed by Frykberg and colleagues in 1989. This landmark article detailed the potential healing properties of this new class of minimal injuries when followed with nonoperative management and serial arteriograms. This new approach revealed the natural history to be somewhat benign in that the vast majority (up to 89%) would either resolve spontaneously or remain unchanged. Approximately 11% would deteriorate and require surgical repair, but this could be done safely and with no increase in morbidity or limb loss when performed on a delayed basis. A larger series published almost 2 years later confirmed the earlier results, by showing 87% of minimal injuries would heal if treated conservatively (Dennis and colleagues, 1990) (Table 3–2). Other trauma centers soon reported similar experiences when nonoperative management of these minimal injuries was employed (Francis and colleagues, 1991; Itani, 1991; Trooskin, 1993;

Gahtan, 1994). The ability to resolve these minimal injuries in nonextremity arteries was also first demonstrated by Frykberg and colleagues (1991) in a series that included injuries of the torso and neck.

The data consistently illustrated that different types of minimal injuries behaved differently over time. Smooth arterial narrowings would almost uniformly resolve on their own and are the most benign of the minimal injuries (Figs. 3–1B and 3–2B). Intimal flaps or irregularities would deteriorate into pseudoaneurysms approximately 10% of the time. The morphology of the intimal disruption did not reliably predict the possibility of it worsening. Even the fact that a flap might be large or directed "upstream" into the prograde flow of blood did not seem to be a particularly ominous sign (Fig. 3–3B). Also, cases in which there appeared to be little intimal damage were later found to worsen into pseudoaneurysms. The long held view that these types of injuries would soon lead to acute arterial occlusions was also proven to be false. To date, there have been no documented cases of these types of minimal injuries ever deteriorating in such a fashion. Of note, no heparin or any type of antiplatelet agent was ever used in these studies.

Small (<2-cm) pseudoaneurysms are much less common, and as a result, a much smaller number of these lesions have been followed. Older series had demonstrated their potential to thrombose, embolize, become infected, and even rupture (Linde-nauer, Thompson, and Kraft, 1969; Bole, Munda, and Purdy, 1976). More current studies have also shown them to be more likely to worsen over time if watched expec-tantly than smooth narrowings or intimal flaps (Dennis and colleagues, 1990). Approximately 40% will eventually require surgical repair, and the remaining 60% will either remain stable or improve (Fig. 3–4B). Even those pseudoaneurysms diagnosed on a delayed diagnosis basis carry an amputa-tion rate reported to be zero (Feliciano and colleagues, 1987; Richardson, Vitale, and Flint, 1987). This indicates a more flexible approach is possible than mandatory repair.

Small AV fistulas are the rarest of the minimal injuries and similarly may or may not resolve over time. Smaller AV fistulas tend to close spontaneously, and larger ones will more often remain patent and become symp-tomatic (Shumacker and Waysson, 1950; Fryk-berg and colleagues, 1991). Due to the small numbers involved, the exact chance of resolution is difficult to determine. Initial observation of small fistulas has proven to be benign and late repair can also be undertaken with no increase in morbidity.

Over the past decade, no center has been able to demonstrate any conclusive data con-trary to these studies. Anecdotal reports have described cases of delayed presentations of arterial injuries (Perry, 1993; Tufaro, 1994). These reports generally lack detailed accounts of the initial presentation, initial management, overall incidence, and consistent follow-up by an experienced surgeon. Despite this lack of any substantial conflicting evidence, many surgeons expressed concern that over the long-term follow-up of these patients, some of these minimal injuries would eventually lead to vascular-related problems. This argument was put to rest with a 5- to 10-year study showing no negative long-term sequelae (Dennis and colleagues, 1998). Two groups of patients were studied. The first group of 39 patients had doc-umented minimal injuries on arteriograms between the years 1986 and 1989. Twenty-three of these patients (58%) were re-evaluated by history, physical examination, and ultrasound at a mean follow-up interval of 9.1 years (range, 8.6 to 11.1 years). All were

asymptomatic, all had normal physical exam-ination results, and only one had a residual mild narrowing by ultrasound. A second much larger group of 287 patients with penetrating proximity injuries who were seen between the years 1989 and 1991 and not evaluated by arteriography was also con-sidered. Four had required delayed surgery, all within the first week of the injury. Seventy-eight patients representing 90 injuries (29%) could be contacted. All patients within this group reported no long-term complications from any missed injury that later developed into a significant vascular problem. No patient at this institution (including those outside this study) has been found to have any deteriora-tion after 3 months following the initial trauma if they are compliant with follow-up. Based on these long-term data, it appears that nonoperative management can now be con-sidered the standard of care of these minimal injuries when identified by arteriography or ultrasound. Follow-up of these patients is extremely important both within the initial hospitalization and for up to 3 months after the injury. This component of the man-agement may limit the application of this approach in small nondesignated trauma centers with limited personnel and resources.

APPLICATION TO PENETRATING PROXIMITY EXTREMITY TRAUMA

The rationale behind obtaining arteri-ograms in all penetrating trauma to the extremities in which the penetrating agent or missile trajectory was determined to be in proximity to major arteries was the 10% to 20% chance of a clinically occult injury that would otherwise escape detection by physical examination. The new emerging data that documented these minimal injuries had a benign clinical course led to the next step of no longer obtaining arteriograms, because their detection would not alter any manage-ment decisions. A summary of 15 studies using this approach documents the overall missed injury rate to be 1.4% (Table 3–3). This rate is not significantly different than the 0.3% to

TABLE 3–3
PROFILE OF ASYMPTOMATIC PENETRATING INJURIES IN PROXIMITY TO EXTREMITY ARTERIES*

Author	No. of Proximity Wounds	No. of Occult Vascular Injuries (%)	No. of Occult Vascular Injuries Requiring Surgery (%)[†]
Dennis and colleagues, 1990[‡]	254	25 (10)	2 (0.8)
Francis and colleagues, 1991[‡]	160	17 (11)	7 (4.4)
Gahtan, 1994	394	37 (9.4)	7 (1.8)
Gomez and colleagues, 1986	72	17 (24)	1 (1.4)
Hartling and colleagues, 1987	36	5 (14)	0
Itani and colleagues, 1992	1712	216 (14)	28 (1.6)
Kauffman, 1992[‡]	92	22 (24)	0
Lipchik, 1987	59	3 (5)	1 (1.7)
McCorkell and colleagues, 1985	57	7 (12)	0
McDonald, Goodman, and Weinstock, 1975	85	5 (6)	0
Rose and Moore, 1988	97	Not Given	0
Smyth, 1991	65	2 (3)	1 (1.5)
Tohmeh, 1990	58	1 (1.7)	0
Trooskin, 1993[‡]	153	7 (4.6)	1 (1.3)
Weaver and colleagues, 1990[‡]	157	17 (11)	1 (0.6)
Total	3451	381 (11)	50 (1.4)

*Including only published cases in the extremity proper, excluding shotgun and thoracic outlet injuries.
[†]Percentage of all proximity wounds, excluding negative explorations.
[‡]Prospective study.
From Dennis JW, Frykberg ER, Veldenz HC, et al: Validation of nonoperative management of occult vascular injuries and accuracy of physical examination alone in penetrating extremity trauma: 5-10 year follow-up. J Trauma 1998;44:243-253.

6% missed injury rate reported for arteriography (Sclafani and colleagues, 1986; Feliciano, 1987). In addition, arteriography carries the small but real risk of contrast allergy and local complication such as hemorrhage, pseudoaneurysms, and thrombosis. Depending on the location and extent of the examination, the cost of arteriography will approach $2000 to $3000 per patient. The time involved in obtaining any imaging study may also delay the definitive treatment of other serious associated injuries.

Some trauma centers, however, have been reluctant to base treatment on physical examination results alone and have advocated duplex ultrasound or Doppler pressure measurements as alternatives (Bynoe, 1991; Johansen and colleagues, 1991; Knudson and colleagues, 1993). Though accurate, these tests require time, equipment, and skilled personnel. In addition, no study has ever demonstrated them to be significantly more accurate than physical examination alone. Again, emphasis must be placed on the importance

of close observation of these patients to identify the small group that will eventually deteriorate and require surgery. This should be done for the first 24 hours after the injury and for the first 3 months after discharge. Careful instructions must be given to patients concerning the possible development of significant vascular symptoms and the need to return immediately to the hospital should they develop at home. The current management algorithm for penetrating extremity injuries at the University of Florida, Jacksonville, is shown in Figure 3–5 (Dennis and colleagues, 1998).

APPLICATION TO PENETRATING NECK INJURIES

Early military and civilian experience first led surgeons to adopt the practice of mandatory neck exploration for any penetrating injury deep to the platysma (Hughes,

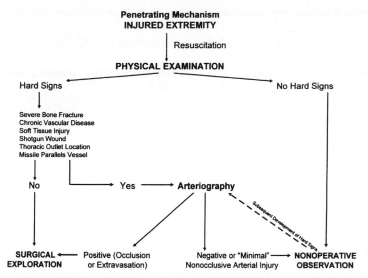

Penetrating Mechanism
INJURED EXTREMITY

Resuscitation

PHYSICAL EXAMINATION

Hard Signs   No Hard Signs

Severe Bone Fracture
Chronic Vascular Disease
Soft Tissue Injury
Shotgun Wound
Thoracic Outlet Location
Missile Parallels Vessel

No   Yes ——→ Arteriography

Subsequent Development of Hard Signs

SURGICAL ←— Positive (Occlusion   Negative or "Minimal" ——→ NONOPERATIVE
EXPLORATION   or Extravasation)   Nonocclusive Arterial Injury   OBSERVATION

■ FIGURE 3–5
Algorithm for evaluation and management of penetrating extremity trauma used at University of Florida, Jacksonville. (From Dennis JW, Frykberg ER, Veldenz HC, et al: Validation of nonoperative management of occult vascular injuries and accuracy of physical examination alone in penetrating extremity trauma: 5-10 year follow-up. J Trauma 1998;44:243-253.) ■

1954; Fogelman, 1956). Penetrating neck injuries were later divided and classified in the 1960s according to anatomic zones, and management was based on the zone in which the injury occurred (Monson, Saletta, and Freeark, 1969). Patients with penetrating injuries to zones 1 and 3 were recommended to undergo arteriography because of their difficult exposure, and patients with zone 2 injuries would continue to be explored, regardless of the physical findings.

Similar to the history of managing penetrating extremity trauma, the high number of negative explorations led surgeons to consider arteriography as an alternative. An extended review by Merion in 1981 analyzed 27 articles in the literature concerning this topic and found no significant difference in the morbidity or mortality rates between the two treatment groups (Merion, 1981). These results subsequently led most trauma centers to replace routine exploration with arteriography (Massac, 1983; Hiatt, Busuttil, and Wilson, 1984; Carducci, 1986). As experience grew, it was soon noted that similar to extremity arteriography, cervical arteriography began to identify minimal injuries in the carotid and vertebral arteries. Initially, surgical dogma stated that any abnormality seen on arteriogram required surgical repair. In the late 1980s and early 1990s, however, having observed the benign natural history of these minimal injuries in the extremities, some

centers began challenging the need to obtain any imaging study (Rivers, 1988; Menawat and colleagues, 1992). Careful analysis revealed that minimal injuries of the cervical arteries occurred in approximately 5% of the patients in this situation and could be safely observed. This was particularly helpful in zone 3 and vertebral arteries, because of their difficult surgical access. Also noted were other abnormalities such as asymptomatic vertebral artery occlusions, which did not need to be treated either. Mean follow-up time was 6 months for the entire study group.

These retrospective studies formed the basis on which prospective studies could be performed (Atteberry and colleagues, 1994; Biffl and colleagues, 1997; Sekharan and colleagues, 2000). The rationale was similar to that in the extremities: If minimal injuries do not have to be treated, then arteriography is not needed to identify them. It then follows that physical examination alone is adequate to determine whether a patient needs surgical repair after penetrating trauma to zone 2, which is amenable to it. Prospective studies appear to support this hypothesis (Table 3–4). The combined false-negative or missed injury rate using this approach is 0.6%, which is equal to or better than that of arteriography or ultrasound without the added time and cost (Table 3–5). Some reluctance still appears to linger by surgeons to accept this management approach to zone 2 neck injuries. Many

TABLE 3–4

PENETRATING NECK TRAUMA: MANAGEMENT BY MECHANISM AND LOCATION OF INJURY

		Observed				Explored		
		−	+	Missed Injury (%)	−	+	Negative Exploration (%)	Significant Injury (%)
Zone 1	GSW	6	0	0	0	8	0	57
	SW	23	0	0	1	3	25	11
Zone 2	GSW	19	0	0	3	20	13	55
	SW	109	1	0.9	12	44	21	27
Zone 3	GSW	12	0	0	1	5	17	18
	SW	37	0	0	0	8	0	29
Total		206	1	0.5	17	88	16	29

GSW, gunshot wound; SW, stab wound.
From Biffl WL, Moore EE, Rehse DH, et al: Selective management of penetrating neck trauma based on cervical level of injury. Am J Surg 1997;174:678-682.

trauma centers still obtain arteriograms or ultrasounds in these patients (Demetriades, 1995; Ginzburg, 1996). This is probably because of a persistent yet unfounded concern over causing a stroke by missing a significant injury, a complication considered more serious than a missed injury of the extremity. Published long-term follow-up data are somewhat lacking at this time also.

APPLICATION TO HIGH-RISK ORTHOPEDIC INJURIES

Generally, much less evidence is known concerning minimal arterial injuries and blunt trauma. Although the overall risk of arterial injury with bone fractures is between 0.3% and 6.4% (depending on the definition),

TABLE 3–5

STUDIES RECOMMENDING PHYSICAL EXAMINATION ALONE IN THE MANAGEMENT OF PENETRATING ZONE 2 NECK INJURIES

	No. of Penetrating Zone 2 Injuries			
Study	Total	With Hard Signs or Explored	With No Hard Signs	No. of Missed Injuries (%)
Biffl and colleagues, 1997*	208	80	128	1 (0.9)
Beitsch, 1994	178	42	136	1 (0.7)
Jarvik, 1995	111	45	66	0
Demetriades, 1993*	335	66	269	2 (0.7)
Gerst, 1990	110	52	58	0
Byers, 1990	106	62	44	0
Rivers, 1988	23	1	22	0
Sekharan and colleagues, 2000*	145	31	114	1 (0.8)
Totals	1216	379	837	5 (0.6)

*Prospective study.
From Sekharan J, Dennis JW, Veldenz JC, et al: Continued experience with physical examination alone for evaluation and management of penetrating zone 2 neck injuries: Results of 145 cases. J Vasc Surg 2000;32:483-489.

several orthopedic injuries have been well documented to carry an increased risk up to 20% of the time (Lange and colleagues, 1985; Bassett, 1986; Cone, 1989). These include posterior knee dislocations, supracondylar humerus fractures, first rib fractures, and proximal tibia and distal femur fractures. The devastating consequences of a missed arterial injury in these cases (limb loss risk up to 60%) have led many surgeons to obtain arteriograms in all patients with these fractures or dislocations. This practice would identify minimal arterial injuries on approximately 15% to 30% of the arteriograms obtained in the patients with no clinical signs, a rate somewhat higher than that seen in penetrating proximity injuries (Dennis, 1993; Atteberry and colleagues, 1996). Furthermore, despite having a different etiology of these minimal injuries, the little information to date indicates these to have a similar benign natural history.

Particularly ominous has been arterial injuries associated with knee dislocations. This is due to results of early series in which the incidence of limb loss was over 50%, although more recently this risk has been reduced to less than 5% (Bishara and colleagues, 1986). The question whether minimal injuries found in the popliteal artery following knee dislocation could be watched was answered in two studies in 1992 and 1993 (Treiman and colleagues, 1992; Dennis, 1993). These are the two largest studies reported, and when their data are combined, 16 minimal injuries (all intimal irregularities and smooth narrowings) were observed nonoperatively without a single adverse outcome. Strict follow-up immediately after any orthopedic manipulation and for several weeks after an injury is essential for this type of management to be successful.

The use of physical examination alone to determine whether immediate significant vascular injury has occurred with these high-risk types of orthopedic injuries has been advocated (Treiman and colleagues, 1992; Atteberry and colleagues, 1996). The presence of hard signs of vascular injury mandates surgery or arteriography, depending on the exact type of clinical picture. Patients with a bruit or thrill, distal ischemia, active

hemorrhage, or absent pulses are generally treated with immediate exploration. Those with non-life-threatening bleeding or expanding hematomas should undergo arteriography, because up to 70% of these cases will not have significant arterial injury requiring repair. Often, single hand-injected arteriograms in the operating room before the orthopedic manipulation are the simplest and most expeditious means to evaluate the arterial status. Arteriograms are essential if there are multiple sites of potential arterial injury because of more than one orthopedic injury. If minimal injuries are detected, they may be safely observed with careful follow-up. Recent analysis has shown this approach to be both safe and accurate when evaluating patients with knee dislocations (Miranda, 2001).

SUMMARY

Information gathered to date indicates minimal injuries tend to follow a similar natural history regardless of the trauma etiology. Smooth narrowings are extremely benign and can be watched with the assurance that almost all will resolve spontaneously. Intimal irregularities or flaps will also generally heal, although it must be recognized that 10% to 15% will deteriorate and require definitive treatment. This change will almost always occur within the first 3 months after an injury, and patients should always be followed for this amount of time as a minimum. Those injuries that deteriorate may be repaired on a delayed basis with no proven adverse effect on morbidity or mortality. Careful instructions must be given to patients upon discharge, to help them recognize if their particular arterial injury is worsening. Small pseudoaneurysms (<2 cm) may also be safely watched but have a far greater tendency to progress to needing direct repair. This probably happens 40% to 50% of the time. In addition, small AV fistulas need not always be fixed immediately unless symptomatic. Evidence shows that clinical follow-up is adequate in most instances; however, duplex ultrasound can be an adjunct in some difficult or particularly worrisome injuries.

Knowing this natural history allows physicians treating trauma patients to use physical examination as the definitive basis on which to manage penetrating injuries to the extremities and neck, as well as knee dislocations from blunt trauma. The algorithm in Figure 3–4 may be used in these situations. The only difference in using this approach with neck injuries is that distal ischemia may be manifested by focal neurologic deficits such as a stroke or transient ischemic attack.

Once patients are identified as to having a deteriorating minimal injury, they can usually be repaired on an urgent, elective basis dependent on the presenting symptoms. Standard surgical techniques may be used in almost all cases. Depending on the experience and expertise of the treating surgeons, endovascular techniques are also proving to be very useful in these situations (Marin, Veith, and Panetta, 1994; Weiss and Chaikoff, 1999). The placement of a stent graft across these lesions on a planned basis either in the operating room or in the endovascular suite has become standard treatment in some trauma centers. Long-term studies will be needed to ensure the durability of endovascular repair in these situations and compare their outcome with proven surgical techniques.

REFERENCES

Penetrating extremity trauma and minimal arterial injuries

Dennis JW, Frykberg ER, Crump JM, et al: New perspectives on the management of penetrating trauma in proximity to major limb arteries. J Vasc Surg 1990;11:84-93.

Dennis JW, Frykberg ER, Veldenz HC, et al: Validation of nonoperative management of occult vascular injuries and accuracy of physical examination alone in penetrating extremity trauma: 5-10 year follow-up. J Trauma 1998;44:243-253.

Frykberg ER, Crump JM, Dennis JW, et al: Nonoperative observation of clinically occult arterial injuries: A prospective evaluation. Surgery 1991;109:85-96.

Frykberg ER, Crump JM, Vines FS, et al: A reassessment of the role of arteriography in penetrating extremity trauma: A prospective study. J Trauma 1989;29:1041-1052.

Weiss VJ, Chaikof EL: Endovascular treatment of arterial injuries. Surg Clin North Am 1999;79:653-665.

Penetrating neck injuries and minimal arterial injuries

Biffl WL, Moore EE, Rehse DH, et al: Selective management of penetrating neck trauma based on cervical level of injury. Am J Surg 1997;174:678-682.

Menawat SS, Dennis JW, Laneve LM, et al: Are arteriograms necessary in penetrating zone II neck injuries? J Vasc Surg 1992;16:397-401.

Sekharan J, Dennis JW, Veldenz JC, et al: Continued experience with physical examination alone for evaluation and management of penetrating zone 2 neck injuries: Results of 145 cases. J Vasc Surg 2000;32:483-489.

Orthopedic injuries and minimal arterial injuries

Atteberry LR, Dennis JW, Russo-Alesi F, et al: Changing patterns of arterial injuries associated with fractures and dislocations. J Am Coll Surg 1996;183:377-383.

Bishara RA, Pasch AR, Lim LT, et al: Improved results in the treatment of civilian vascular injuries associated with fractures and dislocations. J Vasc Surg 1986;3:707-711.

Initial Care, Operative Care and Postoperative Care

DAVID B. HOYT
RAUL COIMBRA

Mechanical Ventilation

Antibiotics

Assessment and Determination of Take Back

    Bleeding

    Vascular patency

    Abdominal compartment syndrome

    Extremity compartment syndrome following prolonged ischemia

  ● SUMMARY

INTRODUCTION

The prehospital and the initial in-hospital management of trauma patients with vascular injuries remain a challenge. Specific maneuvers or techniques can be used in the prehospital setting to control external hemorrhage, but rapid transport to a trauma center is of utmost importance.

Vascular injuries following blunt trauma are considered a marker of severe trauma and as such should be treated in the context of multisystem trauma. Penetrating mechanisms cause vascular injuries more often than blunt trauma, and depending on the injury location, patients may present with external hemorrhage, internal hemorrhage, ischemia, or more rarely, a pulsating hematoma or a traumatic arterio-venous fistula.

GENERAL GUIDELINES: INITIAL CARE

The initial evaluation and management of patients with vascular injuries follow the guidelines established by the advanced trauma life support (ATLS) course of the American College of Surgeons-Committee on Trauma (ACS-COT).

The history should include details about the mechanism of injury (e.g., blunt vs. penetrating, position of the patient at the time of injury, position of the extremity observed by prehospital providers, blood loss at the scene, and previous injuries).

Primary Survey

The assessment of airway is the first priority even with evidence of obvious hemorrhage. Penetrating wounds of the face, neck, and chest may be accompanied by airway obstruction from bleeding or hematomas. The airway should be controlled as soon as possible in this circumstance and may require direct transport to the operating room for definitive control with access to complete instrumentation, excellent light, and anesthesia.

Many penetrating vascular wounds may present with entrance wounds at the lower neck or upper abdomen. The wound trajectory may be such that the chest is involved. There may be a pneumothorax, hemathorax, or tension pneumothorax, which will present as difficulty with breathing and will require appropriate diagnosis and decompression with a chest tube. This may often be difficult to distinguish from airway obstruction or may present with airway obstruction in the same patient. Systematic evaluation and treatment is the best course.

The occasional patient will present with difficulty breathing caused by hypovolemic shock. Control of the airway before assessment and treatment of the circulation remains the priority, even in this circumstance.

After assessment of the airway and breathing and definitive airway control, the hemodynamic status is assessed. Initially, palpation of pulse gives a rapid assessment. The presence of a radial pulse correlates with a blood pressure of at least 90 mm Hg. The absence of radial pulse with the pressure of a carotid pulse suggests a blood pressure of 60 mm Hg. Overall hemodynamic assessment should include direct blood pressure measurement, but caution should be exercised in the patient with a "stable blood pressure." Systolic blood pressure can be maintained in the normal range until almost 30% of circulating blood volume is lost (class I and II hemorrhage). Reliance on blood pressure alone can overlook a patient with significant hypovolemia. As such, measurement of the base deficit will also give an initial estimate of the total volume of hemorrhage and guide subsequent volume resuscitation and assessment of response to resuscitation (Table 4–1).

Recent changes in the ATLS protocols have suggested that bleeding control is a priority when evaluating the circulation, before fluid resuscitation. This is important in patients with vascular injuries, because they may present with external hemorrhage, for which external compression should suffice to control bleeding. They may also present with intracavitary hemorrhage in the chest or abdomen, requiring an operation to control active hemorrhage, as part of the resuscitation phase of care. Always keeping control of bleeding as an early priority will shift priorities to early operation. This is best for vascular injuries.

Although the ideal fluid therapy (type of solution, volume given, and timing of infusion) for the bleeding patient still remains a matter of controversy, it seems reasonable to avoid over-resuscitation, particularly in the subgroup of patients in whom the index of suspicion for the presence of a major vascular injury is high.

The two major goals in the management of traumatic shock during initial assessment and resuscitation are to arrest hemorrhage and to restore blood volume to provide adequate tissue oxygen delivery. Delayed resuscitation has been proposed to avoid rapid increases in blood pressure, clot dislodgement, and consequently, increased hemorrhage. Avoidance of over-resuscitation before surgical control is obtained is certainly prudent. However, whether all trauma victims would benefit from delayed fluid resuscitation is not clear.

Rapid cannulation of large veins is essential for adequate fluid therapy. Care should be taken when cannulating upper or lower extremity veins in patients with proximal penetrating injuries. To achieve adequate fluid resuscitation, one should use large-bore tubing. Warmed fluids should be infused to prevent or minimize heat loss and subsequent hypothermia. Rapid infusion systems (such as the level I) have the ability to infuse large volumes of warmed solutions per minute. Most practitioners agree that the initial resuscitation should be with crystalloids (Ringer's lactate or normal saline); however, a small but very important subset of patients will also require blood transfusion. This will be true if the estimated blood loss is greater than 30% of the total circulating blood volume. Availability of type-specific or O-negative blood is an essential component of the resuscitation of the severely injured patient.

Resuscitative or emergency department (ED) thoracotomy can be used as an adjunct to resuscitation in the severely injured patient. However, not all patients are candidates for

TABLE 4–1
QUANTIFICATION OF BLOOD LOSS (ATLS, 1993)

	Class I	Class II	Class III	Class IV
Blood loss (mL)	≤750	750-1500	1500-2000	>2000
Blood loss (%)	≤15	15-30	30-40	>40
Heart rate	<100	>100	>120	>140
Respiratory rate	14-20	20-30	30-40	>35
Urinary output	>30	20-30	5-15	Absent
Level of consciousness	Anxious	Agitated	Confused	Confused/lethargic
Blood pressure	Normal	Normal	Decreased	Decreased

this procedure. In general, survival rates are higher for patients presenting with vital signs than for patients presenting only with signs of life. Victims of penetrating trauma benefit more than patients with blunt trauma.

In general, ED thoracotomy is indicated in patients with penetrating wounds to the chest who develop sudden cardiac arrest or loss of vital signs during transport, persistent hypotension with signs of cardiac tamponade, or intrathoracic hemorrhage. Patients with penetrating injuries to the abdomen and refractory hypotension may benefit from ED thoracotomy and aortic cross clamping before exploratory laparotomy is performed; however, this is often a matter of individual preference. Blunt trauma victims with cardiopulmonary resuscitation (CPR) in progress and no cardiac electrical activity upon arrival are not candidates for this procedure.

A rapid neurologic assessment should be done. A depressed level of consciousness may be due to shock, associated blunt head injury, drugs or alcohol, or occasionally direct injury to the carotid artery. Abnormal or asymmetrical motor function should raise suspicion of an intracranial mass lesion and consideration of evaluation with a computed tomographic (CT) scan should be an early priority.

Particularly in victims of penetrating trauma, it is also important to examine the whole body surface area, undressing the patient completely because small gunshot or stab wounds may be hidden between the buttocks, gluteal folds, in the back, in the axilla, or in the folds of the neck. With complete exposure, the ongoing concern for hypothermia should be initiated and the patient adequately covered with warm blankets while keeping the ambient temperature warm as well.

Secondary Survey

The secondary survey should include a detailed examination of the vascular system in the extremities. The documentation of distal pulses is important and will guide further investigations and the use of specific diagnostic tools. The presence of a distal pulse,

TABLE 4–2
HARD AND SOFT SIGNS OF ARTERIAL INJURY

Hard Signs	Soft Signs
Signs of ischemia	Diminished distal pulses
Pallor	Penetrating injury in the proximity of major artery
Pain	Fracture in the proximity of major artery
Pulselessness	History of external bleeding at the scene
Paresthesia	Peripheral neurologic deficit
Paralysis	
Poikilothermia	
Pulsatile bleeding	
Palpable thrill/audible bruit	
Expanding hematoma	

however, does not rule out a proximal arterial injury. On the other hand, bilateral absence of distal pulses in a patient in shock with poor tissue perfusion does not indicate an arterial injury.

Clinical signs of arterial injury are divided into "hard" and "soft" (Table 4–2). According to the physical examination findings, patients can be stratified according to the risk of having an arterial injury. Patients with hard signs have high-risk injuries, those with soft signs have intermediate-risk injuries, and those with no soft or hard signs have low-risk injuries. Accuracy of this classification system for the lower extremities is improved when the ankle-brachial index (ABI) is added.

A thorough and ongoing neurologic evaluation of the victim with penetrating extremity trauma is mandatory. Changes in the neurologic examination results may indicate aggravation of ischemia or a developing compartment syndrome, and changes in priorities and management might be necessary in these circumstances.

The diagnosis of a vascular injury in the multi-injured patient depends on the mechanism, clinical signs at presentation, and the type of arterial injury (Fig. 4–1).

ETIOLOGY, INCIDENCE AND CLINICAL PATHOLOGY

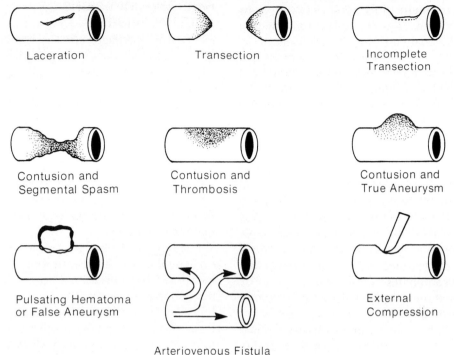

■ FIGURE 4–1
Common types of arterial injury. (From Rich NM, Spencer FC: Vascular Trauma. Philadelphia, WB Saunders, 1979.) ■

NECK VASCULAR INJURIES

Penetrating neck injuries generally present with external bleeding, a significant hematoma, or airway obstruction. Surgical access is limited and determined by surface landmarks that correlate with surgical accessibility. Monson's zones define the limits of surgical exposure. Zone III injuries (above the angle of the mandible) may not be surgically accessible and angiography can help define this possibility with a suspicious wound or hematoma. Zone II wounds (between the angle of the mandible and the cricoid cartilage) are directly accessible through the standard sternocleidomastoid approach. Zone II wounds (below the cricoid cartilage or adjacent to the thoracic inlet) may require thoracic exposure, and hemodynamically stable patients should undergo angiography to allow surgical planning.

Blunt carotid or vertebral injuries may be suspected because of neurologic abnormalities detected, but not confirmed, on CT scan. Generally a mechanism of extension and external rotation can be elicited. Any suspicion or evidence of blunt neck trauma should raise the possibility of carotid injury and duplex scanning will screen for this possibility.

THORACIC VASCULAR INJURIES

Penetrating thoracic vascular injuries usually present with hemothorax or ischemia. Chest tube output will determine whether a thoracotomy is necessary for bleeding control and definitive repair of the arterial injury. If upper extremity or cerebral ischemia is the predominant clinical sign, a preoperative angiogram will help operative planning in the hemodynamically stable patient. Recent experience with thoracic wounds that traverse the chest has used fine-cut CT scans to define superficial wounds in hemodynamically stable patients. Further experience is needed to better define the indications.

The aorta or its thoracic branches may be injured after blunt thoracic injuries. Most patients who bleed from these injuries die at the scene or during transport. The majority of patients with blunt thoracic aortic injury will present to the ED hemodynamically stable and will have a widened mediastinum on initial chest x-ray films. The predominant sign accompanying injuries to the thoracic aortic main branches is upper extremity or cerebral ischemia. The diagnosis is confirmed by angiography or high-quality helical CT scans. Patients with isolated blunt injuries to the thoracic aorta should undergo operative repair. However, many of these patients have associated closed head injuries, and the management of the aortic tear (operative vs. nonoperative) will depend on the severity of the head injury.

ABDOMINAL VASCULAR INJURIES

Blunt abdominal vascular injuries are rare. The astute physician should suspect a major intra-abdominal injury secondary to penetrating trauma when the patient does not respond to initial fluid resuscitation. These patients should be quickly transported to the operating room, and the diagnosis is usually made intraoperatively. Line placement in the lower extremity should be avoided in patients with a high index of suspicion for major intra-abdominal vascular, particularly inferior vena caval injuries.

EXTREMITY INJURIES

In general, patients presenting with significant external hemorrhage or limb ischemia caused by an isolated penetrating injury to the extremity do not pose any difficulty in the diagnosis and management. These patients require no additional diagnostic tests and should be promptly transported to the operating room. Patients with multiple penetrating injuries to the extremity presenting with ischemia also should be promptly operated on; however, a preoperative angiogram may be useful in determining the exact location of the most proximal injury, thus helping with operative planning.

Angiography is the "gold standard" test to evaluate the arterial tree. In some instances, hemodynamic instability, associated life-threatening injuries, or the need to perform other surgical procedures, moving the patient to the angiography suite is not feasible. In cases of prolonged ischemia or in which the decision to perform "damage-control" surgery on the injured extremity by placement of an intravascular shunt is necessary, an intraoperative on-table angiogram can be obtained.

Trauma surgeons should be familiar with this procedure, because it may save enormous amounts of time and may expedite reperfusion of an ischemic limb. For the lower extremity, an 18-gauge needle is inserted into the femoral artery, below the inguinal ligament. An x-ray plate is placed under the thigh and 20 mL of contrast is injected under pressure. Compression of the femoral artery above the needle site will limit contrast dilution, and the dye should be injected as rapidly as possible. Flow through the Luer lock connector will prevent injecting too rapidly. The initial film will give the surgeon an idea when to expose the film to x-ray after the end of the injection to demonstrate the vessels in the area of interest. Subsequent films are obtained distally.

For the upper extremity, on-table angiograms are useful if one wants to evaluate the proximal axillary artery and the subclavian artery. This can be done by inserting an 18-gauge needle in the brachial artery and inflating the cuff of a blood pressure manometer over the forearm. An x-ray plate is positioned under the upper extremity and upper chest, and 20 mL of contrast is injected under pressure. Further films are obtained depending on the area of the arterial tree to be studied.

Blunt arterial injuries are usually caused by significant forces applied to the extremities, also leading to fractures or dislocations. The classic fracture or dislocation sites associated with arterial injuries are listed in Box 4–1. Alignment and immobilization of fractures is mandatory to decrease bleeding, avoid further injury to soft tissues, and eventually restore distal flow.

In general, vascular injuries are just one component of a multitude of injuries, and adherence to the priorities set forth by the ATLS will facilitate initial management and diagnosis. The management of life-threatening injuries takes precedence over limb-threatening injuries. In the presence of multiple injuries, the management of peripheral vascular injuries may be delayed, although trauma surgeons should keep in mind that duration of ischemia greater than 6 hours is, in general, associated with poor functional outcome and should be avoided.

COMPLEX ISSUES WITH CONCOMITANT INJURIES

Blunt Trauma

In patients with concomitant blunt thoracic or abdominal trauma and peripheral vascular injuries with ischemia, the initial priority is to stop the bleeding in the chest (chest tube placement and eventually thoracotomy) or abdomen (exploratory laparotomy). If the anticipated ischemia time is greater than 6 hours, consideration should be given to concomitant operations (exploratory laparotomy and/or thoracotomy and vascular exploration) by two separate surgical teams, as well as fasciotomy and use of temporary antra-arterial shunts.

For patients with peripheral vascular injuries and associated long bone fractures or dislocations, best care is provided by a combined approach, taking into account the duration of ischemia. Usually the vascular injury can be approached first and the decision to use an antra-arterial shunt and perform orthopedic fixation followed by definitive repair of the vascular injury versus primary

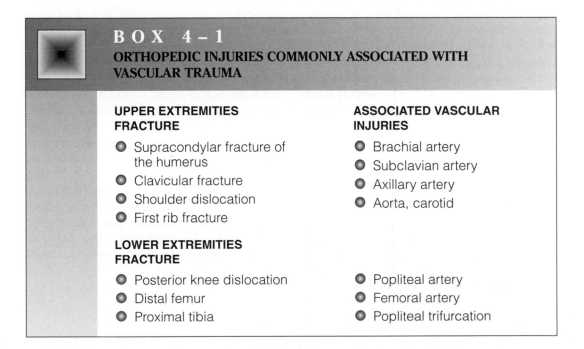

BOX 4 – 1

ORTHOPEDIC INJURIES COMMONLY ASSOCIATED WITH VASCULAR TRAUMA

UPPER EXTREMITIES FRACTURE	ASSOCIATED VASCULAR INJURIES
● Supracondylar fracture of the humerus	● Brachial artery
● Clavicular fracture	● Subclavian artery
● Shoulder dislocation	● Axillary artery
● First rib fracture	● Aorta, carotid
LOWER EXTREMITIES FRACTURE	
● Posterior knee dislocation	● Popliteal artery
● Distal femur	● Femoral artery
● Proximal tibia	● Popliteal trifurcation

repair of the vascular injury followed by orthopedic fixation is made intraoperatively based on objective assessment of the duration of ischemia and the degree of bony instability. Adequate communication between the surgeon and orthopedist is key to a successful management of these complex patients.

Penetrating Trauma

The decision-making process in patients with penetrating injuries in multiple body areas is far less complicated than in blunt trauma. The principles of management, however, remain the same.

In patients with penetrating thoracic and abdominal injuries, the priority is to treat thoracic conditions first (hemothorax or pneumothorax), because in the ABCs breathing (or *B*) comes before circulation (or *C*). As with blunt chest trauma, most patients with penetrating chest injuries will not require a thoracotomy and tube thoracentesis will suffice. Once pleural problems have been addressed, abdominal bleeding should then be addressed by means of an exploratory laparotomy.

In patients with penetrating neck and abdominal wounds, the initial priority is to obtain a patent airway. If there is active bleeding from the neck wound, a two-team approach should be considered in the hypotensive patient, and a concomitant neck and abdominal exploration should be performed. If that is not feasible, then applying gentle pressure to the neck wound, opening the abdomen, and packing to control major bleeding should be done before the formal neck exploration is performed, because the likelihood of one dying from exsanguination is higher with abdominal bleeding than cervical bleeding. The same principles (ABCs) apply to penetrating neck, thoracic, and abdominal injuries.

In patients with chest or abdominal injuries and extremity vascular injuries, the priority is to rule out intrathoracic hemorrhage, pneumothorax, and cardiac tamponade. Then, attention is paid to the abdomen. Most patients will require an exploratory laparotomy. Lower extremity vascular injuries are the last priority in this scenario. Depending on the necessity, an on-table angiogram to determine the location of the arterial injury, and eventually, intra-arterial shunt placement can be done as described previously. Patients with multiple penetrating injuries of the extremity and signs of ischemia should undergo an angiography to help with surgical planning, and this can be done in the operating room.

PERIOPERATIVE CARE

Initial Anesthesia and Intraoperative Monitoring

The multi-injured patient with a vascular injury usually presents with hypovolemia caused by hemorrhage. Two factors are of utmost importance when initially assessing such patients and while in the operating room: the evaluation of the circulating blood volume deficit and the prediction of additional losses.

Oxygenation and ventilation, maintenance of an adequate perfusion pressure, infusion of warm fluids, and serial monitoring of urinary output, temperature, hematocrit, blood gases, base deficit, and coagulation studies are the intraoperative priorities in the multi-injured patient. More sophisticated and invasive monitoring techniques may not be feasible during the resuscitative and operative phases of care but should be implemented during the critical care phase.

Ketamine or etomidate are appropriate for induction of anesthesia in hypotensive, hypovolemic patients. Fentanyl and nitrous oxide are also adequate for anesthesia and analgesia, but care should be taken when hypovolemia is profound. Volatile agents, benzodiazepines, and barbiturates should be avoided.

All patients receive antibiotics preoperatively. Antibiotics should be chosen to achieve broad coverage but limit toxic side effects, particularly when aggravated by associated shock. A second-generation cephalosporin is ideal.

Volume Therapy

One of the main goals of perioperative care is to achieve hemodynamic stability. After traumatic hemorrhage has been controlled, other factors may interfere with hemodynamic stability. Hemostasis is impaired by the development of hypothermia coagulopathy and acidosis.

Initially, maintenance of adequate intravascular volume is achieved by fluid resuscitation (with crystalloid and blood) during the operative phase and extended into the initial critical care phase. Although more sophisticated devices may be available for intraoperative monitoring of the cardiovascular system, large-bore intravenous (IV) lines, a central line (internal jugular or subclavian), and an arterial line will generally be adequate.

Following massive bleeding and shock, profound acidosis can be concerning because of the perceived risk of low pH level. Acidosis will resolve with control of bleeding and adequate volume resuscitation. Use of $NaHCO_3$ should be limited because rapid formation of increased CO_2 can cause precipitation of intracellular acidosis and make things worse. The overuse of bicarbonate can lead to diminished oxygen delivery by shifting the oxygen disassociation curve so that oxygen is more tightly bound. Acidosis should never be treated with HCO_3 unless the pH level is less than 7.1 to 7.2. The bicarbonate deficit should be calculated and only 50% should be replaced until it can be reassessed. Calculation of the HCO_3 deficit is according to the formula: base deficit × body weight × 0.2. The space of distribution of HCO_3 is considered to be 20% of the total body.

A great deal of confusion and controversy regarding the indications for urgent or emergent blood transfusion in the severely injured patient exists. Several factors should be considered before the decision to transfuse is made, including degree of hemorrhage, hemoglobin level, intravascular volume status, and chronic diseases. The goal of blood transfusion is to enhance oxygen delivery to the tissues.

Communication between the surgery team and the anesthesiologist is important to avoid over-transfusion and under-transfusion intra-operatively. Similarly, the use of too much crystalloid can occur particularly if one is not watching simple parameters. It can be easy to over-resuscitate with crystalloid if the patient initially has no urine output because of shock-induced acute tubular necrosis (ATN). Continuous surveillance of the correction of the base deficit should be a reliable guide to volume resuscitation in this circumstance, and pushing fluid until urine output returns will overload the patient.

Uncross-matched type O blood is immediately available for patients with blood loss greater than 30% to 40% of total circulating blood volume with hypotension. If the patient's blood type is known, transfusion of type-specific uncross-matched blood is appropriate. If time is not a cause for concern, type-specific cross-matched blood should be used. In an emergency situation, there is often not enough time to perform all compatibility testing.

Autotransfusion is an excellent alternative or adjunct to massive blood transfusion in the hypotensive trauma patient. It is primarily useful in patients with a large hemothorax. The blood accumulated in the reservoir connected to the chest tube can be transfused. Intraoperative blood salvage using cell-saver devices is effective in reducing transfusion of stored autologous blood, even in the presence of bacterial contamination, because the red blood cells are washed before transfusion. Most people will not use contaminated blood however. Complications of autotransfusion include coagulopathy resulting from excessive amounts of anticoagulants or infusion of activated products of coagulation and fibrinolysis leading to disseminated intravascular coagulation (DIC).

The use of heparin in the acute setting of vascular trauma is controversial. Because of a multitude of injuries and in view of massive fluid and blood resuscitation, heparin should primarily be used locally in vascular trauma, and systemic heparinization should be avoided until the patient is in the intensive care unit (ICU). After 24 hours when hypothermia and coagulopathy have been corrected, and if no brain or spinal cord injury has been identified, if needed, systemic heparin might be appropriate.

Platelets are used when the platelet count drops to less than 50,000 cells/mm³ associated with microvascular bleeding. Prophylactic platelet administration after massive transfusion is not indicated. Fresh frozen plasma (FFP) contains all coagulation factors and is used in the severely injured patient who has continuous bleeding after transfusion of approximately one blood volume or when an intraoperative coagulopathy is identified as measured by a partial thromboplastic time (PTT) of more than 1.5. FFP should not be used as a volume expander during the resuscitation phase and is not indicated for general coagulopathy prophylaxis after massive transfusion.

Cryoprecipitate contains fibrinogen, factor VIII, factor XIII, and von Willebrand's factor. In the acute setting, it is indicated only in severe fibrinogen deficiency, or when the serum fibrogen level is less than 100 mg%.

Hypothermia

Hypothermia in the severely injured massively resuscitated trauma patient is multifactorial and may occur at any phase of care. In patients experiencing hypoperfusion and shock, heat production is decreased. Rapid infusion of large amounts of unwarmed crystalloid and stored blood also contributes to hypothermia.

Normal production is 315 kJ per day and normal loss is about the same. Body temperature drops by 1°C for each additional 315 kJ lost. Each liter of crystalloid at 21°C can cause 67.2 kJ of heat loss and each unit of 4°C blood can cause 30°C heat loss. Even with modest resuscitation, this compounded heat loss can rapidly cause significant hypothermia.

Hypothermia affects coagulation by decreasing platelet function, altering enzymatic kinetics in the coagulation cascade, and increasing fibrinolysis. Oxygen consumption and cardiovascular oxygen demand are increased in mild hypothermia, and moderate to severe hypothermia can lead to arrhythmias, hypotension, and sudden cardiac arrest. Other effects of hypothermia include depression of the respiratory center, bronchospasm, decreased cerebral blood flow, altered level of consciousness, fluid shifts, prolonged drug metabolism, decreased intestinal motility, hyperglycemia, and increased affinity of hemoglobin for oxygen.

Rewarming can be passive or active. Passive external rewarming is indicated for mild hypothermia and is achieved by increasing room temperature and using blanket coverage to prevent further heat loss. Complications associated with passive rewarming may include metabolic acidosis and increased lactic acid production. Active external rewarming includes the use of heating or convective air blankets and radiant warmers. Active core rewarming is indicated for hypothermic patients with severe vasoconstriction. Methods include warmed IV fluids, body-cavity (pleural, peritoneal) lavage with warm fluids, airway rewarming, and extracorporeal circulatory rewarming (cardiopulmonary bypass). The latter is the most effective rewarming method. Prevention by avoiding transfusion of unwarmed crystalloid and refrigerated blood is important, to avoid the problem during the first several hours after injury.

Damage Control

The surgical management of the severely injured massively bleeding trauma patient has changed dramatically in the last decade. The concept of staged laparotomy or damage-control operation has emerged from the observation that prolonged operations to repair all injuries will lead to physiologic exhaustion, associated with hypothermia, acidosis, coagulopathy, and death.

By definition, it is a phased approach to the critically injured patient. The indications include patients with hypothermia (temperature <35°C), nonmechanical bleeding, pH level less than 7.15, and significant retroperitoneal and visceral swelling due to massive fluid resuscitation. Eligible patients are those with major solid organ injury, pelvic fractures, major abdominal vascular injury, bleeding injuries in more than one body area, or multiple competing injuries. The goal of the initial operation is to control bleeding and gross contamination of the peritoneal cavity with intestinal contents. This can be achieved by shunting or ligating injured vessels, packing solid organs (particularly the liver), and closing or resecting bowel injuries en bloc, using staplers.

The definitive reconstruction is left to a second operation while performing a temporary closure of the abdomen. The second phase or stage occurs in the critical care unit, where the patient will continue to be resuscitated and rewarmed and will receive coagulation factors to correct coagulopathy. The goal of this phase is to restore some of the patient's physiologic reserve by correcting the base deficit, restoring intravascular volume, and achieving adequate oxygenation. Once stable (i.e., mechanical bleeding stopped, the base deficit corrected, and the body temperature near normal), the patient is taken back to the operating room for definitive repair of all injuries. This is an approach described for abdominal trauma but has been extended to chest and pelvic and/or extremity injuries associated with other competing injuries.

If the abdomen is closed during the first or second operation, continuous surveillance is necessary to identify an early complication associated with this approach abdominal hypertension, and its most severe form, the abdominal compartment syndrome.

POSTOPERATIVE PRIORITIES

Hemodynamic Monitoring and Transfusion in the Postoperative Phase

Postoperative placement of a Swan-Ganz catheter to monitor cardiac output and pulmonary capillary pressure in persistently unstable patients or in patients with preexisting illnesses in the ICU is appropriate. Nonetheless, it has been ours and others experience that analysis of base-deficit trends is as helpful as more sophisticated methods to monitor effectiveness of resuscitation. If used, physiologic parameters should not replace the use of metabolic endpoints such as base deficit.

Postoperatively, the decision to transfuse is not as simple, because clear guidelines do not exist and the "10/30 rule" (10 g/dL of hemo-globin or 0.30 hematocrit) is no longer widely accepted. The young adult trauma patient without comorbid conditions and with a near-normal intravascular volume usually tolerates a hematocrit level as low as 0.20. Elderly patients with limited cardiopulmonary reserve may need blood transfusion to maintain a hematocrit level of more than 0.25, but no good data are available to define this endpoint.

Recently, signs and symptoms of anemia and oxygen delivery measurements have been used as transfusion triggers; however, in the immediate post-traumatic or postoperative period, most trauma patients will be sedated and intubated in the ICU, making it difficult to evaluate symptoms of anemia. Tachycardia and hypotension may reflect anemia but may also occur secondarily to inflammatory mediator release and the systemic inflammatory response and are, therefore, not relatable transfusion endpoints.

Measurements of oxygen delivery and consumption are probably more reliable in predicting transfusion requirements. It seems reasonable to transfuse blood to patients with a hemoglobin concentration of 7 g/dL or less, provided the intravascular volume is normal and there are no associated chronic illnesses. It is also common practice to transfuse blood to patients with hemoglobin concentrations between 7 and 10 g/dL who have coronary artery disease, are older than 60 years, and have congestive heart failure.

Recent National Institutes of Health (NIH) recommendations for perioperative blood transfusion state that no single criterion for transfusion such as a hemoglobin concentration less than 10 g/dL should be used and that clinical judgment cannot be replaced by any single measurement. Perioperative transfusion of homologous blood carries documented risk of infectious and immune changes. Recent availability of alternatives to autologous blood transfusion should be carefully evaluated.

Coagulation Monitoring

As in the operating room, functional evaluation of coagulation includes platelet number and function, activity of coagulation factors, and clot breakdown.

Procoagulant activity is evaluated by quantifying the prothrombin time (PT) and the activated partial thromboplastin time (APTT). In the operating room, the time required to perform these test may limit their usefulness, but postoperatively this should not be a problem. Platelet function is evaluated by the bleeding time and can be used at the bedside to indicate efficacy of coagulation therapy. Thromboelastography is a measure of whole blood coagulation, and it seems to correlate well with other tests of platelet function. It has been shown to be useful in the operating room to make the diagnosis of factor deficiency, DIC, platelet dysfunction, and others, although its use is not widespread.

In the ICU setting, serial monitoring of PT, PTT, fibrinogen, fibrin degradation products, and platelet count should be done in the severely injured patient who has received significant amounts of blood products intraoperatively or in patients in whom temporary hemostatic measures (e.g., packing) were used because of diffuse bleeding associated with hypothermia, acidosis, and intraoperative coagulopathy. Transfusion of clotting factors and platelets, treatment of underlying shock and hypothermia, and adequate oxygenation constitute the basis of therapy in patients with post-traumatic coagulopathy. This must be done by a constant effort, with both nurses and physicians collaborating until the goal is accomplished. Less than a full effort will often be met with failure.

Complications following Massive Blood Transfusion

Box 4–2 lists the most common complications after multiple blood transfusions. The incidence of these complications varies with the amount of blood units transfused. Metabolic abnormalities are common following transfusion. Hyperkalemia may be due to potassium being released from destroyed red blood cells. Acidosis may occur as a result of the accumulation of lactic and pyruvic acids in stored blood; however, metabolic alkalosis occurs more commonly, because of the conversion of citrate to bicarbonate in the liver.

Citrate intoxication may induce refractory hypotension, particularly following massive transfusion or continuous infusion at high rates. Acute lung injury (ALI) is rare but may be eventually seen in the postoperative period as a result of complement activation induced by the presence donor antibodies interacting with recipient granulocytes. Coagulopathy following massive transfusion is usually due to dilution of platelets and consumption of coagulation factors. Microvascular bleeding in the setting of massive transfusion and major blood loss occurs when platelet counts drop to less than 50,000 cells/mm^3, and fibrinogen level is less than 100 mg%. DIC may develop postoperatively, secondary to prolonged shock, acidosis, and hypoxia. Treatment of DIC should focus on the underlying cause and replacement of coagulation factors and platelets.

After massive transfusion of citrated blood, hypocalcemia may develop. Hypocalcemia may lead to cardiac dysfunction and hypotension; however, coagulopathy rarely occurs, unless serum calcium levels are less than 0.2 mg/dL. Mobilization of Ca^{2+} is usually adequate after infusion of large amounts of citrate. Calcium replacement should be based on measured levels and should not given prophylactically.

Patients with normal liver function should not receive empirical calcium supplementation. Iatrogenic hypercalcemia leads to arrhythmias and hypotension. The only patients who should receive supplemental calcium following massive transfusion are those with severe liver disease.

Mechanical Ventilation

The routine management of ventilation has changed significantly over the last decade. For the uncomplicated patient who undergoes surgery with no anticipated postoperative problems, weaning and extubation should follow a standard protocol relying on the rapid shallow breathing index as an indicator for extubation success.

A considerable number of severely injured patients will develop ALI and acute respira-

BOX 4 – 2
COMMON COMPLICATIONS AFTER BLOOD TRANSFUSION

TRANSFUSION TRANSMITTED DISEASES
- Hepatitis
- Human immunodeficiency virus
- Bacterial infections
- Viral infections

HYPOTHERMIA

COAGULATION DYSFUNCTION
- Factor dilution
- Disseminated intravascular coagulation
- Thrombocytopenia

ACID-BASE IMBALANCE

ELECTROLYTE IMBALANCE

HEMOLYTIC REACTIONS

ALLERGIC (NONHEMOLYTIC) REACTIONS

TRANSFUSION-RELATED ACUTE LUNG INJURY

CITRATE INTOXICATION

tory distress syndrome (ARDS). Early ALI/ARDS usually follows massive fluid resuscitation and its occurrence depends at least on the injury severity and hyper-inflammation in the post-traumatic period. Late ARDS is usually caused or accompanied by sepsis.

New mechanical ventilation strategies have recently been developed to provide adequate oxygenation and to decrease the risk of barotrauma and ventilator-induced lung injury. A protective strategy can be defined as low tidal volumes and the elimination of inspiratory plateau pressure while maintaining positive end-expiratory pressure (PEEP) above the lower inflection point of the pressure-volume compliance curve. This can be done with a volume ventilator or a pressure ventilator, and the recent use of pressure-control ventilation has gained popularity because of the relative ease in achieving this protective strategy.

The use of permissive hypercapnia often becomes a necessary by-product of this protective strategy and has become acceptable practice. Multiple studies have suggested this strategy is associated with lower mortality. Recently, several studies evaluated protective strategies and compared them to traditional strategies in the treatment of ARDS. Taken together, a lung protective strategy including lower tidal volumes, permissive hypercapnia, and the use of PEEP above the inferior inflection point while limiting inspiratory plateau pressure seems preferable and probably is associated with improved survival. Because an actual increase in oxygenation does not explain the difference in outcome, the reduction in sheer stress and inflammation accompanies a lung protective strategy could conceivably account for the observed effect. Those who follow an evidence-based strategy in caring for their patients should consider the routine use of a protective strategy. In general, most patients will do well if they are placed on initial tidal volume of 4 to 8 mL/kg, with plateau pressures not to exceed 35 mL H_2O.

Another technique used to improve oxygenation is called *prone ventilation*. The rationale for prone ventilation is to decrease the volume loss that accompanies patients lying on their back and thereby correct ventilation/perfusion mismatch. Most believe that recruitment of previously atelectatic areas induced by altered gravitational forces accounts for redistribution of blood flow and improvement in ventilation/perfusion and oxygenation. Although the evidence is still being assessed, this remains an important adjunct to patients who are difficult to ventilate. Several techniques that allow this to be done safely in most patients have emerged, including turning devices and protective padding.

Once a patient's ALI or ARDS is resolved, all patients must go through a weaning process; recent studies suggest that using a strategy of a once-daily trial of spontaneous breathing is associated with more rapid extubation than intermittent mechanical ventilation (IMV) or pressure support weaning. Most importantly, a consistent protocol, if used by physicians, nurses, and respiratory therapists together, seems to be critical to rapid successful weaning.

Antibiotics

The use of antibiotics should be guided by the general principles of the use of antibiotics in trauma patients. In general, these should be limited to a preoperative dose and 24 hours of postoperative antibiotics. No good data exist about whether prolonged antibiotics in patients in whom a vascular graft is placed reduces the incidence of postoperative infection; however, many practitioners will extend antibiotic coverage for several days. When there is gross contamination and a vascular graft needs to be placed (a colon injury and iliac artery injury), trying to cover the graft or route the graft through uncontaminated

tissue is best, thereby trying to avoid the problem altogether. The use of antibiotics in this situation will be user dependent, and even here, prolonged antibiotics have some attendant risks.

Antibiotics should be limited to second-generation cephalosporins and the use of multiple antibiotics and in particular amino glycosides should be avoided. Recently surveillance data have documented dramatic increases in the incidence in infections caused by *Staphylococcus aureus*, coagulase-negative *S. aureus*, *Streptococcus pneumoniae*, and *Enterococcus*. These organisms are associated with a rapid increase in resistance to many available antimicrobial agents, and prolonged use of antibiotics in the initial phase of treatment will select out resistant organisms and subsequently cause resistant infection, which may be ultimately untreatable.

Equally important to antibiotics is the provision of good graft and anastomosis coverage with local tissue. The use of adjacent muscle, omentum, or even the rotation of a nonadjacent muscle to get adequate coverage and sealing of a graft is essential for avoiding infection.

Once in the postinjury period, antibiotics should be targeted to a specific diagnosis, and if started for empirical therapy, they should be stopped as soon as cultures direct specific therapy or indicate that therapy is not needed. The length of treatment should be restricted to a defined period and the antibiotics stopped. Patients should be re-cultured if they develop new symptoms. Recent strategies to overcome antibiotic resistance include the use of rotation of various antibiotics for empirical therapy. This avoids the "antibiotic pressure" that allows resistant organisms to emerge. This may be a useful strategy, but it will require further study.

Assessment and Determination of Take Back

Ongoing assessment of vascular injuries involves the evaluation of bleeding, assessment of peripheral pulses, and the development of compartment syndromes of the abdomen and extremity.

BLEEDING

Following massive bleeding and coagulopathy, the assessment of bleeding involves critical judgment. On the one hand, until the coagulopathy has been reversed and the patient warmed, reoperation for bleeding may be unsuccessful. Similarly, in the presence of profound shock, primary hemostasis may have prevented small vessels from bleeding, thereby avoiding surgical hemostasis only to subsequently vasodilate and bleed in the ICU. This dilemma is solved only by careful bedside surveillance, concerted correction with coagulation factors, and continuous monitoring of output (e.g., chest tube and drains), abdominal distention, hematocrit, and coagulation indicators.

Once a reasonable attempt and success with rewarming and factors and platelet repletion has occurred, one has to decide whether the possibility of unchecked bleeding exists. If there is concern and the rate of drain output or hematocrit is falling, or if ongoing blood replacement does not seem better or continually gets worse, then returning to the operating room and re-exploration is the most appropriate course of action. Reapplication of damage control and temporary closure may also be appropriate after re-exploration.

VASCULAR PATENCY

After vascular repair or reconstruction, particularly if accompanied by shock, assessment of peripheral pulses may be difficult in the cold vasoconstricted patient. The initial presence of adequate perfusion can be reassuring and the presence of symmetrical pulses detectable by Doppler flow studies will provide initial evidence of patency. With warming, distal perfusion should progressively improve with brisk capillary refill and good venous filling. As resuscitation improves, pulses should return or suspicion should be raised that there is a problem. Use of segmental Doppler flow studies may help, but if there is any question about thrombosis, re-exploration or angiography should be immediately pursued.

ABDOMINAL COMPARTMENT SYNDROME

The abdominal compartment syndrome usually occurs in patients undergoing damage-control operations, intra-abdominal packing, massive fluid resuscitation, and visceral swelling. It is characterized by the presence of a distended tense abdomen, hypoxia, carbon dioxide retention, oliguria, hypotension, and high peak inspiratory pressures. The diagnosis is suspected on the basis of physical findings and is confirmed by measurement of intra-abdominal pressure indirectly as bladder pressure. Patients with a bladder pressure higher than 25 to 30 cm H_2O should return to the operating room for decompression and the abdomen should be left open.

EXTREMITY COMPARTMENT SYNDROME FOLLOWING PROLONGED ISCHEMIA

Extremity compartment syndrome is the result of trauma or reperfusion following severe prolonged ischemia, leading to increased swelling within a closed fascial compartment. It may also occur after massive fluid resuscitation, and continuous surveillance is required to avoid delays in diagnosis. This contained swelling results in an elevation in tissue pressure up to the point that blood flow is compromised and no longer provides enough oxygen to the cells. If left untreated or undiagnosed, it will result in myonecrosis and limb dysfunction or limb loss.

The most commonly involved areas are the anterior compartment in the lower leg and the volar compartment in the forearm. Because nerve tissue is more susceptible to ischemia than other tissues in the extremity (e.g., muscle, bone, and tendons), initial symptoms are paresthesia and pain. On palpation, the muscles are tense, and if the patient is awake and able to cooperate with physical examination, pain may be severe and eventually increased with passive movement of the extremity and contraction of the involved muscles. Pulses are usually palpable, even in advanced stages, and its presence does not rule out this diagnosis. The diagnosis is based on physical findings, although a high index of suspicion is necessary in the subgroup of patients with associated injuries in other body areas with competing pain or those sedated on mechanical ventilation. Once the diagnosis of compartment syndrome is suspected, compartment pressure should be measured. Fasciotomy is generally indicated when compartmental pressure is greater than 30 mm Hg.

SUMMARY

The management of vascular injuries can be one of the most challenging injuries in the severely injured patient. They will often be accompanied by airway obstruction or troubled breathing caused by penetrating adjacent wounds and will often present in hypovolemic shock. As such, decision making and prioritization, decision making in the operating room, and limiting operative surgery initially and staging it subsequently are complex decisions that when made correctly will save lives.

Because of the nature of these injuries, these patients are at the highest risk for postoperative/post-traumatic complications including aspiration, ARDS, renal failure, and coagulopathy. The trauma surgeon must be equipped to anticipate each of these problems and stay ahead of their subsequent deterioration by aggressive management.

REFERENCES

Battistella FD: Ventilation in the trauma and surgical patient. Crit Care Clin 1998;14:731-742.

Cosgriff N, Moore EE, Sauaia A, et al: Predicting life-threatening coagulopathy in the massively transfused trauma patient: Hypothermia and acidosis revisited. J Trauma 1997;42:857-862.

Davis JW, Parks SN, Kaups KL, et al: Admission base deficit predicts transfusion requirements and risk of complications. J Trauma 1996;41:769-774.

Gentilello LM, Pierson DJ: Trauma critical care. Am J Respir Crit Care Med 2001;163:604-607.

Ham AA, Coveler LA: Anesthetic considerations in damage control surgery. Surg Clin North Am 1997;77:909-919.

Hirshberg A, Mattox KL: Planned reoperation for severe trauma. Ann Surg 1995;222:3-8.

Ivatury RR, Diebel L, Porter JM, et al: Intraabdominal hypertension and the abdominal compartment syndrome. Surg Clin North Am 1997;77:783-800.

Jurkovich GJ, Greiser WB, Luterman A, et al: Hypothermia in trauma victims: An ominous predictor of survival. J Trauma 1987;27:1019-1024.

McFarland JG: Perioperative blood transfusions: Indications and options. Chest 1999;115:113-121.

Price JA, Rizk NW: Postoperative ventilatory management. Chest 1999;115:130-142.

Rotondo MF, Zonies DH: The damage control sequence and underlying logic. Surg Clin North Am 1997;77:761-777.

Shackford SR, Rich NH: Peripheral vascular injury. In Mattox KL, Feliciano DV, Moore EE (eds): Trauma. New York, McGraw Hill, 2000.

Diagnosis of Vascular Trauma

JOHN T. ANDERSON
F. WILLIAM BLAISDELL

- ● PATHOPHYSIOLOGY
  - Classification
  - Mechanism
  - Ischemia
  - Reperfusion Injury
  - Compartment Syndrome
- ● DIAGNOSIS
  - History
  - Physical Examination
  - Hard and Soft Signs of Vascular Injury
  - Ancillary Tests
- ● SUMMARY

Diagnosis and management of vascular injury has evolved dramatically over the past century. Early experience during combat demonstrated that prompt identification and repair of injured arteries resulted in improved functional outcome and decreased rates of amputation. Military experience supported routine operative exploration of gunshot wounds of the extremities because of a high incidence of vascular injury following high-velocity gunshot wounds in proximity to major vessels. Application of these principles to civilian trauma that typically involves low-velocity gunshot wounds, shotgun wounds, or stab wounds resulted in unacceptably high rates of negative explorations. Arteriography was promulgated as an alternative to mandatory exploration in patients without obvious vascular injury (i.e., no findings of pulselessness, arterial bleeding, or expanding and/or pulsatile hematoma). However, the yield of routine application of arteriography, especially for proximity alone, is also low. Further, not all arterial injuries identified by arteriography require surgical treatment. Recently, the goal has shifted toward the identification of those injuries that require operative intervention. To this end, algorithms varying from use of physical examination alone or in combination with duplex ultrasonography and/or selective arteriography have been promoted. The ideal diagnostic approach that will maximize accurate detection of vascular injury while minimizing morbidity and cost is still a matter of debate and active research.

PATHOPHYSIOLOGY

Classification

Although a wide variety of individual injury types may result from trauma (see Fig. 4–1), they essentially fall into three basic categories. The arterial wall can be completely transected, partially transected, or injured without transection. The patient with a completely transected artery will frequently have a history of initial active bleeding but present without overt hemorrhage. The media of the normal artery is capable of significant vasoconstriction that promotes clot formation and hemostasis. If the involved artery is a conduit vessel, distal pulses will be absent. In certain circumstances, hemostasis may not be achieved. Iliac and intercostal arteries may continue to bleed as tethering of the vessels by surrounding structures prevents retraction. Also, in older patients and those with diseased

vessels due to atherosclerosis, the artery may be incapable of adequate vasoconstriction and bleeding may continue unabated.

Partial transection of an artery limits vasoconstriction and the injured area tends to gape open. Active external bleeding will continue if not contained by surrounding tissues. A pseudoaneurysm will form if the tissues prevent active external bleeding. Acutely, this may be manifest as a pulsatile hematoma at the site of injury. Pulses may continue to be palpable distal to the site of injury. At times, the initial arterial injury is not apparent and an expanding pseudoaneurysm may later present with pain, a pulsatile mass, or symptoms of nerve impingement. Veins run in proximity to arteries and are frequently injured along with the artery. An arteriovenous (AV) fistula may result as blood decompresses from a partially transected artery into an adjacent injured vein. The AV fistula often is not apparent on initial presentation. Typically, the fistula enlarges over time and may ultimately result in high-output cardiac failure or chronic arterial or venous insufficiency.

Finally, the arterial wall can be injured without full-thickness transection. The intima of the artery is relatively inelastic in comparison to the media and the adventitia. Stretch or compression of an artery may disrupt the intima and tunica interna of the media while leaving the tunica externa of the media and the adventitia of the artery intact. Thrombosis of the artery may result from clot formation following exposure of the highly thrombogenic media or from a mechanical obstruction as a result of an intimal flap. Alternatively, small clot fragments may form and embolize distally. More severe degrees of stretch or compression may weaken or disrupt an additional layer of the arterial wall so that a pseudoaneurysm may form; extreme degrees of stretch will result in complete disruption. The use of the term *spasm* is mentioned only to be discarded. True arterial spasm, defined as constriction of the media in an otherwise uninjured vessel, is rarely present. Spasm identified on arteriography invariably represents an intimal injury or embolic clot from a more proximal arterial injury.

Mechanism

Penetrating mechanisms are responsible for most vascular injuries, even in rural centers that generally care for a predominately blunt trauma population. Civilian penetrating trauma is almost exclusively from low-velocity mechanisms such as handgun, knife, or shotgun injuries. Less common injuries can occur from penetration by sharp objects such as glass, metal, or wood splinters. These mechanisms typically cause partial or complete transection of the artery as a result of direct trauma. Occasionally, the vessel is indirectly injured as a result of an associated fracture. High-velocity (>2500 feet per second) gunshot wounds can directly and indirectly injure arteries. Even a trajectory in proximity to a major artery may cause arterial damage as the kinetic energy of the high-velocity projectile is transferred to the tissues. Extensive soft tissue and skeletal damage and collateral circulation disruption also occur.

Blunt trauma generally causes vascular injury as a result of stretch or compression. Usually, arterial thrombosis results. The arteries are particularly susceptible to injury at sites of arterial fixation and around joints, for example, the popliteal artery, which may be injured following knee dislocation (Fig. 5–1). At times, bony fragments can puncture the vessel directly, as with a supracondylar femur fracture (Fig. 5–2).

Associated injuries, many of which are life threatening and require immediate inter-

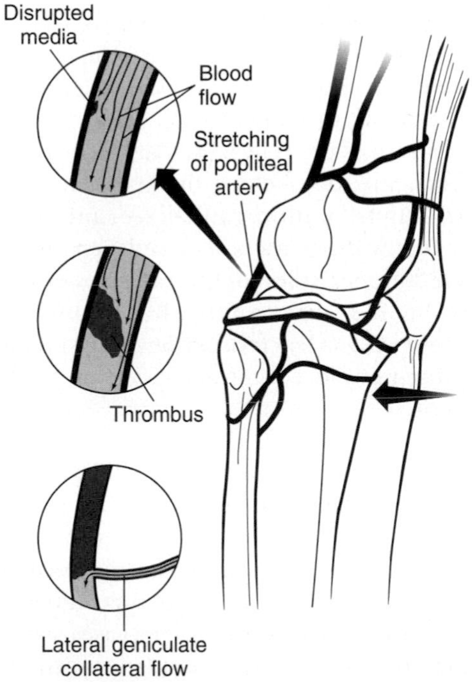

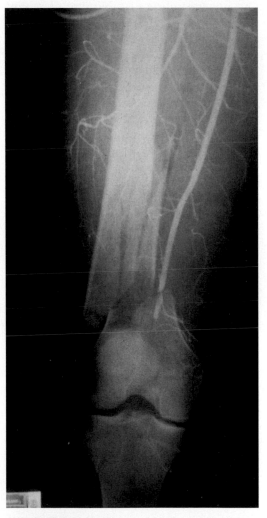

■ **FIGURE 5–1**
Mechanism of popliteal artery injury following posterior knee dislocation. (Redrawn from American College of Surgeons: ACS Surgery: Principles and Practice. New York: WebMD, 2003.) ■

■ **FIGURE 5–2**
Injury to the distal superficial femoral artery associated with a supracondylar femur fracture. ■

vention, are frequently present in combination with penetrating and blunt vascular injuries. Damage due to penetrating trauma is generally confined to the area of the trajectory of the penetrating object, although multiple injury sites are common. Blunt trauma results in a wider distribution of affected structures. Overall, mortality and amputation are more common following blunt trauma.

Ischemia

As a general rule, re-establishing perfusion within a "golden period" of 6 hours from the time of injury is a desirable goal to ensure optimal functional outcome. Warm ischemia less than 4 hours generally will not lead to muscle necrosis, whereas delays beyond 6 hours may be associated with significant muscle damage. Clinical decisions should not be made with strict adherence to these time limit guidelines because some degree of collateral circulation is often present and reperfusion even beyond 6 hours following injury may result in successful functional outcome. In blunt trauma, associated tissue trauma may interrupt collaterals to a greater extent then penetrating trauma and likely accounts in part for the increased severity of ischemia and the higher rate of amputation following blunt trauma. An exception to this generalization may be seen with high-velocity bullet wounds in which associated soft tissue injury and collateral disruption may be significant.

The peripheral nerves are especially susceptible to ischemia. This is the consequence of a high basal metabolic rate and a general lack of significant glycogen stores. Dysfunction of the nerves due to ischemia results in a "stocking-glove" distribution sensory deficit. This finding portends progression to gangrene if perfusion is not re-established promptly. This should be distinguished from direct peripheral nerve injury that will present with a neurologic deficit in the distribution of the nerve. Paralysis associated with an anesthetic limb carries a bad prognosis. Restoration of blood flow in such a limb, even within the golden period cited earlier, may result in limb loss.

Reperfusion Injury

"Reperfusion injury" is the damage caused locally (i.e., to skeletal muscle and peripheral nerves) and systemically following re-establishment of blood flow to an ischemic body region. Ischemia sets into process a number of biochemical alterations that cumulate in cellular damage following reperfusion. The severity of the reperfusion injury is correlated with the volume of ischemic tissue (i.e., lower limb vs. upper limb) and duration of ischemia. A variety of substances are released including superoxide anion, a highly reactive free radical. Reperfusion results in microvascular endothelial membrane damage, neutrophil activation, platelet aggregation, and decreased nitric oxide production. Ultimately, microvascular perfusion is compromised resulting in progression of the original ischemic injury. Release of metabolic products into the systemic circulation may cause hyperkalemia, acidosis, and myoglobulinemia. Additionally, the inflammatory and coagulation systems are activated. Cardiac arrhythmias, acute respiratory distress syndrome, renal failure, multiorgan failure, and death may follow if not identified and aggressively treated. Reperfusion of the entire lower limb may be life threatening. Reperfusion of the lower leg is less morbid but can still have life-threatening consequences in the older patient.

Compartment Syndrome

Compartment syndrome results from swelling of soft tissues enclosed within a relatively rigid fascial space. As pressure increases within the compartment, microvascular perfusion is limited, and ultimately, tissue necrosis results. Most commonly, compartment syndrome occurs in the lower leg or forearm, however, additional locations can be involved. Swelling may result from hemorrhage into the soft tissues, from tissue edema as a result of venous occlusion, from ischemic or dying muscle, or from external causes such as tight casts or circumferential burn eschars.

The diagnosis of compartment syndrome is clinical and based on clinical findings of the four *P*s: pressure, pain, paresthesia, and intact pulses. Increased pressure is manifested as a tense compartment to palpation and can be confirmed by direct pressure measurement. Pain is out of proportion to that expected from the extremity injury. Also, passive stretching of the ischemic muscle aggravates the pain. Paresthesia, which may progress to complete anesthesia and paralysis, is a late finding in compartment syndrome. Distal pulses are often intact, a finding that when present serves to distinguish compartment syndrome from arterial insufficiency.

Compartment pressures are readily measured with either handheld devices (e.g., Stryker pressure monitor) or with a side-port catheter attached to an arterial pressure transducer. Blood flow to muscle is cut off when compartment pressures exceed venous pressure. Criteria based on an absolute compartment pressure value are of limited utility in hypotensive patients. Several investigators have advocated calculation of a gradient between the measured compartment pressure and either the mean arterial pressure or the arterial diastolic pressure. A gradient of less than 10 to 30 mm Hg below the diastolic or less than 30 to 40 mm Hg below the mean arterial pressure has improved specificity in the diagnosis of extremity compartment syndrome. Of note, patients with venous injury or obstruction are particularly susceptible to subsequent compartment syndrome and should be closely monitored.

An effort should be made to determine the cause of the compartment syndrome. The ultimate functional outcome of fasciotomy depends on the etiology of the compartment syndrome and the extent of muscle necrosis. Increased compartment pressures due to either hemorrhage into the compartment or venous obstruction, especially with underlying viable muscle, are clear-cut indications of the need for fasciotomy. Controversy regarding the utility of fasciotomy arises in patients who have compartment syndrome on the basis of ischemia alone (e.g., compartment syndrome of the calf following prolonged femoral

artery occlusion). Release of the fascial envelope will not result in recovery of necrotic muscle. Subsequent infection, nonhealing, and need for amputation generally result. These patients are best served without fasciotomy. The muscle will become fibrotic; however, the patient may be left with a functional limb.

DIAGNOSIS

Identification and management of life-threatening injuries and treatment of shock should be the first priority. Advanced Trauma Life Support (ATLS) guidelines should be followed. Initial treatment and evaluation should proceed simultaneously. It is important to recognize and control external hemorrhage. Generally, direct pressure is effective. Patients should be promptly resuscitated as the presence of shock itself may lead to diminished pulses in the extremities and confusion about the presence of vascular injury. Associated fractures and dislocations may compromise vascular patency and should be reduced. Frequently, there are associated injuries to the abdomen, chest, or head that require immediate intervention. Prompt resuscitation and identification and management of vascular injuries should be the goals to limit warm ischemia and ensure optimal functional outcome.

History

The patient and prehospital personnel should be questioned about the mechanism of injury. With penetrating trauma, information such as the length of the knife, the number and direction of bullets fired, and the body position at the time of injury should be sought. With blunt trauma, the severity of the injury mechanism (e.g., distance of fall, vehicle speed, and damage) and evidence of fracture, dislocation, or altered perfusion of extremities should be elucidated. Further, certain mechanisms such as "car bumper" injuries or posterior knee dislocations may be associated with vascular injury and their occurrence should be sought. The amount and character of blood loss should be ascertained. Bright red pulsatile bleeding is suggestive of an arterial injury, whereas dark blood suggests a venous origin. Evidence of shock must be sought from the prehospital personnel, as well as the volume of fluid administered. The use of a tourniquet and duration of its application should be determined. Information about neurologic symptoms including sensory and motor deficits should be obtained. Also, the patient should be questioned regarding a history of peripheral vascular disease, diabetes, or other conditions such as coronary artery disease that carry a high incidence of associated vascular disease.

Physical Examination

The patient should be adequately exposed and thoroughly examined. Deformity due to fracture or dislocation should be identified. Careful attention should be directed to skinfolds in the axilla or perineum and buttocks that may hide wounds due to penetrating trauma. In the case of penetrating trauma, the trajectory of the wounding object should be estimated, particularly with reference to major arteries. Wounds should be inspected for evidence of active bleeding or hematoma formation. The character of the bleeding, pulsatile bright red blood, or a steady ooze of dark blood should be noted. A tense or expanding hematoma indicates the presence of an arterial injury with bleeding contained by surrounding soft tissues. Finally, the opposite uninjured extremity should be inspected for evidence of chronic peripheral vascular disease. Absent pulses in the non-injured leg markedly decreases the likelihood of vascular injury in the traumatized extremity.

The pulse examination should include palpation of pulses proximal and distal to the injury. Skin temperature and capillary refill distal to the injury should also be assessed as indexes of perfusion. A difference in the character of the pulse or skin perfusion should prompt additional workup. Of note, pulses may be palpable and normal in up to one third of patients with a vascular injury. Comparison of skin perfusion and pulses of the injured extremity to that of the non-injured extrem-

ity is very helpful. Hypoperfusion and diminished peripheral pulses due solely to shock will be similar on both sides. Further, diminished or absent pulses as a result of peripheral vascular disease are generally symmetrical between the extremities. Occasionally, patients may have a congenital absence of the dorsalis pedis pulse.

AV fistulas may be identified by auscultation of a bruit over the involved arterial segment; a thrill, palpable evidence of an AV fistula, is rarely present in acute injury. A glove should be placed over the bell of the stethoscope to keep the stethoscope free of blood when there is an open injury. Thrills and bruits may not be obvious, particularly early after injury. AV fistulas generally progress over time and bruits that were not initially present may appear the next day.

Complete preoperative evaluation and documentation of neurologic function is important, as ultimate functional outcome largely depends on intact sensory and motor function. As mentioned, a "stocking-glove" distribution sensory deficit indicates neurologic dysfunction due to ischemia. Development of gangrene will ensue if flow is not promptly re-established.

Hard and Soft Signs of Vascular Injury

Findings identified on history and physical examination may be divided into two categories, hard signs and soft signs, each with a varying degree of association with arterial injury (Table 5–1). Hard signs are strong predictors of the presence of an arterial injury and the need for operative intervention. Obvious examples are pulsatile bleeding or an expanding hematoma. Evidence of ischemia manifested with the six *P*s: Pulselessness, pallor, pain, paralysis, paresthesia, and poikilothermia are further strong evidence of arterial injury. A thrill, palpable evidence of an AV fistula, is not as commonly noted as is a bruit. An arterial pressure index (API) of less than 0.90 is included as a hard sign. The API is determined by dividing the systolic pressure of the injured limb by the systolic pressure of the non-injured limb.

TABLE 5–1
HARD VERSUS SOFT SIGNS OF VASCULAR INJURY

Hard Signs	Soft Signs
Active arterial bleeding	Neurologic injury in proximity to vessel
Pulselessness/evidence of ischemia	Small to moderate-sized hematoma
Expanding pulsatile hematoma	Unexplained hypotension
Bruit or thrill	Large blood loss at scene
Arterial pressure index < 0.90 pulse deficit	Injury (due to penetrating mechanism, fracture, or dislocation) in proximity to major vessel

trauma to look for foreign bodies or evidence of fracture or dislocation. Radiopaque markers should be placed on all penetrating wounds for identification on subsequent radiographs. The number of bullets visualized should be correlated with the number of wounds. The sum of the number of bullets and the number of wounds should equal an even number. If the sum results in an odd number, the possibility of a missile embolism should be entertained. The bullet may travel within the vascular system to the heart and pulmonary system if the bullet gains access to the venous system (Figs. 5–3 and 5–4) or the distal artery if the bullet gains access to the arterial system. Additional x-ray films, including fluoroscopy, should be obtained and the

Johansen and colleagues (1991) found that an API of less than 0.90 had 95% sensitivity and 97% specificity for identification of occult arterial injury. Further, an API of more than 0.90 had a 99% negative predictive value for an arterial injury. However, an API may be normal in patients who have injuries to non-conduit vessels such as the femoris profunda. Also, API can be unreliable in the evaluation of penetrating injuries in the region of the groin. Nonetheless, the API is readily obtained at bedside and is a useful extension of the physical examination, particularly when the pulse strength is questionably diminished.

Soft signs are suggestive of an arterial injury, though with a much decreased sensitivity and specificity than hard signs (see Table 5–1). The incidence of arterial injury varies with the specific finding. When proximity is the only indicator of possible vascular injury, evaluation with arteriography generally finds identifiable injuries in fewer than 10% of patients, and many do not require additional specific treatment other than observation alone. Much of the controversy of vascular trauma evaluation centers on the workup of patients with soft signs.

Ancillary Tests

Plain x-rays of the injured extremity should be obtained in both penetrating and blunt

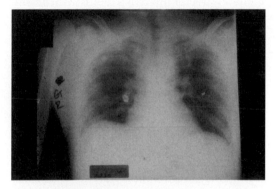

■ **FIGURE 5–3**
Bullet embolism to pulmonary artery from iliac vein injury. (From What's Your Diagnosis: Photographic Case Studies in General Surgery. Greenwich, Conn: Cliggott Publishing, 1994.) ■

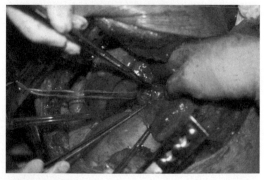

■ **FIGURE 5–4**
Extraction of bullet embolism to right pulmonary artery. (From What's Your Diagnosis: Photographic Case Studies in General Surgery. Greenwich, Conn: Cliggott Publishing, 1994.) ■

patient re-examined until the discrepancy is resolved. Occasionally, folds in the axilla and perineum may hide additional wounds. Finally, the foreign body image should be scrutinized. Blurring of the edges of the bullet suggests movement that could be the result of an intimate relationship with a pulsatile artery.

Application of routine operative exploration of penetrating extremity trauma to civilian trauma proved to result in a large number of negative explorations. In a landmark paper, Snyder and colleagues (1978) validated the use of arteriography to accurately detect vascular lesions. They evaluated 177 patients with 183 penetrating extremity injuries using arteriography and subsequent operative exploration. They identified 1 false-negative and 14 false-positive arteriograms. Arteriography is generally not required in patients with obvious arterial injury (e.g., active arterial bleeding, pulselessness, and/or expanding hematoma). However, arteriography is invaluable in patients in whom the diagnosis is less clear or the extent or location of vascular injury is not readily apparent (Table 5–2). Arteriography is generally well tolerated. Complications can occur in 2% to 4% of patients. Usually, these are minor, most frequently limited groin hematomas. Major complications such as iatrogenic pseudoaneurysms, AV fistulas, or embolic occlusion are uncommon. In part, this may reflect the younger population typical for trauma.

Patients who require urgent operation either for an obvious vascular injury or for life-threatening associated injuries should have any necessary arteriograms performed in the operating room to minimize warm ischemia time. Arteriograms are obtained with percutaneous cannulization of the artery proximal to the site of suspected injury. Contrast is then injected into the artery, and plain films are obtained. Fluoroscopy can be used as an alternative to plain radiographs to minimize the amount of contrast required and to aid with timing of the contrast injection. If visualization of the axillary artery is necessary, outflow occlusion with a cuff can be performed to allow filling of the axillary artery proximal to the site of contrast injection as described by O'Gorman and colleagues (1984). Of note, O'Gorman and colleagues (1984) described the use of surgeon-performed angiography in the emergency room to exclude significant vascular injury. They were subsequently able to discharge some patients from the emergency room.

Duplex ultrasonographic scanning has been shown by several investigators to have a sensitivity and specificity approaching 100% for the investigation of penetrating extremity trauma. The modality combines real-time two-dimensional imaging with guided Doppler insonation. Flow to or from the point of Doppler investigation can be represented on a color scale. Duplex ultrasonography is more sensitive than an API evaluation. Further, nonconduit arterial injuries, which do not alter the API, can be evaluated.

Evaluation of the patient with penetrating extremity trauma who presents with only soft signs of arterial injury continues to be a subject of debate. Routine use of arteriography on patients with proximity injuries will identify abnormalities in up to 10% of cases. Several series report the need for vascular repair in between 0.6% and 4.4% of patients with proximity penetrating injuries (Dennis, 1998). Dennis, Frykberg, and colleagues (1998) has championed physical examination alone in this group, arguing that patients those patients who need operative intervention will ultimately develop identifiable hard signs. A number of investigators have promulgated duplex ultrasonography as a noninvasive alternative between routine arteriography and physical examination alone. The lesions missed on initial physical examination that ultimately require operative intervention are

TABLE 5–2
INDICATIONS FOR ARTERIOGRAPHY: EXTREMITY TRAUMA

Unclear location or extent of vascular injury
Extensive soft tissue injury
Fracture or dislocation
Trajectory parallel to an artery
Multiple wounds
Shotgun injuries
Peripheral vascular disease

injuries to the profunda femoris artery, pseudoaneurysms, and AV fistulas. Both of these lesions progress with time and delayed operative repair is technically more challenging. Further, many investigators have documented the poor follow-up possible in the trauma population. Duplex ultrasonography is capable of detecting these lesions at the time of initial presentation. The major limitations are that the modality is technician dependent and often not readily available during off-hours when most patients are injured. However, even proponents of physical examination alone advocate admission and observation for 24 hours. Moreover, more than 43% of patients with proximity penetrating extremity trauma at University of California–Davis required physical therapy, and 46% required complex wound care. Thus, admission during which duplex ultrasonography can be obtained is easily justified. Ultimately, the choice is a balance between the need to promptly diagnose all arterial injuries requiring treatment and prevent unnecessary morbidity on the one hand and the cost, availability, and morbidity of diagnostic modalities on the other hand.

Patients with suspected vascular injury fall into three basic priorities: (1) Patients with evidence of pulselessness/ischemia, active bleeding, or a pulsatile hematoma, (2) patients with hard signs and a palpable pulse, and (3) patients with soft signs or an injury known to be associated with vascular injury. In all patients, life-threatening injuries take priority and should be addressed immediately. The patient should be resuscitated and shock managed appropriately. Fractures and dislocations should be reduced and the pulse examination and skin perfusion evaluated. Hard and soft signs should be specifically elicited (Fig. 5–5).

Patients who are pulseless or show evidence of ischemia or those who have active bleeding manifested with either external bleeding or an expanding pulsatile hematoma should be taken promptly to the operating room. Often, the location of the injury can be identified from the history and physical examination and operative intervention can proceed directly. However, in certain circumstances, the exact location or extent of injury may be unclear (see Table 5–2). In these patients, on-table arteriography, performed in the operating room, is used to assess vascular injury and minimize warm ischemia time.

Patients who have hard signs but have a palpable pulse and no evidence of ischemia can generally undergo a more deliberate workup. Usually information required to guide intervention is obtained from formal arteriography in the radiology suite. In general, the quality of formal arteriograms is better than that of those obtained in the operating room. Additionally, therapeutic endovascular procedures such as embolization of bleeding muscular branches, pseudoaneurysms, or AV fistulas can be performed in the radiology suite. Occasionally urgent operation is required for associated injuries, such as intra-abdominal injury. In these patients, on-table arteriography provides a means to promptly identify arterial injuries to guide subsequent operative or nonoperative management.

Patients who have soft signs or who have a mechanism suggestive of an arterial injury, such as a posterior knee dislocation, can be evaluated in various ways. Viable options, each with their ardent advocates and literature support, include routine arteriography or duplex ultrasonography and/or serial physical examination. Vascular abnormalities identified by duplex ultrasonography are subsequently evaluated with arteriography as a diagnostic and possibly therapeutic intervention. Development of hard signs in patients followed by physical examination is generally evaluated by formal arteriography.

Patients with injury in the region of the groin, thoracic outlet, or neck should undergo arteriography. Duplex ultrasonography of the subclavian, axillary, and iliac vessels is limited. Further, consequences of missed injuries in these areas, such as exsanguination from intrapleural hemorrhage, may be catastrophic. At times, the vascular lesion may be amenable to treatment with endovascular techniques.

Once arterial injuries are identified and delineated, management proceeds as appropriate.

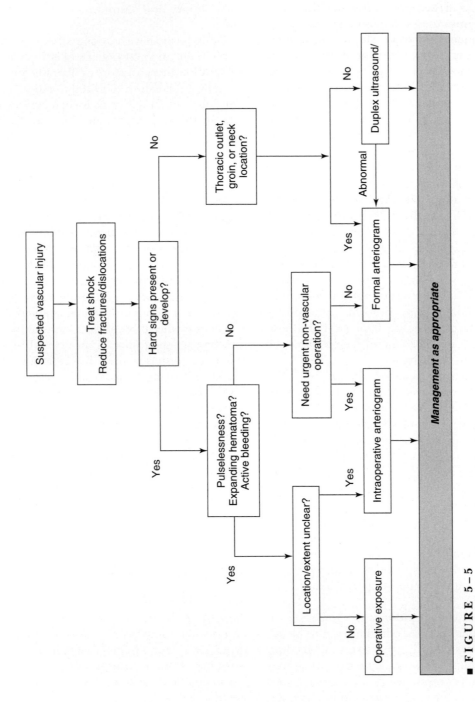

■ **FIGURE** 5–5
Evaluation of suspected extremity vascular injury. ■

SUMMARY

Diagnostic modalities and algorithms have evolved as treatment paradigms have progressed over the past century from expectant management, to repair of all arterial injuries, to the repair of selected arterial injuries practiced today. Continued refinements are to be expected with ongoing clinical research and patient follow-up.

REFERENCES

Dennis JW, Frykberg ER, Veldenz HC, et al: Validation of nonoperative management of occult vascular injuries and accuracy of physical examination alone in penetrating extremity trauma: 5- to 10-year follow-up. J Trauma 1998; 44(2):242-252.

The authors present long-term outcome data to validate safety and efficacy of physical examination alone to determine the treatment of penetrating extremity trauma. Two groups of patients are presented, the first during a period of liberal use of arteriography, and the second with the use of physical examination alone. Group 1 had 43 patients with 44 clinically occult injuries subsequently demonstrated on angiography. Four (9%) had deterioration within a month and required operative repair. Follow-up, with a mean of 9.1 years, was possible in 58% of the remaining patients; all were asymptomatic. Group 2 had 287 patients with 309 asymptomatic proximity injuries evaluated by physical examination alone. Four (1.3%) deteriorated and required surgery. Follow-up, with a mean of 5.4 years, was possible in 29%; no patient reported vascular symptoms.

Fry WR, Smith RS, Sayers DV, et al: The success of duplex ultrasonographic scanning in diagnosis of extremity vascular proximity trauma [see Comments]. Arch Surg 1993;128(12):1368-1372.

Study of the use of duplex ultrasonographic scanning in the evaluation of penetrating extremity vascular trauma. Two-hundred patients with 225 penetrating extremity injuries were evaluated with duplex ultrasonography for either vascular proximity injury or diminished pulse strength. Arteriograms were obtained in the first 50 patients. The sensitivity and specificity were both 100% in this initial cohort. Duplex ultrasonography was used in the remaining 175 injuries.

Eighteen injuries were identified, seventeen of which were confirmed by either arteriography or operative exploration. The remaining patient had spasm of the superficial femoral artery on arteriography, which did not require treatment. Seven unsuspected venous injuries were identified.

Johansen K, Lynch K, Paun M, Copass M: Noninvasive vascular tests reliably exclude occult arterial trauma in injured extremities. J Trauma 1991;31(4):515-522.

Follow-up study to validate the use of arterial pressure index (API) to exclude significant arterial damage in patients with extremity trauma. Overall, a value of 0.90 was found to have a sensitivity and specificity of 95% and 97%, respectively, for the presence of significant arterial injury. A value of more than 0.90 had a negative predictive value of 99%. Arteriography was advocated for those limbs with an API of less than 0.90. The authors argue the API is safe, accurate, and cost-effective in the evaluation of extremity vascular trauma.

O'Gorman RB, Feliciano DV, Bitondo CG, et al: Emergency center arteriography in the evaluation of suspected peripheral vascular injuries. Arch Surg 1984;119(5):568-573.

Description of a surgeon-performed arteriography in a group of 488 patients with suspected vascular injuries. The majority of arteriograms were obtained for proximity (353/488); 76 arteriograms were performed for a diminished pulse. Overall, 20% of the patients were found to have a vascular injury requiring subsequent operative intervention. Only one false-normal and four false-abnormal arteriograms were reported. The authors conclude that the method is simple, sensitive, and cost-effective in patients with potential peripheral vascular injuries.

Richardson JD, Vitale GC, Flint LM Jr: Penetrating arterial trauma. Analysis of missed vascular injuries. Arch Surg 1987;122(6):678-683.

Classic article describing an experience of 677 patients with penetrating wounds to the upper and lower extremity and neck with suspected vascular injury. Patients were evaluated with a combination of surgical exploration and/or arteriography. Long-term follow-up for an average of 5.1 years was obtained in 33% of the patients. Missed vascular injuries were identified in patients undergoing either surgical exploration alone or arteriography alone. No missed injuries were identified in patients who underwent both arteriography and surgical exploration.

Snyder WH III, Thal ER, Bridges RA, et al: The validity of normal arteriography in penetrating trauma. Arch Surg 1978;113(4):424-426.

Landmark paper comparing arteriography to operative vessel exploration. One hundred seventy-seven patients with 183 penetrating extremity wounds were evaluated with arteriography and subsequent operative exploration. Compared to operative exploration, arteriography had 36 true positives, 132 true negatives, 14 false positives, and 1 false negative. The authors conclude that arteriography is sensitive enough to exclude arterial injury in patients with equivocal clinical signs of vascular injury.

6

Vascular Diagnostic Options in Extremity and Cervical Trauma

KAJ JOHANSEN

INTRODUCTION

Sometimes the diagnosis of extremity arterial trauma is straightforward: Torrential hemorrhage, acute limb ischemia, a pulsatile hematoma, or other such urgent problems generally require little attention to diagnostic maneuvers other than immediate operation. However, a large proportion of peripheral vascular injuries may not be immediately apparent, presenting in subtle, confusing, or obscure fashion. Alternatively, vascular injuries may be entirely silent, discovered only during a general diagnostic survey of the trauma patient. This chapter elucidates currently accepted "best practices" for the diagnosis of extremity and cervical vascular trauma.

PENETRATING AND BLUNT TRAUMA TO THE EXTREMITIES

Injury to the major arteries of the extremities may result in severe bleeding or in immediate or delayed ischemia—in either case, a

125

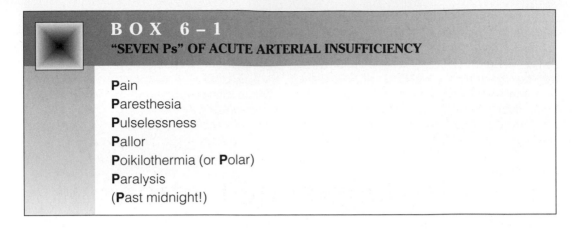

BOX 6–1

"SEVEN Ps" OF ACUTE ARTERIAL INSUFFICIENCY

Pain
Paresthesia
Pulselessness
Pallor
Poikilothermia (or Polar)
Paralysis
(Past midnight!)

threat to limb viability. Further, as is noted later, technically successful revascularization of the traumatized extremity may threaten extremity viability anew by producing an ischemia-reperfusion phenomenon, manifested clinically by compartment syndrome.

Patients with substantial ongoing external bleeding, rapidly expanding hematoma, evidence for acute arterial insufficiency—the "Seven Ps" (Box 6–1)—or other less common objective signs of major arterial injury (e.g., the presence of a large arteriovenous [AV] fistula) almost always warrant immediate operation as the first diagnostic test. Other diagnostic tests such as arteriography are dilatory and rarely add useful decision-making information (occasional patients, such as those with shotgun injuries or with extremity fractures at multiple levels, may require imaging studies preoperatively to define the precise anatomic site of arterial disruption). The need for immediate operation is obvious in patients with exsanguinating hemorrhage, and equivalent urgency is present in patients with acute arterial insufficiency, in whom experimental and clinical data as well as long-established clinical observation document at most a 6-hour "grace period" to restore perfusion before a substantially increased likelihood of postoperative tissue infarction and limb loss can be anticipated. This acceptable "golden period" may be even shorter if shock, crush injury, or other comorbidities complicate the clinical picture.

Unfortunately, most patients with extremity trauma do not have "hard" signs of vascular injury but only "soft" indications that arterial or venous injury has occurred. Alternatively, they may have no evidence to support the possibility that a vascular injury is present, but only clinical suspicion based on the mechanism of injury or on proximity of the injury tract to important vessels.

A Historical Perspective

The "gold standard" for making the diagnosis of occult extremity injury has changed substantially during the professional lifetime of many still-active clinicians. Wound exploration was the norm in the 1950s and 1960s and had even been mandated in the battlefield setting. However, the morbidity of this approach (including the extremely low yield of mandatory wound exploration) became clear and resulted in a switch to the use of contrast arteriography (usually by a transfemoral arterial approach) in the 1970s and 1980s. This approach was fueled by the general belief (promoted by experienced trauma surgeons at several major trauma centers) that physical examination is inadequately accurate for the assessment of vascular status in injured extremities (Perry, Thal, and Shires, 1971). Contrast arteriography proved relatively rapid and extremely sensitive and specific for the identification of arterial disruption in trauma victims; several studies documented false-positive and false-negative rates of less than 2% in contrast arteriography performed to rule out arterial injury in the extremities (Snyder and colleagues, 1978; Rose and Moore, 1988).

However, contrast arteriography generally requires transfer of the patient out of the emergency department (ED) to a site in which ongoing surveillance, volume resuscitation, and management of secondary injuries are difficult to conduct. Contrast arteriography is invasive and expensive and has a small but definite risk of contrast dye reactions or arterial puncture-site complications. Most importantly, it became clear that the real clinical yield of contrast arteriography, when performed as the screening technique of choice in injured extremities, is extremely low. In several series, fewer than 5% of patients actually required operative intervention for arterial injuries discovered by means of contrast arteriography (Frykberg and colleagues, 1989; Anderson and colleagues, 1990).

Noninvasive Physiologic Vascular Tests

In the 1980s, some clinicians began to use several noninvasive diagnostic techniques in the acute setting, which had previously been found to be of major diagnostic value in the assessment of chronic arterial occlusive disease. These included measurement of Doppler-derived arterial pressure indexes (APIs) and the use of duplex sonography. These two techniques have proven extremely useful as initial screening tests for patients thought potentially to harbor an occult extremity arterial injury.

Lynch and Johansen (1991) initially demonstrated that among 100 injured limbs in 93 patients, in whom both Doppler APIs and contrast arteriography were carried out, a Doppler API of 0.90 had a sensitivity of 87% and a specificity of 95% for arterial injury. Because two (2%) of the contrast arteriograms were actually falsely positive in circumstances in which the ultimate outcome had been accurately predicted by the Doppler API, the sensitivity and specificity of the Doppler API technique was actually even higher—95% and 97%—when clinical outcome was used as the comparison standard. The negative predictive value for an API of more than 0.90 was 99%.

In a subsequent study, Johansen and colleagues (1991) evaluated 100 consecutive limbs in 96 vascular trauma victims by screening Doppler API; arteriography was reserved for patients in whom Doppler API was less than 0.90. In this series, 83 limbs had a normal API (>0.90) and 17 limbs had an abnormal API and underwent contrast arteriography. The patients with a normal Doppler API were followed up clinically and by duplex sonography; none required further vascular intervention, and all (except for two patients who underwent normal arteriograms as a protocol violation) had been spared contrast arteriography. Among the 17 limbs undergoing contrast arteriography, 16 (94%) arterial abnormalities were found and seven underwent operative intervention.

These studies demonstrated that use of Doppler API could substantially reduce the number of "exclusion" contrast arteriograms performed in our trauma center (an 80% reduction compared with the 12-month period before the trial, $P < .01$), markedly increase the diagnostic "yield" when contrast arteriography was required, facilitate the overall management of most patients not requiring contrast arteriogram, and save a substantial sum in hospital charges (Lynch and Johansen, 1991; Johansen and colleagues, 1991).

Many of the trauma victims in the studies in which Doppler API was validated were the victims of penetrating trauma. For this reason, some trauma specialists—especially orthopedic surgeons—were reluctant to accept Doppler API as a screening test for proximal extremity injuries in blunt trauma—fractures, dislocations, and crush injuries. Accordingly, Cole and colleagues (1999) recently conducted a study of 70 trauma victims (75 limbs) who had suffered fractures and dislocations around the knee. Among these patients, Doppler API was normal in 57 limbs and abnormal in 18. By clinical outcome (including duplex scan in about one third of the patients), no late abnormalities were identified in the individuals who had an initially normal Doppler API. In those with a Doppler API of less than 0.90, contrast arteriography was performed in 16 (88%) and was positive in 14 (87% of arteriograms); operative repair was performed in 6 (33%). The negative predictive value of a normal Doppler API in these bluntly traumatized lower extremities was 100% (Cole and colleagues, in press), suggesting that Doppler API is as accurate and useful a screening tool in blunt extremity trauma as it is for penetrating injury.

Studies from other trauma centers regarding the utility of Doppler API in screening through the extremities for a potential arterial injury came to similar conclusions (Schwartz and colleagues, 1993; Frykberg, 1995). Schwartz and colleagues (1993) use a higher threshold Doppler API of 1.0, thereby slightly increasing sensitivity at the expense of a substantially higher number of negative contrast arteriograms.

The limitations of Doppler API as a screening tool for occult arterial injury in the extremities must also be made clear. The technique does not accurately diagnose damage in branch arteries (e.g., the profunda femoris or profunda brachii arteries), cannot accurately detect small intimal flaps, AV fistulas or pseudoaneurysms, and will not, of course, discover significant venous injuries. This diagnostic technique is clearly much less accurate in the interrogation of arteries proximal to the inguinal or axillary crease, for example, the iliac or subclavian/axillary arteries; such vessels are best evaluated by contrast arteriography. The Doppler API technique can be "fooled" (as can contrast arteriography) by arterial spasm and may not detect arterial lacerations.

Accordingly, Doppler API has been validated as an accurate, rapid, inexpensive, and noninvasive bedside screening examination for the purposes of initial screening of a bluntly or sharply injured extremity for occult arterial injury.

The excellent diagnostic capabilities of duplex sonography—pulsed wave Doppler ultrasound—became clear in the mid 1980s, again in the evaluation of carotid (and other types of) atherosclerosis. This technology has been thoroughly assessed as being portable, rapid, and noninvasive in the evaluation of trauma victims.

Panetta and colleagues (1992) demonstrated, in a carefully performed comparative study of duplex sonography and arteriography among different types of experimental arterial injuries, that when evaluated by blinded observers, duplex sonography was overall more accurate than contrast arteriography in diagnosing arterial disruption ($P < .02$), especially for arterial lacerations ($P < .001$).

Among 89 patients with 93 sites of extremity or cervical trauma, Meissner, Paun, and Johansen (1991) demonstrated that duplex sonography resulted in only four false positives and no false negatives for significant arterial injury. A similar study in 198 trauma patients by Bynoe and colleagues (1991) from the University of South Carolina found only two false-positive and one false-negative study. In this study, sensitivity was 95% and specificity was 99% for arterial injury.

These studies might appropriately be criticized because arteriography control was not consistently carried out. Fry and colleagues (1993) conducted a trial in patients with extremity trauma in which the first 50 subjects who were studied by Doppler ultrasound also underwent contrast arteriography (or operative exploration). When perfect agreement was discovered between ultrasonographic and arteriographic diagnostic modalities in these patients, a subsequent 175 patients were studied by duplex scan alone, with arteriography reserved for patients with an abnormal ultrasonographic study. This trial of duplex scan showed 100% sensitivity and 97% specificity for major arterial trauma; only one false-positive study resulted. In addition, the investigators reported discovery of seven major venous injuries by means of duplex sonography, which they asserted would not have been identified had only contrast arteriography been performed as a diagnostic tool (Fry and colleagues, 1993).

The advantages of duplex scanning as a screening examination for arterial injury in a patient with extremity trauma are obvious; it can be brought to the bedside in the ED and is noninvasive, rapid, easily repeated, and inexpensive. In addition, certain injuries not readily identified by other means—for example, major venous disruptions—may potentially be identified by this technique.

The limitations of duplex sonography must also be emphasized. These include potentially reduced access because of open wounds, dressings, splints, or casts; relatively lesser accuracy in identifying truncal vascular injury; and a substantial "learning curve" for technologists and interpreting physicians. In addition, at a time of continued economic retrenchment by urban trauma hospitals, it has become increasingly difficult to sustain night/weekend vascular laboratory coverage, obligatory for evaluation of trauma victims in the ED.

Do all arterial injuries need to be repaired? Although some continue to adhere to the traditional tenet that any arterial disruption warrants operative exploration (Stain and colleagues, 1993), more contemporary studies, based on the excellent natural history data which can be accumulated from repeated duplex ultrasonograms of various arterial injuries, have suggested that many "minor" arterial injuries—small intimal flaps, pseudoaneurysms, and AV fistulas—resolve on their own without intervention. The observation that most intimal injuries that result from catheter arteriography go on to "heal" without operation certainly predicts such a conclusion. Stain and colleagues (1993) observed 80 "minimal" pseudoaneurysms, intimal flaps or dissections, and AV fistulas with serial duplex ultrasound examinations; at the end of 12 months, only 4 (5%) of the lesions had required operative repair.

Thus, the noninvasive vascular physiologic examinations of Doppler API measurement and duplex sonography can be employed with accuracy and cost-effectiveness in the evolution of extremity arterial injuries. We have developed an algorithm (Fig. 6–1) that incorporates these modalities.

Limb Swelling and Pain following Extremity Revascularization

The unwary clinician may ignore the fact (or fail to recall) that prolonged or severe limb ischemia followed by successful revascularization can result in the ischemia-reperfusion phenomenon, manifested clinically as compartment syndrome. This may be seen particularly after crush injuries, combined arterial and venous trauma, closed fractures of the

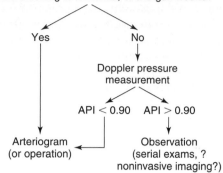

■ **FIGURE 6–1**

Algorithm for diagnostic management of patients potentially harboring an extremity vascular injury. ■

extremity, and ischemia complicated by systemic hypotension or shock. Compartment syndrome, if not recognized and treated in a timely fashion, is associated with a substantial risk of myonecrosis and limb loss.

In the otherwise uncomplicated trauma victim, the diagnosis of compartment syndrome is usually straightforward. Such patients have pain out of proportion to what would be expected, as well as inexorably worsening neurologic dysfunction of the extremity as characterized by both numbness and extensor weakness. Calf or forearm muscles (for practical purposes, the only two sites where compartment syndrome normally presents) will be unnaturally tight, swollen, and tender. Thus, the diagnosis of compartment syndrome is not difficult, given the appropriate clinical scenario and the symptoms and signs noted earlier.

However, relevant symptoms and signs may be obscured by one or more of a constellation of comorbid conditions. These may include intoxication with alcohol or other drugs, closed head injury, general or neuraxial anesthesia, spinal cord injury resulting in paraplegia or quadriplegia, or obscuration of the examination by casts, splints, or dressings. In such patients, the diagnosis of compartment syndrome may be obscured or ignored until muscle necrosis has already occurred.

One approach, espoused by many, is to adopt a liberal posture toward the performance of prophylactic fasciotomy when even the possibility of compartment syndrome is contemplated. I am a proponent of such a view. However, in certain clinical settings, such an approach might be imprudent or unwarranted, and alternative dependable means of making the diagnosis of compartment tissue hypertension are required.

The time-honored technique is that of tissue manometry, using various commercially available devices to transduce tissue pressure after insertion of a needle into a given compartment of the calf or forearm. This technique, in use since the mid 1970s (Whiteside and colleagues, 1975; Matsen, 1978) is both sensitive and specific for compartmental hypertension; its only drawbacks are its invasive nature (thus making it difficult to do repeat studies) and the fact that devices for measuring may occasionally be unavailable, out of commission, or unfamiliar to the clinician. Tissue pressures higher than 40 mm Hg or higher than 30 mm Hg for longer than 3 hours have been considered diagnostic of compartmental hypertension and are an indication for immediate fasciotomy (Matsen, 1978). A more contemporary understanding of the pathophysiology of compartmental hypertension compares the measured compartment pressure to either the diastolic or the calculated mean arterial pressure, with compartmental hypertension being characterized by a pressure differential of less than 30 mm Hg (Matava and colleagues, 1994).

Other techniques, such as the measurement of somatosensory evoked potentials (Present and colleagues, 1993), the use of near-infrared spectrophotometry (Giannotti and colleagues, 2000), and the objective measurement of tissue hardness (Steinberg and Gelberman, 1994) have been assessed.

A clever conceptual leap by Jones, Perry, and Bush (1989), experimentally validated by Ombrellaro and colleagues (1996), permits the assessment of effects of tissue pressure on calf or forearm venous hemodynamics by use of venous duplex scanning. Arterial pressures and flows should clearly be only minimally (if at all) impacted by changes in ambient tissue pressure. However, venous hemodynamics should be exquisitely sensitive to local tissue pressure: Normal venous pressures in the calf

and forearm are virtually identical to tissue pressures (5 to 10 mm Hg). Whereas the sensitivity of duplex scanning of the calf or forearm veins for compartment syndrome may not be particularly high (i.e., abnormal venous hemodynamics might be due to crush injury, hematoma, splints or dressings, or compartmental hypertension), the specificity of examination should be quite close to 100% (i.e., normal tibial venous respiratory variation and phasicity in a particular calf compartment indicate that compartmental hypertension cannot be present). Duplex scanning of tibial or forearm veins is the screening test of choice at my medical center in patients in whom the diagnosis of compartment syndrome is entertained.

PENETRATING OR BLUNT INJURIES TO THE BRACHIOCEPHALIC VESSELS

Among many other complications of trauma to the head, neck, and upper chest is the possibility of injury to the large arteries and veins of the head and upper extremities. Not only is early or delayed exsanguination a risk, but the late implications of arterial thrombosis or embolization secondary to dissection, intimal flap, or pseudoaneurysm include the risk of disabling or even lethal stroke. An ongoing controversy attends the question of the proper diagnostic pathway to be followed in patients with penetrating cervical trauma—mandatory exploration or selective operation based on the results of a panel of diagnostic tests (arteriography, triple endoscopy, barium swallow). This dispute remains undecided despite careful ongoing evaluation over the last 4 decades.

As for other anatomic sites in the body, signs of significant hemorrhage (pulsatile external or oropharyngeal bleeding, expanding/ pulsatile hematoma) mandate immediate operation. In addition, it has become increasingly clear that cervical vascular injury associated with any degree of neurologic deficit warrants emergency extracranial carotid (or vertebral) arterial reconstruction as well (Richardson and colleagues, 1992). Although the results of such surgical repair in patients with carotid artery injury associated with coma are generally dismal, case reports suggest that even in this desperate setting, occasional cerebral salvage can occur by timely carotid arterial repair (Robbs and colleagues, 1983).

As elsewhere, much more major controversy attends the management of patients with "soft" signs of cervical carotid (or vertebral) arterial injury or in whom there is concern about an occult arterial injury based on the sounding mechanism or the location of the injury tract. Because such wounds potentially also involve the airway or (as seriously) the esophagus or the oropharynx, either routine operative exploration as the first diagnostic test or a series of radiographic, endoscopic, and arteriographic studies is obligatory in this setting. As noted already, no clear consensus has been achieved in defining the superiority of one diagnostic approach over the other.

Detection of occult cervical arterial injuries is assisted by now well-established means of categorizing such potential injuries by anatomic site. It is generally agreed that injuries below the sternal notch (zone 1) will likely require median sternotomy or thoracotomy for management; accordingly, preoperative contrast arteriography is generally considered necessary. Injuries above the angle of the jaw (zone 3), because they are surgically remote, may require craniotomy or (potentially) even more complex vascular exposure; contrast arteriography is thus indicated in this setting as well. Arteriography for lesions in zone 3 also occasionally identifies lesions surgically inaccessible enough (e.g., in the carotid siphon) so that treatment by catheter-directed means (e.g., coil embolization of carotid artery-cavernous sinus fistula) is the preferred therapeutic choice.

In zone 2 penetrating injuries to the neck, duplex sonography has been found to play a highly dependable diagnostic role. Fry and colleagues (1994), using control arteriography "run-in" for the first 15 patients in a series of 100 patients, demonstrated equivalent 100% sensitivities and specificities for duplex sonography in examining cervical carotid injuries. Demetriades and colleagues (1995) compared contrast arteriography, duplex sonography, and simple serial physical examination in 82 patients with penetrating neck trauma. As previously demonstrated with peripheral arterial injuries in the extremities, contrast arteriography was "hypersensitive" for arterial injuries; 11 arterial disruptions were discovered, but only 2 required operation. Physical examination was accurate for all clinically significant injuries but missed six minor vascular injuries. Duplex sonography found 10 of the 11 injuries detected by contrast arteriography, and sensitivity and specificity for clinically relevant injuries were 91% and 99%, respectively.

Blunt cervical arterial injuries are even more complicated to diagnose, because unlike penetrating trauma (which usually involves the common carotid artery), blunt trauma more commonly involves the internal carotid artery. Closed head injury, basilar skull fractures, various forms of deceleration motor-vehicle accidents resulting in injuries to the head and neck, and the increased use of shoulder-lap restraints have resulted in a sharply increased recent incidence of blunt carotid injury (Kerwin and colleagues, 2001). Because these patients frequently present without initial symptoms only later developing neurologic deficits related to thrombosis or dissection of the internal carotid artery, a screening technique that is accurate and rapid would clearly be of use in this clinical scenario.

Duplex sonography may play a substantive role as a screening tool in this setting. As demonstrated in the landmark animal studies by Panetta and colleagues (1992), duplex scanning is as accurate as contrast arteriography in the diagnosis of dissections, intimal flaps, and arterial lacerations. In a large series of patients with blunt cervical trauma, Fabian and colleagues (1996) demonstrated the diagnostic value of duplex sonography in detecting occult arterial injuries. Because logistic regression analysis of the data in this study demonstrated independent survival benefit associated with heparinization in those patients not requiring operation, the value of early diagnosis of such initially silent injuries (either by sonography or by contrast arteriography) is abundantly clear.

Contrast-enhanced cervical computed tomographic (CT) scanning with fine cuts at the cervical level was demonstrated by Zeman and colleagues (1995) at the University of Vermont to be more accurate even than ultrasonography or arteriography in determining whether a bluntly traumatized or dissected carotid artery is patent or not. Indeed, because many such patients undergo head CT scans to rule out concurrent cerebral injuries, an effective strategy might potentially be to continue the scan down to the level of the carotid bifurcation, thereby demonstrating in a few extra minutes whether the internal carotid arteries are intact and obviate the need to perform either duplex sonography or four-vessel cerebral arteriography.

Transcranial Doppler (TCD) studies have been used only rarely in the trauma setting. However, conceptually this technology may play a useful role in selected patients with actual or potential cerebrovascular trauma, on either a blunt or a penetrating basis (Rae-Grant and colleagues, 1996). For example, TCD studies can demonstrate the adequacy of intracranial arterial flow and can contribute to a decision about whether extracranial carotid (or vertebral) revascularization needs to be performed. In addition, information regarding whether temporary carotid shunting during arterial reconstruction should be used can be derived from TCD studies. Finally, in patients with devastating head injuries (or in whom irreversible brain injury is suspected), TCD is an acknowledged means of demonstrating (based on intracranial arterial flow arrest) that the patient is brain dead (Wejdiecks ejection fraction, 2001).

Physical Examination

The simplest diagnostic tool is a careful physical examination. As previously intimated, the adequacy of physical examination in the diagnosis of vascular trauma has been heavily debated over the past 3 to 4 decades. Experienced trauma surgeons at Parkland Hospital in Dallas, in a series of reports in the 1970s, suggested the relative inaccuracy (or at least inadequacy) of physical examination alone in patients potentially harboring an arterial injury and were in the vanguard of those promoting the use of routine "exclusion" arteriography in patients with extremity trauma

(Perry, Thal, and Shires, 1971; Snyder and colleagues, 1978).

However, it has subsequently become clear that physical examination has an important role to play, at least as a screening tool for various forms of penetrating and blunt extremity and cervical trauma. I consider measurement of Doppler arterial pressure in injured extremities and calculation of Doppler API to be a simple extension of palpation and other aspects of the physical examination; Doppler API has been found, in studies in which I as well as others have participated, to be highly sensitive and specific in the diagnosis of important forms of flow-limiting lesions of extremity arteries (Lynch and Johansen, 1991; Johansen and colleagues, 1991; Cole and colleagues, in press; Schwartz and colleagues, 1993; Frykberg, 1995).

Physical examination has also been found to be accurate for important extracranial carotid artery injuries in a controlled trial comparing serial physical examination with duplex sonography and contrast arteriography (Demetriades and colleagues, 1995). Coming full circle, Francis and colleagues (1991) from Parkland Hospital confirmed the validity of serial physical examination by an experienced surgeon in ruling in or out extremity vascular injury.

SUMMARY

The morbidity and mortality associated with major central or peripheral vascular injury mandate diagnostic measures that are rapid (or at least timely) and accurate. Because of the invasiveness and morbidity of contrast arteriography and operative exploration, such diagnostic maneuvers are optimally rapid, portable, noninvasive, repeatable, and inexpensive.

Contrast arteriography continues to be the "gold standard" for establishing the presence and anatomic location of arterial injuries within the chest or abdomen and in zones 1 and 3 for penetrating neck trauma. However, widespread use of contrast arteriography in the diagnosis of vascular injury is hampered by its invasiveness, expense, the time taken to perform such studies, and the necessity in most cases to carry such studies out in a site remote from the ED or the operating room.

Prospective studies in trauma victims have demonstrated the validity of Doppler arterial pressure measurement as a sensitive and specific screening tool for both penetrating and blunt arterial injuries that are axial and flow limiting. Duplex sonography subsequently has been found to be as accurate as contrast arteriography in the diagnosis of extremity arterial injury, and the technique has the additional benefit of being able to diagnose major venous injuries of the extremities. Duplex ultrasonography has been demonstrated to have diagnostic accuracy equivalent to that of contrast arteriography in penetrating zone 2 injuries of the neck and has equivalently excellent diagnostic accuracy in blunt trauma to the extracranial carotid and vertebral arteries. Detection of patency of the internal carotid artery following blunt trauma and subsequent dissection is accurately made with contrast-enhanced cervical CT scanning, a more accurate means of assessing flow than either contrast arteriography or duplex sonography.

Although compartment syndrome may be best averted by adoption of a liberal policy of prophylactic fasciotomy in trauma victims at significant risk of developing this complication, alternative diagnostic methods may include a series of minimally invasive or noninvasive techniques measuring tissue pressure or hardness, neurologic function, or compartment venous hemodynamics.

Finally, after being long discounted as a valid means of diagnosing occult arterial injury, serial physical examination has been resurrected as an accurate diagnostic technique by well-performed prospective clinical trials.

REFERENCES

Abou-Sayed H, Berger DL: Blunt lower-extremity trauma and popliteal artery injuries: Revisiting the case for selective arteriography. Arch Surg 2002;137(5):585-589.

Anderson RJ, Hobson RW, Padberg FT, et al: Reduced dependency on arteriography for penetrating extremity trauma (PET): Influence of wound location and non-invasive vascular studies. J Trauma 1990;30:1059-1065.

Barnes CJ, Pietrobon R, Higgins LD: Does the pulse examination in patients with traumatic knee dislocation predict a surgical arterial injury? A meta-analysis. J Trauma 2002;53(6):1109-1114.

Bynoe RP, Miles WS, Bell RM, et al: Noninvasive diagnosis of vascular trauma by duplex ultrasonography. J Vasc Surg 1991;14:346-350.

Cole P, Campbell R, Swiontkowski M, Johansen K: Doppler arterial pressures reliably exclude occult arterial injury in blunt lower extremity trauma. J Orthop Trauma (in press).

Demetriades D, Theodorou D, Cornwell E, et al: Penetrating injuries of the neck in patients in stable condition: Physical examination, angiography or color flow Doppler imaging. Arch Surg 1995;130:971-975.

Fabian TC, Patton JH Jr, Croce MA, et al: Blunt carotid injury: Importance of early diagnosis and anticoagulant therapy. Ann Surg 1996;223:513-522.

Francis H III, Thal ER, Weigelt JA, Rodman HC: Vascular proximity: Is it a valid indication for arteriography in asymptomatic patients? J Trauma 1991;31:512-514.

Fry WR, Dort JA, Smith RS, et al: Duplex scanning replaces arteriography and operative exploration in the diagnosis of potential cervical vascular injury. Am J Surg 1994;168:693-695.

Fry WR, Smith RS, Sayers DV, et al: The success of duplex ultrasonographic scanning in the diagnosis of extremity vascular proximity trauma. Arch Surg 1993;128:1368-1372.

Frykberg EP: Advances in the diagnosis and treatment of extremity vascular trauma. Surg Clin North Am 1995;75:207-215.

Frykberg ER, Crump JM, Vines FS, et al: A reassessment of the role of arteriography in assessing acute vascular injuries. J Trauma 1989;29:1041-1052.

Giannotti G, Cohn SM, Brown M, et al: Utility of near-infrared spectroscopy in the diagnosis of lower extremity compartment syndrome. J Trauma 2000;48:397-399.

Johansen K, Lynch K, Paun M, Copass MK: Non-invasive vascular tests reliably exclude occult arterial trauma in injured extremities. J Trauma 1991;31:515-522.

Jones WG II, Perry MO, Bush HL Jr: Changes in tibial blood flow in the evolving compartment syndrome. Arch Surg 1989;124:801-804.

Kerwin AJ, Bynoe RP, Murray J, et al: Liberalized screening for blunt carotid and vertebral artery injuries is justified. J Trauma 2001;51:308-314.

Lynch K, Johansen KH: Can Doppler pressure measurements replace "exclusion" arteriography in extremity trauma? Ann Surg 1991;214:737-741.

Matava MJ, Whiteside TE Jr, Seiler JG III, et al: Determination of the compartment pressure threshold of muscle ischemia in a canine model. J Trauma 1994;37:50-58.

Matsen FA III: Compartmental syndrome: a unified concept. Clin Orthop 1978;113:8-13.

Meissner M, Paun M, Johansen K: Duplex scanning for arterial trauma. Am J Surg 1991;161:552-555.

Ombrellaro MP, Stevens SL, Freeman ML, et al: Ultrasound characteristics of lower extremity venous flow for the early diagnosis of compartment syndrome: An experimental study. J Vasc Technol 1996;20:71-75.

Panetta TF, Hunt JP, Buechter KJ, et al: Duplex ultrasonography versus arteriography in the diagnosis of arterial injury: An experimental study. J Trauma 1992;33:627-635.

Perry MO: Complications of missed arterial injuries. J Vasc Surg 1993;17:399-403.

Perry MO, Thal ER, Shires GT: Management of arterial injuries. Ann Surg 1971;173:403-408.

Present DA, Nainzedeh NK, Ben-Yishay A, Mazzara JT: The evaluation of compartmental syndromes using somatosensory evoked potentials in monkeys. Clin Orthop 1993;287:376-285.

Rae-Grant AD, Eckert N, Barbourt PJ, et al: Outcome of severe brain injury: A multimodality neurophysiologic study. J Trauma 1996;40:401-407.

Richardson R, Obeid FN, Richardson JD, et al: Cerebrovascular injury: Neurologic consequences. J Trauma 1992;32:755-760.

Robbs JV, Human RR, Rajaruthnam P, et al: Neurological deficit and injuries involving the neck arteries. Br J Surg 1983;70:220-222.

Rose SC, Moore EE: Trauma angiography: The use of clinical findings to improve patient selection and care preparation. J Trauma 1988;28:240-245.

Schwartz MR, Weaver FA, Yellin AE, et al: Refining the indications for arteriography in penetrating extremity trauma: A prospective analysis. J Vasc Surg 1993;17:166-170.

Snyder WH III, Thal ER, Bridges RA, et al: The validity of normal arteriography in penetrating trauma. Arch Surg 1978;113:424-426.

Stain SC, Yellin AE, Weaver FA, et al: Selective management of nonocclusive arterial injuries. Arch Surg 1989;124:1136-1140.

Steinberg BD, Gelberman RH: Evaluation of limb compartments with suspected increased interstitial pressure: A non-invasive method for determining quantitative hardness. Clin Orthop 1994;300:248-253.

Wejdiecks EF: The diagnosis of brain death. N Engl J Med 2001;344:1215-1221.

Whiteside TE Jr, Haney TC, Morimoto K, Harada H: Tissue pressure measurements as a determinant for the need of fasciotomy. Clin Orthop 1975;113:43-51.

Zeman RK, Silverman PM, Vieco PT, Costello P: CT angiography. AJR Am J Roentgenol 1995;165:1079-1088.

PRINCIPLES OF OPERATIVE CARE

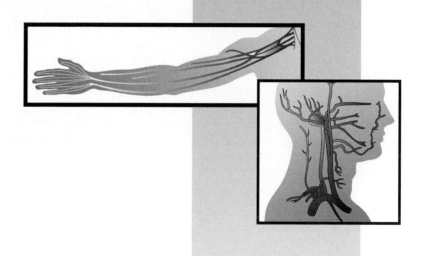

Access, Control and Repair Techniques

KENNETH L. MATTOX
ASHER HIRSHBERG

137

The repair of vascular injuries is one of the most challenging aspects of trauma for the surgeon. In the massively bleeding patient with a major vascular injury, rapid and effective exposure and control of the bleeding vessel often mark the difference between a spectacular save and on-table death from exsanguination. Despite recent advances in trauma systems, prehospital care, operative techniques, and critical care, many critically injured patients still die in the operating room (OR) from uncontrolled hemorrhage from major vessels. Vascular trauma is especially demanding also because there is a very narrow margin for technical and judgment errors. Compared with gastrointestinal injuries, for example, vascular repairs are much less forgiving and less tolerant of technical imperfection.

The operative sequence in vascular trauma consists of access, exposure, control, and repair. While the specific techniques used in addressing individual injuries are described in other chapters in this book, this chapter addresses the general principles underlying the operative approach to injuries to blood vessels. Our purpose is therefore to provide, in one location, a single comprehensive reference to operative principles in vascular trauma, with special emphasis on universal considerations that form the foundation for the control and repair of vascular injuries.

POSITIONING

Correct positioning of the injured patient on the operating table and an accurate definition of the operative field are the keys to a smooth operative procedure. Incorrect positioning can turn a straightforward operation into a technical nightmare, severely limits the surgeon's options, and reflects lack of understanding of the ramifications and potential scenarios into which the procedure may evolve.

The "generic" position of the trauma patient in the OR is in the supine position, with both arms fully extended (Fig. 7–1). One of the cardinal principles in trauma surgery is that the surgeon must be prepared to rapidly shift his or her attention to another visceral cavity, so the potential operative field for truncal trauma extends from the chin to below the knees and as far laterally as the posterior axillary lines on both sides, even if the initial procedure is

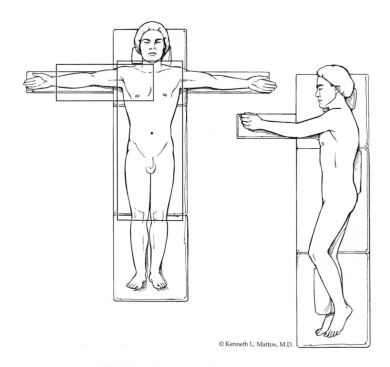

■ **FIGURE 7–1**
Drawing depicting supine and right decubitus (left chest up) positions. ■

© Kenneth L. Mattox, M.D.

focused on the abdomen or the chest. When the operative procedure is limited to an extremity, the surgeon must still be prepared for an unexpected deterioration that may require access to the chest (for chest tube placement) or the groin (for insertion of a line). Thus, for example, it would be a bad mistake to attempt to use the posterior approach to the popliteal artery in the trauma patient, because with the patient in the prone position, the surgeon's options for interventions in other anatomic locations are severely limited.

A left posterolateral thoracotomy, which is performed with the patient in a right lateral decubitus position, is a notable exception. Because gaining access to the posterior mediastinal structures (such as the descending thoracic aorta or the esophagus) through an anterolateral thoracotomy is difficult, it may occasionally be necessary to place the injured patient in the right lateral decubitus position, thus limiting access not only to the contralateral chest but also to the abdomen or the extremities. Choosing the right lateral decubitus position in the trauma patient is therefore a calculated risk that is typically undertaken only after injuries to other visceral compartments have been ruled out.

When positioning the patient for a peripheral vascular repair, the surgeon must keep in mind several important principles: The potential operative field extends at least one joint above and below the injured segment. An uninjured lower limb must be included in the field to enable rapid harvesting of the saphenous vein. For injuries in proximity to the groin or axilla, considerations of proximal control dictate that the abdomen or chest, respectively, be included in the operative field. Lastly, full mobility of the injured extremity within the operative field is mandatory to enable the surgeon to adjust the position of the relevant vascular segments as the operation unfolds.

In summary, when positioning the patient with vascular trauma, it is a good general principle to always consider the "worst-case scenario." This means not only optimizing exposure of the relevant anatomic area but also being fully prepared either for a large extension of the incision or for an urgent intervention in another visceral compartment (Box 7–1).

INITIAL HEMORRHAGE CONTROL

Initial control of external hemorrhage, whether in the field, emergency department, or OR, is one of the first priorities addressed during the primary survey of the injured patient according to Advanced Trauma Life Support principles. Control of external hemorrhage (typically from an injured extremity) is usually achieved by simple digital or manual compression, which will almost invariably control bleeding without damaging adjacent elements of the neurovascular bundle. In unusual circumstances, such as combat trauma care or a mass casualty scenario, an arterial tourniquet may be lifesaving, albeit at the price of compromising both the collateral circulation and venous drainage from the injured extremity.

The classic error in temporary control of external hemorrhage is an attempt to use surgical instruments (such as hemostats) instead of digital pressure to obtain control in the field or in the emergency department. Blind groping with hemostats in the face of ongoing torrential hemorrhage is not only ineffective but also likely to result in iatrogenic damage to the adjacent structures of the neurovascular bundle and convert a simple partial injury into a complete transection with a crushed arterial wall.

Manual compression of the bleeding site (usually by a member of the trauma team other than the surgeon) should be continuously maintained into the OR, until proper proximal and distal control is obtained. The compressing hand should then be prepared in the operative field. While the surgeon makes the incision to obtain proximal and distal control and expose the injured vessel, the first assistant should maintain external manual pressure. Selective clamping of the vessel should thus be performed under optimal conditions in the OR, away from the site of injury and using appropriate vascular instruments and technique.

B O X 7 – 1
INCISIONS USED FOR CONTROL, EXPOSURE, AND REPAIR OF VASCULAR INJURY

Anterior neck, anterior to the sternocleidomastoid muscle
Supraclavicular
Infraclavicular
Combined supraclavicular/infraclavicular
Axillary
Inner arm
Antecubital fossa
Forearm
Anterior left second interspace
Left fourth or fifth posterolateral thoracotomy
Median sternotomy with anterior cervical or supraclavicular extension
Midline laparotomy
Low transverse lateral abdominal (kidney transplant incision)
Groin incision
Medial distal thigh
Medial proximal calf
Fasciotomy incisions of the extremity

Balloon catheter tamponade is a very useful adjunct to initial control of external hemorrhage, especially for penetrating injuries to the groin, clavicular fossa, and axilla, where manual pressure is not as effective and a tourniquet cannot be applied. A Foley balloon catheter is rapidly inserted into the actively bleeding tract of a bullet or a stab wound and then is inflated. This simple maneuver creates local extraluminal compression of the injured vessel, which temporarily controls hemorrhage and frees the compressing hand of the assistant (Fig. 7–2).

General Principles of Vascular Control

Definitive control of a major vascular injury is the accurate placement of vascular clamps on both the inflow and the outflow tract of the injured vessel. This cardinal principle of obtaining proximal and distal control before approaching the injured segment is one of the fundamentals of surgery for vascular trauma, and its importance cannot be overstated.

Most vascular injuries exhibit some degree of tamponade, be it from a hemostatic plug, surrounding tissues, local pressure, spasm of the injured vessel, or a combination thereof. Entering the hematoma without first obtaining proximal and distal control away from the site of injury is the worst mistake a surgeon can commit, a mistake that often leads to unnecessary blood loss, a disorganized attempt to regain control, and sometimes exsanguination and death.

Proximal control is obtained outside the hematoma surrounding the injured segment. This frequently requires extension of the surgical incision and dissection through virgin tissue planes. An important principle in obtaining proximal control is to try and go beyond an anatomic structure that serves as a natural barrier to the expansion of the hematoma. For example, dissection in the groin to gain control of an injured common

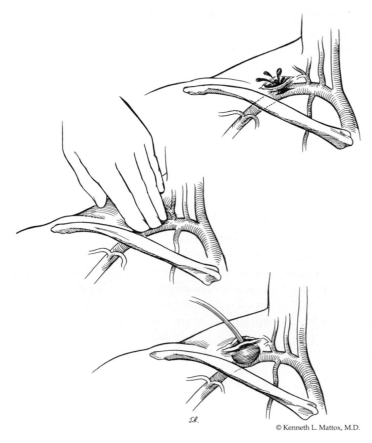

■ **FIGURE 7–2**
Drawing depicting the insertion of a balloon catheter through the site of a lower neck penetrating wound to control hemorrhage. ■

© Kenneth L. Mattox, M.D.

femoral artery is difficult and fraught with danger. If the surgeon extends the incision cranially and dissects above the inguinal ligament, he or she discovers that the ligament serves as a natural barrier to the expansion of the hematoma, and the tissue planes above it are much easier to identify. Similarly, the pericardium is a barrier to the extension of a mediastinal hematoma from an innominate artery injury, and the parietal pleura is a barrier to the extension of an axillary hematoma.

Occasionally, precise definition of the injured vessel is impossible and vigorous bleeding presents an immediate and grave danger to the patient's life. Under these circumstances, an alternative "last-resort" technique is application of a large noncrushing vascular clamp to the total gross area of active hemorrhage, including adjacent structures. Once "global" proximal and distal vascular control has been achieved, the clamp can either be removed or be gradually advanced toward the site of the specific injury as dissection proceeds in a relatively bloodless field.

Another important adjunct is the use of intraluminal Fogarty balloon catheters. When the proximal or distal segment of the injured vessel is inaccessible to direct clamping (e.g., deep in the pelvis), a useful alternative is the insertion of a Fogarty balloon catheter connected to a three-way stopcock into the orifice of the bleeding vessel. Inflation of the balloon inside the vessel lumen achieves direct intraluminal hemostasis and obviates the need for time-consuming and difficult dissection to define the vessel from the outside.

ADJUNCTS TO HEMORRHAGE CONTROL

An important aspect of hemorrhage control is fluid resuscitation. The trauma team must direct the resuscitative efforts toward controlled rather than overaggressive fluid administration. A crucial part of initial hemorrhage control is creation of a hemostatic plug, a soft clot that is formed at the site of injury by the hemostatic mechanisms of the body. Dislodgment of this clot is now presumed to occur at a lower systemic blood pressure than previously appreciated. The resuscitating team should therefore avoid attempts to achieve a blood pressure at "normal" preinjury levels and remember that a systolic pressure in the range of 80 mm Hg is actually in the bleeding patient's best interest. Aggressive resuscitation that leads to rebleeding and the need for additional fluids (the so-called "cyclic hyper-resuscitation") creates a dilutional coagulopathy, activates inflammatory mediators, and promotes further bleeding. Avoiding hypothermia and dilution, both of which directly contribute to a coagulopathic state, is also very important in enabling effective hemostasis by the coagulation cascade.

The surgeon may elect to use an intravascular temporary shunt (see Chapter 8) as a hemorrhage control technique. When inserted into an injured vessel and held in place proximally and distally, the shunt effectively controls hemorrhage while preserving distal flow. Topical hemostasis has been an aid to hemorrhage throughout history using a wide variety of hemostatic agents ranging from cellulose, thrombin-like products, and fibrin glue. The common denominator of all these topical measures is reliance on the body's physiologic hemostatic mechanisms. The benefit of the topical device is not always clear, and in the context of vascular trauma, it is never a substitute for a carefully placed vascular suture. It may however serve as a hemostatic adjunct near a vascular repair, to help control oozing from the suture line or from adjacent raw surfaces. During the last decade, topically applied "fibrin glue" has been used in liver, spleen, and raw surface bleeding. A dry fibrin dressing technology, based on thrombin powder, is under development, which has shown promise in the laboratory as being able to stop bleeding even from medium-size arteries and veins.

Recent research focuses on enhancing the body's physiologic clotting mechanism in areas of endothelial disruption. Recombinant activated factor VIIa, a hemostatic product used in the treatment of hemophilia, recently has been successful in treating coagulopathic bleeding in critically injured patients. Several case reports have led to laboratory studies in animal models. If proven effective in controlled clinical trials, this agent may represent a paradigm shift from external control to initiating focused clotting "from within."

EXPOSURE AND CONTROL OF SPECIFIC INJURIES

Gaining access and exposure to perform precise reconstruction is a surgical art form made possible by a detailed knowledge of surgical anatomy, experience, and judgment, as well as an intuitive ability to rapidly access difficult areas without adding iatrogenic injury. In vascular trauma, there are times when aggressive blunt dissection is necessary to achieve access and control, while other situations demand the most delicate touch in dissecting, exposing, and repairing a complex injury. Nowhere else in surgery is this dichotomy of the surgical craft more obvious than in a patient with a vascular injury. Some injuries pose special problems of access and hemorrhage control, primarily because the injury is not in a body area commonly operated on and familiar to the surgeon (Box 7–2).

Incisions for vascular trauma are selected with the goal of control, exposure, and repair. Some incisions are those routinely used for elective vascular reconstruction, and others have been specifically adapted for vascular trauma. Over the years, some incisions have declined in use or become obsolete. For example, the "trapdoor" incision (whereby a left supraclavicular incision is connected to an anterolateral thoracotomy incision by means of a partial median sternotomy) was found to add very little to the exposure of a vascular injury in the thoracic outlet while leading to significant chronic causalgia-like pain. The anterior thoracoabdominal incision was found to be too time consuming in the trauma setting, did not allow for adequate

BOX 7-2

LIST OF INJURIES THAT POSE SPECIAL DIFFICULT ACCESS AND HEMORRHAGE CONTROL CHALLANGES

High carotid injury
Vertebral artery hemorrhage
Thoracic outlet vascular injury
Azygous vein
Axillary artery injury
Proximal abdominal aorta
Intrathoracic inferior vena cava
Suprarenal inferior vena cava
Deep pelvic iliac vascular injury
Complex groin vascular injury
Distal popliteal/tibial vascular injury

exposure of the thoracic aorta or other thoracic vasculature, and had significant long-term healing complications (Box 7–3).

Neck

Access to virtually all vascular injuries in the neck is accomplished via an incision along the anterior border of the sternocleidomastoid muscle. The patient is positioned with the head rotated as much as possible away from the operated side and extended, with the shoulders supported. The operative field always includes the anterior chest and an uninjured lower extremity.

A typical incision for neck exploration for trauma extends from the suprasternal notch upward toward the ear lobe. Slightly curving the upper part of the incision away from the jaw will prevent inadvertent damage to the marginal mandibular branch of the facial nerve. During an exploration for penetrating trauma, and particularly in the presence of

BOX 7-3

INCISIONS THAT ARE INFREQUENTLY OR NO LONGER USED FOR VASCULAR TRAUMA

Collar neck incision
Across the clavicle incision
"Trapdoor" or "book" thoracotomy
Anterior thoracoabdominal
Posterior thoracoabdominal
Combined midline abdominal extending across the groin
Posterior popliteal
Transverse abdominal
Abdominal paramedian

active hemorrhage, many anatomic landmarks in the neck are obscured or distorted, and the surgeon has to rely on rapid identification of three key landmarks: the anterior border of the sternocleidomastoid, the internal jugular vein immediately behind it, and the facial vein.

After division of the platysma the incision "opens up," allowing identification of the anterior border of the sternocleidomastoid. Lateral retraction of the muscle and further dissection in the middle cervical fascia exposes the jugular vein (Fig. 7–3). Dissection along the anterior border of the jugular vein allows the surgeon to identify, isolate, and divide the common facial vein between ligatures. This vein, a major branch of the internal jugular, is the "gateway to the neck" because free access and exposure of the common carotid artery and its bifurcation hinges upon division of the facial vein. Furthermore, the facial vein is frequently at the level of the carotid bifurcation.

The sequence of dissection in the neck depends on the operative findings. In most cases, the focus of interest is the content of the carotid sheath, in which case dissection proceeds medial to the internal jugular vein, with special care being taken to identify and

protect the vagus nerve. However, when arterial bleeding emanates lateral to the carotid sheath, the entire neurovascular bundle (including the internal jugular vein, the carotid artery, and the vagus) should be retracted medially, and dissection lateral to this anatomic compartment will allow access to the transverse processes of the cervical vertebrae and hence to the vertebral artery, an uncommon but life-threatening source of hemorrhage.

The cardinal principle of obtaining proximal and distal control before entering the injured segment applies in the neck. Occasionally, this will entail extending the neck incision into a median sternotomy to gain proximal control at the thoracic outlet for injuries to the proximal common carotid artery (zone 1). On rare occasions with simultaneous bilateral injury, especially with a bullet across the neck ("transcervical" trajectory), a *U*- or *H*-shaped incision coming across the trachea caudally to the thyroid cartilage facilitates bilateral neck exploration or exposure of both carotid sheaths and the anterior airway.

THORACIC OUTLET

The thoracic outlet is a transitional anatomic area between the neck and the chest, where vascular injuries are difficult to access. Most surgeons infrequently operate in this area; therefore, deciding on the correct incision can be problematic.

A patient with a thoracic outlet injury may be hemodynamically stable, thus allowing a precise angiographic localization of the injury. Under these circumstances, the location of the injury dictates the incision and the operative approach. However, when the patient is actively bleeding from a vascular injury in the thoracic outlet, the decision has to rely on the clinical presentation. A penetrating injury around the distal clavicle that is bleeding externally can initially be controlled with a Foley balloon tamponade inserted into the missile tract (Fig. 7–2). An incision above and parallel to the clavicle will expose the injured vessel (see later discussion). On the other hand, a

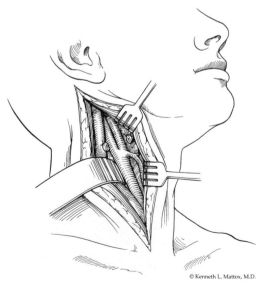

© Kenneth L. Mattox, M.D.

■ FIGURE 7–3
Drawing depicting a "standard" neck incision, anterior to the sternocleidomastoid muscle with division of the anterior facial vein. ■

hemothorax is usually associated with a more medial injury, which may require proximal control of the subclavian artery through a high anterolateral thoracotomy on the left, or a median sternotomy on the right. For a patient with a thoracic outlet hematoma evident on the chest radiograph and without supraclavicular or neck hematoma, a median sternotomy is the incision of choice.

Access to the innominate artery, proximal left carotid, intrathoracic superior vena cava, and innominate vein is via a median sternotomy. The key landmarks to performing a safe median sternotomy is to identify the sternal notch, the xiphoid, and the sternal midline, extending the incision a few centimeters below the xiphoid and opening the linea alba. A probing finger bluntly develops the space under the sternum both from below and from above behind the manubrium. One should be careful with the use of electrocautery at the manubrial notch when dividing the retrosternal ligament attachment to the anterior neck fascia, because iatrogenic injury to the innominate artery and carotid may occur. This blunt dissection just beneath the sternum is relatively easy and proceeds in a bloodless plane. The sternal saw divides the sternum from the xiphoid to the manubrium, taking care to always stay in the midline. A partial sternotomy usually does not yield appropriate exposure and should therefore be avoided. Bleeding from the edge of the sternum can be impeded by the use of electrocautery. Only in the coagulopathic patient will bone wax be required for hemostasis from the marrow of the sternum. The sternal retractor is gradually opened as dissection continues. If one immediately opens the sternal retractor to its full extent, an area of vascular injury can be "opened" more widely during forceful retraction of the sternum. In addition, excessive and over-retraction of the sternum can create rib fractures, sternal fracture, and stretch injury to the brachial plexus. The pericardium is sharply entered in the midline and the dissection is carried cephalad to the area of an injury or to the innominate vein that crosses in front of the aortic arch. This opening of the pericardium allows for the sternal retractor to be opened more widely for more exposure.

Access to the extrathoracic left subclavian artery may be difficult, especially if the arm is extended. It is best achieved with the arm prepared free and initially placed at the patient's side. Exposure of the extrathoracic portion of the subclavian artery requires an incision about one fingerbreadth above and parallel to the clavicle from the sternal notch extending laterally. After division of the platysma muscle, the clavicular portion of the sternocleidomastoid is either retracted medially or more conveniently divided. The scalene fat pad is encountered and removed, exposing the clavicular head of the sternocleidomastoid muscle and the anterior scalene muscle. The phrenic nerve crosses in front of the anterior scalene muscle and must be isolated and carefully preserved. The more posteriorly located brachial plexus should also be protected while dividing the anterior scalene muscle. It is at this point that the subclavian artery first comes into view. It can now be carefully dissected and exposed. *Care must be taken, because this is one of the most fragile arteries in the body.* Only on rare occasions where the injury is proximal to the insertion of the scalene anticus muscle will the head of the clavicle need to be removed.

In the presence of an expanding hematoma in the supraclavicular area, often it is difficult to define the anatomic landmarks. Under these circumstances, the artery can be rapidly exposed through the bed of the clavicle. The incision is made along the clavicle itself, and the bone is rapidly exposed. A periosteal elevator is used to peel off the periosteum around the clavicle and thus separate the bone from the adjacent muscles. The bone is rapidly divided as laterally as possible, lifted from its bed by grasping it with a towel clip, and the head is separated from the sternoclavicular joint and removed. The subclavius muscle is sharply divided along the bed of the clavicle, providing access to the anterior scalene muscle and the phrenic nerve.

For an extrathoracic left subclavian artery injury, a short anterior thoracotomy above the nipple (in the left second or third interspace) may facilitate looping of the intrathoracic portion of the left subclavian artery proximal to the injury (Fig. 7–4). A clamp or a snare tourniquet is then applied, which can be tightened as the subclavian injury is exposed through a separate clavicular incision. Because of rich collateral circulation, this mode of proximal control does not stop bleeding completely but does help to make the situation more amenable to repair.

An innominate artery injury may present intraoperatively as a large superior mediastinal hematoma. Blind dissection in such a hematoma is fraught with danger, because vascular structures (e.g., the innominate vein) are difficult to identify. Under these circumstances, it is often prudent to deliberately enter the pericardium, which serves as a natural barrier to the extension of the hematoma. The vessels can be identified and controlled proximally, and a bypass graft can be inserted before dissection within the hematoma itself is undertaken (Fig. 7–5).

Chest

The chest is composed of three separate visceral compartments, each accessible through different incisions. In the presence of massive

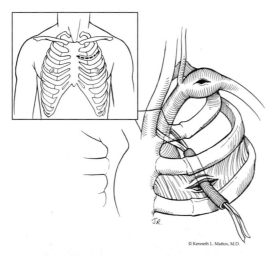

■ FIGURE 7–4
Drawing depicting an extrathoracic hematoma around the left subclavian artery and a left second interspace anterolateral thoracotomy, picking up the proximal left subclavian artery, encircling it with a ligature tourniquet (snare), to be used if necessary for vascular control when the hematoma is entered from a supraclavicular approach. ■

hemothorax, the utility incision is an anterolateral thoracotomy, because it is and easy to perform and it does not require special positioning. An anterolateral thoracotomy is performed in the fourth or fifth intercostal space on the side of the presumed injury, that is, below the nipple in the male patient or the manually retracted breast in the female patient. The incision extends from just lateral to the sternum to the midaxillary line. In the female patient, it is made in the inframammary crease. The pectoralis muscle is divided by dissection and the ribs are exposed. The intercostal muscles are divided along the upper aspect of the rib to avoid the neurovascular bundle, and the pleura is entered. A rib spreader is inserted with the handle pointing toward the axilla. Once inside the pleural cavity, the surgeon's first act is to mobilize the lung by dividing the pulmonary ligament up to the level of the inferior pulmonary vein. The lung is retracted anteriorly and the posterior mediastinum is thus exposed. In the left hemithorax, this incision provides good exposure of the descending thoracic aorta, left subclavian artery, left pulmonary artery, and pulmonary veins. In the right side of the chest, the intrathoracic inferior vena cava (IVC), right pulmonary artery, azygous vein, and superior vena cava can be seen. A transsternal bilateral anterolateral incision (clamshell) is accomplished by joining left and right anterolateral thoracostomies across the sternum using a Gigli saw, large-bone cutters, or an electric saw. Care must be taken to make the transsternal incision in the midportion of the body of the sternum, and not at the xiphoid, so a firm osseous closure will be possible at the end of the operation. Care must also be taken to identify and ligate the divided internal mammary arteries. This clamshell incision is the only one that provides access to all three thoracic cavities, albeit at the cost of slight increased morbidity.

A patient with precordial penetration who is not in extremis and whose bullet trajectory appears to be through the mid upper mediastinum is best approached via a median sternotomy. With some difficulty, this incision affords access also to the azygous vein, right main pulmonary artery, and left proximal subclavian artery.

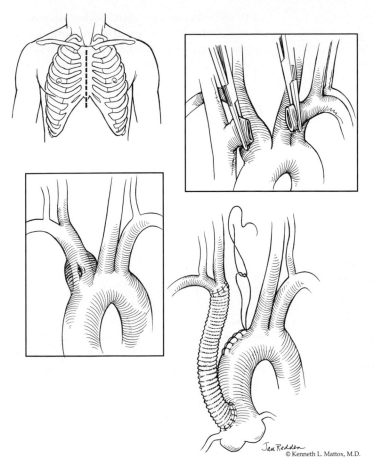

Jan Redden
© Kenneth L. Mattox, M.D.

■ **FIGURE 7–5**
Drawing of a hematoma around the innominate artery and proximal left carotid artery with a median sternotomy and ligation of the innominate vein covering this area. Also shown is a "bypass" technique from the ascending aorta (end to side) to the distal innominate artery (end to end), with oversewing of the stump of the innominate artery at the aortic arch. ■

Although a resuscitative thoracotomy is usually performed via an anterolateral thoracotomy, when a descending thoracic aortic repair is planned, a posterolateral thoracotomy is preferable. In either case, the posterior mediastinum is exposed by rotating the lung anteriorly (Fig. 7–6). Division of the parietal pleura over the posterior mediastinum and mobilization of the hilum of the lung will assist in this exposure. The esophagus is located just anterior to the aorta and the recurrent laryngeal nerve recurs around the ligamentum arteriosum. It is important not to injure these structures during access, exposure, or reconstruction.

If the surgeon performs an anterolateral thoracotomy and discovers a posterior injury (e.g., to the esophagus or the descending aorta), he or she is better advised to close the anterior incision and put the patient into a right lateral decubitus position. A left posterolateral fourth interspace incision is performed and the chest entered.

Approaching a thoracic aortic injury in its usual location just distal to the ligamentum arteriosum, the lung is retracted anteriorly. The distal thoracic aorta, well away from the hematoma is encircled first, followed by the subclavian artery as it exits the chest. At this point, the transverse arch is dissected free from the pulmonary artery and the aortic arch between the left carotid artery and the left subclavian artery is encircled. This "control" is achieved well away from the undisturbed hematoma. If the surgeon elects to use cardiopulmonary bypass or active shunting, the cannula for this adjunct can be inserted at this point.

An injury to the azygous vein is usually serendipitously discovered at emergency thoracotomy. Anterior incisions make exposure and ligation of a bleeding azygous

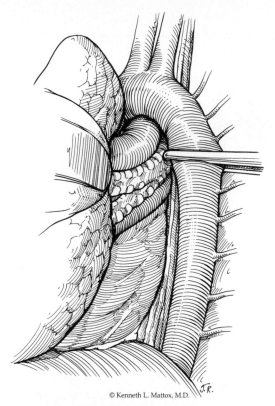

© Kenneth L. Mattox, M.D.

■ **FIGURE 7–6**
Exposure of the proximal descending thoracic aorta, by rotating the lung anteriorly and demonstrating that the esophagus is anterior to the aorta. Vascular clamp on the descending thoracic aorta as a temporary attempt to impede the rate of distal hemorrhage. ■

difficult and may require cardiopulmonary bypass, with double caval cannulation and repair of the caval injury from within the opened right atrium.

Upper Extremity

AXILLARY ARTERY

The first and second parts of the axillary artery are approached through an infraclavicular incision that extends from the mid-clavicle to the deltopectoral groove. The fibers of the pectoralis major are separated bluntly, revealing the clavipectoral fascia medial to the pectoralis minor muscle. Opening the clavipectoral fascia and dissection in the axillary fat reveals first the axillary vein and then deep and superior to it, the axillary artery with the adjacent elements of the brachial plexus. The second part of the axillary artery is exposed by hooking up and then taking down the insertion of the pectoralis minor muscle as close as possible to the coracoid process using the electrocautery (Fig. 7–7). In the presence of an axillary hematoma, it may be advisable to first obtain proximal control on the subclavian artery through a supraclavicular incision and then perform a separate axillary incision or alternatively transect the clavicle to join the incisions.

Other axillary exposures that are sometimes used in elective situations are rarely if ever used in the trauma situation. These include a lateral approach to the distal artery through a vertical incision along the lateral border of the pectoralis major or the deltopectoral groove approach. Lastly, endovascular control is possible when active extravasation is noted from the subclavian–axillary complex at angiography. A pair of occluding balloons, proximal and distal to the site of injury, will provide temporary control and minimize blood loss.

BRACHIAL ARTERY

The proximal brachial artery is usually approached via a medial upper arm incision placed in the groove between the biceps and

vein very difficult, contributing to the high mortality of this injury. Using an extra long needle holder and approaching the injury from the left side of the operating table provides the surgeon with the greatest chance for achieving suture ligation of a bleeding azygous vein.

The thoracic IVC is entirely within the pericardium and very difficult to expose. The surgeon may encounter an injury to this structure, digitally control the bleeding deep within the right lower pericardium, and then have great difficulty exposing the area for repair. Should bleeding be controlled, the trauma surgeon should call for a thoracic surgeon for assistance before attempting to proceed, because repair is exceedingly

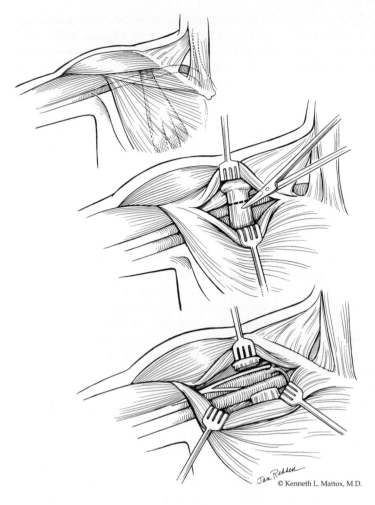

Jan Redden
© Kenneth L. Mattox, M.D.

■ **FIGURE 7–7**
Drawing of exposure of the axillary artery by division of the muscle fibers between the clavicular and pectoral portions of the pectoralis major muscle and detachment of the insertion of the pectoralis minor on the coracoid process of the scapula. ■

triceps muscles. Care should be taken in an arm with a large hematoma, as the neurovascular bundle is closer to the surface than one might expect and iatrogenic injury is to be avoided. Care must also be taken to identify any concomitant injury to the brachial vein and adjacent nerves. Dissection in the groove between the triceps and biceps muscles reveals the neurovascular bundle, and the first structure that is encountered is the median nerve, which should be carefully preserved.

A distal brachial artery injury often requires exposure at the antebrachial fossa, through a sigmoid incision that avoids crossing in the antecubital skin crease. The artery is located immediately below the biceps tendon, which can be divided with impunity. The sigmoid incision may be carried upward along the medial part of the upper arm or distally to expose the brachial artery bifurcation.

Access to vascular injuries in the extremities is based on the Henry principle of extensile exposure. Every incision can be extended proximally or distally or joined with an incision exposing a more proximal or distal vessel. Thus, the subclavian and axillary exposures can be joined by dividing the clavicle. The axillary and brachial incisions can be joined by extending the former in the deltopectoral groove across the shoulder.

Abdomen and Pelvis

Abdominal vascular injuries account for the majority of truncal vascular trauma seen in a civilian practice. These injuries are approached via a midline laparotomy incision, one of the most commonly used incisions in trauma. After incision of the skin and subcutaneous tissue using the xiphoid process and umbilicus as markers, the linea alba is gained by identifying the midline decussation of the fibers of the anterior rectus sheaths on both sides. In a trauma laparotomy, time is typically not wasted on superficial hemostasis and the entire incision is rapidly performed with a scalpel. The peritoneum is typically entered immediately above the umbilicus, where rapid atraumatic penetration of the peritoneum is usually possible. Very rarely will the surgeon choose a different incision. In a patient who is in shock and has had multiple previous operations through a midline incision, it may be wise to avoid the dense and time-consuming adhesions by rapidly performing a subcostal ("chevron" or "rooftop") incision instead.

When considering definitive control and repair of intraabdominal vascular injury, the surgeon has several distinct patterns of retroperitoneal hematoma to guide him or her to specific vascular injuries. An upper abdomen (supramesocolic) midline retroperitoneal hematoma is associated with injury to the suprarenal aorta, celiac axis, and the superior mesenteric artery. The midabdominal midline retroperitoneal (inframesocolic) hematoma is associated with proximal renal artery and infrarenal aortic or vena cava injury. A perinephric hematoma may be associated with renal or renal vascular injury. A pelvic midline hematoma is most often associated with a pelvic fracture or bladder injury, and a large or expanding lateral pelvic hematoma is associated with iliac vascular injury. A right lateral retroperitoneal hematoma suggests an IVC injury that may be infrarenal or retrohepatic. Finally, a hematoma presenting in the porta hepatis indicates an injury to the portal venous system.

Currently, initial vascular control of intraabdominal hemorrhage is achieved in the abdomen alone, initially by using laparotomy pads or manual/digital pressure.

Rapid evisceration of the small bowel will allow the surgeon to define the area of major hemorrhage. In the presence of profuse bleeding from a midline retroperitoneal hematoma, the first assistant digitally occludes the aorta at the esophageal hiatus. Use of various aortic occluding instruments is much less effective than simple digital occlusion. Virtually all abdominal venous bleeding can initially be controlled by pressure packs.

Temporary control of gross bleeding in the area of the celiac trunk often presents a difficult technical situation to the surgeon because visibility in this area is very limited without elaborate dissection. Hemostasis can sometimes be achieved with a large gross ligature, using rather large suture material, such as 1 or 0 suture on a large needle (Fig. 7–8). Although intended as a temporary

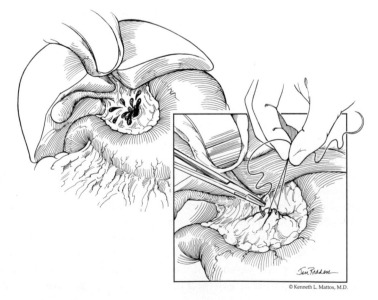

■ **FIGURE 7–8**
Drawing depicting a gross ligature of an area of gross bleeding such as in the area of the celiac axis. This suture should be rather large suture material, such as 1 or 0 suture on a large needle. This is a temporary tactic and might be removed later after other control techniques. ■

© Kenneth L. Mattox, M.D.

hemostatic maneuver, if the maneuver is effective and the surgeon is satisfied that mesenteric and hepatic injuries have not resulted from this "blind" suturing, this temporary suture may be left in place permanently.

Cross clamping of the aorta has traditionally been viewed as an important maneuver in trauma surgery. Such clamping is performed both to control exsanguinating hemorrhage in the abdomen or pelvis and as a resuscitative maneuver. Historically, this has been done by cross clamping the descending thoracic aorta in the chest, away from the site of intraabdominal bleeding (Fig. 7–6). Unfortunately, this addition of a thoracic incision in a patient with a complex abdominal injury who is already coagulopathic, acidotic, and hypothermic serves only to aggravate this often fatal triad and should therefore be avoided. The aortic cross-clamp maneuver is performed for several reasons, the most common one being to preserve the residual blood volume for vital perfusion of the heart, brain, and lungs during resuscitative emergency department thoracotomy. However, when performed for proximal control of an injury to the abdominal aorta or its visceral branches, the inexperienced surgeon rapidly discovers that because of very rich collateral circulation, this does not dry up the operative field. However, digital occlusion of the abdominal aorta at the esophageal hiatus will markedly reduce bleeding (Fig. 7–9). Numerous complications have occurred after thoracic or abdominal aortic cross clamping, especially when the procedure is performed by an inexperienced surgeon. If clamping of the supraceliac aorta is required, the safest technique is either to take down the left triangular ligament of the liver or to bluntly enter the lesser omentum and then perform a blunt digital separation of the fibers of the diaphragmatic crus immediately above and behind the origin of the abdominal aorta, as described by Veith, Gupta, and Daly (1980). The surgeon's index finger is then insinuated through the diaphragmatic crus on each side of the aorta, to create just enough space for the clamp on both sides of what is in fact the lowermost part of the thoracic aorta. Using this technique, the surgeon avoids the

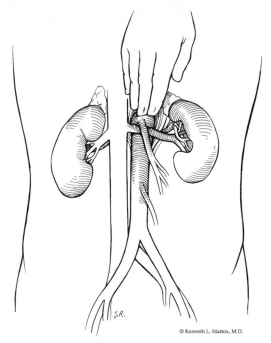

■ **FIGURE 7–9**
Drawing depicting the right hand of the first assistant (left-hand side of the patient's body), compressing the abdominal aorta, with a hematoma around the aorta at the level of the mesenteric vessels and achieving vascular control. ■

hazardous and frustrating dissection in the thick periaortic tissue that surrounds the first part of the visceral aortic segment.

Access to the injured suprarenal aorta is one of the greatest operative challenges in abdominal trauma. An anterior approach would require the stomach and pancreas to be either retracted or transected, and the dense periaortic nerve and fibrous tissue make dissection in this area difficult. A medial rotation of all the intraabdominal viscera to the patient's right from a dissection plane lateral to the left colon and going behind the spleen, kidney, and tail of the pancreas allows a lateral and relatively easy approach to the aorta. This intraoperative maneuver has been called the "Mattox maneuver" for the past 2 decades (Fig. 7–10). This dissection plane is on top of the psoas muscle and can be rapidly achieved by rapid blunt dissection that begins with the peritoneal reflection lateral to the distal descending colon and is carried upward

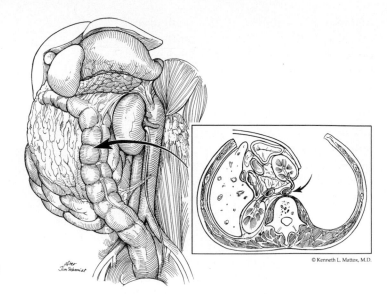

© Kenneth L. Mattox, M.D.

■ **FIGURE 7–10**
Rightward visceral rotation from the left side from the diaphragm to the iliac arteries ("Mattox maneuver"). ■

lateral to the spleen and up toward the diaphragmatic hiatus, rotating all left-sided abdominal viscera medially and exposing the abdominal aorta from the esophageal hiatus to where the external iliac arteries exit the abdomen to the groin. In most situations where this maneuver is needed, the retroperitoneal hematoma itself already achieves a significant separation of the relevant dissection planes, thus greatly facilitating the maneuver. The left lateral diaphragmatic crux can be divided and a lateral incision in the diaphragm can further expose the distal thoracic aorta for proximal control even as high as the T6 vertebra without having to open the chest. A thick fascial layer separates the aorta from the dissection plane and must be carefully incised to cleanly define the aortic wall in preparation for clamping. In the presence of proximal vascular control, the aorta loses its pulse and is a flaccid tube that is not always easy to identify in a large hematoma. As soon as the aorta is exposed, vascular clamps are then precisely placed on the injured vessel for control and reconstruction.

The infrarenal aorta is exposed by eviscerating the small bowel to the patient's right and upward, mobilizing the ligament of Treitz, and then longitudinally dividing the posterior peritoneum between the duodenum and the inferior mesenteric vein. The pitfall in this exposure is failure to identify the left renal

vein in the presence of a large infrarenal hematoma, which may lead to an iatrogenic injury and additional blood loss.

The most complete and extensive access to the mid and lower retroperitoneal structures is by performing the Cattell-Braasch maneuver, an extensive mobilization of the peritoneal structures off the aorta, vena cava, and their major branches (including the renal and iliac vessels) (Fig. 7–11). This maneuver involves division of the peritoneal attachments of the duodenum, right colon, and mesentery of the small bowel from the posterior abdominal wall. The line of incision is a triangle that begins at the lateral edge of the hepatoduodenal ligament (adjacent to the common bile duct), is carried downward to the cecum, and then upward along the insertion of the small bowel mesentery to the ligament of Treitz. This allows full rotation of the midgut from the duodenum to the transverse colon with its accompanying mesentery, up onto the anterior chest. The extended Kocher maneuver is mobilization of the duodenum and right colon only, a limited version of the full Cattell-Braasch maneuver that is often sufficient to expose vena cava injuries.

The renal vessels can be controlled either proximally ("midline looping") or by mobilizing the kidney itself and clamping across the renal hilum. Midline looping conforms to the principle of proximal control and

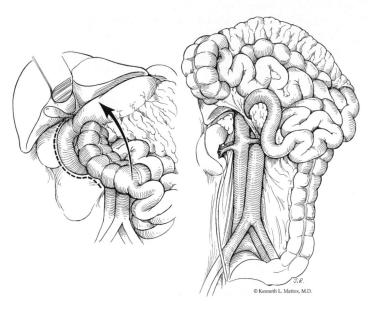

■ **FIGURE 7–11**
Drawing depicting the combined Kocher and Cattell-Braasch maneuvers showing that the movement of the duodenum, small bowel, and right colon to the left exposes the entire inferior vena cava, right renal vessels, and the right iliac vessels. ■

involves identification and isolation of the left renal vein as it crosses the aorta, and then identification and looping of the right or left renal artery as it comes off the aorta. In the presence of an actively bleeding perinephric hematoma, it is sometimes quicker to simply mobilize the entire kidney from its bed in a manner akin to a splenectomy and place a vascular noncrushing clamp en masse across the entire hilum.

Control of the portal vein between the top of the pancreas and the liver is aided by a Pringle maneuver, which consists of placing a vascular clamp across all of the structures of the porta hepatis. Under rare conditions, a "double Pringle" maneuver is performed by placing vascular clamps on either side of an injury in the hepatoduodenal ligament.

The control of portal venous injuries behind the pancreas is often challenging and can be aided by deliberate division of the neck of the pancreas (Fig. 7–12. Control by direct pressure or application of large vascular clamps is accomplished preparatory to this division. Dissection in the hepatoduodenal ligament and identification and division of the gastro-duodenal artery is the most time-consuming part of this elaborate (but sometimes lifesaving) maneuver. This procedure is the only practical way to gain access to the confluence of the splenic and superior mesenteric veins to form the portal vein.

The suprarenal retrohepatic IVC is another area of difficult exposure. A contained hematoma in this location is best left undisturbed because there are no major retrohepatic arterial structures, so the injury is invariably venous and can often be controlled with local pressure. If free bleeding from this

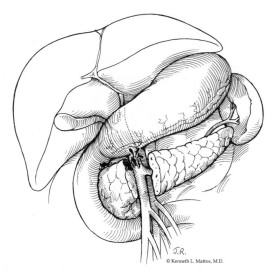

■ **FIGURE 7–12**
Drawing depicting exposure of the portal vein and proximal superior mesenteric vein, by dividing the mesenteric root and deliberately dividing the neck of the pancreas, showing the confluence of the superior mesenteric vein, and splenic vein to form the portal vein. ■

area is encountered, containment with laparotomy packs is the goal, with atrial caval shunts reserved for uncontrolled hemorrhage from the retrohepatic IVC.

Injury to the iliac vasculature, either at the confluence of the iliac veins to the IVC or at the inguinal ligament, poses several exposure and control challenges (Fig. 7–13). After opening the abdomen and discovering a hematoma in the pelvic retroperitoneum, hemorrhage control might require initially local pressure using folded sponges on a "sponge stick." This is mainly because "blind" clamping of the iliac arteries in a hematoma is likely to result in injury to the immediately underlying iliac veins or the overlying ureters. On rare occasions, large vascular occluding clamps are required to gain control en masse of both the iliac artery and the iliac vein.

A careful technique for gaining control of an iliac vascular injury in a gradual fashion has been described by Burch and colleagues (1990). Initially, the distal aorta and vena cava are clamped away from the pelvic hematoma, and the distal external iliac artery is controlled by "towing in" with a large Deaver retractor over the lower edge of the abdominal incision, thus globally compressing the external iliac vessels against the pelvic brim. As dissection proceeds into the pelvis, the upper clamps are gradually advanced distally to selectively control the injured arterial or venous segment of the iliac vasculature, a technique called "walking the clamps." On very rare occasions, the groin must be opened to gain control of backflow by occluding the common femoral artery and the deep femoral vein.

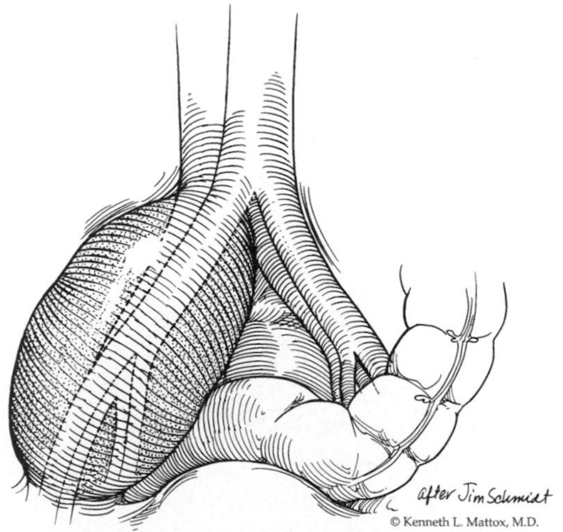

Lower Extremity

Three areas in the lower extremity are the focus of the surgeon considering a vascular injury: the groin, distal thigh, and proximal calf. At the groin, access is achieved via a routine groin incision, exposing the common femoral artery and its branches. The distal superficial femoral and proximal popliteal arteries are approached via a distal medial thigh incision.

GROIN

In the emergency department, active bleeding from the groin is often controlled by direct pressure. This challenging bleeding can also be controlled by balloon tamponade. The dilemma is whether to go into the abdomen for proximal control or to approach the injury directly in the groin. If a penetrating wound such as a gunshot injury also obviously enters the abdomen, then rapid proximal control in the abdomen is indicated because there is an independent indication for laparotomy. However, if the injury appears to be limited to the groin, options are either to do a vertical utility incision over the femoral triangle with an extension unto the inguinal ligament and then divide the ligament and gain proximal control or to first gain proximal control through an oblique incision above and parallel to the inguinal ligament and expose the external iliac vessels in this extraperitoneal location. In our experience, it is almost always possible to gain proximal control of femoral injuries in the groin. A useful trick is to identify the inguinal ligament and instead of incising it to just separate the fibers of the ligament approximately 1 to 2 cm above its shelving edge, and thus bluntly

■ FIGURE 7–13
Drawing depicting a lateral lower abdominal hematoma suggesting an injury to the iliac vasculature. ■

"penetrate" through the ligament into the retroperitoneum. This small opening is usually enough to insert a narrow and deep retractor, to feel the external iliac pulse, and to clamp the artery safely.

The technical key to a safe dissection in the groin in the presence of a vascular injury is to identify the common, superficial, and deep femoral arteries and their accompanying veins before clamping, to avoid troublesome back bleeding and to preserve the deep femoral artery. The lateral circumflex iliac vein crosses the deep femoral artery very close to its origin and is easily injured when looping of the profunda femoris is attempted in the presence of a large hematoma and hostile groin anatomy. The specific location of the injury to the femoral vessels has profound implications on the repair options. Often the surgeon must extend the initial incision to create a broader exposure than was initial thought to be sufficient.

DISTAL SUPERFICIAL FEMORAL ARTERY

A medial distal thigh incision is the "utility" approach to the distal superficial femoral artery, deep femoral vein, and proximal popliteal artery. The sartorius muscle is reflected upward or downward and Hunter's canal is opened. Proximal control can be achieved by a proximal tourniquet, proximally occluding the distal femoral artery, or control from a groin incision with exposure of the proximal superficial femoral artery. Care should be taken not to iatrogenically injure the saphenous vein or its accompanying nerve that in the thigh travels in proximity to the superficial femoral artery.

POPLITEAL ARTERY AND BRANCHES

A difficult area for vascular access is the popliteal artery. Injuries at the popliteal bifurcation are best exposed by a liberal incision below the knee, which in the presence of a large hematoma, fractures, or soft tissue destruction may begin proximal to the knee in an uninjured area and extend distally according to the principle of extensile exposure. Often adjacent nerves and veins are also injured. Although it is acceptable to cut across the pes anserinus at the medial aspect of the knee, it is less morbid to make two incisions (one above the knee and the other below the knee) if the popliteal artery injury is in the proximal or mid segment of this artery. A pneumatic tourniquet in place at the groin may assist access to the proximal tibial arteries during dissection and identification of the injured vessels.

Care must be taken to *not* injure the greater saphenous vein at the time of the skin incision so that it can serve as a collateral venous outflow tract should the popliteal vein require ligation. The contralateral leg is prepared and draped so that this uninjured site can be used for a substitute conduit if necessary.

As a useful general guideline, the major neurovascular bundles of the lower extremity are always located immediately behind the bone. This is especially important to remember in the presence of hematoma and gross anatomic distortion. Thus the distal superficial femoral artery and the popliteal artery will be found immediately behind the femur, and the popliteal bifurcation and tibioperoneal trunk will be found immediately behind the tibia. One often encounters the accompanying vein before the artery during the dissection.

The incision to expose the tibioperoneal trunk and its branches is made just posterior to the medial edge of the tibia. It is carried down to the medial head of the gastrocnemius muscle that is sharply divided off the tibia (Fig. 7–14). Often the attachments of the soleus muscle must also be detached to expose the posterior tibial and peroneal vessels. In the presence of a hematoma, it is often advisable to begin the dissection far proximally, identify and isolate the uninjured proximal popliteal segment, and then gradually advance distally toward the injury.

The medial approach affords only proximal control of the origin of the anterior tibial artery. The vessel itself is best exposed through an anterolateral incision placed approximately two fingerbreadths lateral to the anterior edge of the tibia and carried past the fascia and between the tibialis anterior and the extensor hallucis longus muscles.

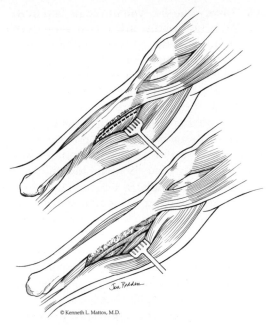

© Kenneth L. Mattox, M.D.

■ **FIGURE 7–14**
Drawing depicting a long below the knee
medial incision, division of the medial head of
the gastrocnemius muscle to expose the distal
popliteal and tibial vessels. ■

REPAIR PRINCIPLES
AND TECHNIQUES

For both vascular trauma and elective vascular reconstruction, a number of basic principles apply to all areas of vascular surgery. These
principles especially apply to the injured
vessel that may be surrounded by a hematoma,
may be actively bleeding, or may be in an area
of disrupted or "hostile" anatomy. Before any
vascular procedure, the surgeon should ascertain the availability of any special instruments,
equipment, assistants, imaging devices, or
other devices that might be required during
the procedure. After making the decision to
explore an area, gaining access and control,
and then discovering a vascular injury, the progression through repair is as follows:

Ensure proximal and distal control.

Explore the injury.

Carefully enter the hematoma.

Assess the extent of the injury or injuries.

Decide whether "vascular damage control" is
required.

Determine the amount of debridement
required.

Determine the type of repair required.

Set up the vessels for evaluation and repair by
placement of "stay sutures."

Pass Fogarty catheters to ensure the proximal
and distal clot has been removed.

Instill local heparin into the open vessels.

Apply local vascular occluding devices.

Perform the suture line.

Flush proximally and distally before completion of the suture line.

Complete the suture line.

Remove the clamps.

Assess the distal circulation.

Consider the need for fasciotomy.

Determine special post-repair requirements.

Each of these steps are not covered in detail,
but the major points of interest to the trauma
surgeon are covered.

1. **Ensure proximal and distal control.**
   To enter a hematoma without the ability
   to have proximal and distal control will
   cause the trauma surgeon to have considerable difficulty with the vascular injury
   and add to the potential for additional
   iatrogenic injury.

2. **Explore the injury.**
   The area of the hematoma or the trajectory of a wounding agent is evaluated
   and explored. Associated injuries are
   tabulated and the surgeon determines
   priorities. Because of the potential for
   exsanguinating hemorrhage and distal
   ischemia, vascular injury usually takes the
   highest priority.

3. **Carefully enter the hematoma.**
   Anatomy is often distorted following
   trauma. The surgeon enters the area of

specific vascular injury and assesses the extent of the vascular injury. Although proximal and distal control has been obtained, local control is often required, by direct digital pressure, movement of vascular clamps closer to the vascular wound, application of a partially occluding vascular clamp, and/or the use of intraluminal balloons.

4. **Decide whether "vascular damage control" is required.**
   The patient with a vascular injury presents in a hemodynamically unstable condition, often acidotic, coagulopathic, and hypothermic, thus differing considerably from the patient requiring elective vascular surgery. It is at this point that the surgeon should consider options for "vascular damage control." This might include ligation of this specific vascular injury for local hemorrhage control and performing an extra-anatomic bypass for distal perfusion. Vascular damage control might also entail the insertion of a temporary intraluminal shunt. Finally, a damage control tactic of ligation might become the final procedure if hemorrhage is controlled and distal circulation is intact.

5. **Determine the amount of debridement required.**
   The extent of an "adequate" debridement of an injured vessel is a matter of judgment. With simple lacerations and penetrations from low-velocity missiles, debridement should be to the extent to demonstrate a normal-appearing intima. With extensive arterial destruction, such as with high-velocity gunshot wounds, blast injury, and crush injury, more extensive debridement is necessary. Detection of a normal-appearing arterial wall, including an intact intima, is usually satisfactory evidence of sufficient debridement. The surgeon should closely observe the quality of both inflow and outflow because this gives some indication of problems proximal to the repair and on the adequacy of collateral circulation.

6. **Determine the type of repair required.**
   It is at this point that the surgeon determines whether the injury can be repaired by simple lateral repair, apply a patch angioplasty, perform an end-to-end anastomosis, or insert a substitute conduit. This decision might require another member of the operative team to obtain a saphenous vein from the previously prepared leg donor site.

7. **Set up the vessels for evaluation and repair by placement of "stay sutures."**
   The vessel to be repaired is "set up" for the reconstruction. This often entails the application of lateral stay sutures and establishment of a new clean operative field.

8. **Pass Fogarty catheters to ensure the proximal and distal clot has been removed.**
   A surgeon who uses Fogarty catheters only occasionally should be reminded of a number of caveats (Box 7–4). Overinflation of the balloon will cause it to rupture and potentially cause intimal injury at the site of rupture. In addition, there is a risk of remote perforation of the vessel and an increased risk to the intima with each repeated pass of the catheter. Much of the art form of using Fogarty balloon catheters is in the feel and touch of pressure or resistance felt by the surgeon at the time of advancing the catheter, inflation of the balloon, and extraction of the catheter. At least two "clean" passes should be made before declaring that an artery is free from distal clots. The operating surgeon should control three items simultaneously: the pressure on the syringe connected to the Fogarty balloon catheter, the pull of the catheter extracting any clots, and the orifice of the vessel. Many surgeons will infuse a small amount of heparinized saline after the final pass of the catheter as the clamp is reapplied to the vessel.

9. **Instill local heparin into the open vessels.**
   Systemic anticoagulation is rarely used in patients with acute trauma, especially with

BOX 7–4
CAVEATS IN THE USE OF FOGARTY CATHETERS
IN VASCULAR TRAUMA

Choose the smallest balloon that will accomplish the task required.

Estimate the size of the most distal site to which the balloon is to be inserted in determining the size of the balloon to be used.

Always read the volume of liquid required to inflate the balloon.

Put *only* the volume of liquid required to inflate the balloon in the syringe used for inflation.

Test the balloon inflation before insertion into the artery to ensure that the balloon is functional and to see the diameter of the inflated balloon.

Always advance the ballooned catheter with the balloon deflated.

Always advance the balloon with the surgeon's fingers, not an instrument.

Should resistance be met, further advancement should *not* be attempted.

Remember that the Fogarty catheter can perforate an artery if forced.

The surgeon who advances the catheter should inflate the balloon, and if resistance is met, the balloon should not be inflated further.

With the balloon inflated, the catheter should be withdrawn. During the withdrawal if the surgeon meets resistance, the balloon should be allowed to deflate slightly before beginning the withdrawal anew.

Remember that an overinflated Fogarty balloon can tear the intima of an artery and forcibly extract long segments of intima, denuding the interior of the artery.

Should clot be removed, a second pass should be accomplished.

Passes to the distal artery should continue until no clot remains to be removed.

multisystem acute trauma. The trauma and/or vascular surgeon is always concerned about coagulopathies and worried that with systemic heparinization, hemorrhage at the sites of injury will compound those injuries, especially the head and orthopedic trauma. Furthermore, many trauma patients often are already somewhat, if not frankly, coagulopathic by the time they get to the OR. Aggressive crystalloid fluid resuscitation of as little as 750 mL of fluid results in a statistically difference in the clotting studies compared with matched patients who received little or no resuscitative fluid. The first concern of a trauma surgeon is that no new factors are introduced that would contribute to a coagulopathy. Hypother-

mia, dilution of clotting factors, and addition of drugs that alter clotting all contribute to a coagulopathy.

Except for patients who are placed on total cardiopulmonary bypass, systemic anticoagulation is avoided acutely in the trauma patient. However, under certain circumstances, systemic heparinization may be in the patient's best interest. When the arterial injury is the result of a single penetrating injury (such as a stab wound to the brachial artery), the risk of bleeding is minimal, and in a teaching situation or when the reconstruction is very time consuming, systemic heparinization may be considered. Similarly, in the presence of severe and prolonged distal ischemia (e.g., when a first reconstruction is unsatisfactory and an immediate redo is required), when there is concern about clotting of the microcirculation and irreversible damage, again systemic heparin may be considered provided that no other injuries are likely to bleed.

Most patients with vascular injury undergo operation in this acute period. Many trauma patients with vascular trauma have undergone a series of arteriograms in the angiographic suite, where repeated aliquots of heparin have been administered. Should an early operation follow, the surgeon would be well served to determine the level of anticoagulation by an intraoperative determination of the activated clotting time.

Many surgeons will consider the administration of heparin to patients with an acute, totally occluded artery, to preserve distal function, with the theory being that collaterals and venous return are preventing from thrombosing. Whether this is true for trauma patients, who are already relatively coagulopathic, is unknown. Because many of the coagulation profiles available in many hospitals report a result at least 1 to 2 hours after the blood was obtained and the patient's coagulation status may have changed considerably in that period, tests that demonstrate concurrent status are preferred. Most trauma centers also have either cardiac or vascular surgical capability and have equipment to measure an activated clotting time available in the ORs; this test is preferred. The activated clotting time is well recognized by cardiac surgeons to be an excellent determinant of the effect of heparin on clotting activity.

Many surgeons elect to inject through the open ends of an injured vessel proximally and distally small aliquots of heparinized saline. These solutions contain a variable number of units of heparin, depending on the local recipe. Often these "local" injections result in a "systemic" heparinization dose, which literally occurs within minutes of the infusion.

10. **Apply local vascular occluding devices.**
   The locally applied vascular occluding device should be noncrushing and gentle to the vessel. A vascular clamp should *not* be maximally applied but closed only to the extent required to prevent bleeding from the open ends of the vessel. In some locations, a customized snare tourniquet allows for the occlusion to be complete but keeps the instruments out of the operative field. In other instances, intraluminal balloon catheters serve as the occluding device.

11. **Perform the suture line.**
   Anastomoses must be tension free and carefully constructed to create an everted, smoothly coapted layer of intact and healthy intima. The surgeon should wear magnifying loupes if necessary, especially for small vascular reconstructions. Several options exist for vascular trauma reconstruction.

   a. **Simple vascular repair techniques**
      Any vascular reconstruction in vascular trauma should be tailored to both the patient's condition and the particular injury encountered. There is no single "practice guideline" that is applicable to every injury. A large number of acceptable standards of practice exist. For instance, for an unstable patient with extensive truncal injury, an extremity arterial injury may be left unreconstructed to focus on a critical life-threatening truncal injury. In such an omission or delay, an amputation might be the ultimate outcome in a patient who is now alive because the truncal and cerebral injuries were addressed. Several simple approaches to vascular reconstruction exist.
      A "simple" vascular repair technique is a lateral venorrhaphy or arteriorrhaphy. Should lateral arteriorrhaphy or venorrhaphy be accomplished without narrowing the vessel and without tension on the suture line, this technique is the preferred approach over more complex vascular

repair techniques. Lateral repair is sometimes performed in a linear and at other times in a horizontal manner. In principle, the axis of the suture line should be oriented perpendicular to the axis of the vessel, to avoid narrowing. However, in special circumstances when the vessel is large (such as the IVC) and a perpendicular repair is impossible, a suture line parallel to the axis of the vessel is an acceptable second-best approach.

The choice relates to the size of the vessel and the surgeon's preference. Surgeons choose the smallest suture material possible to accomplish the closure safely, most often using polypropylene suture material.

Ligation of a bleeding vessel has been a form of vascular control/repair, because the word *suture* was used in the Edwin Smith Surgical Papyrus. The ancient and modern literature aptly demonstrates the natural history following ligation (or thrombosis) of major arteries and some major veins, that being distal ischemia and loss of the distal organ, often expressed as an amputation. Ligation is an option in almost all venous injuries and in a number of arterial injuries when the patient's condition and overall trauma burden preclude a reconstruction. Examples of arteries that can be ligated include subclavian, internal iliac, superficial femoral, one of the tree distal vessels in the lower arm or calf. In other instances, ligation (e.g., external iliac artery) may be required for hemorrhage control in a very complex injury, where a secondary reconstruction outside the major injury is accomplished (a femoral-femoral arterial crossover graft). Ligation of one of paired arteries (brachial and ulnar arteries, anterior and posterior tibial arteries) is tolerated provided distal crossover collateral circulation exists (as in the case of an intact palmar arterial arch). If ligation is used as a procedure of choice for vascular hemorrhage

control, the surgeon must early and frequently assess the viability and function of the circulation distal to the ligature and make a decision if secondary procedures are indicated.

b. End-to-end repair
If a lateral arteriorrhaphy or venorrhaphy is not possible, an end-to-end repair is preferable if possible. Such an anastomosis must be tension free. When debridement has occurred, it may be very difficult to bring the vessel ends together into a tension-free anastomosis. Mobilization of an artery by tying off branches in order to "gain length" is time consuming and often leads to the need for revision. Our preference is, when an artery is completely transected and debrided, to consider the insertion of a substitute conduit. Often a microscope or magnifying loupes are used for very small vessels. For very small vessel anastomoses, an interrupted suture line has greater long-term patency. Precision in the performance of a vascular anastomosis is paramount to immediate and long-term patency. The smaller the vessel, the more unforgiving of lack of precision and attention to detail. As with the use of Fogarty balloons, a number of principles exist relating to the performance of a vascular anastomosis (Box 7–5). With an exercise of precision and abiding by these principles, the surgeon should expect a high degree of success from the vascular anastomosis. Reasons for failure include lack of distal flow, lack of inflow, narrowed anastomosis, presence of distal clot, and kinking of the conduit, among others.

For a continuous anastomosis, the surgeon should use "triangulation" or lateral "stay" suture techniques to ensure that the anastomosis is not narrowed. The first assistant must be vigilant to ensure that the continuous anastomosis is not "purse stringed" by the assistant pulling to tightly on the suture as he or she follows for the

BOX 7-5

PRINCIPLES RELATING TO THE PERFORMANCE OF A VASCULAR ANASTOMOSIS

The anastomosis must be tension free.

Consideration must be given to the various positions of the adjacent and distal anatomy after repair.

Consideration should be made for redundancy to allow for full extension of an extremity after reconstruction.

Consideration must be made regarding coverage of the repair.

The suture material must be nonabsorbable.

The finest suture material to accomplish a permanent anastomosis should be selected.

The needle size and shape should be chosen to maximize an ideal anastomosis.

The needle must enter the vessel at a right angle.

The rotation on the needle should follow the curve of the needle.

The needle should be grasped with the needle driver somewhere between the middle of the curve and the tip.

The suture material should not be used to "pull" the anastomosis together but lie together without tension.

surgeon. Another consideration is to spatulate the anastomosis to make the anastomosis actually larger than the repaired vessel. Some end-to-end anastomoses are accomplished using vascular staples. Some appropriately chosen techniques should be used to determine the adequacy of the anastomosis at the completion of the procedure. Some surgeons choose Doppler ultrasound, and others will use arteriography, depending on the size of the vessel.

c. Insertion of a substitute conduit

A substitute interposition conduit has been used extensively in vascular trauma. An interposition (end-to-end, end-to-side, or side-to-side) conduit is used when extensive destruction exists and one of the other reconstruction options does not exist. Considerable discussion, debate, and research have focused on the synthetic versus autogenous conduits. This concern basi-

cally comes down to a consideration in only two locations, the superficial femoral and the subclavian arteries. In the trunk, use of PTFE or Dacron prostheses are an issue of size match and durability. Long-term favorable results have been extensively reported. In the neck, distal extremities, and smaller truncal arteries, the size match of currently available prostheses is unacceptable and use of the scavenged saphenous vein is most appropriate. Currently, for vessels 5 mm or smaller, the use of the saphenous vein is the preferred conduit.

Debate has also occurred regarding which graft material to use in the presence of potential infection. One option would be to use ligation and extra-anatomic routing around the area of infection when potential or real infection occurs. In some instances, such as reconstruction of an injured abdominal aorta, it is virtually impossible to avoid reconstruction in an area of potential infection. In other instances, infection is not a consideration until a graft is later exposed, or a secondary infection or abscess occurs in an area of infection. Another argument has been whether venous or arterial autografts are "living" at the time that the conduit is scavenged and repositioned elsewhere, devoid of its vasovasorium. A case can be made that this (foreign body) collagen tube becomes "living" after it has become re-endothelized at a later date. If this is correct, all substitute conduits— regardless of being autologous, homologous, frozen, xenographic, or manufactured—the infectious risk should be similar. Despite the use of Dacron substitute conduits in the injured abdominal aorta for almost all reported successfully managed cases and a high rate of enteric contamination at the time of implantation, no infected aortic grafts in these cases have been documented in the literature. Other synthetic grafts, such as those constructed with PTFE, have been percutaneously punctured and yet have a suggested "resistance to infection." More than 30 laboratory studies have been reported in which purposeful infections have been created around grafts, comparing synthetic with autogenous material. The infectivity is almost identical, but the complications are different, both in the laboratory and in people. With synthetic conduits, perigraft infections result in either suture line aneurysms, thrombosis of the graft, or occasionally sepsis from chronic graft infection. With "autogenous" conduits, periconduit infections result in dissolution of the collagen tube, distal embolization, and often exsanguinating hemorrhage, sometimes uncontrollable.

Although end-to-end anastomoses are often used at both ends of the substitute conduit, consideration for an end-to-side reconstruction at either end or both ends of the conduit war-

rants consideration. In some instances, such as injury to the popliteal artery, immediately behind the knee, this variation offers an additional option with long-term favorable results.

d. Patch angioplasty
Patch angioplasty using autogenous venous material is actually used very infrequently in vascular trauma. When it is used, it is often as a secondary procedure to correct a narrowing at a previous reconstruction. With current technology, a catheter-based interventional dilation and stenting would precede a secondary open procedure to widen a previously constructed vascular repair.

12. **Flush proximally and distally before completion of the suture line.**
Before the completion of the suture line, the proximal and distal clamps are temporally removed to ensure that prograde and retrograde back bleeding occurs. If there is *no* back bleeding from the distal suture line, one might consider another pass of the Fogarty catheter.

13. **Complete the suture line/clamp removal.**
When the surgeon is ensured that inflow and outflow are adequate, the suture line is completed and the clamps are removed.

14. **Assess the distal circulation.**
After completion of a vascular reconstruction, the surgeon must evaluate the adequacy of the anastomosis for any stenosis, kinking of the prosthesis, and patency of the distal outflow tract. This is best accomplished using completion arteriography, which despite the availability of Doppler and ultrasound technologies still remains the "gold standard." However, in the critically injured patient, there may not be time for a completion study. When dealing with large arteries, such as the iliac, subclavian, and femoral vessels, a good distal pulse and a normal triphasic Doppler signal are often taken

as evidence of a technically satisfactory repair. The best time to accomplish any needed re-reconstruction is at the time of the first operation.

15. Consider the need for fasciotomy.

Fasciotomy and compartment syndromes are addressed in Chapter 23. In cases of an ischemic limb for more than 4 hours, the surgeon is well advised to consider performing a fasciotomy before a vascular reconstruction. In cases of ligation of an outflow vein, especially the iliac, axillary, deep femoral, or popliteal veins, a postrepair fasciotomy is strongly encouraged. If there be any concern for the performance of a fasciotomy, compartment pressures can be measured. Although debate exists concerning the exact pressures where a fasciotomy must be performed, compartment pressures of more than 30 cm H_2O should cause the surgeon to strongly consider the procedure.

16. Ensure appropriate coverage.

A cardinal principle in vascular trauma is that a vascular reconstruction must always be covered with viable soft tissue; otherwise, failure with catastrophic bleeding is all but certain. Coverage can be achieved using various techniques, but in the presence of massive soft tissue destruction, covering an arterial graft with viable soft tissue can be both challenging and time consuming. Most often, coverage is with the tissue within the operative field, which in the normal closure adequately covers the vascular repair. On occasion, special flaps will be necessary to bring vascularized pedicles over the reconstruction. In extremely rare situations, use of porcine xenograft or homograft material might be neces-sary to temporarily cover a vascular reconstruction.

The trauma surgeon undertaking a vascular reconstruction must keep in mind the importance of soft tissue coverage because occasionally an unusual or unorthodox extra-anatomic route will be selected for the graft just because the conventional anatomic route is exposed or will present a cover problem.

SUMMARY

This chapter is intended to communicate the fundamentals required by a general surgeon approaching a patient with a suspected or proven vascular injury upon arrival in the OR. The principle of initial control of external hemorrhage is followed by considerations for positioning on the OR table and determination of incision placement.

Fundamental in approaching a vascular injury is initially obtaining access and control *away* from the area of suspected injury so no additional injury ensues as the area of specific injury and hemorrhage is dissected. An area-by-area review of some general access and control suggestions is provided for specific injuries.

Finally, some general repair techniques are presented, which are standard for the reconstruction of any vascular injury.

REFERENCES

Buckman RF, Miraliakbari R, Badellino MM: Juxtahepatic venous injuries: A critical review of reported management strategies. J Trauma 2000;48:978-983.

Burch JM, Richardson RJ, Martin RR, Mattox KL: Penetrating iliac vascular injuries: Recent experience with 233 consecutive patients. J Trauma 1990;30:1450-1459.

Feliciano DV, Burch JM, Mattox KL, et al: Balloon catheter tamponade in cardiovascular wounds. Am J Surg 1990;160:583-587.

Henry AK: Extensile Exposure, 2nd ed. Baltimore: Williams & Wilkins, 1957.

Hoyt DB, Coimbra R, Potenza BM, Rappold JF: Anatomic exposures for vascular injuries. Surg Clin North Am 2001 Dec;81(6):1299-1330.

Martin RR, Barcia PJ, Johnson EA: Making matters worse: Complications of initial evaluation, treatment and delayed diagnosis. In Mattox KL (ed): Complications of Trauma. New York, Churchill Livingstone, 1994, pp 139-154.

Mattox KL: Red River anthology. J Trauma 1997; 42:353-368.

Mattox KL, Hirshberg A: Vascular trauma in vascular surgery. In Haimovici H, Ascer E, Hollier LH, et al (eds): Haimovici's Vascular Surgery—

Principles and Techniques, 4th ed. Cambridge, Mass, Blackwell Scientific, 1995.

Mattox KL, McCollum WB, Jordan GL Jr, et al: Management of penetrating injuries of the suprarenal aorta. J Trauma 1975;15:808-815.

Rutherford RB: Atlas of Vascular Surgery. Basic Techniques and Exposures. Philadelphia, Harcourt Brace Jovanovich, 1993.

Surgical exposure of vessels. In Haimovici H, Ascer E, Hollier LH, et al (eds): Haimovici's Vascular Surgery—Principles and Techniques, 4th ed. Cambridge, Mass, Blackwell Scientific, 1995, pp 351-420.

Veith FJ, Gupta S, Daly V: Technique for occluding the surpaceliac aorta through the abdomen. Surg Gynecol Obstet 1980;151(3): 426-428.

Wind GG, Valentine RJ: Anatomic Exposures in Vascular Surgery. Baltimore, Williams & Wilkins, 1991.

Damage Control for Vascular Trauma

ASHER HIRSHBERG
BRADFORD G. SCOTT

INTRODUCTION

"Damage control" is a surgical strategy for the staged management of multivisceral trauma that represents a major paradigm shift in trauma surgery. With this approach, the traditional single definitive operation is replaced by a staged repair, whereby a rapid "bailout" operation (to control hemorrhage and spillage) is followed by a delayed reconstruction after the patient's physiology has been stabilized. In the last decade, this approach has become part of the standard repertoire of trauma surgeons when operating on their most critically wounded patients.

Major vascular trauma is often part of the injury complex in patients with exsanguinating hemorrhage in whom the damage-control approach is the patient's only hope. Therefore, a detailed acquaintance with this strategy and its application to the management of arterial and venous injuries is mandatory for every surgeon involved in trauma care.

Damage control for vascular injuries is particularly challenging because of the inherent conflict between the need for a precise and time-consuming vascular reconstruction on

165

the one hand and the urgency of an abbreviated procedure on the other. However, the futility of attempting a complex arterial repair in the presence of diffuse coagulopathy should be quite obvious even to a surgeon who is unacquainted with the damage-control strategy.

The concept of staged repair in emergencies is not new to vascular surgeons. For example, the current operative management of infected intra-abdominal aortic grafts often consists of a two-stage operation whereby an extra-anatomic bypass is inserted first, and removal of the infected graft is delayed for a subsequent procedure. The reason for this is not technical, but it is the desire to avoid a huge physiologic insult in a compromised patient. Similarly, a staged repair of a bleeding aortoduodenal fistula (the first operation consisting of temporary control of bleeding and of the duodenal perforation much like in a damage-control procedure) has been advocated as a more effective approach than the traditional one-stage operation because the results of the latter carry a prohibitive mortality.

This chapter presents the general philosophy of damage control and the underlying physiologic considerations that form the rationale for employing the strategy. This will then serve as a background for a discussion of the application of damage-control principles to the modern management of vascular trauma, and a detailed description of specific "bailout" techniques for the management of major arterial and venous injuries.

EVOLUTION OF THE DAMAGE-CONTROL CONCEPT

During the past 2 decades, civilian trauma surgeons have encountered new wounding patterns characterized by high-energy transfers (from automatic weapons and fast motor vehicles) causing extensive damage to multiple organs and massive blood loss. These exsanguinating patients, who previously would have died before reaching the hospital, are now rapidly transferred to trauma centers by efficient prehospital systems, presenting surgeons with an unusual array of challenges. The conventional operative sequence for trauma, consisting of rapid access, bleeding control, and reconstruction, is inappropriate in these exsanguinating patients. Such definitive repair usually requires lengthy and complex procedures, which these critically ill patients will not tolerate. The result of heroic attempts at definitive repairs has typically been early postoperative death due to "irreversible shock," diffuse coagulopathic bleeding or multiple organ system failure. These considerations have led to the development of the damage-control approach, a modified operative sequence whereby only immediately life-threatening visceral injuries are addressed using rapid temporary lifesaving measures. The patient is then transferred to the surgical intensive care unit (ICU) for rewarming and resuscitation, and definitive repair of the injuries is postponed until reoperation can be performed on a nonbleeding, stable patient with restituted physiologic parameters (see Table 8–1).

Damage control represents a profound change in the way trauma surgeons view their role in the operating room. The center of attention has shifted from reconstruction of the anatomy to restitution of the injured patient's physiologic reserves. In other words, the completeness of the anatomic repair is temporarily sacrificed to address the physiologic insult before it becomes irreversible. Herein lies the fundamental difference between the traditional approach of a single definitive procedure and the damage-control approach of a staged repair.

Trauma surgeons were slow to adopt this unconventional strategy because abrupt termination of an "unfinished" operation and acceptance of a temporary and anatomically incomplete repair seemed to contrast with traditional surgical values. This is why almost a decade passed between the original description of the strategy in patients with coagulopathy by Stone, Strom, and Mullins in 1983 and the publication of the first large series in the early 1990s. Gradual adoption of damage control as a valid alternative to the traditional definitive operation evolved slowly (see Table 8–1). In the mid-1990s, the new approach was expanded to the management of urologic, thoracic, vascular, and even limb injuries.

TABLE 8–1
THE EVOLUTION OF "DAMAGE CONTROL"

Period	Key Development	References
1983	Staged approach to coagulopathy	Stone, Strom, and Mullins
1982-1990	Sporadic technical reports Balloon catheter tamponade	Feliciano and colleagues (1990)
1991	Largest series (200 patients) and philosophy explained	Burch and colleagues (1992)
1992	"Damage control" coined	Rotondo and colleagues (1993)
1992-1994	New concept gains acceptance	Morris and colleagues (1993)
1994-1997	Extension outside abdomen	Hirshberg et al (7) Wall and colleagues (1994) Porter and colleagues (1997) Scalea and colleagues (1994)
1997-Present	Attempts to define physiological envelope	Cosgriff and colleagues (1997) Cushman and colleagues (1997) Garrison and colleagues (1996)

The Physiologic Envelope

The concept of the "physiologic envelope" is key to understanding the rationale of damage control. Despite technologic advances, the operating room remains a physiologically unfavorable environment for the severely wounded patient. Extensive peritoneal exposure during a trauma laparotomy results in accelerated heat loss, which is further aggravated by massive transfusion. Hypothermia in turn impairs blood clotting and thus contributes to ongoing hemorrhage. Shock leads to metabolic acidosis and a subsequent need for further transfusion. The most obvious manifestation of the injured patient's physiologic derangement is, therefore, the triad of hypothermia coagulopathy and acidosis. Together these derangements create a self-propagating vicious cycle that eventually leads to an irreversible physiologic insult. This irreversibility may present intraoperatively as diffuse bleeding that cannot be controlled surgically, followed by refractory ventricular arrhythmias and death. More commonly, the patient survives the operation only to exhibit a refractory systolic blood pressure of 60 to 80 mm Hg, oliguria, peripheral vasoconstriction, massive swelling, progressive

hypoxemia, and diffuse oozing from every incision and vascular access site. Death almost invariably ensues within the first few postoperative hours.

Thus, the triad of hypothermia, coagulopathy, and acidosis defines the patient's physiologic envelope, a set of physiologic parameters that together mark the boundary between a survivable physiologic insult and an irreversible derangement. Termination of the operative procedure before this physiologic envelope is breached is the essence of damage control.

Hypothermia has emerged as a central pathophysiologic event in exsanguinating trauma patients. Shocked patients with penetrating torso injuries lose body heat to a mean temperature of 34.5°C by the time they reach the operating room. The ambient temperature in the operating room is around 22°C, and rapid infusion of crystalloids or blood without a warming device contributes to the fast development of hypothermia. The open peritoneal cavity itself is also a major source of accelerated heat loss. It has been clearly shown that in the severely injured patient, hypothermia is harmful and adversely affects survival independent of injury severity. Of the three components of the physiologic envelope, hypothermia is the only one for which there is a well-defined threshold value. In 1987, Jurkovich and colleagues convincingly demonstrated that in severely wounded patients undergoing laparotomy, a core temperature less than 32°C is associated with 100% mortality. Based on this observation, a mathematical model of intraoperative heat loss during laparotomy for exsanguinating hemorrhage predicts a window of opportunity of no more than 60 to 90 minutes before this threshold is reached.

Coagulopathy typically presents as diffuse oozing inside and outside the operative field. Attention has focused on hypothermia as the cause of coagulopathy in trauma. Hypothermia affects clotting through alteration of platelet function and inhibition of the coagulation cascade. In the hypothermic patient, platelets are sequestered in the liver and spleen and exhibit marked morphologic changes. Platelet activation is inhibited resulting in prolongation of the bleeding time and other abnormal platelet function test results. The enzymes of the coagulation cascade are temperature sensitive and therefore are inhibited during hypothermia. However, both platelet dysfunction and enzyme inhibition become clinically important only when the core temperature drops to less than 32°C, which is well below the usual range seen in the severely injured.

Hemodilution is another important cause of coagulopathy in exsanguinating patients. Extensive blood loss and massive replacement with packed cells and crystalloids combine to produce rapid "washout" of platelets and clotting factors. Because many of the patients undergoing damage-control operations require massive transfusion, and because the actual blood volume of these patients changes rapidly and is difficult to quantify, dilution is probably an underestimated contributor to coagulopathy. Hypothermia and dilution also have been clearly shown to have an additive effect in causing clotting abnormalities.

Coagulopathy in the critically injured patient is a clinical and not a laboratory diagnosis. Standard coagulation tests often fail to reflect the full magnitude of the clotting disorder in these patients because they are routinely conducted at 37°C and often take too long to be useful guides for real-time replacement of clotting factors in the exsanguinating patient.

Lactic acidosis is the result of anaerobic glycolysis and reflects inadequate tissue perfusion. Acidosis adversely affects myocardial contractility and cardiac output in animal models, but the full scope of its physiologic and metabolic effects remains unclear. Acidosis is a useful measure of the severity of shock and a reliable predictor of survival. Serum lactate levels, base deficit, and the time interval to normalization of the serum lactate have all been shown to closely correlate with mortality from severe trauma in both animal and clinical studies. However, no well-defined threshold value for lactic acidosis can serve as a marker of irreversible shock.

Several attempts were made to better define the physiologic envelope. Cosgriff and colleagues (1997) analyzed prospectively collected physiologic data from 58 injured patients who received massive transfusions, and they identified four significant risk factors that predict the onset of coagulopathy: pH < 7.10, temperature <34°C, Injury Severity Score >25, and systolic blood pressure <70 mm Hg. About one in four severely injured patients requiring massive transfusion developed coagulopathy, but when all four risk factors were present, the probability of developing coagulopathy was 98%. In another study, Cushman and colleagues (1997) attempted to quantify the physiologic envelope in a series of 53 patients with iliac vascular injuries. Their study showed that an initial pH level of less than 7.1 and a final operating room temperature of less than 35°C were the best predictors of imminent death.

Practical Application of "Damage Control"

The damage-control sequence consists of three phases: initial operation, surgical ICU resuscitation, and planned reoperation. The initial operation is typically a rapid "bailout" procedure in which the surgeon does only the absolute minimum necessary to save the patient's life. Rapid temporary techniques are used to control bleeding, prevent spillage of intestinal content or urine, restore blood flow to vital vascular beds, and achieve rapid closure of the abdomen or chest. Time-consuming formal resections and reconstructions are deliberately avoided.

Bleeding from solid organs (such as the liver) or diffusely oozing cavities (such as the retroperitoneum) is controlled by packing. Spillage of intestinal content is controlled by ligation or stapling of bowel injuries without resection, or by external tube drainage of duodenal, pancreatic, and common bile duct injuries. Similar spillage-control techniques have been applied to injuries of the urinary tract. In the chest, stapled nonanatomic lung resection and laying open a bullet tract through the lung parenchyma to control bleeding (instead of resection) enable rapid termination of the operative procedure in accordance with damage-control principles.

Closure of the injured cavity is performed rapidly using temporary measures, such as skin-only closure by a running monofilament suture. In the presence of massive visceral edema that precludes skin closure without tension, plastic silos or absorbable mesh is used to temporarily accommodate and protect the edematous viscera.

The second phase of the sequence is resuscitation in the surgical ICU. Aggressive correction of hypothermia is the most important consideration in the early postoperative period. This can usually be achieved using vigorous external rewarming, but arteriovenous rewarming can greatly expedite the process in severely hypothermic patients. Empirical replacement of blood, plasma, and platelets is equally important to restore normal hemostasis. Support of the cardiovascular system focuses initially on volume replacement. The early use of invasive cardiovascular monitoring (a soon as the patient's coagulopathy is corrected) may be a useful adjunct. To achieve a favorable outcome, these patients require a direct and massive investment of bedside time and continuous direct involvement of the trauma team in the early postoperative period.

Not uncommonly, patients may require an urgent (unplanned) reoperation during the second phase of the damage-control sequence. The main indication for urgent reoperation is ongoing hemorrhage. This is usually the

result of either failed hemostasis during the "bailout" procedure, a missed injury, or an iatrogenic trauma. Other indications for an urgent reoperation are intra-abdominal hypertension and limb ischemia distal to an indwelling temporary intraluminal shunt.

Planned reoperation is undertaken in a stable patient, usually within 2 to 3 days of the initial "bailout" procedure. The aims at this stage are to perform a definitive repair of the injuries and to accomplish formal closure of the visceral cavity.

Although most trauma cases are effectively managed using the traditional approach of a single definitive operation, the damage-control approach is indicated only in a small group of the most critically injured patients, and one of the major problems facing the surgeon is deciding when to employ it.

Formally stated, *damage control* is indicated when the magnitude of the visceral damage is such that definitive repair of all injuries is likely to exceed the patient's physiologic limits. However, this is a simplified definition of a complex and multidimensional dilemma. Making the decision early, within a few minutes of entering the injured cavity, is one of the keys to successful damage control. Garrison and colleagues (1996) have shown that an early decision to perform packing is an important determinant of survival in abdominal trauma, because deterioration in coagulation, low pH level, and long duration of hypotension are all associated with a decreased chance of survival.

Because no good qualitative definition of the point at which the physiologic insult becomes irreversible is available, an early decision to "bail out" must rely on recognition of typical injury patterns that require damage control rather than on physiologic parameters. The combination of a major intra-abdominal vascular injury with hollow or solid-organ damage is a class injury pattern in which an early decision to "bail out" is often lifesaving. However, isolated major vascular injuries can usually undergo a definitive repair even in a patient who has sustained a massive amount of blood loss because bleeding is controlled, resuscitation can be accomplished intraoperatively, and the definitive repair can be accomplished relatively quickly. Other patterns include destruction of the pancreaticoduodenal complex, a high-grade hepatic injury, retroperitoneal or pelvic bleeding, and injuries to multiple visceral compartments.

VASCULAR REPAIR TECHNIQUES

The application of damage-control principles to vascular trauma hinges on a clear distinction between two categories of vascular repairs: simple and complex. Simple repairs are rapid and straightforward and include lateral repair, ligation, and temporary intraluminal shunt insertion. These techniques are not time consuming, do not create long suture lines, and can be used even in the presence of diffuse coagulopathic bleeding or unfavorable physiology. Complex repairs include vascular reconstructions such as end-to-end anastomosis, patch angioplasty, and graft interposition. These techniques are usually poor options in the hypothermic coagulopathic patient not only because they result in ongoing oozing from the suture lines but also because they are time consuming and significantly prolong the "bailout" procedure. This unorthodox approach represents a sharp deviation from the standard principles of vascular reconstruction but is eminently applicable to the damage-control scenario, in which not everything that is technically possible is in the patient's best interest.

Lateral repair is feasible in the absence of complete transection or extensive destruction of the arterial wall. It is important to maintain the orientation of the repair perpendicular to the axis of the vessel, to avoid stenosis.

Ligation is an underused option in the severely injured patient, especially when the injured vessel is relatively inaccessible or a complex repair is required. All limb veins can be ligated with impunity, and certainly in the context of damage control, reconstructing a peripheral vein is unjustified. The subclavian and iliac veins and the inferior vena cava can be rapidly ligated with the acceptable price of postoperative limb edema. Ligation of the portal and superior mesenteric veins is a valid option in the patient *in extremis*, but this results in massive third spacing that requires very aggressive fluid resuscitation in the postoperative phase.

Many injured arteries can also be ligated with impunity. The external carotid artery is an obvious example. In the context of penetrating trauma, injury to the inaccessible retromandibular part of the internal carotid artery (in zone 3) is managed by ligation or balloon tamponade, with the calculated risk of a neurologic deficit weighted against the necessity of obtaining rapid hemostasis. In most patients, ligation of the subclavian artery does not result in critical ischemia of the upper extremity because of the ample collateral circulation around the shoulder. The amputation rates following ligation of the femoral arteries were 81% for the common femoral and 55% for the superficial femoral artery, based on data from World War II (before the advent of fasciotomy). When a major limb artery is ligated during a damage—control procedure, it is usually prudent to proceed with an immediate fasciotomy.

Ligation of the proximal suprapancreatic superior mesenteric artery has been reported as a valid technical alternative in critically injured patients who are unlikely to tolerate a lengthy reconstruction because the rich collateral blood supply from the inferior mesenteric and celiac arteries will maintain midgut viability. The celiac axis can be ligated with impunity, and complex repair of renal artery injury in the exsanguinating patient with multiple injuries should not be attempted.

An effective alternative to ligation in inaccessible sites is balloon catheter tamponade, a simple and effective vascular damage-control technique. A Foley or large Fogarty balloon catheter is inserted into the tract of the injuring missile, and the balloon is inflated until hemorrhage is controlled. Balloon tamponade can be either a temporary hemostatic maneuver or even a definitive management of an inaccessible injury (Fig. 8–1). Balloons have been successfully used to control bleeding from the carotid artery high in the neck, from inaccessible pelvic vessels, or from a transfixing liver injury.

Another useful hemostatic technique is packing. Although traditionally employed to achieve hemostasis from high-grade liver

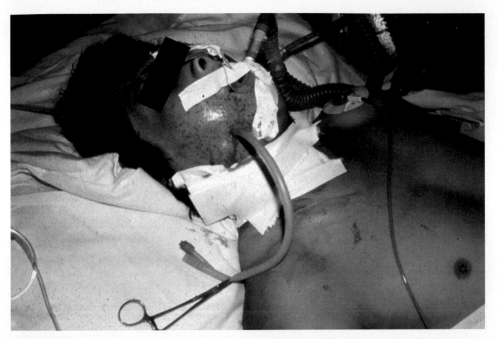

■ **FIGURE 8-1**
Balloon catheter tamponade of the distal internal carotid artery in zone 3 of the neck. ■

injuries, packing is a very useful adjunct in a coagulopathic patient with a limb injury and ongoing hemorrhage from multiple muscular bleeders that cannot be controlled directly.

TEMPORARY SHUNTS

Intraluminal shunts are prosthetic conduits placed within the vessel lumen across an injured segment to temporarily reestablish blood flow until a definitive vascular reconstruction can be performed. Vascular surgeons have used temporary shunts for at least 3 decades. In 1971, Eger and colleagues described the use of a shunt in a series of popliteal artery injuries to maintain limb perfusion while the bones are aligned before vascular repair. This series was the first modern report of the use of shunts in vascular trauma. It has recently been shown in an experimental study that a temporary shunt provides approximately half the blood flow of the intact vessel and that increased oxygen extraction compensates for the lower flow.

The choice of shunt material is a matter of personal preference, because any rigid smooth synthetic tube of appropriate caliber can serve as a temporary vascular conduit. The original description by Eger and colleagues (1971) was of a polyethylene tube with a side port. The side port facilitates access for monitoring of flow or flushing of the lumen. Others have used commercially available carotid shunts (such as a Javid or a Sundt shunt) or a heparin-bonded catheter or have improvised with a segment of a suction catheter or small Argyle's catheter cut to the appropriate length.

Temporary shunts remained functional for as long as 24 hours in an animal model. In clinical practice, temporary shunts remain functional for many hours, and patency as late as 36 hours after insertion has been observed. The presence of coagulopathy in the critically injured usually prevents clotting of the shunt during the first postoperative hours, so early postoperative failure is usually the result of a technical error during insertion. Temporary shunt insertion is an excellent damage-control option because it is rapid, controls hemorrhage from the injured vessel, and preserves

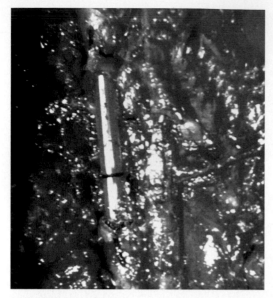

■ **FIGURE 8-2**
A temporary intraluminal shunt (Argyle's tube)
maintaining flow across a transected brachial
artery. ■

distal flow while keeping all future reconstructive options open for the surgeon
(Fig. 8–2).

Shunts are also used in the surgical repair
of combined orthopedic and vascular injuries.
Here the preferred sequence would be to
achieve bone alignment before arterial reconstruction, but often the extremity is grossly
ischemic and requires immediate restoration
of distal flow. Shunt insertion allows fracture
fixation to proceed and allows a subsequent
vascular reconstruction once the bones are
properly aligned.

Temporary shunts have been used in the
management of brachial, iliac, femoral, and
popliteal arterial injuries. A single case of
the successful use of a temporary shunt for
superior mesenteric artery injury has been
reported. Several attempts have been made
to use an Argyle chest tube as a temporary
shunt across an injury to the abdominal aorta
in patients *in extremis,* none of whom survived
beyond the immediate postoperative period.
Insertion of a temporary intraluminal shunt
begins with proximal and distal control of the
injured segment. Typically, the injured artery
will be completely or almost completely transected. The injury should be carefully assessed

and the inflow and outflow tracts to the
damaged segment should be cleared by a
Fogarty balloon thrombectomy. A shunt of the
appropriate diameter is then gently inserted
distally, flushed retrograde, and then inserted
proximally. Special care is taken to avoid
raising an intimal flap or causing additional
injury to the vessel. The shunt can be secured
in place either with heavy silk ligatures or vessel
loops held in place by a Rummel tourniquet.
The former technique is simpler but more
traumatic to the arterial wall. A central heavy
silk ligature placed around the mid-body of
the shunt is helpful for manipulation and
serves as a marker for proximal or distal migration of the conduit. Once the shunt is in place,
distal perfusion should be confirmed by palpation of a distal pulse or obtaining a Doppler
signal distal to the injured segment. Systemic
heparin is not administered.

The two major postoperative concerns are
shunt dislodgment and thrombosis. Dislodgment of the shunt is rare and usually results
from inadequate fixation of the shunt in place.
There is sudden gross swelling of the involved
extremity with oozing between the skin
sutures, indicating the presence of a rapidly
expanding hematoma. Immediate reexplo-
ration is indicated to obtain hemostasis and
reinsert the shunt.

Early shunt failure is usually caused by a
technical problem, and much like with early
postoperative failures of arterial reconstructions, the cause is poor inflow, a problem with
the shunt itself, or inadequate outflow. Poor
inflow or outflow can be the result of an intimal
flap, a more proximal or distal injury, or a
residual thrombus (proximal or distal to the
shunt). The shunt itself can also be occluded
by tying the ligatures that fix it in place too
tightly, by angulation from excessive length,
or by migration of the shunt into a distal arterial branch.

POSTOPERATIVE LIMB ISCHEMIA

Limb ischemia is the major concern after
damage-control procedures that include a vascular component. Ischemia may be the result

of intentional ligation of the injured artery, a clotted temporary shunt, a failed repair, or a missed injury. The major considerations in the management of limb ischemia in the damage-control context are the same regardless of the etiology. The first obvious step is the diagnosis of limb ischemia. Normal peripheral pulses are rarely palpable in these patients, even in the absence of an arterial injury. Hypotension, hypothermia, peripheral vasoconstriction, and edema of the injured extremity all combine to make the diagnosis of limb ischemia quite difficult in the critically wounded. Therefore, it is vital to establish reliable vascular follow-up parameters in the injured extremity immediately upon the patient's arrival in the surgical ICU.

Such a parameter can be a Doppler signal, the presence of capillary refill, or even a pulse oximeter that is applied to a toe in the relevant extremity. The diagnosis of acute postoperative ischemia is based on a change in this follow-up parameter and on a difference between the perfusion of the two extremities that gradually becomes apparent as the patient's hypothermia and hypovolemia is corrected.

Because an ischemic extremity is not an imminent threat to life, immediate reoperation is usually not undertaken. Instead, the surgeon should assess the patient's overall physiology, clinical trajectory, and the feasibility of a vascular repair, and then formulate a plan of action. For example, undertaking a vascular reconstruction in the presence of clinically obvious coagulopathy is futile and often leads to further deterioration in the patient's already precarious condition. When the circumstances are unfavorable for an urgent complex arterial reconstruction, acceptable options may include watchful waiting to see whether the collateral circulation sustains limb viability, performing a fasciotomy at the bedside, or thrombectomy with reinsertion of a temporary shunt until the patient is stable enough to undergo a definitive arterial reconstruction. Late (>12 hours) occlusion of the shunt usually indicates that the patient's coagulopathy has been corrected and that it is time for a definitive repair.

On rare occasions, an urgent reconstruction is required for limb salvage in a patient

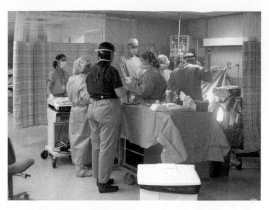

■ **FIGURE 8–3**
Bedside surgery in the surgical intensive care unit. An urgent vascular reconstruction can occasionally be undertaken at the bedside in unstable patients with limb-threatening ischemia following damage-control surgery. ■

whose physiology is so unstable that making a trip to the operating room is extremely risky. Under these unusual circumstances, simple peripheral arterial reconstruction can be undertaken at the bedside in the surgical ICU. This entails a serious logistic effort to mobilize operating room technology and create an appropriate sterile work environment at the bedside (Fig. 8–3). However, in the critically ill patient on high-dose inotropic support and severe acute respiratory distress syndrome on a nonconventional ventilatory mode, this may be the safer option. A classic example is a bedside crossover femorofemoral bypass in a critical patient whose iliac artery has been ligated or whose iliac shunt has clotted off.

PLANNED REOPERATION

The vascular damage-control sequence ends with a planned reoperation in which definitive reconstruction of the injuries is undertaken. The timing of a planned reoperation depends on the clinical circumstances, but in general the patient should be stable, warm, and with normal coagulation. If possible, a planned repeated laparotomy should be postponed until the patient has attained a negative fluid balance because the presence of swollen edematous bowel and a noncompliant abdominal wall typically precludes definitive abdominal closure. If the required vascular reconstruction is in the abdomen, it is undertaken before depacking of solid organs because the removal of packs may result in rebleeding and the need for repacking and rapid "bailout."

Peripheral arterial reconstructions are performed in the standard fashion. The extreme circumstances of patients undergoing damage-control procedures often preclude formal angiographic imaging of the injured arterial tree before reoperation, and the surgeon may, therefore, elect to begin the vascular reoperation with an on-table angiogram to precisely delineate the anatomic conditions before reconstruction and to ascertain that there are no missed injuries proximally or distally. If a temporary intraluminal shunt is in place, the shunt is removed and a Fogarty balloon catheter is passed proximally and distally. The arterial wall is then trimmed so the sites of the ligatures or Rummel tourniquets securing the shunt in place are not incorporated into the suture line because the arterial wall is presumed to be compromised. The injury is carefully assessed and dÈbrided, and a decision is made regarding the optimal reconstructive technique. In the femoral segment, the choice of conduit for definitive reconstruction (either vein or PTFE) is a matter of controversy, and despite concerns about an increased risk of infection following reoperation in the same site, there are no data to support preference of one option over the other. Fasciotomy, if not previously performed, should be considered under these circumstances, because it extends the tolerance of the limb to ischemia and protects against the swelling that occurs with reperfusion after a prolonged ischemic insult.

The definitive vascular repair is often performed in conjunction with operative procedures in other visceral compartments. If the various planned repairs are performed in a serial fashion, the operative time is prolonged in a patient who is still critically ill. Thus, every effort should be made to shorten the operative time by planning a multiteam simultaneous operation. With correct planning of the operative sequence, the vascular team can work in parallel with other teams addressing abdominal, thoracic, or head injuries.

REFERENCES

Accola KD, Feliciano DV, Mattox KL, et al: Management of injuries to the superior mesenteric artery. J Trauma 1986;26(4):313-319.

Aucar JA, Hirshberg A: Damage control for vascular injuries. Surg Clin North Am 1997;77:853-862.

Bickell WH, Wall MJ Jr, Pepe PE, et al: Immediate versus delayed fluid resuscitation for hypotensive patients with penetrating torso injuries. N Engl J Med 1994;331:1105-1109.

Ballard RB, Salomone JP, Rozycki GS, et al: "Damage control" in vascular trauma: A new use for intravascular shunts. Paper presented at the Twenty-Eighth Annual Meeting of the Western Trauma Association, Feb 22-28, 1998, Lake Louise, Alberta, Canada.

Burch JM, Ortiz VB, Richardson RJ, et al: Abbreviated laparotomy and planned reoperation for critically injured patients. Ann Surg 1992;215:476-484.

Coburn M: Damage control for urologic injuries. Surg Clin North Am 1997;77:821-834.

Cosgriff N, Moore EE, Sauaia A, et al: Predicting life-threatening coagulopathy in the massively transfused trauma patient: Hypothermia and acidoses revisited. J Trauma 1997;42:857-862.

Cushman JG, Feliciano DV, Renz BM, et al: Iliac vessel injury: Operative physiology related to outcome. J Trauma 1997;42:1033-1040.

Dawson DL, Putnam AT, Light JT, et al: Temporary arterial shunts to maintain limb perfusion after arterial injury: An animal study. J Trauma 1999;47:64-71.

DeBakey ME, Simeone FA: Battle injuries of the arteries in World War II. Ann Surg 1946;123:534-579.

Eger M, Golcman L, Goldstein A, Hirsch M: The use of a temporary shunt in the management of arterial vascular injuries. Surg Gynecol Obstet 1971;132(1):67-70.

Feliciano DV, Burch JM, Mattox KL, et al: Balloon catheter tamponade in cardiovascular wounds. Am J Surg 1990;160:583-587.

Garrison JR, Richardson JD, Hilakos AS, et al: Predicting the need to pack early for severe intra-abdominal hemorrhage. J Trauma 1996;40:923-929.

Gentiello LM, Jurkovich GJ, Stark MS, et al: Is hypothermia in the victim of major trauma protective or harmful? A randomized, prospective study. Ann Surg 1997;226:439-447.

Gubler KD, Gentiello LM, Hassantash Maier RV: The impact of hypothermia on dilutional coagulopathy. J Trauma 1994;36(6):847-851.

Hirshberg A, Mattox KL: "Damage control" in trauma surgery. Br J Surg 1993;80:1501-1502.

Hirshberg A, Mattox KL: Planned reoperation for severe trauma. Ann Surg 1995;222:3-8.

Hirshberg A, Sheffer N, Barnea O: Computer simulation of hypothermia during "damage control" laparotomy. World J Surg 1999;23:960-965.

Hirshberg A, Stein M, Adar R: Reoperation: Planned and unplanned. Surg Clin North Am 1996;77:897-907.

Hirshberg A, Walden R: Damage control for abdominal trauma. Surg Clin North Am 1997; 77:813-820.

Hirshberg A, Wall MJ Jr, Mattox KL: Planned reoperation for trauma: A two year experience with 124 consecutive patients. J Trauma 1994;37:365-369.

Hirshberg A, Wall MJ Jr, Ramchandani MK, Mattox KL: Reoperation for bleeding in trauma. Arch Surg 1993;128:1163-1167.

Husain AK, Khandeparker JMS, Tendolkar AG, et al: Temporary intravascular shunts for peripheral vascular trauma. J Postgrad Med 1992;38:68-69.

Johansen K, Bandyk D, Thiele B, Hanser ST Jr: Temporary intraluminal shunts: Resolution of a management dilemma in complex vascular injuries. J Trauma 1982;22(5):395-402.

Jurkovich GF, Greiser WB, Luterman A, Curreri PW: Hypothermia in trauma victims: An ominous predictor of survival. J Trauma 1987;27:1019-1024.

Majeski JA, Gauto A: Management of peripheral arterial vascular injuries with a Javid shunt. Am J Surg 1979;138:324-325.

Mattox KL, Hirshberg A: Vascular trauma. In Haimovici's Vascular Surgery: Principles and Techniques, 4th ed. Cambridge: Blackwell Science, Inc, 1996.

Michelson AD, MacGregor H, Barnard MR, et al: Reversible inhibition of human platelet activation by hypothermia in vivo and in vitro. Thromb Haemost 1994;71(5):633-640.

Morris JA Jr, Eddy VA, Blinman TA, et al: The staged celiotomy for trauma. Issues in unpacking and reconstruction. Ann Surg 1993;217:576-586.

Patt A, McCroskey BL, Moore E: Hypothermia-induced coagulopathies in trauma. Surg Clin North Am 1988;68:775-785.

Porter JM, Ivatury RR: In search of the optimal end points of resuscitation in trauma patients: a review. J Trauma 1998;44:908-914.

Porter JM, Ivatury RR, Nassoura ZE: Extending the horizons of "damage control" in unstable trauma patients beyond the abdomen and gastrointestinal tract. J Trauma 1997;42(3):559-561.

Pourmoghadam KK, Fogler RJ, Shaftan GW: Ligation: An alternative for control of exsanguination in major vascular injuries. J Trauma 1997; 43:126-130.

Reed RL II, Johnson TD, Hudson JD, Fischer RP: The disparity between hypothermic coagulopathy and clotting studies. J Trauma 1992;33:465-470.

Reilly PM, Rotondo MF, Carpenter JP, et al: Temporary vascular continuity during damage control: Intraluminal shunting for proximal superior mesenteric artery injury. J Trauma 1995;39:757-760.

Rohrer MJ, Natale AM: Effect of hypothermia on the coagulation cascade. Crit Care Med 1992;20:1402-1405.

Rotondo MF, Schwab CW, Gonigal MD, et al: "Damage control": An approach for improved survival in exsanguinating penetrating abdominal injury. J Trauma 1993;35:375-383.

Rotondo MF, Zonies DH: The damage control sequence and underlying logic. Surg Clin North Am 1997;77:761-777.

Scalea TM, Mann R, Austin R, Hirschowitz M: Staged procedures for exsanguinating lower extremity trauma: An extension of a technique [case report]. J Trauma 1994;36:291-293.

Sriussadaporn S, Pak-art R: Temporary intravascular shunt in complex extremity vascular injuries. J Trauma 2002 Jun;52(6):1129-1133.

Stone HH, Febian TC, Turkleson ML: Wounds of the portal venous system. World J Surg 1966;6: 335-341.

Stone HH, Strom PR, Mullins RJ: Management of the major coagulopathy with onset laparotomy. Ann Surg 1983;197:532-535.

Walker AJ, Mellor SG, Cooper GJ: Experimental experience with a temporary intraluminal heparin-bonded polyurethane arterial shunt. Br J Surg 1994;81:195-198.

Wall MJ Jr, Hirshberg A, Mattox KL: Pulmonary tractotomy with selective vascular ligation for penetrating injuries to the lung. Am J Surg 1994;168: 665-669.

Wall MJ Jr, Soltero E: Damage control for thoracic injuries. Surg Clin North Am 1997;77:863-878.

Watts DD, Trask A, Soeken K, et al: Hypothermic coagulopathy in trauma: Effect of varying levels of hypothermia on enzyme speed, platelet function, and fibrinolytic activity. J Trauma 1998;44:846-854.

DIAGNOSTIC AND INTERVENTIONAL RADIOLOGY

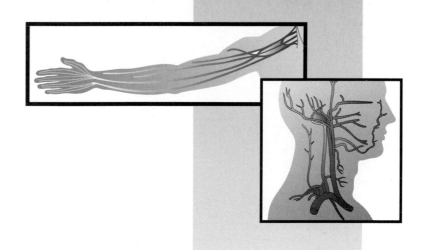

9

Imaging and Interventional Radiology of Vascular Trauma

SALVATORE J. A. SCLAFANI

I maging has long been a key component in the care of patients with vascular injury. Originally used to map out chronic complications of trauma such as arteriovenous fistulas (AVFs), it eventually became an alternative to mandatory exploration of extremity penetrations in proximity to major vascular structures and the main diagnostic modality for suspected major truncal vascular injuries.

New angiographic modalities using computed tomography (CT) and magnetic resonance (MR) may well replace conventional angiography in the future.

Interventional radiology for vascular injury was described more than 30 years ago. Initially used to treat vascular injury within the kidney, it has since become the definitive therapeutic option for hemorrhage from pelvic fractures and is accepted as an alternative to operative hemostasis for a variety of other injuries. Recent developments in stent graft technology will lead to an expanded role for endovascular procedures.

This chapter describes the accepted and future roles of imaging in the management of patients with suspected vascular injury. We shall first elaborate on the technical and methodologic aspects of angiography for trauma and then describe the angiographic findings of injuries to specific vessels. Finally, the role of endovascular techniques are elucidated.

INDICATIONS AND CONTRAINDICATIONS FOR ANGIOGRAPHY

In determining need for angiography, the surgeon must balance the value of the information that the study will provide against the risks and the time expended to attain it. The clinical condition of the patient, management priorities in trauma, and the patient's ability to tolerate transport to vascular imaging areas and the time of the procedure must all be factored into the decision. The surgeon must also be aware that the value of vascular imaging is highly dependent on the anatomic location and the mechanisms of injury. Vascular imaging has its most important role in the detection and treatment of vascular injuries in inaccessible locations. The specific indications for angiography in the various anatomic compartments are discussed in detail in respective chapters.

The major contraindications to vascular imaging are clinical. In general, hemodynamic instability is such a contraindication, although in certain circumstances (such as a pelvic fracture) angiography is the modality of choice for control of hemorrhage in hemodynamically unstable patients. An urgent laparotomy or thoracotomy has precedence and usually obviates the use of preoperative angiography, especially when angiography must be performed in a location other than the operating room.

Other contraindications are related to the use of contrast agents. A previous serious allergic reaction to contrast media is a relative contraindication, although a previous reaction does not predict the occurrence or severity of another reaction. Anaphylactic reactions cannot be predicted.

A history of asthma should raise awareness to the possibility of an allergic reaction, but asthma in itself is not a contraindication to the administration of contrast media.

The risks of renal failure are increased in patients who are dehydrated, have diabetes, preexisting renal disease, or multiple myeloma. This is especially true of patients with both preexisting renal failure and diabetes. Although these conditions do not constitute a contraindication to a contrast study, they often influence the decision to perform it, how it is done, and which contrast agents are used.

Contrast Media–Related Risks

Modern contrast media, both low osmolar and iso-osmolar, have a very low risk of adverse effects. These contrast reactions usually occur with venous injections that result in histamine release from pulmonary mast cells. The most common reaction is vomiting, which used to be seen in as many as 1 in 10 patients who received intravenous injections of contrast. True allergic reactions, including urticaria, angioneurotic edema, bronchospasm, and anaphylactic shock, are reported in about 1 in 8000 administrations of nonionic contrast media and about 1 in 4000 administrations of ionic contrast. These reactions rarely occur when the contrast is injected through an arterial catheter. I have seen no major allergic reactions and two cases of urticaria in 30 years and more than 40,000 procedures.

Premedication with prednisone is a strategy to decrease the risks of allergic reaction in patients who are asthmatic or highly allergic. However, the 2-day administration of prednisone is not feasible in most acute trauma situations. I have empirically used methylprednisolone in acute emergencies, but this is not based on proven scientific evidence.

Nephrotoxicity does not occur unless risk factors such as diabetes, preexisting renal failure, sickle cell anemia, or multiple myeloma are present. My impression is that most trauma patients who are young and healthy and who are usually managed by aggressive fluid resuscitation resulting in diuresis are unlikely to develop renal failure unless there is some other reason for this, such as prolonged shock or other cause of renal failure. These renal effects can be blunted by adequate hydration or premedication with acetylcysteine.

When there is preexisting renal failure, contrast agents can be avoided by performing MR imaging (MRI) or MR angiography (MRA) using gadolinium, which is not nephrotoxic. Another alternative contrast agent is carbon dioxide.

Technical Complications

Recent technological advances have made catheter-related complications a relatively rare entity, especially in the young trauma patient with normal vessels. Vasospasm is common in children and young adults. I have found that administering calcium channel blockers before the procedure is helpful in preventing spasm.

The pathologic state of the vessels of the elderly with tortuosity and advanced atherosclerotic plaques and stenoses makes catheterizations more difficult and may result in dissections, perforations, embolization, and thromboses.

Femoral access site complications, such as hematoma, AVF, and false aneurysm, occur infrequently but usually can be avoided by attention to detail during catheter removal. Manual compression of the puncture site for a minimum of 15 minutes is usually satisfactory to avoid the development of false aneurysms and groin hematomas. Sandbags are not recommended because they do not provide focal compression and a hematoma may be hidden by the sandbag. Prolonged compression is necessary in patients with hypertension or obesity. I always compress over the arterial puncture site rather than over the skin puncture site, which is left visible to assess adequacy of compression. If coagulopathy is present, the physician is advised to correct the coagulopathy before removal of the sheath. It is safer to leave the catheter in place until then.

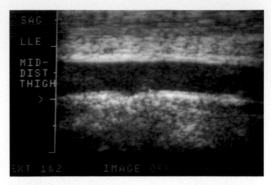

■ **FIGURE 9–1**
Ultrasound of brachial artery injury. This patient sustained a gunshot wound of the arm. Asymptomatic, an arteriogram was performed because the trajectory was in proximity to the brachial artery. Arteriography (not shown) revealed a partial wall injury with an intimal flap. Ultrasound was performed immediately after the arteriogram so that the injury would be followed noninvasively. Despite the marking of the exact site of the injury, the ultrasonographer had considerable difficulty identifying it. There is a slight decrease in echo along the intimal lining. The lumen is slightly bulged at that area. ■

ALTERNATIVE IMAGING

Catheter-based angiography is the gold standard for the diagnosis of vascular injuries. Although the images may not always reflect that pathologic state of the injured vessel, it is highly accurate in detecting the presence of injuries. However, alternative imaging modalities exist and are rapidly gaining important roles in the management of patients with suspected vascular injury, mainly because they are less invasive than angiography and sometimes involve much less elaborate logistics. These modalities are often used as screening studies to determine the need for angiography.

Ultrasound

Color flow duplex imaging can identify false aneurysms as collections of pulsatile flow with a forward and backward color signal seen in the aneurysm sac. Duplex has also been reported as capable of detecting minimal injuries, such as intimal tears and small pseudoaneurysms. However, my attempt to correlate angiographic "minimal injuries" with ultrasound was not successful (Fig. 9–1).

Computed Tomographic Angiography

CT (Fig. 9–2) has improved in speed and resolution in the past 5 years while becoming less expensive and allowing more sophisticated manipulation of the acquired data using current computer technology. The new multidetector scanners also allow real-time coronal and sagittal two- and three-dimensional images, which may in some cases resemble angiograms. Virtual angioscopy is also possible. Indeed there are now strong arguments suggesting that CT angiography (CTA) may be satisfactory for the screening and diagnosis of various vascular diseases including

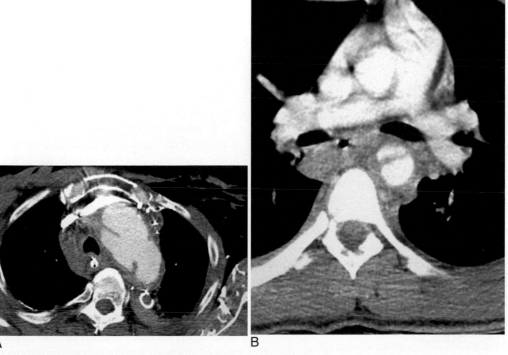

■ FIGURE 9–2

Computed tomography of arterial injury. *A,* Computed tomographic (CT) arteriography at the aortic arch level illustrates quite clearly the disruption of the aortic wall on the medial side of the arch in this 79-year-old unrestrained driver. Intimal flaps are also visible. Aortography was performed after this CT because the surgeon desired further analysis. Aortography was difficult because the guidewire and the catheter advanced out of the lumen into the pseudoaneurysm. *B,* A CT scan of another patient reveals a filling defect, which could be misinterpreted as an dissection. However, aortic trauma rarely results in extensive dissection. Rather, this appearance is the result of volume averaging of the pseudoaneurysm and the aortic lumen. The intimal tear is seen between them. ■

pulmonary embolism and some types of arterial trauma.

CTA has high sensitivity and specificity in blunt aortic injury. A normal CT scan rules out an injury and thus obviates the need for aortography in most circumstances. An abnormal CTA scan may require aortography for confirmation and precise delineation of the findings.

In the abdomen, there should be a delay of 70 to 90 seconds between contrast injection and scanning. This time window can be used to investigate the thoracic aorta before scanning the abdomen. Thus, no additional contrast media or time is necessary for screening the thoracic aorta using CTA.

Magnetic Resonance Angiography

MRI is another noninvasive alternative for diagnosing vascular pathology, using time-of-flight imaging and contrast-enhanced MRA. The use of MR for traumatic conditions has not received much attention. Difficulties in questioning patients about the presence of metallic artifacts and the incompatibility of standard resuscitation and monitoring equipment with MRI technology are obstacles in the use of MR in the trauma situation.

ANGIOGRAPHIC FINDINGS IN VASCULAR TRAUMA

Angiography demonstrates abnormalities of the arterial contrast column and does not correlate with surgical findings or with the pathologic study results. Many of the alterations in the contrast column are nonspecific and the natural history of these findings is unpredictable. Vascular trauma is typically associated with six angiographic findings.

Extravasation (Fig. 9–3) is defined as the presence of extravascular contrast. Extravasations are coarse, irregular accumulations of contrast media that persist into the venous phase. Extravasation may not be visible on the early arterial films (Fig. 9–3A). The density is highest at the beginning of the sequence, comparable to the density of the injected arterial opacification, and may fade slightly toward the end of the sequence (Fig. 9–3B).

Extravasation must not be confused with the appearance of veins seen at the end of the series. These gradually become visible as the sequence progresses and are most pronounced toward the end of the series. The density never reaches that of arterial contrast media. Different oblique views facilitate this distinction.

The size of the extravasation does not necessarily correlate with the degree of bleeding (Fig. 9–3C). The appearance is often a reflection of the "dead space" created by the traumatic lacerations. Extravasation may give the appearance of a "false aneurysm" (Fig. 9–3D), which may be lobulated or round. Extravasations are seen with both lacerations and transactions of arteries.

Narrowing of the contrast column (Fig. 9–4) is a nonspecific finding that may be caused by intimal, mural, and extrinsic etiologies. Narrowing can be physiologic and reversible or result in a permanent stricture.

The most common form of narrowing is vasospasm caused by contraction of the media in response to a noxious stimulus such as stretching or guidewire manipulation (Fig. 9–4A). It is most pronounced in children and young adults, particularly women, and in patients who abuse cocaine. It is seen more commonly in injuries to muscular arteries than in those to visceral vessels. The appearance is that of single or multiple areas of narrowing. The narrowing is concentric and may involve varying lengths. Vasospasm may be so intense that the appearance of the vessel may be indistinguishable from that of thrombosis.

Vasospasm can be differentiated from other causes of narrowing if it can be reversed by vasodilators. In some patients, intra-arterial transcatheter administration of 100 to 200-µg boluses of nitroglycerin is effective in reversing or decreasing vasospasm. Nifedipine administered 24 hours in advance of arteriography may prevent vasospasm in young people undergoing elective arteriography.

Luminal narrowing can also be caused by an intramural hematoma, either in the subintima or beneath the adventitia. The appearance is that of asymmetrical and eccentric narrowing (Fig. 9–4B and C).

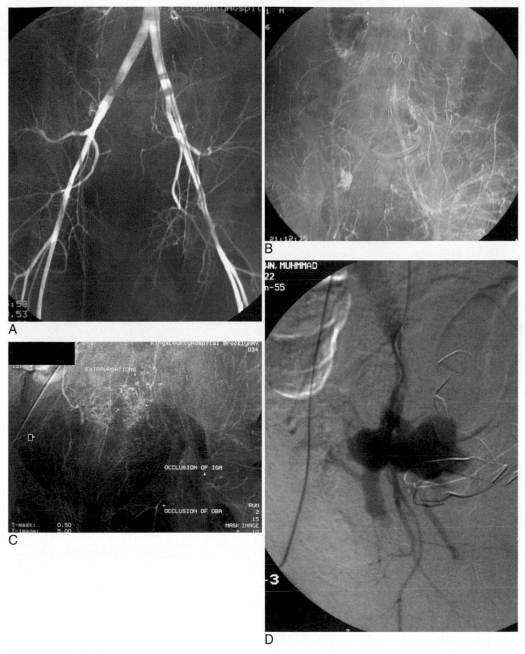

■ **FIGURE 9-3**

Extravasation. *A,* Early-phase image of a pelvic aortogram failed to identify any significant abnormality except vasospasm. No extravasation is seen. *B,* Venous-phase film in the same study shows multiple areas of arterial density contrast persisting after the arteries have emptied. *C,* Multiple small dots of contrast are seen over the sacrum. The small size of these extravasations does not reflect the massive blood loss that has resulted in hemodynamic instability. *D,* Large extravasation from the internal iliac artery is associated with early opacification of the common iliac vein. ■

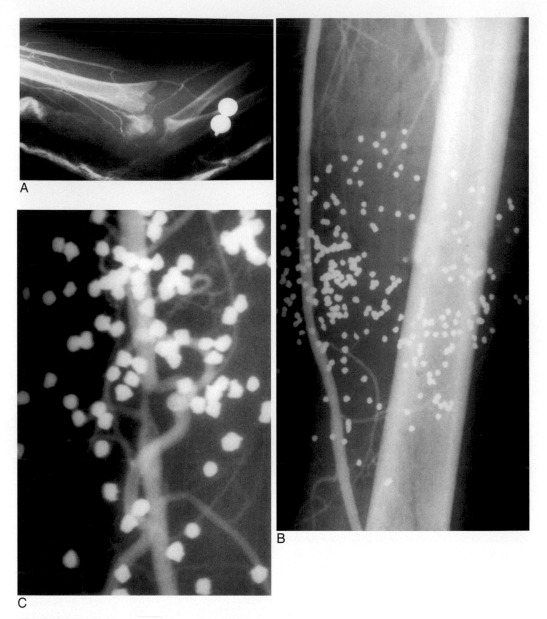

■ **FIGURE 9-4**

Luminal narrowing. *A,* Vasospasm. The brachial artery is markedly narrowed over the region of the transcondylar fracture of the humerus. Initially thought to be occluded. Exploration revealed only vasospasm. *B,* There is an eccentric focal narrowing of the superficial femoral artery resulting from this shotgun blast. This is consistent with a mural hematoma. *C,* Close-up 9 months later shows high-grade stenosis secondary to stricture.

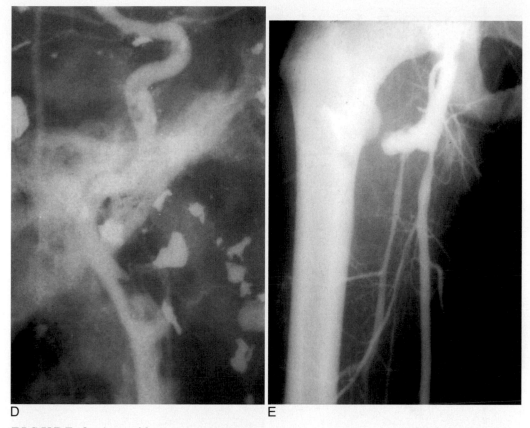

D   E

■ **FIGURE 9–4**, cont'd

D, There is narrowing of the internal carotid artery as the vessel enters the carotid canal. This narrowing is the result of thrombus filling the lumen of the vessel. Note also the filling defects in the cavernous portion of the carotid. These represent emboli. *E,* There is narrowing of the superficial femoral artery by a false aneurysm of the deep femoral artery. After embolization of the profunda injury, the superficial femoral arterial lumen will return to normal caliber. ■

Mural thrombus, a soft clot attached to the wall of an injured vessel, may also appear as a narrowing on angiography. Injury to the wall, exposing media to the circulation, initiates a cascade of platelet attraction, adherence, and thrombus formation (Fig. 9–4D). Laminar flow can make this appear smooth and gently tapering, but such a lesion is always asymmetrical. Finally, extrinsic pressure can result in luminal narrowing. This may be caused by a false aneurysm in an adjacent artery or by pressure from a displaced bony fragment or a bullet (Fig. 9–4E).

Luminal dilatation (Fig. 9–5) is another typical angiographic finding and is the result of intimal disruption. Stretch injuries of the arterial wall, such as occurs in deceleration aortic injuries or from the temporary cavitation of high-velocity missiles, result in disruption of the intima and part of the media while the remaining portions of the wall remain intact. Active bleeding does not occur initially because the outer portions of the arterial wall remain as a barrier. Arterial pressure now exerts its effect on the remaining elastic layers and this results in expansion of the arterial lumen. This results in the formation of a pseudoaneurysm (Fig. 9–5A). Dilatation of the vessel also occurs in chronic AVFs. In this condition, high-flow and arterio venous (AV) shunting results in degeneration of the arterial wall. These factors lead to increased diameter of the vessel (Fig. 9–5B).

There are several causes of *intraluminal filling defects* (Fig. 9–6). These include intimal flaps, emboli, intramural hematoma,

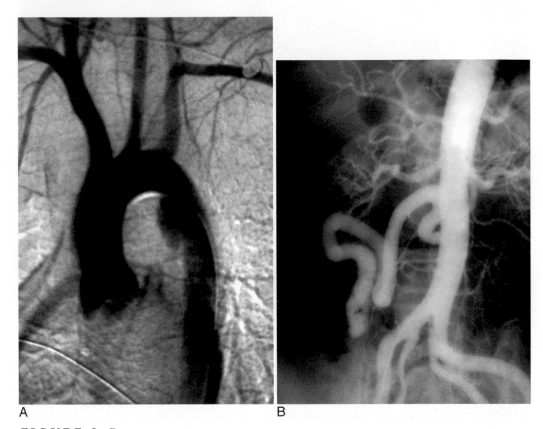

A B

■ **FIGURE 9–5**
Luminal dilatation. *A,* There is luminal dilatation at the region of the aortic isthmus. This dilatation is a pseudoaneurysm, resulting from unrestricted dilation of the aorta because of intimal/medial rupture. *B,* This large and tortuous vessel is the ovarian artery, which has dilated to the diameter of the common iliac artery because of a chronic arteriovenous fistula resulting from trauma many years previously. ■

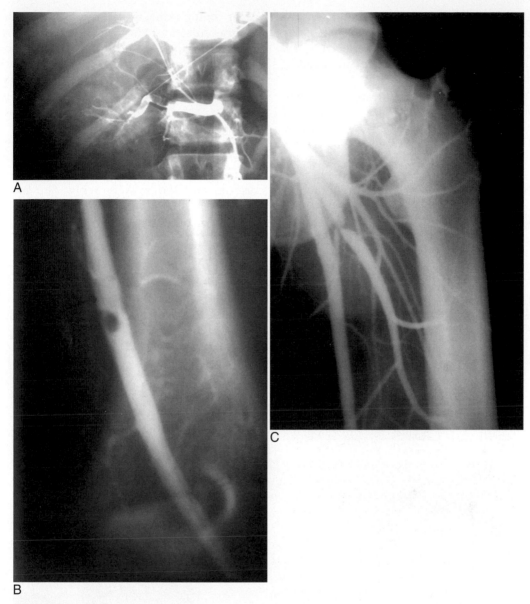

■ FIGURE 9–6
Luminal filling defects. *A,* The filling defect within the right renal artery represents thrombus secondary to stretch injury of the renal artery. Slight amounts of contrast media pass around the thrombus. *B,* A rounded filling defect in the brachial artery represents thrombus attaching to a brachial artery damaged by a knife wound. Extravasation is prevented because the thrombus seals the hole. *C,* An intimal flap of the deep femoral artery has resulted in a filling defect. The defect is sharp and linear. ■

intraluminal thrombus, and intravascular foreign bodies such as bullet fragments. Streaming and incomplete replacement of unopacified blood with the contrast column also creates an appearance of a filling defect that must be differentiated from true filling defect. Similarly, misregistration artifacts may also create what appear to be filling defects on arteriography.

Intraluminal thrombus (Fig. 9–6*A* and *B*) is usually focal, resulting in an unopacified area within the contrast column. These thrombi can appear as linear defects or as a mound narrowing the vessel. In some cases, a wavy linear filling defect trails from this larger mural defect. This represents a trailing thrombus.

Intimal flaps (Fig. 9–6C) appear as sharp and well-defined linear filling defects that may be seen both proximal and distal to the injury. They appear to originate at the edge of the arterial injury and will typically change orientation and appearance from image to image in a sequence. Intimal flaps are often associated with dilatation of the vessel wall or extravasation.

Streaming artifacts may result from poor contrast injection. These can be identified by changes in appearance on multiple projections, and an increase in flow rate and volume of the contrast injection will abolish them and clear up the confusion. Misregistration artifacts can be excluded by viewing the angiogram without subtraction.

Disruption of contiguous hollow structures sometimes results in *AVF* (Fig. 9–7), a persistent communication between high-pressure arteries and low-pressure veins. The most common of these findings are AVF between systemic arteries and systemic veins of the

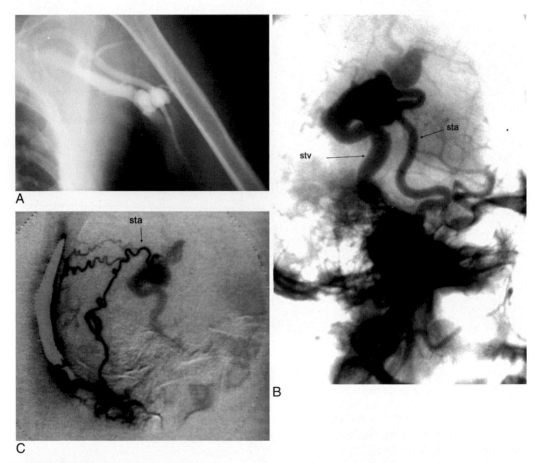

■ **FIGURE 9–7**

Arteriovenous fistula. *A*, Acute axillary arteriovenous fistula secondary to a gunshot wound. Note the absence of enlargement of the distal artery and the lack of peripheral venous filling. These findings indicate an acute process. *B* and *C*, Chronic superficial temporal artery arteriovenous fistula. The patient sustained a blow to the head as a child. She now presents with pulsating tinnitus. On the superficial temporal arteriogram *(B)*, the superficial temporal artery is enlarged and very tortuous. A false aneurysm is interposed between the superficial temporal artery and superficial temporal vein. Selective occipital arteriography *(C)* was used to assess the distal aspect of the superficial temporal artery. Flow is retrograde back to the fistula. Again tortuous ecstatic branches are seen. ■

extremities because of the close proximity of the vena comitantes and the inflow arteries. Angiographically the findings are usually straightforward with denser than normal opacification of venous structures occurring within 2 to 4 seconds of the injection of the contrast. Occasionally, these fistulas will be demonstrated only on follow-up angiography rather than during the acute phase (Fig. 9–7A). The angiographic appearance of chronic AVFs is more complex (Figs. 9–5B and 9–7B and C). Because of chronic high-volume and high-pressure inflow, numerous collateral circuits will be recruited to send blood flow to the low-pressure veins. These appear as highly tortuous hypertrophied vessels. The primary inflow vessel also dilates. Venous distention usually results in venous incompetence and the development of varicosities.

Determining the site of the fistulous communication is sometimes very difficult because of the very rapid filling of numerous arteries and veins. Very rapid filming sequences, superselective catheterization, and multiple oblique views are helpful in determining the site of the fistula (see Fig. 9–7B and C).

Occlusion (Fig. 9–8) is defined as the absence of flow beyond a focal point in a vessel. An occlusion may present as nonvisualization of the occluded vessel or as slow filling with an abrupt stop (Fig. 9–8A). The occluded column of contrast may have a tapered end, appear as an abrupt horizontal ending, or have a meniscoid appearance. Delayed images may show the distal end of the vessel filling through collateral circulation (Fig. 9–8B). There are four main reasons for occlusion: preexisting atherosclerotic disease, vasospasm, thrombo-

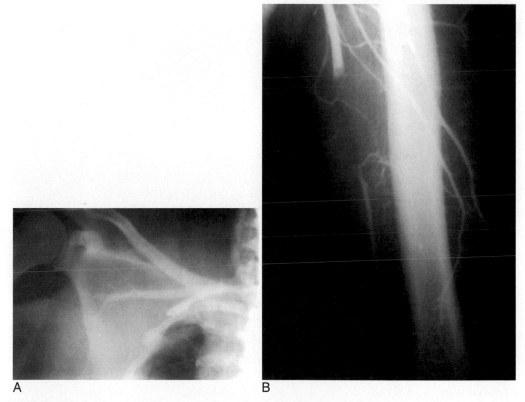

A   B

■ **FIGURE 9–8**
Occlusions. *A,* Scapulothoracic dissociation. The shoulder has been pulled and stretched. The scapula has been wrenched from the chest wall and the sternoclavicular joint has been ruptured. The axillary artery has been stretched and the intimal disrupted. Thrombosis is the result. *B,* Gunshot wound has resulted in thrombosis of the superficial femoral artery. The exact site of the injury cannot be presumed as prograde and retrograde thrombosis will occur to points of intact branches. ■

sis, and distal embolism. It is often difficult to differentiate spasm from the other causes of occlusion. An embolism may have a characteristic appearance with a meniscus at the end of the contrast column resulting from outlining the top of the embolism. However, vasospasm and thrombosis may be impossible to differentiate.

ENDOVASCULAR INTERVENTIONS IN ARTERIAL TRAUMA

Temporary Hemostasis

Temporary angiographic control can be used as an adjunct to operative repair (Fig. 9–9).

The aim is to minimize dissection and facilitate the operation by obtaining control of the injured vessel preoperatively using an occluding balloon. This technique is most useful when active extravasation from a major artery is seen on angiography.

The technique is straightforward. First, selective catheterization is accomplished with a directional catheter. Then a guidewire is advanced through the catheter to a position distal to the site of injury (Fig. 9–9A). After removal of the directional catheter, a balloon catheter is advanced to a position proximal to the injury. Through this primary balloon catheter a second balloon catheter is coaxially advanced distal to the injury. When both balloons are inflated, the injury site is isolated between the two balloons (Fig. 9–9B).

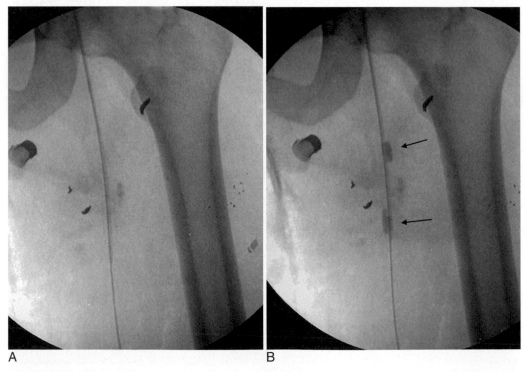

A   B

■ **FIGURE 9–9**
Temporary balloon occlusion. A 22-year-old man sustained multiple gunshot wounds of the thigh resulting in a tense hematoma. Because there were multiple injuries, arteriography was requested to determine where the injury was. The study (not shown) revealed transection of the superficial femoral artery in the upper thigh and bleeding worsened during arteriography. Temporary balloon occlusion was employed for hemostasis en route to the operating room. *A,* A guidewire has been advanced distal to the injury site. *B,* Balloons have been inflated proximal and distal to the site of bleeding. ■

Embolization

Transcatheter embolization is indicated for injury to arteries that are inaccessible such as the intraparenchymal renal vessels, which cannot be selectively exposed without risk of losing the entire kidney. Embolization is also indicated for vessels that are not necessary for tissue perfusion, such as muscular branches.

Embolization techniques can be divided into two general categories: conduit occlusion (Figs. 9–10 and 9–11) and parenchymal or tissue bed occlusion (Figs. 9–3 and 9–12). Coils are used to occlude conduits of 2 to 15 mm in diameter when the vascular bed is intact. The goal of coil embolization is to focally occlude an injured vessel but spare the uninjured distal vascular distribution. Coil embolization is used to treat false aneurysms, lacerations, transections, and AVFs of conduits rather than for stopping tissue bed bleeding. Coil occlusion may also be used to selectively decrease flow and pressure to an injured organ to effect hemostasis while avoiding infarction by allowing collateral flow (Fig. 9–10).

Coils are constructed of stainless steel helical wire with cotton or Dacron threads attached to the coil. The coil has a fixed diameter and will not migrate distally in a vessel of comparable size. The threads result in platelet aggregation and thrombus formation at that site. Intimal damage ensues and occlusion propagates proximally and distally to the coil

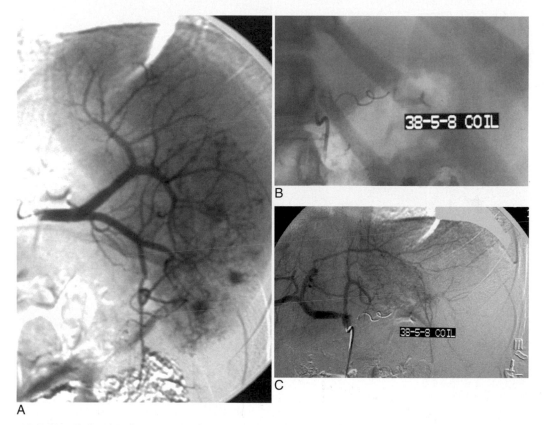

■ **FIGURE 9–10**
Coil embolization for selective hypotension. A 32-year-old motorcyclist sustained injury of the spleen, which was diagnosed on computed tomography. *A,* Splenic arteriography was performed. There are multiple areas of contrast extravasation that are predominantly localized to the lower pole of the spleen. *B,* Coils have been deployed in the midsplenic artery. Occlusion results in diminished perfusion pressure and flow into the organ. *C,* Arteriography repeated after coil occlusion illustrates collateral perfusion of the distal splenic artery via gastric and pancreatic collateral vessels. This maintains viability of the spleen while hemostasis is achieved. ■

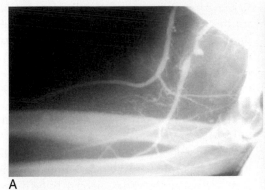

A

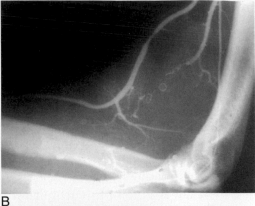

B

■ **FIGURE 9–11**
Proximal and distal coil occlusion of the
brachial artery. *A,* Arteriography of the elbow
demonstrates that there is a high origin of the
ulnar-interosseous artery. The brachial
(radial) artery is lacerated with extravasation
surrounded by areas of luminal narrowing.
Coils were placed proximal and distal to the
site of injury. *B* and *C,* Arterial phase and
venous phase images illustrated occlusion of
the vessel and reconstitution of the radial
artery through collateral vessels. Retrograde
bleeding is prevented by the distal coil. ■

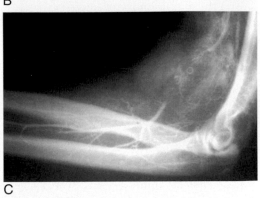

C

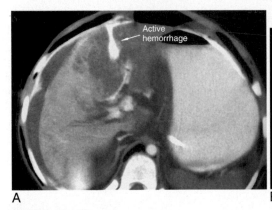

A

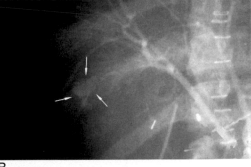

B

■ **FIGURE 9–12**
Gelfoam pledget embolization of intrahepatic arterial bleeding. *A,* Computed tomography reveals a
laceration of the liver with active hemorrhage extending into the peritoneal cavity. *B,* Arteriography
shows active bleeding from the right hepatic artery. Selective embolization was tedious. Therefore,
small pledgets of surgical gelatin were flow directed from a more proximal location. Hemostasis was
achieved. ■

to points where there are patent arterial branches. Coils must be properly sized, as delivery of a coil too small will result in distal embolization and potential distal infarction, and delivery of too large a coil may prevent re-formation into the coiled shape or may result in deployment that is too proximal and in errant emboli. The aim is to place coils both proximal and distal to the injury site when possible, to avoid recurrence of hemorrhage from retrograde flow.

For an arterial laceration, it is usually possible to advance a guidewire into the artery distal to the site of injury because the vessel ends remain aligned (see Fig. 9–11A). The catheter is then advanced over the wire into the distal vessel. The tip of the catheter is placed beyond the injury but proximal to the first distal branch. The size of the vessel is measured and a coil 1 to 2 mm larger in diameter than the vessel is pushed through the catheter with a guidewire. When the coil exits the catheter, it will reform into its memorized helical shape. Coils are delivered until there is no flow distal to them. Then the catheter is withdrawn into the vessel proximal to the injury and positioned distal to the branch closest to the injury site. Additional coils are introduced and this isolates the arterial disruption (see Fig. 9–11B and C).

The placement of coils across a transected vessel is more problematic because the vessel ends may retract and misalign or the distal segment may thrombose. In these situations, the disrupted end is gently probed with a guidewire or glidewire in an attempt to advance it directly into the distal part of the artery. This is successful in about 40% of cases. When this is not possible, several alternative methods can be used to reach the distal vessel such as cannulating collateral pathways or a retrograde puncture of the distal vessel. If the distal end of an injured artery is thrombosed, it may be unnecessary to advance the catheter distally.

Vascular Bed Occlusion

Parenchymal disruptions and muscular injuries result in damage to small vessels (1 to 3 mm in size) (see Figs. 9–3B and C and

9–12). These injuries are very distal and often multiple. Selective catheterization is difficult and time consuming. Control of this type of hemorrhage is accomplished by particulate embolization that reduces blood flow to the entire vascular bed rather than focal conduit embolization.

The material of choice for this type of vascular occlusion in pledgets of surgical gelatin, cut into cubes of approximately 1 to 2 mm. The Gelfoam reaches its target by flow direction (rather than superselective catheterization) and scatters into multiple small branches, which diminish but do not obliterate blood flow. This is followed by thrombosis. Surgical gelatin works by causing mechanical obstruction and intimal damage resulting in further thrombosis. Mechanical obstruction is temporary because surgical gelatin is digested by macrophages. Depending on blood flow, Gelfoam may last a few days or weeks. However, the thrombosis that occurs may be permanent.

Stents and Stent Grafts

Uncovered stents are wire meshes that remain expanded after deployment. They either are stretched out by balloon or are self-expanding. Stents provide a framework to maintain luminal diameter and patency of vessels with partial wall injuries such as intimal tears and they can be used to reexpand arteries that have developed strictures from trauma. They have also been used as a trap through which coils can be delivered into false aneurysms without risk of the coils falling out of the false aneurysm and embolizing into normal distal vessels (Figs. 9–13 and 9–14).

Covered stents are wire meshes that are covered with an impermeable or semipermeable membrane such as Dacron or vein. They can be created in the angiography suite from available components. Recently a prepackaged stent covered with Dacron has been approved for use in the bronchial tree. This has also been used with success in arterial injuries. They can provide a conduit that seals the hole in the artery from within the vessel and can be delivered to remote sites from the femoral access site. However, the

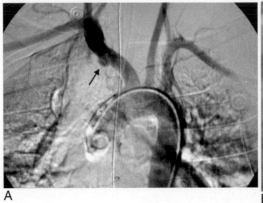

A

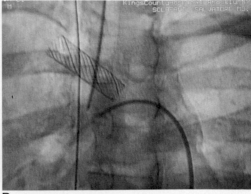

B

■ **FIGURE 9–13**
Stent graft repair of a laceration of the
innominate artery. A 19-year-old man
sustained a transmediastinal gunshot wound
but was hemodynamically stable. Computed
tomography revealed evidence of injury of a
great vessel. *A,* Arch aortography revealed a
false aneurysm on the right side of the
innominate artery. *B,* A wall graft was
deployed over the area of the injury. *C,* Post-
deployment aortography shows coverage of
the area and maintenance of blood flow. ■

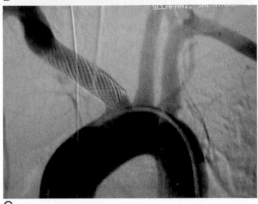

C

long-term durability of covered stents has not
been determined yet.

TREATMENT OF SPECIFIC VASCULAR INJURIES

Neck

INTERNAL CAROTID ARTERY

Three endovascular procedures—transcatheter embolization, covered stent deployment, and temporary balloon occlusion—are
available for the management of internal
carotid artery (ICA) injuries (Fig. 9–15).

Transcatheter embolization should be
considered if the location of the injury is
inaccessible to operative repair. The exact
site considered "inaccessible" varies considerably between surgeons. Most surgeons
will not be able to repair an injury located

above the inferior endplate of the second
cervical vertebral body as seen on a lateral
arteriogram.

Transection of the ICA above the angle of
the mandible with poorly controlled bleeding or AVF from the proximal vessel and no
prograde intracranial flow warrants angiographic embolization. External hemorrhage
is difficult to control in this area because the
bleeding often comes from the throat, nose,
or ear. Packing of these orifices often diminishes but does not effectively stop the hemorrhage. The time needed to operatively
explore and occlude this vessel is greater than
that needed for coil occlusion.

Patients with prolonged coma who have
arteriographic evidence of thrombosis of the
ICA should undergo transcatheter embolization. This is also true if thrombus has propa-
gated into the petrous and cavernous portions
of the carotid. Asymptomatic patients with
carotid occlusion may be considered candidates for embolization despite the absence
of bleeding. Vasospasm may be causing the

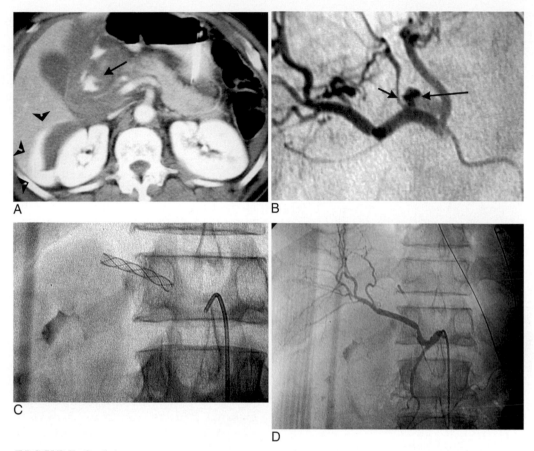

■ **FIGURE 9-14**
Stent graft of hepatic hilar arterial injury. The patient fell 15 meters from a roof. He was hypotensive on admission, but vital signs improved after resuscitation. *A,* Computed tomography revealed extrahepatic extravasation into the subhepatic space. The hepatic artery was ill defined, enlarged, and irregular. This was interpreted as a hepatic hilar injury. *B,* Proper hepatic arteriography shows an area of extravasation from the hepatic artery distal to the origin of the left hepatic artery. *C,* A 6-mm wall graft was deployed. *D,* Follow-up arteriography 1 month later shows flow through the stent and no extravasation. ■

occlusion and resolution may dislodge proximal thrombus into the brain. Additionally, occlusion, caused by vasospasm, may hide a true mural injury that will subsequently result in an AVF or pseudoaneurysm.

The decision to embolize the ICA in a patient who has a nonocclusive ICA injury is difficult, because the ideal aim is the restoration of flow, not the termination of flow. Many injuries that are not accessible should be observed with antiplatelet protective therapy before resorting to embolization. If follow-up imaging shows deterioration requiring endovascular treatment, then further evalua-

tion of its occlusion is needed to ensure that embolization itself will not result in a neurologic deficit. Provocative testing by temporary balloon occlusion is warranted to determine whether the patient will tolerate occlusion before embolization is undertaken.

Temporary balloon occlusion should also be considered when active bleeding is identified on arteriography from a portion of the ICA that is believed by the surgeon to be accessible to repair.

For distal ICA injuries at the upper limits of operability above the angle of the mandible, control of the distal vessel is the major pro-

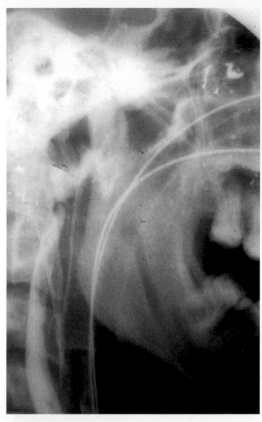

■ **FIGURE 9–15**
Coil embolization of the internal carotid artery.
Arteriography demonstrates active
extravasation into the nasopharynx. There was
no flow distally after transection of the internal
carotid artery. Active hemorrhage from
transection of the high cervical or the petrous
portions of the carotid is an indication for
embolization of the vessel. ■

blem. Back-bleeding from the petrous portion
of the ICA can be difficult to control operatively because the distal vessel cannot be identified or because it retracts into the carotid
canal and cannot be clamped. Therefore,
control of the distal end of the vessel by temporary balloon occlusion is extremely helpful
in expanding the possibilities for repair.

Intimal injuries of the ICA may result from
stretch injuries related to hyperextension,
basilar skull fractures, or penetrating trauma.
Such intimal flaps are life threatening due to
secondary embolism of intraluminal thrombus (see Fig. 9–4*D*). The treatment of such
injuries is currently undergoing analysis.
Antiplatelet therapy is used by many practi-

tioners to avoid such complications. The augmentation of angioplasty by the placement of
an expandable stent has become a standard
therapy for intimal flaps resulting during
angioplasty. Such an approach has been used
for ICA intimal injuries. The reader is cautioned to take into consideration the potential for intracranial embolization after stent
placement. Anticoagulation is strongly recommended as part of this procedure.

Covered stents have also been deployed in
ICA injuries and may have some role to play
in the future. Although these devices have
been used for trauma to the iliac artery,
the subclavian artery, and the femoral artery,
a number of issues must be addressed
before their use can be recommended in the
ICA.

EXTERNAL CAROTID ARTERY AND
ITS BRANCHES

Bleeding from the external carotid artery and
its branches can be quite problematic. Massive
external hemorrhage from the external
carotid artery and its facial, lingual, maxillary,
occipital, and auricular branches can be
massive. Ligation of the external carotid
artery may be ineffective as extensive collateral networks occur to all of these vessels. (See
Fig. 9–7*B* and *C*.)

Arteriography is very helpful in detecting,
identifying, and controlling hemorrhage from
these vessels. Hemostasis of lacerations and
transactions and control of AVFs of the larger
conduits requires selective and precise proximal and distal coil occlusion. Peripheral small
branch bleeding can usually be managed by
flow directed particular embolization using
surgical gelatin pledgets. Caution to avoid
inadvertent intracranial embolization and
stroke requires precise and secure catheter
placement.

VERTEBRAL ARTERY

Embolization is the treatment of choice for
most transmural injuries of the vertebral
artery. The vessel is expendable because of
the dual blood supply of the basilar artery.

The use of angiographic embolization in nonocclusive and nonbleeding vertebral artery injuries is less clear. The maintenance of prograde blood flow is always desirable. Therefore, some have treated these injuries by observation. Observation is not without risks as embolic strokes and occlusions have been reported. I suggest that observed patients be administered platelet inhibitors such as aspirin during observation. Test occlusion with a temporary occlusion catheter can help make the decision. If this test shows that occlusion is well tolerated, embolization of the vertebral artery can be considered to avoid the subsequent development of false aneurysms or AVFs. If test occlusion results in neurologic deficit, embolization is not recommended.

Coils are the preferred material for embolization of the vertebral artery because it is a conduit vessel. Particulate embolization is contraindicated. Proximal embolization alone may be insufficient because of the direct line contralateral flow created by the vertebrobasilar junction. Delayed development of AVFs supplied by an untreated distal segment filling from the basilar artery is well known. Furthermore, proximal embolization limits the approach to the distal segment.

Direct balloon occlusion of the mouth of a false aneurysm or an AVF of the vertebral artery without obliteration of the lumen of the artery and coil occlusion of pseudoaneurysms has also been described. A detachable balloon is advanced through the hole in the vessel and inflated. The advantages of these techniques are that prograde flow is maintained and the hole in the wall is closed. Although most patients can tolerate embolization of one vertebral artery because collateral circulation is sufficient, this procedure is particularly valuable in those circumstances in which the contralateral vertebral artery is atretic or hypoplastic. The incidence of hypoplasia of one of the vessels is 15% and atresia occurs in about 5%.

When vertebral artery injury results in occlusion of the proximal segment, proximal coil embolization occlusion has been recommended because occlusion secondary to vasospasm may be transient. In these cases, the catheter should never be advanced

through thrombus because this maneuver may dislodge the clot and result in intracranial embolization. Therefore, the coils should be delivered just proximal to the site of occlusion.

There are occasions when the proximal segment has thrombosed but the distal segment remains patent by retrograde flow from the contralateral vertebral artery through the basilar artery. This is an extremely challenging situation. A microcatheter or flow-directed balloon catheter can be advanced from the contralateral vertebral artery into the basilar artery and then directed downward into the distal end of the injured vertebral artery. Another option is to try to access the vessel through venous communications when there is an AVF. Finally, percutaneous puncture of the second or third portion of the vertebral artery can be attempted.

Thoracic Vascular Injuries

Endovascular stent grafts may change and expand the role of the interventional radiologist in the treatment of thoracic vascular trauma. They may be useful as a temporary bridge or a permanent implant. However, it is too early to make predictions regarding the ultimate place of this rapidly emerging technology in the treatment of large vessel injuries.

The close proximity of large central veins to the arterial structures in the chest makes mediastinal AVFs fairly common, especially after penetrating injury. The high flow and low resistance of the central veins make these fistulas particularly high-output lesions that are difficult to visualize arteriographically. Interventional techniques can obviate the need for operative exploration in many instances when arteriography demonstrates fistulas of noncritical vessels, which can be treated by angiographic embolization or stent and/or graft placement.

BRACHIOCEPHALIC VESSELS

Several endovascular techniques have been described for subclavian injuries. Angioplasty has been used to tack down the intimal flap. An alternative to simple angioplasty is the deployment of a stent to compress the damaged intima against the wall during the healing process. However, rupture of a partial thickness injury during these maneuvers is a potential risk. The radiologist must be prepared to inflate the balloon to control hemorrhage in such situations while the patient is rapidly prepared for surgery. (See Fig. 9–13.)

Interventional techniques also have a role in the management of transmural subclavian injury because they may allow the surgeon to avoid a sternotomy for proximal control. Maneuvers include stent placement, covered stent placement, and temporary placement of an occlusion balloon before surgery.

A covered stent can be considered for both intimal injuries and transmural injuries. Temporary balloon occlusion is a more conventional technique for radiologists that can be particularly helpful in subclavian arterial injuries. Balloon occlusion will provide the surgeon with proximal control of the vessel without the time or morbidity of a sternotomy. The injury can be approached through a supraclavicular incision with the knowledge that proximal control has been obtained from within the lumen. A double balloon device can provide proximal and distal control. It is often helpful to advance the catheter tip into one of the small branches of the subclavian artery, such as the thyrocervical trunk or costocervical trunk, to provide an anchor for the catheter.

Small Branch Injuries

The costocervical trunk and the thyrocervical trunk originate from the subclavian artery. For injuries to these vessels and their branches, angiographic embolization is the primary method of hemostasis. Damage to the thyrocervical trunk itself should be treated by isolation using large vessel occlusives. The trunk is usually short and may be tortuous. Extreme care should be taken to avoid reflux of a coil into the subclavian. If embolization cannot be performed safely, one should consider operative ligation as an alternative.

There are numerous small branches that may be injured in addition to the trunks themselves. These may be difficult to reach because of the tortuosity of the trunk. Proximal coil occlusion of the proximal trunk may not be adequate because of the rich collateral network. Flow directing small pledgets of surgical gelatin into the area of bleeding is usually effective.

Arteries that have been treated by transcatheter techniques include the intercostal arteries, the internal mammary arteries, the bronchial arteries, thoracic wall arteries, and small intrathoracic pulmonary arteries.

Abdominal Vascular Injury

AORTA

There are limited applications of endovascular techniques in patients with abdominal aortic injury. These patients are usually injured by penetrating trauma and their critical condition generally obviates the use of less direct methods of management. Rarely an aortic injury that has gone unrecognized during operation can be identified by angiography. Stent grafts have been used with success for aortic aneurysms. There may be a role for these devices in the treatment of abdominal aortic injury.

LUMBAR ARTERY

Lumbar artery injuries are encountered when pelvic fractures are associated with lumbar spine fractures. These are usually transverse process fractures, but they may also be seen with compression fractures. They are identified when abdominal aortography is performed as part of the evaluation of pelvic fracture bleeding. Embolization is an effective method of controlling hemorrhage from these vessels. There is a notable anomaly, the artery of Adamkiewicz, which replaces several segmental spinal arteries. This long conduit may originate at any spinal level from T6 to L3. Because this vessel supplies several segments of spinal cord, occlusion of this vessel creates an area of ischemia within the spinal cord. Embolization of the artery of Adamkiewicz is contraindicated.

Pedicle Vascular Injury

Decelerating trauma can result in vascular injuries to the arterial conduits of the abdominal viscera by stretching the artery at points of fixation. The renal artery is the most common of the pedicle injuries, although the celiac, the hepatic, and the splenic and superior mesenteric arteries may all be injured in this manner. Stretch injuries run a spectrum from vasospasm to transection. Intimal tears may be flow limiting and cause thrombosis or they may result in platelet deposition and subsequent distal embolization without thrombosis. Transmural injuries may result in blood loss and expanding perihilar hematomas. (See Fig. 9–14.)

Several direct and indirect signs of arterial injury may lead to invasive imaging and intervention. When peripheral infarcts in an organ are seen on CT scan, one should suspect an intimal injury and platelet emboli from the site of injury. Centrally located hematomas that obscure the region of the hilum also suggest the diagnosis of pedicle injury.

Conduit preservation is usually desirable in liver and kidney hilar injuries because these organs have limited collateral circulation. The spleen has a rich collateral network that maintains perfusion after occlusion of the splenic artery.

Several endovascular techniques can be used to manage these stretch injuries. Balloon catheters can be inflated to press the intimal flap back against the media. Since the rate of re-endothelialization depends on the cross-sectional area of intimal defect, decreasing the overall dimension of the intimal defect should increase the rate of healing. When this maneuver is not successful in improving intimal coverage and reducing resistance to flow, a bare metal stent may be used to maintain the reduction of the intimal flap.

If the injury is a transmural laceration or transection, then bare stenting may be insufficient to prevent blood loss because the defect may be kept open by the stent.

The use of covered stents to maintain flow while covering the hole in the vessel is an attractive innovation that is now available. This may be the most expeditious method of revascularization.

Injury to the splenic artery carries more management options. In addition to those mentioned earlier in this chapter, the splenic conduit can be sacrificed by coil occlusion without causing splenic infarction. The excellent collaterals allow rapid return of splenic blood flow (see Fig. 9–10).

Pelvis

Vascular injuries associated with blunt pelvic fractures are usually to the small branches of the internal iliac artery. Pelvic hemorrhage associated with penetrating pelvic trauma is more commonly caused by injuries to the larger conduit vessels of the aortoiliac and the iliocaval systems. (See Fig. 9–3.)

The indications for embolization are based on the hemodynamic status and the degree of blood loss, that is, the same as those for pelvic arteriography. Therefore, embolization should be performed whenever arterial extravasation is seen. Indeed, angiography should not be performed unless the angiography technician is prepared to embolize when signs of arterial injury are identified.

It is not possible to diminish pelvic and hypogastric venous flow by arterial embolization. The practice of "empirical embolization" in the absence of arterial injury is not recommended. Instead, other possible sources of blood loss should be considered.

Hemorrhage associated with pelvic fracture hemorrhage typically originates from multiple and bilateral small vessels supplying or adjacent to muscles, tendons, ligaments, nerves, and bone (see Fig. 9–3B and C). This requires small embolic material. The emboli must reach into the distal small vessels and bypass the numerous and extensive peripheral and central collateral circulation. Although these collaterals maintain adequate perfusion to the tissues supplied by the embolized vessels, they also increase the risks of recurrent bleeding as these collaterals enlarge. This is the reason that bilateral hypogastric artery ligation is unsuccessful in controlling pelvic hemorrhage. Surgical gelatin is the preferable embolic material for hemorrhage associated with pelvic fractures. Pledget size is dependent on the size of the vessels that are injured, but one must consider the effects of vasospasm and hypovolemia in determining the size of the vessels. The ideal size is generally between 2 and 4 mm^3; this allows collateral flow to reach the tissues while direct flow to the bleeding site is terminated. Smaller pledgets are not recommended because they may reach too far distally and result in ischemia or infarction.

The optimum site of embolization is to the artery in the distribution of bleeding. However, superselective catheterization of these multiple small vessels is more difficult and time consuming. It is not warranted in hemodynamically unstable patients. It is more practical to place the catheter more proximally and allow blood flow to carry the emboli to the site of bleeding. The advantages of a more central location in the hypogastric artery are the avoidance of vasospasm, a more expeditious and less complicated embolization, and flow direction of the emboli. This "spray" of emboli creates multiple sites of occlusion that diminish direct flow to the zone of hemorrhage.

The disadvantage of this nontarget embolization is that emboli may flow to areas of the pelvis, which are not bleeding and this may result in ischemia of normal tissues. However, nontarget embolization has not been a problem as long as the pledgets are not made too small. Bilateral hypogastric embolization has been well tolerated by my patients with minimal complications.

"Coil blockade" can be used to prevent embolization of uninjured pelvic vascular beds. This technique occludes the origins of normal vascular beds with coils that act in a fashion as "filters" to block the flow of pledget emboli into normal vascular beds. Embolization with Gelfoam through a catheter placed proximally allows flow of the small particulate emboli to the area of bleeding. The endpoint of embolization is stasis within the bleeding vessel. It is vital that pelvic aortography and bilateral hypogastric angiography be performed after embolization to assure that bleeding does not persist through collateral circulation. Hypogastric arteriography alone may not visualize the collaterals from the femoral arteries.

Upper Extremity

Particulate embolization is appropriate when hemorrhage results from laceration of terminal vessels of axillary artery such as the thoracoacromial and the circumflex humeral arteries. These vessels are often too small and too tortuous to allow superselective catheterization with standard catheters and the effort and time needed to use coaxial microcatheters is not worth it. Large vessel occlusives such as coils are inadequate for these terminal branches. Embolization with small particles of Gelfoam in the range of 1 to 2 mm^3 can be injected. The catheter should be placed in a larger more proximal vessel so blood flow can be maintained around the catheter allowing the emboli to flow into the small vessels. When the catheter is placed too distally, there may be inadequate flow to advance the emboli into the periphery. The emboli should be introduced in small aliquots slowly and with little injection pressure to avoid reflux of emboli into the axillary artery and down into the hand vessels. Larger aliquots of pledgets tend to clump near the site of injection and this diminishes the likelihood that the emboli will reach the peripheral bleeding site.

Coil occlusion is more appropriate for injuries of the larger axillary conduits such as the subscapular and lateral thoracic branches. These larger longer and less tortuous conduit vessels arborize at some distance from their origin. Using microcatheters coaxially, often it is possible to isolate the area of the torn vessel without damaging the vascular bed. If that is not possible, particulate embolization is an acceptable alternative. Postembolization arteriography requires careful attention to all potential collateral circulation to the shoulder, including subclavian branches and chest wall vessels.

THE ARM

The brachial artery is the most commonly injured blood vessel of the upper extremity.

The diagnosis of brachial artery injury is usually obvious by physical examination: External hemorrhage is common, and loss of palpable pulses is likely. Diagnostic arteriography is rarely necessary.

There are some circumstances when arteriography has value. The propensity of the brachial artery to develop vascular spasm after any trauma may result in loss of pulses without any true transmural vascular injury. Fractures or direct contusion of the vessel without definitive transmural injury may result in pulse deficit. When pulses are diminished but not absent, arteriography can sometimes be used to differentiate spasm from traumatic occlusion or intimal disruption (see Fig. 9–4A).

Revascularization is preferable to embolization. Endovascular techniques have few indications in the management of vascular injuries of the arm. When vasospasm is identified, intraarterial vasodilators such as nitroglycerine in 200 microgram doses sometimes restore pulses. Vasodilator infusion therapy can differentiate true vascular injury from pure spasm. When a vessel appears normal without other signs of vascular injury after vasodilator therapy, one can be fairly confident that true arterial injury is not present. On the other hand, when narrowing resolves, underlying signs of true vascular injury, such as intimal flaps, extravasation and AVFs may be better seen.

There is rarely indication for permanent transcatheter occlusion of the brachial. When the radial or ulnar artery originates aberrantly from the proximal brachial or axillary artery, the brachial artery is expendable and embolization with coils can be used to treat brachial artery injury (see Fig. 9–11).

Embolotherapy of branches of the brachial arterial can be considered when the patient can tolerate the time necessary to complete the diagnostic evaluation and selective catheterization and when embolization can be done safely without significant risk of distal errant embolization. It is not an essential procedure and it is often easier and safer to directly control these vessels operatively. However, if branch injuries are found in stable patients without external blood loss, and the catheter can be seated securely within the injured vessel, an attempt at transcatheter occlusion can be made.

THE ELBOW, FOREARM, HANDS, AND WRISTS

The clinical presentation of vascular injuries in the forearm usually is evident on physical examination, resulting in hematomas, external bleeding, or pulse deficits. The approach to the treatment of these wounds differs considerably from that of the brachial artery. The presence of three arterial conduits and the rich network of collateral arteries around the wrist make each of the vessels expendable. In contradistinction to the brachial artery of which repair is usually attempted, the forearm branches are usually ligated. Therefore, transcatheter arterial embolization can be considered as an alternative for either the radial, the ulnar, or the interosseous arteries. Occlusion of any of these vessels can be considered for transmural injury when the viability of the hand is not placed in jeopardy by occlusion, when the catheter can be safely and expeditiously placed at the site of injury, and when vasospasm has not occurred. If the catheter cannot be securely positioned selectively within the injured vessel, embolization should not be attempted. If subselective catheterization proves to be time-consuming, the procedure should be aborted and the patient sent to the operating room.

Embolization of branches of the radial and ulnar vessels is rarely indicated since the necessary superselective catheterization is laborious and filled with risk of errant emboli and occlusion resulting from catheter spasm and stasis. Control of bleeding from these vessels can be accomplished with less risk by direct pressure and, if necessary, operative ligation.

Lower Extremity

THE HIP AND GROIN

Iatrogenic vascular injury is the most common injury since procedures that damage these vessels, including angiography, cardiac catheterization, femoral arterial and venous access, and vena caval filter placement, are so common.

Clinical signs of arterial injury are often readily apparent because of the superficial location of injuries, but occult injuries may also occur, especially if the wound results in AVF, arterial occlusion, or intimal damage. The collateral circulation of the hip is rich. Distal pulses can sometimes be palpated in the presence of major vascular injury.

Common Femoral and Superficial Femoral Arteries

Patients with clinically evident signs of arterial injury in the groin do not require diagnostic arteriography. Interventional techniques, however, can be useful in some arterial injuries in the groin. Transcatheter arterial embolization can be used to control muscular branch bleeding. Temporary balloon occlusion can be used to obtain proximal and distal vascular control of the external iliac and femoral arteries before exploration, and iatrogenic false aneurysm resulting from iatrogenic puncture of the superficial femoral artery (SFA) can be managed nonoperatively by compression techniques. The use of covered stents placed percutaneously has also been described.

The common femoral artery (CFA) and SFA are not expendable as conduits. Therefore, embolization is not indicated for acute transmural injury of these arteries vital to lower extremity viability. Operative revascularization is the procedure of choice for transmural injury. The placement of a covered intravascular stent across a transmural laceration of the CFA or SFA is a potential application of this new technology. Limited data at the present time prevents recommendation of widespread use of this technique, but maintenance of flow has been reported.

If arterial extravasation of the CFA or SFA is seen at angiography, preoperative hemostasis can be achieved by placement of a temporary occlusion balloon at or above the site of injury (see Fig. 9–9). This can allow a more orderly preparation of the operating suite and the patient before definitive repair. Operative exposure of the injured segment can proceed without arterial blood loss.

Profunda Femoris Artery

The origin of the profunda femoris artery (PFA) is often amenable to operative repair. As a major collateral circuit in atherosclerotic disease of the iliofemoral system, maintenance of the PFA is desirable but not essential. Embolization of the origin of the PFA can be performed as an alternative, especially for chronic AVFs, grossly contaminated wounds, and patients with other mitigating circumstances that make further operation and anesthesia undesirable (see Fig. 9–4E).

Coils are the embolization material of choice for occlusion of lacerations and AVFs. They should be placed proximal and distal to the site of laceration or fistula because the rich collateral networks of the thigh and hip will allow the fistula to persist if an incomplete isolation of the injury is accomplished. Proximal PFA lesions may require occlusion of the origin of the circumflex branches to adequately exclude collateral circulation. Care in sizing and positioning of coil emboli in the proximal PFA should be exercised. Placement of a coil that is too long or too wide in diameter risks retrograde positioning of the coil across the origin of the PFA into the SFA or CFA. One should choose a length of coil shorter than the distance to the origin of the PFA so the coil does not extend into the common femoral artery if incomplete coiling occurs. Coil diameter should be slightly larger or equal in size to the diameter of the PFA at the site of embolization. Gelfoam and other particulate emboli are not desirable for the main conduit.

The medial circumflex and the lateral circumflex femoral arteries are expendable vessels of the groin that are both amenable to embolization when injured. Vascular injuries to the terminal branches of these vessels can be occluded with particulate matter. The particles should be 1 to 2 mm in diameter and introduced slowly and gently through a catheter located near the origin of the circumflex artery. This will allow the particles to flow into the periphery where they will lodge beyond many of the collateral circuits and so prevent recurrent bleeding or pseudoaneurysm. Coaxial catheters can be used to place the emboli as close as possible to the injury site; however, there is really no advantage to this more tedious method.

Embolization of the circumflex femoral arteries proper is best accomplished by coil occlusion unless there is also related small vessel branch bleeding. Gelfoam is undesirable because it must also result in occlusion of small vessels and compromise of the vascular bed, which is not injured.

THE THIGH

As a rule, SFA injury is treated by restoration of prograde flow. Proximal and distal vascular control is followed by resection and replacement of damaged vessel. There are rare indications for endovascular procedures on this essential conduit of the lower leg. When a bleeding SFA injury is identified during angiography, temporary double balloon occlusion proximal and distal to the injury site, providing preoperative vascular control, may result in less blood loss during transit to the operating room and during exposure of the injury. Percutaneous endografts may have a role in limited theoretical situations such as when infections preclude operative exposure. Because the injury site is not dissected, there is no loss of tamponade of the associated venous injury during repair. Diminished blood loss would be advantageous. Further clinical trials are necessary.

Other injuries, such as those to the PFA and its branches, can be managed more easily and less invasively by endovascular procedures than by operative methods. Thigh hematoma resulting from PFA and perforating branch lacerations and transections can be controlled by embolization. These vessels are difficult to expose operatively because they extend posteriorly through the adductor magnus muscle. The unnecessary blood loss from these and the associated venous injuries during operative exposure is a compelling reason to attempt embolization.

THE KNEE AND CALF

Popliteal Artery

Trauma about the knee that results in vascular injury rarely warrants endovascular procedures. The critical nature of the popliteal artery makes it nonexpendable. Embolization does not have any advantage over revascularization. To my knowledge, intentional occlusion of the popliteal artery by embolization techniques has not been reported, although I have performed embolization of a isolated popliteal segment that had become a conduit for a chronic AVF. Treatment of traumatic thrombosis by intra-arterial thrombolytic agents is not indicated. Exacerbation of bleeding and the delay necessary for lysis make this an impractical concept.

Popliteal Artery Branches

The geniculate and sural branches of the popliteal artery, on the other hand, are vessels that can be sacrificed when damaged in the absence of injury of the popliteal artery. Microcatheterization of these branches using coaxial catheters is possible and embolization using coils or Gelfoam pledgets can attain hemostasis. As with embolization of branches of the SFA, errant embolization is a risk because of the difficulties with selective catheterization.

The anterior tibial, posterior tibial, and peroneal arteries and their branches are expendable. In most young trauma patients, patency of one vessel is usually sufficient to maintain viability of the calf and foot. Certainly, occlusion of a single vessel is well tolerated by most patients. Revascularization of these injuries is technically challenging and usually not worth the time necessary to repair them. The use of endovascular techniques of injuries of the trifurcation vessels is well established as a therapeutic option for injuries of the calf.

Diagnostic arteriography of the calf is indicated when there is a history of active pulsating hemorrhage or when hard signs of vascular injury and the limb do not appear to be immediately threatened. Antegrade access with a "downhill" puncture is warranted when there are signs of arterial injury. This allows a more precise positioning of the catheter and allows for a more direct method of delivering embolization materials.

Treatment of injuries of the three major branches of the popliteal artery requires isolation of the damaged segment from arterial flow. This usually requires embolization proximal and distal to the site of injury. The embolic material preferred for this isolation is the coil, although surgical gelatin can also be used.

REFERENCES

Agolini SF, Shah K, Jaffe J, et al: Arterial embolization is a rapid and effective technique for controlling pelvic fracture hemorrhage. J Trauma 1997;43:395-399.

Janicek MJ, Van den Abbeele AD, DeSisto WC, et al: Embolization of platelets after endothelial injury to the aorta in rabbits. Assessment with [111]indium-labeled platelets and angiography. Invest Radiol 1991;26:655-659.

Kantor A, Sclafani SJ, Scalea T, et al: The role of interventional radiology in the management of genitourinary trauma. Urol Clin North Am 1989;16:255-265.

Ohki T, Veith FJ, Marin ML, et al: Endovascular approaches for traumatic arterial lesions. Semin Vasc Surg 1997;10:272-285.

Sclafani AP, Sclafani SJ: Angiography and transcatheter arterial embolization of vascular injuries of the face and neck. Laryngoscope 1996;106:168-173.

Sclafani SJ, Panetta T, Goldstein AS, et al: The management of arterial injuries caused by penetration of zone III of the neck. J Trauma 1985;25:871-881.

Trooskin SZ, Sclafani S, Winfield J, et al: The management of vascular injuries of the extremity associated with civilian firearms. Surg Gynecol Obstet 1993;176:350-354.

10

Endovascular Grafts for Traumatic Vascular Lesions

NICHOLAS J. GARGIULO, III
TAKAO OHKI
NEAL S. CAYNE
FRANK J. VEITH

INTRODUCTION

The advent of endovascular grafting to treat abdominal aortic aneurysms (AAAs) by Parodi, Palmaz, and Barone (1991) has expanded to include arterial occlusive disease, occluded grafts, peripheral aneurysms, and traumatic arterial lesions (Marin and colleagues, 1995a, 1995b; Parodi, 1995). The past decade has marked a new enthusiasm for the endovascular repair of AAAs. However, the value and long-term outcome have yet to be proven. Endoleaks, arterial injury, and late graft deterioration continue to complicate endovascular graft repair of AAAs. Since standard open aneurysm repair remains a safe and reliable procedure with good long-term outcomes, the role of endovascular graft repair in low-risk patients remains to be determined.

207

On the other hand, the role of endovascular grafts for traumatic arterial injuries appears to be more easily defensible, especially when large central vessels are involved. Vascular trauma within the thorax or abdomen complicates the surgical approach to a vascular injury. Distorted anatomy due to a large hematoma or false aneurysm and venous hypertension secondary to an arteriovenous fistula are just a few of the problems encountered during an open repair of injured vessels. Endovascular repair is more appealing because it can be performed from a remote site and does not require direct surgical exposure of the injury site, thus reducing the morbidity and mortality rates that accompany open repair. Furthermore, endovascular repair is most beneficial for those patients who are critically ill from other injuries or medical comorbidities.

The main endovascular techniques used in the treatment of vascular trauma include coil embolization, intravascular stents, and endovascular stented grafts. Traumatic vascular lesions usually have normal, healthy, proximal, and distal arterial segments or graft fixation zones for endovascular graft deployment. This is in contrast to the complex necks and iliac tortuosity of AAAs. As a result, high technical success rates and low rates of endograft migration or leakage have been reported after endovascular grafting for traumatic vascular lesions.

This chapter describes endovascular techniques that may prove helpful in vascular trauma and reviews our experience with endovascular grafts for traumatic lesions at Montefiore Medical Center in New York. We also discuss the role of endovascular grafts for thoracic aortic vascular injuries.

COIL EMBOLIZATION, INTRAVASCULAR STENTS, AND OTHER ENDOVASCULAR TECHNIQUES

Embolization coils have been used to treat relatively small traumatic arteriovenous fistulas and pseudoaneurysms involving nonessential vessels, such as a lumbar artery, the internal mammary artery, or the branches of the hypogastric or deep femoral arteries (Rosch, Dotter, and Brown, 1972; Panetta and colleagues, 1985). Long-term follow-up results of the use of these coil-treated lesions have proven favorable. Placement of intravascular stents is useful for the repair of intimal flaps. Because of their porous nature, however, uncovered stents are not indicated for treating arteriovenous fistulas or pseudoaneurysms of large vessels. Although coils and stents have proved to be effective in selected cases, most patients with vascular trauma are not amenable to such therapy.

A novel method for obtaining intraluminal balloon control of arteries in difficult circumstances has been previously described by our group (Veith, Sanchez, and Ohki, 1998). This technique is particularly useful when bleeding, scarring, or infection makes dissection of proximal arteries difficult or dangerous. Through an arterial puncture distal to the site where proximal control is required, an 18-gauge needle is inserted into a normal artery. A guidewire is inserted through the needle. Over the guidewire, a 6- or 7-Fr hemostatic sheath and dilator is inserted. Under fluoroscopic guidance, a standard balloon catheter is passed through the hemostatic sheath. Radiopaque contrast is then injected to confirm optimal placement of the balloon catheter for proximal occlusion within the arterial tree. The sheath may then be retracted, and the balloon inflated until arterial inflow is occluded. Alternatively, double-lumen balloon catheters may be passed over a guidewire and angiographic techniques can be used to facilitate proximal balloon control.

ENDOVASCULAR GRAFTS FOR ARTERIAL TRAUMA: BACKGROUND

Endovascular grafts have significantly extended the potential of endovascular therapy for vascular trauma. The concept of endovascular grafting for traumatic arterial lesions was initially proposed by Dotter (1969). Volodos and colleagues (1991) were the first to clinically apply this technology by placing

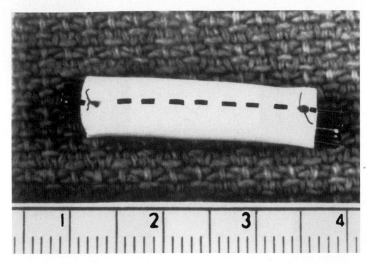

■ **FIGURE 10–1**
Endovascular stented graft. A Palmaz stent is sewn to an expanded PTFE graft. (From Ohki T, Veith FJ, Marin ML, et al: Endovascular approaches for traumatic arterial lesions. Semin Vasc Surg 1997;10:272-285.) ■

a Dacron graft and a self-expanding stent to treat a thoracic aortic pseudoaneurysm in 1986.

Endovascular grafts have been used to treat almost every kind of injury at various locations in the body. Some patients treated with endovascular grafts have been hemodynamically stable. However, some of these grafts have also been used to treat life-threatening acute hemorrhage (Becker and colleagues, 1991; Patel and colleagues, 1996). The types of devices that have been reported are predominantly a combination of a Palmaz stent and an expanded PTFE (ePTFE) graft (Fig. 10–1) (Marin and colleagues, 1993, 1994; Becker and colleagues, 1995; Terry and colleagues, 1995; Zajiko and colleagues, 1995; Gomez-Jorge and colleagues, 1996; Criado and colleagues, 1997; Dorros and Joseph, 1997). The use of a vein graft in combination with a Palmaz stent has also been reported, since the traumatized field is often contaminated. More recently, industry made devices such as the Corvita endovascular graft, the AneuRx graft and the Wallstent graft have become commercially available in the United States. AneuRx grafts have been approved by the Food and Drug Administration for the treatment of AAAs, and the Wallstent for obstructive biliary lesions. Components of the AneuRx include the bifurcated graft and the proximal and distal extension cuffs. Though not approved for the use in traumatic lesions, these grafts have been used in the "off-label" fashion.

The lesion, location, characteristics, site of arterial access, technical success rate, and the outcome of endovascular grafts in the treatment of vascular trauma are summarized in Table 10–1. These results have been encour-

TABLE 10–1
ENDOVASCULAR GRAFTS FOR ARTERIAL TRAUMA

Type	Combination of Palmaz Stent and Various Grafts				Cragg Endopro	Corvita Graft
Stent	Palmaz stent				Nitinol	Self-expanding braided stent
Graft material	PTFE	Dacron	Vein	Silicone	Ultrathin woven polyester fabric	Polycarbonate urethane
Arterial access	1 or 2	2	2	1 or 2	2	2

1, open arteriotomy; 2, percutaneous.
From Ohki T, Marin ML, Veith FJ: Use of endovascular grafts to treat non-aneurysmal arterial disease. Ann Vasc Surg 1997;11:200-205.

TABLE 10–2
CHARACTERISTICS OF LESION AND OUTCOME BY LOCATION OF INJURY

Location of Trauma	Axillary Subclavian Artery	Aorta or Iliac Artery	Femoral Artery
No. of cases	18	15	5
Cause of injury	Bullet: 55%; catheterization: 28%; others: 17%	Surgical: 36%; catheterization: 18%; bullet: 9%; others: 36%	Bullet: 60%; catheterization: 40%
Presence of pseudoaneurysm	61%	67%	80%
Presence of atrioventricular fistula	44%	73%	40%
Arterial access	Brachial arteriotomy: 39%; Brachial percutaneous: 39%; Femoral percutaneous: 22%	Femoral arteriotomy: 64%; Femoral percutaneous: 36%	Femoral arteriotomy: 80%; Femoral percutaneous: 20%
Technical success rate	94% (17/18)*	100%	100%
Complication: Minor	0%	7%	0%
Major	6%†	7%§	0%
Mean length of stay	3.3 days	4 days	5.3 days
Mean follow-up	18mo	10.5mo	17.4mo
Primary patency	85%‡	100%	100%

*One failure due to misdiagnosis.
†Brachial artery injury during device insertion.
‡Two failures due to stent deformity.
§Distal embolization requiring thrombectomy.

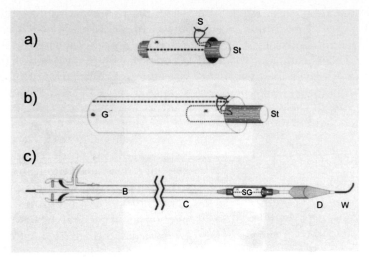

■ **FIGURE 10–2**
A, Schematic drawing of an endovascular stented graft or covered stent. A segment of expanded PTFE is attached to a Palmaz stent (St) using two 5-0 Prolene U stitches (S). *B,* Schematic drawing of a double-stent endovascular stented graft. The proximal stent (St) is sutured to the graft as described in *(A).* The distal end of the graft is marked with gold markers (G) for visualization under the fluoroscope. *C,* The stent graft (SG) is mounted on an angioplasty balloon (B) and placed into a sheath (C) before insertion. Note the presence of a dilator tip (D) at the end of the balloon catheter, which provides a smooth taper within the catheter. W, guidewire. (From Ohki T, Veith FJ, Marin ML, et al: Endovascular approaches for traumatic arterial lesions. Semin Vasc Surg 1997;10:272-285.) ■

aging with a high technical success rate (94% to 100%) and a complication rate of 0% to 7% (Table 10–2), especially when we consider the difficulties that could be encountered in treating these lesions by a direct surgical repair. In addition, the minimal invasiveness and the potential for cost-effectiveness of such endovascular techniques are apparent from the short length of stay (3.3 to 3.5 days) (Table 10–2). Most endovascular grafts are deployed in nonatherosclerotic central vessels of a large caliber and have excellent durability. Mean follow-up at 16 months revealed excellent mid-term patency rates ranging from 85% to 100% depending on where deployment occurred.

The Montefiore Experience with Endovascular Grafts for Arterial Trauma

TECHNIQUE AND DEVICES

At Montefiore Medical Center, we have mainly used the Palmaz stent (Cordis [Johnson & Johnson Company, Warren, NJ]) in combination with a thin-walled ePTFE graft (Fig. 10–1) covering to perform arterial repairs of pseudoaneurysms and arteriovenous fistulas (Marin and colleagues, 1993, 1994, 1995a). Depending on the length of the lesion, either a single stent device or a doubly stented device was used. The stents varied between 2 and 3 cm in length (Palmaz P-204, 294, 308) and were fixed inside 6 mm Gore-Tex grafts (W.L. Gore and Associates, Flagstaff, Ariz) by two U stitches. The stented graft was then mounted on a balloon angioplasty catheter, which had a tapered dilator tip firmly attached to its end (Fig. 10–2). The entire device was contained within a 10- to 12-Fr delivery system for over-the-wire insertion either percutaneously or through an open arteriotomy.

Alternative devices included the Corvita stent graft (Corvita Corporation, Miami, Fla), and the Wallgraft, both of which are fabricated from a self-expanding stent or braided wire. The Corvita stent graft is covered with polycarbonate elastomer fibers, and the Wallgraft is covered with Dacron. The Corvita stent graft may be cut to the desired length in the operating room using a wire-cutting scissors and then loaded into a specially designed delivery sheath. This sheath has a central "pusher" catheter, which is used for maintaining the graft in position while the outer sheath is being retrieved. The Wallgraft comes in various diameters up to 14 mm and lengths up to 7 cm.

RESULTS

Each procedure was performed in the operating room under fluoroscopic (OEC 9800, OEC/GE, Salt Lake City, Utah; Philips, BV 212, Netherlands) guidance. Most cases were performed under local or epidural anesthesia with two cases requiring general anesthesia. A total of 17 stented grafts were used to treat 17 patients with traumatic arterial lesions (Table 10–3). The etiology for these lesions is described in Table 10–3, with the majority comprising gunshot wounds (Figs. 10–3 and 10–4) and iatrogenic injuries (Figs. 10–5 and 10–6).

All injuries except for one were associated with an adjacent pseudoaneurysm (Fig. 10–5). Five patients had an arteriovenous fistula (Fig. 10–6), and eight patients had other associated injuries (Table 10–3).

Procedural complications were limited to one distal embolus, which was treated with suction embolectomy, and one wound hematoma, which resolved without further intervention. Graft patency was 100% with no early or late graft occlusions (mean follow-up was 30 months [range, 6 to 46 months]).

One patient with a left axillary subclavian stent graft developed compression of the stent at 12 months and was treated with balloon angioplasty. This recurred 3 months later but did not require any intervention. At 3-year follow-up, the graft was patent. A second patient developed stenosis at either end of his stent graft and was successfully treated with additional balloon dilation and Palmaz stent placement (Fig. 10–4). A third patient with an axillary pseudoaneurysm repaired with a stent graft required a vein patch to close a small brachial artery insertion site.

Immediate repair of blunt thoracic aortic injuries to prevent rupture of the contained hematoma as previously described may no longer be necessary based on studies by Camp and Shackford (1997) and Maggisano and colleagues (1995). These authors suggest that delayed repair of hemodynamically stable thoracic aortic injuries reduces morbidity and mortality. Delayed repair allows the trauma team to surgically optimize the multi-injured patient before a major surgical insult. These studies have significantly influenced the role of endovascular grafting in the treatment of thoracic aortic injuries. Myriad unique endovascular techniques and grafts have been employed and reported to treat these injuries (White and colleagues, 1997; Lobato and colleagues, 2000; Fontaine and colleagues, 2001; Ruchat and colleagues, 2001).

Endovascular grafting has been employed in blunt and penetrating injuries of the abdominal aorta (White and colleagues, 1997; Fontaine and colleagues, 2001). These include successful exclusion of a posterior aortic pseudoaneurysm between the superior mesenteric artery and the right renal artery following a gunshot wound. A Cooley VeriSoft vascular graft attached to the outer surface of an extra-large Palmaz stent was successfully deployed across the aortic pseudoaneurysm 3 weeks after the initial injury.

In addition to these homemade devices, industry-made devices recently became available. These include the Talent thoracic endovascular graft (World Medical Corporation, Medtronic), the Thoracic Excluder graft (W.L. Gore, Flagstaff, Ariz) and the AneuRx graft (Fontaine and colleagues, 2001; Ruchat and colleagues, 2001). Neither of these has been approved by the FDA for commercialization in the United States; however, some investigators have successfully used these grafts to treat life-threatening thoracic aortic injuries on a compassionate basis. These industry-made devices, especially the Excluder graft, are much more flexible and have a lower insertion profile.

Delayed repair has been reported from 1 week to a mean of 5.4 months after the initial accident. There has been no evidence of endoleak or rupture at approximately 1-year follow-up. Furthermore, although the number

Text continued on p. 218

TABLE 10-3
ENDOVASCULAR GRAFTS FOR TRAUMATIC ARTERIAL LESIONS: MONTEFIORE EXPERIENCE

Sex/Age (Yr.)	Mechanism of Injury	Vessel(s) Involved	PA	AVF	Anesthesia	Associated Injuries	Injury to Repair Time Interval	Stent Graft Length (cm)	Access	Hospital Stay (Days)	Patency (Mo.)	Complications
F/80	Catheterization	RASA	No	No	Local	None	2 days	4†	Right brachial artery	2	1	—
M/21	Surgical trauma	RCIA LCIV	Yes	Yes	Local	None	4 wk	6†	RCFA percutaneous	4	6	—
M/22	Bullet	LSFA	Yes	No	Local	Soft tissue injury; left DVT	12 hr	3	LSFA arteriotomy	6	9*	—
F/85	Surgical trauma	RCIA	Yes	Yes	Local	None	8 yr	5†	LCFA percutaneous	4	11	Distal emboli‡
M/49	Catheterization	RCIA	Yes	Yes	Epidural	None	18 mo	5	RCFA arteriotomy	5	11	Wound hematoma
M/68	Iliac graft disruption	LCIA	Yes	No	Epidural	None	1 mo	9	LCFA arteriotomy	5	9	—
M/66	Aortic graft disruption	Aorta	Yes	No	Epidural	None	1 wk	10	LCFA arteriotomy	5	18	—
M/76	Aortic disruption	Aorta	Yes	No	Epidural	None	3 days	7	LCFA arteriotomy	7	20	—
M/18	Bullet	RASA	Yes	No	Local	None	6 hr	3	Right brachial artery	3	21	—
M/22	Bullet	RASA	Yes	No	Local	Hemothorax	3 hr	3	Right brachial artery	6	21	—
M/18	Bullet	RSA	Yes	Yes	Local	Hemothorax	48 hr	3	Right brachial artery	4	30	—
F/78	Catheterization	RSA	Yes	No	Local	Hemothorax	24 hr	3	Right brachial arteriotomy	8 wk§	37	—
M/78	Catheterization	LCIA	Yes	No	Epidural	None	4 mo	2	LCFA arteriotomy	2	37	—
M/35	Bullet	RASA	Yes	No	Local	Brachial plexus	3 wk	3	Right brachial arteriotomy	4	38	—
M/24	Knife	LASA	Yes	No	General	Pneumothorax; hemothorax	4 hr	3	Left brachial arteriotomy	7	42	Stent compression
M/28	Bullet	RSFA	Yes	No	Local	Left open femur fracture	12 hr	3	RSFA arteriotomy	9	45	—
M/20	Bullet	LSFA LSFV	Yes	Yes	General	Soft tissue buttock	36 hr	3	LSFA percutaneous	5	47	—

*Died 2 months postprocedure (homicide).
†Corvita stent graft.
‡Treated with catheter suction thrombectomy.
§Hospitalized for multiple medical problems.
AVF, arteriovenous fistula; DVT, deep venous thrombosis; LASA, left axillary subclavian artery; LCFA, left common femoral artery; LCIA, left common iliac artery; LSFA, left superficial femoral artery; LSFV, left superficial femoral vein; PA, pseudoaneurysm; RASA, right axillary subclavian artery; RCIA, right common iliac artery; RSA, right subclavian artery; RSFA, right superficial femoral artery.

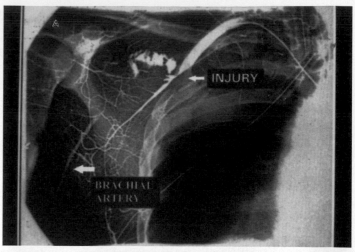

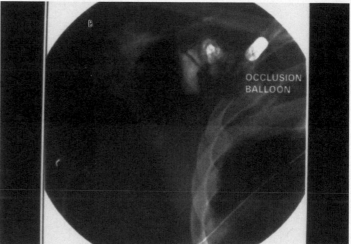

■ **FIGURE 10–3**
Angiographic images of a patient who sustained a gunshot wound to the right chest. *A,* An angiogram performed via a femoral artery puncture shows occlusion of the right subclavian artery and active bleeding. *B,* An occlusion balloon was placed to achieve hemostasis. *C,* Following hemostasis, the patient was taken to the operating room. A guidewire was successfully passed across the injured artery and was repaired by the insertion of a stented graft of polytetrafluoroethylene (expanded PTFE and Palmaz stent). (From Patel AV, Marin ML, Veith FJ, et al: Endovascular graft repair of penetrating subclavian artery injuries. J Endovasc Surg 1996;3:382-388.) ■

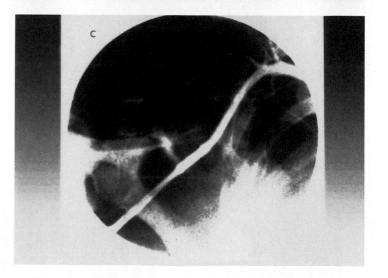

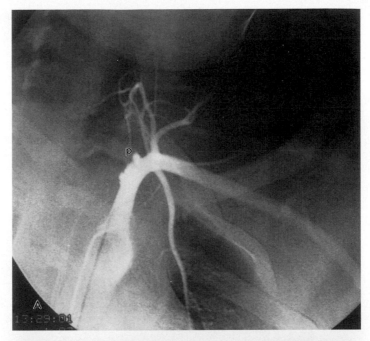

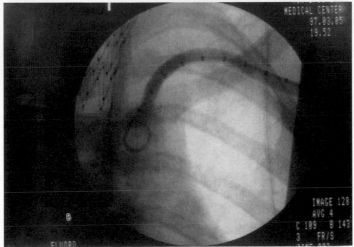

■ **FIGURE 10–4**

The patient is a 19-year-old man status post a gunshot wound to the chest that traversed the mediastinum from right to left, injuring his esophagus, trachea, and left subclavian artery. *A,* The initial angiogram shows occlusion of the left vertebral artery and a small pseudoaneurysm (p) at that site. He was transferred to our institution for endovascular treatment following placement of a covered esophageal stent to repair his tracheoesophageal fistula. *B,* A Corvita endoluminal graft was placed across the lesion and there was excellent flow through it.   *Continued*

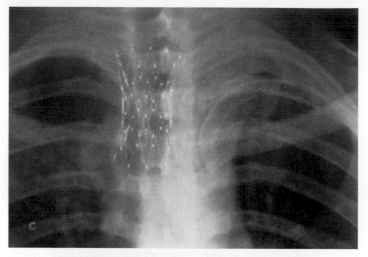

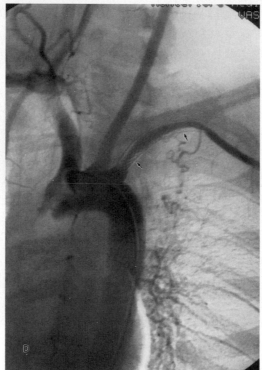

■ **FIGURE 10–4**

cont'd C, A plain x-ray film demonstrates the esophageal stent and the Corvita graft in the left subclavian artery. *D,* At 4 months after graft insertion, his left radial pulse was diminished, although he remained asymptomatic. An angiogram was taken that revealed intimal hyperplasia throughout the graft, more prominent at both ends of the graft *(arrows).* These lesions were angioplastied and a Palmaz stent was placed. After the procedure, the patient had a strong radial pulse. (From Ohki T, Veith FJ, Kraas C, et al: Endovascular therapy for upper extremity injury. Semin Vasc Surg 1998;11:106-115.) ■

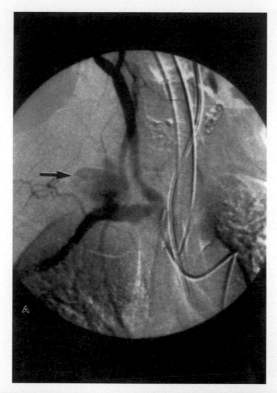

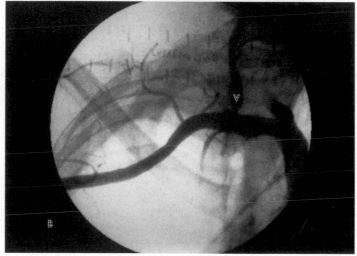

■ **FIGURE 10–5**

A, This arteriogram shows a large pseudoaneurysm of the subclavian artery *(arrow)* just distal to the right vertebral artery that occurred after an attempted subclavian vein catheter insertion. *B,* Following stented graft (expanded PTFE and Palmaz stent) placement through the right brachial artery, the pseudoaneurysm was excluded. Vertebral artery flow was maintained (V). (From Marin ML, Veith FJ, Panetta TF, et al: Transluminally placed endovascular stented graft repair for arterial trauma. J Vasc Surg 1994;20:466-473.) ■

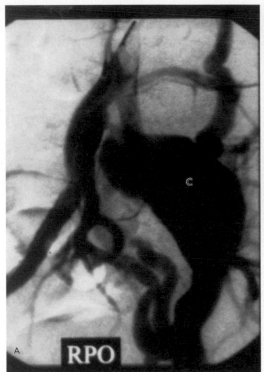
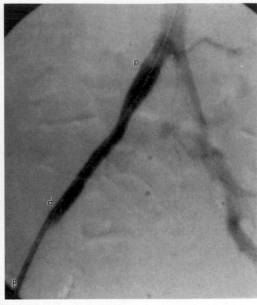

■ **FIGURE 10-6**

A, Preoperative angiogram of an iatrogenic arteriovenous fistula (AVF) following lumbar disk surgery. The patient presented with severe swelling of the left lower extremity. The left common iliac vein (C) is dilated secondary to the fistula. *B,* Completion angiogram. A PTFE graft was fixed proximally (p) and distally (d) with a Palmaz stent to exclude the fistula from the arterial circulation. Coil embolization of the internal iliac artery was performed before stent-graft insertion. (From Ohki T, Veith FJ: Endovascular techniques in the treatment of penetrating arterial trauma. In Yao JST, Pearce WH [eds]. Practical Vascular Surgery, 1st ed. Stamford, Conn, Appleton & Lange, 1999, pp 409-423.) ■

of reported cases is small, there has been no mention of postoperative paraplegia. These limited experiences suggest that endovascular graft techniques will be better than more traditional open techniques of thoracic aortic repair requiring either bypass or the clamp-and-sew technique, which report postoperative paraplegia rates of 4.5% to 16.4%, respectively (Fabian and colleagues, 1997).

SUMMARY

Endovascular grafting for traumatic arterial lesions has become an additional tool for the vascular surgeon. Complex open surgical repair of thoracic or intra-abdominal vascu-

lar injuries may be approached with minimally invasive endovascular techniques. Large hematomas, false aneurysms, and arteriovenous fistulas that often obscure the open surgical field have minimal impact on endovascular repair. This can be performed by accessing vascular lesions from remote sites so that embolization coils, stents, or endovascular grafts may be deployed.

Few vascular injuries may be amenable to coil embolization or stent placement. However, endovascular grafts have greatly expanded endovascular therapy for vascular trauma. These grafts have been used to treat myriad vascular injuries at various locations in the body.

Endovascular grafts have a low morbidity rate, high success rate, reduced anesthetic requirements, and a minimal dissection requirement in the traumatized field. These qualities are particularly advantageous for patients with central arteriovenous fistulas or false aneurysms, especially those critically ill from other coexisting injuries or medical comorbidities.

Endovascular grafts and techniques will continue to evolve and complement traditional open techniques in vascular trauma. Future development of smaller delivery systems, better endografts, operating rooms equipped with improved angiographic imaging systems, and a supply of endovascular equipment will increasingly help vascular surgeons of the future to manage patients with vascular trauma better.

ACKNOWLEDGMENTS

This work was supported by grants from the U.S. Public Health Service (HL 02990), the Manning Foundation, the Anna S. Brown Trust, the New York Institute for Vascular Studies, and the William J. von Liebig Foundation.

REFERENCES

Becker GJ, Benenati JF, Zemel G, et al: Percutaneous placement of a balloon-expandable intraluminal graft for life-threatening subclavian arterial hemorrhage. JVIR 1991;2:225-229.

Becker GJ, Katzen BT, Benenati JF, et al: Endografts for the treatment of aneurysm and traumatic vascular lesions: MVI experience. J Endovasc Surg 1995;2:380-382.

Brandt MM, Kazanjian S, Wahl WL: The utility of endovascular stents in the treatment of blunt arterial injuries. J Trauma 2001;51(5):901-905.

Camp PC, Shackford SR: Outcome after blunt traumatic thoracic aortic laceration: Identification of a high-risk cohort. Western Trauma Association Multicenter Study Group. J Trauma 1997; 43:413-422.

Criado E, Marston WA, Ligush J, et al: Endovascular repair of peripheral aneurysms, pseudoaneurysms, and arteriovenous fistulas. Ann Vasc Surg 1997;11:256-263.

Dorros G, Joseph G: Closure of a popliteal arteriovenous fistula using an autologous vein-covered Palmaz stent. J Endovasc Surg 1995;2:177-181.

Dotter CT: Transluminally-placed coilspring endarterial tube grafts: Long-term patency in canine popliteal artery. Invest Radiol 1969;4:329-332.

Fabian TC, Richardson JD, Croce MA, et al: Prospective study of blunt aortic injury: Multicenter trial of the American Association for the Surgery of Trauma. J Trauma 1997;42:374-380.

Fontaine AB, Nicholls SC, Borsa JJ, et al: Seat belt aorta: Endovascular management with a stent-graft. J Endovasc Ther 2001;8:83-86.

Gomez-Jorge JT, Guerra JJ, Scagnelli T, et al: Endovascular management of a traumatic subclavian arteriovenous fistula. JVIR 1996;7:599-602.

Lobato AC, Quick RC, Phillips B, et al: Immediate endovascular repair for descending thoracic aortic transection secondary to blunt trauma. J Endovasc Ther 2000;7:16-20.

Maggisano R, Nathens A, Alexandrova NA, et al: Traumatic rupture of the thoracic aorta: Should one always operate immediately? Ann Vasc Surg 1995;9:44-52.

Marin ML, Veith FJ, Cynamon J, et al: Initial experience with transluminally placed endovascular grafts for the treatment of complex vascular lesions. Ann Surg 1995a;222:449-469.

Marin ML, Veith FJ, Lyon RT, et al: Transfemoral endovascular repair of iliac artery aneurysms. Am J Surg 1995b;170:179-182.

Marin ML, Veith FJ, Panetta TF, et al: Percutaneous transfemoral insertion of a stented graft to repair a traumatic femoral arteriovenous fistula. J Vasc Surg 1993;18:229-302.

Marin ML, Veith FJ, Panetta TF, et al: Transluminally placed endovascular stented graft repair for arterial trauma. J Vasc Surg 1994;20:466-473.

Marty-Ane CH, Berthet JP, Branchereau P, et al: Endovascular repair for acute traumatic rupture of the thoracic aorta. Ann Thorac Surg 2003 Jun;75(6):1803-1807.

Orend KH, Pamler R, Kapfer X, et al: Endovascular repair of traumatic descending aortic transection. J Endovasc Ther 2002 Oct;9(5):573-578.

Panetta TF, Sclafani SJA, Goldstein AS, et al: Percutaneous transcatheter embolization for arterial trauma. J Vasc Surg 1985;2:54-64.

Parodi JC: Endovascular repair of abdominal aortic aneurysms and other arterial lesions. J Vasc Surg 1995;21:549-557.

Parodi JC, Palmaz JC, Barone HD: Transfemoral intraluminal graft implantation for abdominal aortic aneurysms. Ann Vasc Surg 1991;5:491-499.

Patel AV, Marin ML, Veith FJ, et al: Endovascular graft repair of penetrating subclavian artery injuries. J Endovasc Surg 1996;3:382-388.

Rosch J, Dotter CT, Brown MJ: Selective arterial embolization. A new method for control of acute gastrointestinal bleeding. Radiology 1972;102: 303-306.

Ruchat P, Capasso P, Chollet-Rivier M, et al: Endovascular treatment of aortic rupture by blunt chest trauma. J Cardiovasc Surg 2001;42:77-81.

Terry PJ, Houser EE, Rivera FJ, et al: Percutaneous aortic stent placement for life-threatening aortic rupture due to metastatic germ cell tumor. J Urol 1995;153:1631-1634.

Thompson CS, Rodriguez JA, Ramaiah VG, et al: Acute traumatic rupture of the thoracic aorta treated with endoluminal stent grafts. J Trauma 2002 Jun;52(6):1173-1177.

Veith FJ, Sanchez LA, Ohki T: Technique for obtaining proximal intraluminal control when arteries are inaccessible or unclampable because of disease or calcification. J Vasc Surg 1998;27:582-586.

Volodos NL, Karpovich IP, Troyan VI, et al: Clinical experience of the use of self-fixing synthetic prostheses for remote endoprosthetics of the thoracic and the abdominal aorta and iliac arteries through the femoral artery and as intraoperative endoprosthesis for aorta reconstruction. Vasa 1991;33(suppl):93-95.

White R, Donayre C, Walot I, et al: Endograft repair of an aortic pseudoaneurysm following gunshot wound injury: Impact of imaging on diagnosis and planning of intervention. J Endovasc Ther 1997;4:344-351.

Zajiko AB, Little AF, Steed DL, et al: Endovascular stent-graft repair of common iliac artery-to-inferior vena cava fistula. JVIR 1995;6:803-806.

SPECIFIC
VASCULAR INJURIES

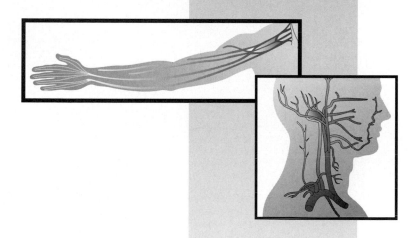

Penetrating Cervical Vascular Injury

RAO R. IVATURY
MICHAEL C. STONER

Injuries to the arteries of the neck are relatively uncommon but are of paramount importance to the trauma and vascular surgeon because of their end organ. The incidence of arterial injury in patients with penetrating neck wounds is 12% to 13%, whereas the incidence of venous injury is 18% to 19% (Asensio and colleagues, 1991, 2001). Mortality attributable to cervical vascular injury has been cited to be as high as 11%. Because of the relatively low overall incidence, it is difficult for any one surgeon to gain extensive experience in the repair and management of these injuries. This underscores the importance of multicenter and registry reviews when determining the proper treatment of these trauma patients. Most of these injuries, and certainly the most significant, are carotid artery injuries.

Ambrose Paré is credited with the first recorded attempt to surgically treat a carotid artery injury more than 400 years ago (Watson and Silverstone, 1939). Paré ligated the carotid artery of a French soldier, saving his life but leaving him with a profound neurologic deficit consisting of left-sided hemiplegia and aphasia. Mr. Flemming (1817), 250 years later, successfully ligated the common carotid artery of a patient aboard the *H.M.S. Tonnant*. The operation was successful in controlling hemorrhage without neurologic consequences.

Simple ligation dominated surgical decision until the last 50 years. The devastating outcome of stroke or death following ligation of the carotid artery led surgeons to adopt a conservative approach to these injuries. Surgery was proposed for those patients with severe hemorrhage, enlarging hematoma, airway compromise, or pseudoaneurysm.

As with most penetrating trauma, military conflicts have provided the bulk of information about penetrating carotid artery injuries. In World War I, Makins (1919) reported that one third of 128 cases of carotid artery injury treated by ligation resulted in irreversible neurologic deficit. During World War II and the Korean conflict, there were a handful of reports of carotid artery repair (Lawrence and colleagues, 1948; Huhges, 1958).

The Vietnam conflict provided a wealth of information about carotid artery trauma.

By this time, improved diagnosis, vascular operative techniques, and instrumentation yielded significantly improved morbidity and mortality. The Vietnam Vascular Registry, a massive project, was instrumental in shaping the modern approach to cervical vascular trauma.

The unfortunate rise in civilian penetrating trauma has been documented in various series. Several factors have led to improved management, probably the most significant of which is expeditious intervention. Fogelman and Stewart (1956) demonstrated a 35% mortality rate in patients with delayed surgical exploration versus 6% for those undergoing immediate operation. The authors advocated prompt exploration of all wounds penetrating the platysma, and this soon became a standard of care. This aggressive approach led to a high rate of negative explorations and caused many surgeons to reconsider the indications for operation. This controversy continues today and is outlined in further detail within this chapter.

SURGICAL ANATOMY

The key landmark to exploration of the neck is the sternocleidomastoid muscle, which defines the anterior and posterior triangles and is invested by the deep cervical fascia. Incision over the anterior aspect of the muscle is the preferred route of exposure for most carotid injuries. Thoracic and cranial extensions are easily adapted to this incision as warranted.

The most superficial layer of the neck musculature is the platysma, a thin confluence of muscle arising from the upper portion of pectorals and inserting onto the skin and subcutaneous tissue of the lower face. As described earlier in this chapter, the platysma is an important landmark of historical significance defining superficial from deep penetrating cervical wounds. The external jugular vein is the only vascular structure between this layer and the deep cervical fascia.

Emerging from the jugular foramen at the base of the skull, the internal jugular vein courses downward within the carotid sheath, along with the carotid artery and vagus nerve. Each component of the carotid sheath is encircled in its own connective tissue investment throughout the cervical region. Because of the considerable distensibility of these connective tissue layers, the carotid sheath tends to be attenuated over the jugular vein. The internal jugular ends at the clavicle where it joins with the subclavian vein to form the brachiocephalic vein. On the left side, an important posterior anatomic relationship is the thoracic duct, which eventually inserts at the confluence of the jugular and subclavian veins.

In most patients, the right carotid arises from the brachiocephalic artery, and the left from the aortic arch. Each artery passes upward to the level of the thyroid cartilage and divides into internal and external branches. Prior to this point, the common carotid is without branches except for the rare anomalous superior thyroid artery or ascending pharyngeal branch. At the bifurcation, the artery dilates, and this region is known as the *carotid bulb*. The carotid bifurcation can be difficult to identify in the presence of an extensive hematoma. An important landmark in identifying the bifurcation is the location of the facial vein and the medial portion of the ansa cervicalis. At their origin, the common carotid arteries are relatively close, separated only by the trachea. As they ascend, thyroid, larynx, and then pharynx intervene between the two arteries. Sternocleidomastoid covers the common carotid artery, the internal carotid artery (ICA), and the external carotid artery throughout their course except for a small window between its anterior border and digastric muscle at the base of the skull (Fig. 11–1).

The ICA is typically larger than the external and supplies the anterior part of the brain and the eye and sends branches to the face and nose. At the origin of the ICA is a pressor receptor, the carotid sinus, stimulation of which results in hypotension and bradycardia. Along the posterior aspect of the artery runs the sympathetic trunk, and the spinal musculature behind that. The esophagus is medial and is of paramount importance when assessing for digestive injury. The hypoglossal nerve courses over the anterolateral aspect and is

an important surgical landmark. A series of important relationships are essential in differentiating the ICA from the external carotid artery: (1) In the vast majority of patients, the ICA has no cervical branches; (2) the ICA usually lies posterolateral to external carotid; and (3) as it ascends, the ICA moves to a medial position relative to external carotid artery (Fig. 11–2).

The external carotid artery, termed *external* because if its extracranial distribution, extends upward to the mandibular neck where it divides into its two terminal branches: the superficial temporal artery and the maxillary artery. The main trunk of the external carotid quickly gives rise to a series of branches: superior thyroid, ascending pharyngeal, lingual, facial, occipital, and posterior auricular. Of note, a portion of the external carotid is encompassed by the parotid salivary gland, an important consideration in exposure and repair.

The vertebral artery is the first and largest branches of the subclavian artery. It ascends behind the common carotid artery to enter the vertebral foramen at the transverse process of the sixth cervical vertebrae. Before entering the base of the skull, the vertebral artery passes behind the lateral aspect of the atlas, in an almost horizontal plane. Once entering the skull through the foramen magnum, the paired vertebral arteries converge, giving rise to the basilar artery and proceed to the circle of Willis as their termination (Fig. 11–3).

It is important for the surgeon to keep in mind the many potential collaterals between the internal and external system, because these collaterals may be able to sustain blood flow after ICA or external carotid artery injury. One significant collateral is between the ophthalmic branch of internal carotid and the facial branch of external carotid artery. Second, the thyrocervical trunk rises up the neck between the jugular vein and the anteromedial boarder of sternocleidomastoid. It is a potential source of collateral flow to the external carotid artery. Perhaps the most important and often misrepresented collateral circulation is the circle of Willis (see Fig. 11–3). Historical autopsy data suggest that up to one half of patients will have "nonstandard" circulation here (Puchades-Orts and

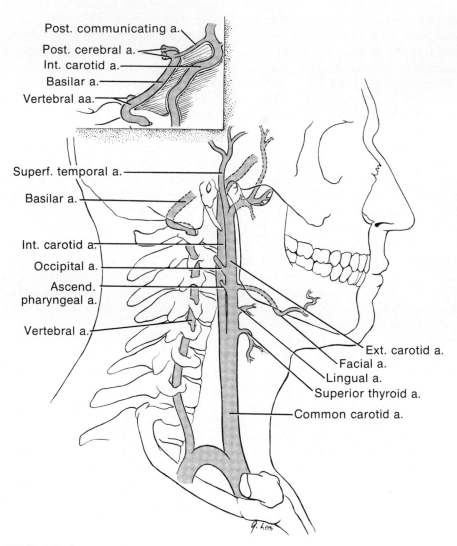

Post. communicating a.
Post. cerebral a.
Int. carotid a.
Basilar a.
Vertebral aa.

Superf. temporal a.

Basilar a.

Int. carotid a.
Occipital a.
Ascend.
pharyngeal a.

Vertebral a.

Ext. carotid a.
Facial a.
Lingual a.
Superior thyroid a.
Common carotid a.

■ **FIGURE 11–1**
Except for the intrathoracic portion of the left common carotid artery, the cervical anatomy of the carotid arteries and the vertebral arteries is bilaterally similar. ■

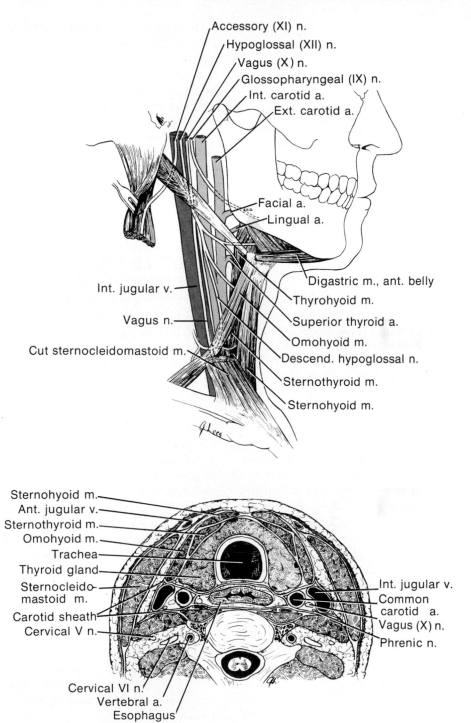

■ **FIGURE 11-2**
The close proximity of important contiguous structures, such as the internal jugular vein and the vagus nerve, is emphasized. The cross section shows the contents of the carotid sheath and the associated surrounding structures. ■

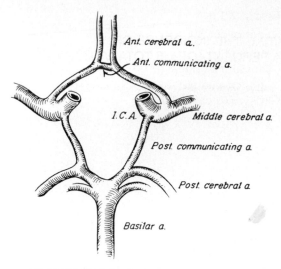

■ FIGURE 11–3
The standard model of the circle of Willis. Although normal variations within the circle are common, hypoplasia of various segments may be particularly significant with interruption of either internal carotid artery. This may result in an inadequate collateral flow. (From Strandness DE Jr. Collateral Circulation in Clinical Surgery. Philadelphia: WB Saunders, 1969.) ■

colleagues, 1976). Because of the redundancy, hypoplasia of an individual component of the circle is rarely a problem, unless carotid flow is interrupted and the segments of the circle are unable to sustain adequate flow. A recent magnetic resonance angiographic study supports this high rate of variance (Krabbe-Hartkamp and colleagues, 1998). The authors noted that only 42% of randomly selected adults had complete circles, with posterior variations being the most common. Other minor collateral circulations exist such as vertebral to vertebral muscular branches, external carotid to external carotid, and vertebral occipital branches.

INCIDENCE AND ETIOLOGY OF CIVILIAN INJURIES

The incidence of carotid artery injuries in civilian series ranges from 12% to 17% of total penetrating neck injuries. Information about the precise anatomic distribution of these injuries is sometimes limited by the presentation of data within a particular study and the lack of a standardized grading system and registry database specific for vascular injury. Recently, Mittal and colleagues (2000) have suggested a grading system to standardize the assessment and reporting of cervical vascular injuries. Compared to military injuries, civilian carotid injury tends to be blunt or stabbing. This must be considered when comparing outcome data between these groups.

INCIDENCE AND ETIOLOGY OF MILITARY INJURIES

Historic military data report that carotid artery injuries represent approximately 5% of all arterial injuries. The most recent and extensive database for modern military traumatic cervical vascular injury is the Vietnam Vascular Registry (Rich and colleagues, 1970). Data from this experience indicate that fragment wounds (projectiles from explosive ordinance, shrapnel, or debris) account for the vast majority of wounds. Gunshot wounds were found to be much less common (especially as compared to civilian trauma) because military weaponry tends to be of high velocity and therefore more likely to be fatal.

The incidence of carotid arterial injury in wartime, based on a total number of arterial injuries, was reported to be highest in a World War I study by Makins (1919) and lowest in a World War II study by De Bakey and Simeone (1946), as indicated in Table 11–1. The Vietnam conflict data indicate that common carotid injury is a more common occurrence than either internal or external carotid injury. Obviously, the vast majority of these injuries are penetrating, because of the nature of weaponry involved.

PATHOLOGY

The patient who survives penetrating neck vascular injury and reaches a surgeon most likely has a laceration or perforation. Complete

TABLE 11-1

COMPILATION OF WARTIME DATA ILLUSTRATING THE INCIDENCE OF
CAROTID ARTERY INJURY EXPRESSED AS A PERCENTAGE OF TOTAL ARTERIAL
INJURIES REPORTED

Study	Total Arterial Injuries	Common Carotid	Internal Carotid	Total Carotid	Percentage
Makins, 1919 (World War I)	120			128	10.7
De Bakey and Simeone, 1946 (World War II)	247			10	0.4
Hughes, 1958 (Korean)	304			11	3.6
Rich and colleagues, 1970 (Vietnam)	100	38	12	50	5.0

disruptions of the carotid artery are almost always fatal, although reports exist demonstrating viable patients with completely transected carotid arteries, with thrombus formation at the severed ends, thus alleviating the hemorrhage (Rich and colleagues, 1970; Harris and colleagues, 1985).

Cerebral vasospasm appears to be an important factor in the pathophysiology of cervical vascular injury. Acute spasm of the cerebral arteries can occur almost immediately after cervical arterial injury and can severely exacerbate ischemia. For the most part, however, spasm seems to play a late role in the potential pathology of carotid or vertebral artery injury, with the peak incidence occurring 5 to 10 days after injury (Kordestani and colleagues, 1997). Acute arteriovenous fistula is an important entity that if improperly identified, will have a high propensity to recur (Marks and colleagues, 1984). Early diagnosis can be difficult on physical examination alone, as the classic murmur may not be audible for several days. Some patients may have a substantial thrill that is palpable along the course of the fistula. Missile trajectory or pattern is very important when one attempts to predict possible fistulas. A report from our own institution described an acute carotid to cavernous sinus fistula after shotgun blast (Fields and colleagues, 2000). Diagnostic modalities for the workup of fistulas and other pathology associated with cervical vascular injury are discussed in the following section.

INITIAL EVALUATION AND MANAGEMENT

A careful history and physical examination should be undertaken. Weapon characteristics are important in predicting the extent of injury, especially for high-velocity missile injury. Trajectory should be assessed from entrance and exit wounds, especially in transcervical wounds because of the high incidence of vital structure damage (Hirshberg and colleagues, 1994). Obvious signs of vascular injury include external hemorrhage, expanding or pulsate hematoma, decreased pulses, and a vascular bruit or thrill. So-called "soft signs" of vascular injury include diminished temporal or facial arterial pulses, signs of hemothorax, or pharyngeal bleeding. Patients with hard signs of vascular injury require emergent neck exploration. A thorough neurologic examination is an integral part of the patient's evaluation. Care should be taken to ascertain for signs of cord injury such as paralysis, paresthesia, and hyperreflexia. Likewise, severe cerebral vascular insufficiency from carotid injury may result in contralateral hemiparesis. Evidence of cerebral infarct is important. This is discussed later in this chapter in the context of vascular repair in a patient with preexisting neurologic deficit.

Initial clinical management begins in the prehospital phase of trauma care. For the patient with penetrating cervical injury, prompt transport to the nearest trauma center with skilled personnel is paramount. Because airway establishment is fraught with a variety of potential problems, patients should probably be intubated only if unresponsive or if their situation is deteriorating and a long transport time is anticipated. External bleeding should be controlled with direct pressure.

When the patient presents to the trauma bay with a penetrating neck injury, airway control should be the foremost concern. Most early deaths in these patients result from either airway compromise or external hemorrhage, both of which can be addressed with fastidious care. The airway management algorithm is straightforward for the unresponsive patient or those presenting in extremis (Rao and colleagues, 1993): rapid establishment of orotracheal or surgical airway. The difficult patient is the agitated patient with obvious severe cervical injury. Establishment of orotracheal or nasotracheal airway may be problematic because of blood or secretions in the oropharynx or the patient's general status.

These patients need the most experienced personnel in the most optimal place possible in the most expeditious way. In our opinion, these patients, if at all possible, should be rushed to the operating room where the most experienced anesthesiologist and surgeon can together manage the airway by carefully individualized interventions: conscious intubation or sedation and a rapid surgical airway.

Once the patient's airway is evaluated and steps are taken to ensure definitive tracheal intubation as required, massive external bleeding needs to be controlled. Precise digital pressure should be applied to any bleeding sites. Nasopharyngeal or oropharyngeal packing may be necessary as a temporary hemostatic aid. During this time, paired large-bore intravenous access should be obtained and secured. Anteroposterior and lateral cervical roentgenograms and chest radiograms are obtained to assess for retained projectile, bony injury, and thoracic or pleural violation.

Outside the context of this chapter, concurrent injury must be assessed and dealt with. The high incidence of aerodigestive tract injury with penetrating neck trauma has been well described and may require rapid diagnosis and treatment. Severe tracheal injury may complicate the establishment of a definitive airway in these patients and can prove fatal. Delay to diagnosis of esophageal or pharyngeal injury is directly related to poor outcome and must be assessed fastidiously (Asensio and colleagues, 2001).

DIAGNOSIS OF VASCULAR INJURIES: ZONES OF NECK AND THE ROLE OF PHYSICAL EXAMINATION

In a landmark 1969 article, Monson and colleagues (1969) arbitrarily divided the neck into three clinical zones (Fig. 11–4). Zone 1 is defined as being below to sternal notch, zone 3 above the angle of the mandible, and zone 2 is the intervening region. This system has become a standard for discussing the diagnostic approach to penetrating neck vascular trauma because of the clinical relevance of injuries to anatomic locations. Zone 2 injuries are accessible via standard cervical approaches and should not present difficulty in obtaining proximal and distal vascular control. Zone 1 injuries by definition involve the thoracic inlet, and proximal control may require thoracotomy or supraclavicular incisions in addition to a cervical dissection. Zone 3 injuries are problematic because of the potential difficulty in obtaining distal control. The widely accepted practice is that zone 2 injuries are explored in the operating room, whereas zone 1 and 3 injuries require angiography because of the more extensive surgical approaches and potential complications.

Surgical access and exposure for symptomatic vascular injuries is relatively easy, and the morbidity from surgical exploration of zone 2 is very low. In addition, several studies have suggested that because zone 2 of the neck is amenable to physical examination, significant vascular injuries in this location are rarely occult. Sekharan and colleagues (2000) reviewed 145 patients with neck penetration; in 30 of these patients, the penetrating trajectory also traversed zone 1 or 3. Thirty-one

ZONES OF NECK FOR TRAUMA

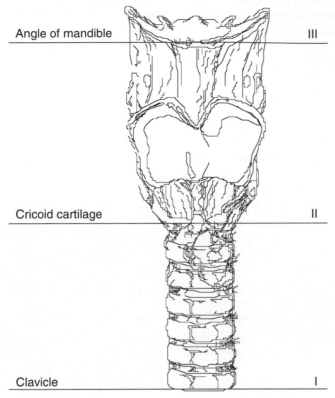

Angle of mandible   III

Cricoid cartilage   II

Clavicle   I

■ **FIGURE 11–4**
Zones of the neck. ■

patients (21%) had hard signs of vascular injury (active bleeding, expanding hematoma, bruit/thrill, pulse deficit, central neurologic deficit) and were taken immediately to the operating room; 28 (90%) of these 30 patients had either major arterial or venous injuries requiring operative repair (the false-positive rate for physical examination thus being 10%). Of the 114 patients with no hard signs, 23 underwent arteriography because of proximity of the injury to the vertebral arteries or because the trajectory included another zone. Of these 23 arteriograms, three showed abnormalities, but only one required operative repair. This case had no complications relating to the initial delay. The remaining 91 patients with no hard signs were observed without imaging or surgery for a minimum of 23 hours, and none had any evidence of vascular injury during hospitalization or during the initial 2-week follow-up period (1/114; false-negative rate for physical

examination, 0.9%). Based on these data, the authors confirmed that patients with zone 2 penetrating neck wounds can be safely and accurately evaluated by physical examination alone to confirm or exclude vascular injury.

Angiography

Four-vessel cervical angiography is the gold standard by which all other modalities are judged. The goal of angiography is to define the exact arterial injury and it anatomic relations, to identify any collateral flow, to look for any arteriovenous communications, and to stratify injuries in the patient with multiple vascular injuries. As angiography became readily available in the last 30 years, this system has become useful to define which injuries require arteriography. The precise indications for arteriography in stable patients, however, remain controversial. Preoperative arteriography is recommended in all patients with zone 1 penetration if they are *hemodynamically stable and do not have evidence of active hemorrhage*. It is recommended because these injuries are frequently clinically occult and their exposure technically challenging. Angiography appears to *be essential in zone 3 neck wounds* because of the potential inaccessibility of distal vascular injuries. The role of angiography in identifying injuries in zone 2 is more controversial, as discussed earlier in this chapter.

Arteriography is more likely to be helpful in low-velocity gunshot wounds than in stab wounds, but *recommendations to eliminate arteriography from a selective management protocol in stab wounds of the neck must await further studies*. High-velocity bullet wounds, shrapnel injuries, and close-range shotgun wounds all have exceptionally high incidences of significant organ injury, and arteriography in the stable patient without exsanguinating hemorrhage may be of considerable assistance.

Azuaje and colleagues (2002) studied 216 patients with penetrating neck injuries (from 1992 to 2001). Excluding 48 emergent explorations and 16 shotgun wounds, the remaining 152 patients had injuries in zone 1 (45 patients), zone 2 (83 patients), and zone 3 (23 patients); 63 patients had a positive physical examination (e.g., hematoma, bruit, thrill, and bleeding) and 40 (68%) also had a positive angiogram. Twenty of these required operative repair. Of the 89 patients with a negative physical examination, only 3 had a positive angiogram and none of these required operative repair. Physical examination had 93% sensitivity and a 97% negative predictive value for predicting the results of angiogram. The authors concluded that with careful physical examination, angiography may not be necessary *irrespective of zone of injury*.

Color Flow Doppler

Recently, color flow Doppler has become an alternative to angiography in the diagnostic workup of vascular trauma. It has been studied to some extent in peripheral arterial injuries, although its use in cervical trauma is ill defined. A study by Fry and colleagues (1994) demonstrated the feasibility of ultrasound for the assessment of vascular injury. A pilot study with 15 patients receiving duplex ultrasonography and concomitant angiography demonstrated equal accuracy of the two techniques. With these pilot data, the study was extended to an additional 85 patients in whom ultrasound was the primary imaging modality. The authors reported that ultrasound was as effective as operative exploration or angiography in their hands. A smaller study in 1996 demonstrated the success of ultrasonography as a screening modality for vascular trauma, with all major injuries being detected by the sonogram (Montalvo and colleagues, 1996). These findings were confirmed by Demetriades and colleagues (1995) in their study of 82 patients. They demonstrated that Doppler imaging identified 10 of the 11 injuries, for a sensitivity of 91% and a specificity of 98.6%. It appears that careful examination coupled with the experienced use of ultrasonography provides results comparable to angiography. Pitfalls with Doppler do exist though, importantly, the difficulty in establishing the exact anatomic relationship with the resolution available to angiography and the difficulty in securing readily available equipment, an experienced technologist, and skilled interpreter.

Computed Tomographic Angiography and Magnetic Resonance Angiography

Currently attracting increasing attention, computed tomographic angiography (CTA) should still be considered unproven. One study looked at 16 patients with suspected traumatic carotid artery injury who underwent CTA. Twelve of these patients had penetrating injuries and four had blunt injuries to the neck. All the CTAs were diagnostic. Positive findings included one complete tear of the right common carotid artery (confirmed by surgery) from a penetrating injury and one bilateral ICA thrombosis after blunt injury to the neck. Negative findings on CTA were confirmed by surgical exploration (Ofer and colleagues, 2001). In a prospective study of 146 arteries (77 carotid, 69 vertebral) studied by means of conventional angiography and helical CTA, conventional angiograms showed arterial injuries in 10 (17%) of 60 patients. These included arterial occlusion ($n = 4$), arteriovenous fistula ($n = 2$), pseudoaneurysm ($n = 3$), pseudoaneurysm with arteriovenous fistula ($n = 1$), and normal arteries ($n = 136$). Nine of ten arterial injuries and all normal arteries were depicted adequately at helical CTA. The sensitivity of helical CTA was 90%, specificity was 100%, positive predictive value was 100%, and negative predictive value was 98%. The sensitivity and specificity of helical CTA, therefore, seem high for detection of major carotid and vertebral arterial injuries resulting from penetrating trauma (Múnera and colleagues, 2000), at least in experienced hands.

Magnetic resonance angiography has been described as an imaging modality in this context as well, but experience with penetrating neck trauma, technical considerations, and limited experience make it difficult to recommend its use (Prabhu and colleagues, 1994; Friedman and colleagues, 1995).

TREATMENT

Innominate and Subclavian Vessel Injuries

Operative exposure of zone 1 vascular injuries are outside the scope of this chapter and are only briefly mentioned for completion. If the patient is hemodynamically unstable with a large hemothorax or excessive bleeding from the chest tube, an anterolateral thoracotomy (high in the third or fourth intercostal space) in the emergency center will allow apical packing and tamponade the bleeding from innominate or proximal subclavian vessels. In the operating room, a median sternotomy will expose the innominate. For the left subclavian artery, the incision may be extended along the sternocleidomastoid or the clavicle. This approach is superior to the "trap-door" incision. The second and third portions of the

subclavian are best approached by an incision along the clavicle with extension along the sternocleidomastoid, if necessary. Subperiosteal resection of the mid or medial one third of the clavicle will allow excellent exposure. Most of these vascular injuries may be managed by simple closure or end-to-end anastomosis. Occasionally, a saphenous vein graft may be necessary. In stable patients with subclavian pseudoaneurysm or intimal injuries, endovascular stent grafts are an evolving option.

Carotid Artery Injuries

The general consensus now is that injuries to the carotid arteries are best approached by surgical intervention and repair, either by end-to-end anastomosis or graft techniques, especially in the accessible portions of the carotid artery (Figs. 11–5 and 11–6). For selected intracranial injuries high in zone 1, endovascular stents are being used with increasing frequency, as discussed later in this chapter.

SURGICAL TREATMENT

The patient should be placed in a prone position with both arms tucked in if possible. As long as there is no concurrent spine injury, a shoulder roll should be placed to extend the neck and the table placed in a semi-Fowler

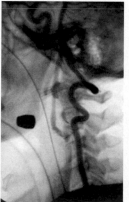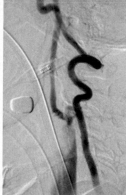

■ **FIGURE 11–5**
Gunshot wound of the neck. Angiogram reveals internal carotid cutoff just distal to its origin. ■

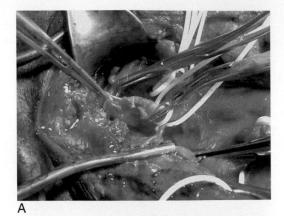

A

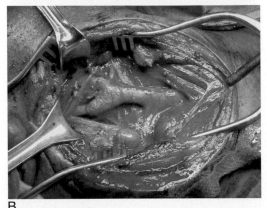

B

■ **FIGURE 11–6**
A and *B,* Carotid artery injury at operation
repaired by a saphenous vein interposition
graft. ■

position to aid in the operative exposure. The
entire thorax and abdomen should be prepared in case of zone 1 injury for accessing
the abdomen for potential multicavitary
injuries. The groin and both thighs are prepared and draped for possible saphenous vein
harvest. Carotid exposure is obtained via a skin
incision made along the anterior border of
the sternocleidomastoid muscle. The carotid
sheath and its contents are readily identifiable.
The venous and lymphatic structures are
retracted in a lateral direction. Proximal and
distal exposure of the carotid arteries is
obtained after identifying the ansa cervicalis
and twelfth cranial nerve. Digital pressure or
a side-biting vascular clamp can be used to
control hemorrhage while obtaining control.
Proximal injury to the carotid at its aortic or
subclavian origin requires more extensive
exposure than the simple neck incision.

Median sternotomy is the most commonly
employed approach. A supraclavicular incision is useful for exposure in some cases, and
dislocation or resection of the clavicle may
improve the exposure, as detailed elsewhere
in this text.

High zone 3 injuries resulting in distal internal carotid laceration or disruption can prove
very problematic in exposure and control.
Anterior subluxation of the mandible can
improve exposure, but only by about 2 cm.
Osteotomy of the mandibular ramus may
provide better exposure and mobility. Placement of a Fogarty balloon catheter to provide
distal vascular control can be lifesaving during
these maneuvers. The carotid artery may
require ligation. Depending on the surgeon's
experience in operating around the base of
the skull, intraoperative assistance from either
a maxillofacial surgeon or a neurosurgeon
is advisable in difficult cases. A recent series
illustrated the management and outcomes of
four consecutive patients, two with pseudoaneurysms and two with acute occlusions, after
injury to the distal cervical/petrous ICA from
gunshot wounds. Preoperative assessment
determined intracranial collateral flow patterns and established the patency of the distal
portion of the petrous ICA. Two patients
underwent cervical-to-petrous ICA vein bypass
grafts without neurologic complications. Both
grafts remained patent without evidence of
emboli at 2 years and 3 months. The two
patients who were managed conservatively
died, one from a massive cerebral infarction
and the other from intracerebral hemorrhage.
These authors concluded that the cervical-
to-petrous ICA vein bypass graft is a valuable
management option that can reduce the
potential morbidity and mortality from acute
ischemic or delayed embolic or hemorrhagic
infarcts (Romily, Newell, and Grady, 2001).
This approach, however, may be of limited
value in the management of the bleeding
patient with a difficult surgical exposure.
In this setting, ligation of the ICA may be
lifesaving.

Once proximal and distal control are
secured, a Fogarty balloon catheter is carefully passed to remove any thrombus and
both proximal and distal ends are flushed
with heparinized saline. A monofilament

polypropylene suture of 5-0 or 6-0 size is used for the repair and handled with appropriate vascular technique. Except for tangential lacerations, primary repair is often difficult, because the transected ends of the artery retract. For a simple, small laceration, interrupted lateral repair is usually possible. Larger lacerations require a running repair, with two separate sutures, each originating in an apex of the injury and is approximated in the middle. Care must be taken to inspect for and repair any intimal flap at this time. This can often be done by incorporating the intimal defect into the laceration repair by using a series of interrupted sutures. Also, the lumen of the artery must not be narrowed by this primary repair; otherwise, vein patch or interposition graft will be required.

Stab wounds or low-velocity missile injuries often result in simple lacerations with minimal devitalized tissue. Most of these arteriotomies can be repaired with simple suture plication or minimal mobilization and primary repair. If there is a considerable destruction of the carotid artery, resection of devitalized tissue may preclude a tension-free primary repair. In these cases, interposition grafting is warranted, preferably using autologous tissue. Saphenous vein is generally accepted to be the ideal conduit. If adequate autologous conduit is not available, synthetic material may be used. The choice between woven Dacron and ethyl polytetrafluoroethylene is based on surgeon's preference, because neither represents an ideal substitute for a vein graft. If anatomy permits, the external carotid artery can be divided at a distal location and transposed to the ICA. The thyroidal and pharyngeal branches should be ligated to provide mobility. The use of a shunt is not mandated by the available data. The Vietnam experience established the safety of carotid artery repair without the use of shunts, even with arterial occlusion lasting up to 60 minutes. In many series, stump pressures (pressure measured in the distal portion of carotid artery after ligation or resection) failed to predict postoperative neurologic deficits after carotid endarterectomy. Even though similar data are not available in civilian trauma series, the use of a shunt or stump pressures is a matter of personal choice.

Recently, percutaneous transluminal placement of endovascular devices has become an alternative option to surgical repair. One series evaluated the potential for using flexible self-expanding uncovered stents with or without coiling to treat post-traumatic pseudoaneurysms involving the extracranial ICA, the subclavian artery, and other peripheral artery (Assali and colleagues, 2001). Three patients with post-traumatic pseudoaneurysms of the carotid (one patient) and subclavian (two patients) were treated by stent deployment (Fig. 11–7). Angiography demonstrated complete occlusion of the pseudo-

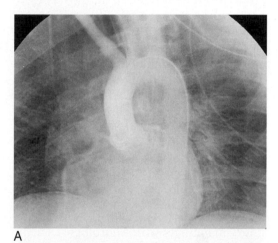

A

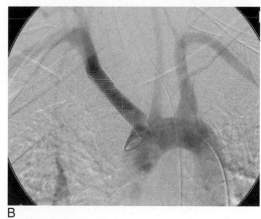

B

■ **FIGURE 11–7**
A and B, Subclavian artery injury just proximal to its origin by a gunshot wound in a patient with severe associated brain injury. This was managed by a stented graft placed by the interventional radiologist. (Courtesy T. Marrone and J. Tisnado.) ■

aneurysms. At long-term follow-up (6 to 9 months), all patients were asymptomatic without flow into the aneurysm cavity by Duplex ultrasound.

Much like in the extremities, minimal injuries to the carotid artery (small pseudoaneurysms or intimal flaps) probably have a benign course, and may *not* necessarily require operative repair. The natural course of many intimal flap injuries is unknown. Considering the nature and importance of the carotid circulation, however, the most judicious course of action may be a serial objective evaluation via duplex color flow ultrasonography or angiography. In a recent experimental study, only up to one third of all intimal injuries resolved without complication, and this figure underscores the need for diligent follow-up (Panetta and colleagues, 1992). There is no definitive information from the literature that elucidates the role of anticoagulation or antiplatelet agents in carotid artery injuries. Some authors, based on elective carotid endarterectomy data, advocate the use of low-dose aspirin or intravenous low-molecular-weight dextran to provide prophylaxis against thrombosis (Robless and colleagues, 1999).

Surgical Treatment of Carotid Artery Injury in Patients with Neurologic Deficits

Bradley in 1973 and Thal and colleagues in 1974 challenged the concept of repairing the carotid artery in the face of an established cerebral infarct and suggested that the repair and establishment of carotid flow may convert an anemic infarct into a hemorrhagic infarct. This concept, however, was refuted by a collective series of 223 patients by Liekwig and Greenfield (1978). Similar data were presented by Unger, Jorgensen, and Hoffman (1990), Lawrence and colleagues (1948), Ledgerwood, Mullins, and Lucas (1980), and Weaver and colleagues (1988). Many of these studies concluded that the outcome was dismal regardless of the type of therapy in the patient with a fixed profound neurologic deficit, but that the patients did better with repair than ligation. It is advisable, therefore, to repair the injury as long as the patient's clinical condition permits.

The prognosis for penetrating carotid artery injuries depends on the neurologic status on admission (Lawrence and colleagues, 1948; Ledgerwood, Mullins, and Lucas, 1980; Demetriades and Stewart, 1985; Asensio and colleagues, 1991; Demetriades and colleagues, 1996a). The mortality rates range from 6.6% to 33%, with an average of 17% (Asensio and colleagues, 1991), mostly related to neurodeficits.

Vertebral Artery Injuries

Vertebral artery injuries fortunately are not common. The first clinical review of vertebral artery injuries is attributed to Rudolph Matas of New Orleans in 1893. In his landmark article, Matas elegantly described the difficulty in diagnosing and surgically managing vertebral artery injuries, "A glance at the surgical anatomy of this vessel as it lies deeply hidden in the skeleton of the neck, only escaping at short intervals from its osseous canal, to become immediately invested by the very important and vital cervical nerves as they issue from the spinal foramina, will at once remind us of the magnitude of the purely technical difficulties in the way of its atypical ligation, and of the errors of diagnosis that must be incurred" (Yee and colleagues, 1995). Reported injuries to the vertebral artery have been exceedingly rare during major conflicts involving the United States. Although three vertebral artery injuries were reported in World War I, none were reported in either World War II, the Korean War, or the Vietnam War (De Bakey and Simeone, 1946).

If identification and exposure of the vertebral artery injury are uncomplicated during neck exploration, proximal and distal surgical ligation of the injured vessel is performed. If encountered at neck exploration, the following steps are indicated: (1) gauze packing at the site of bleeding, (2) exposure of the subclavian artery by dividing the origin of sternomastoid from the clavicle, and (3) proximal control of the origin of the subclavian artery. The neck incision is carried posterior to the ear with division of the attachment of sternomastoid and splenius capitis muscle. Distal ligation may be performed by dividing the splenius capitis and sternomastoid attachments to the mastoid, palpation of the transverse process of the atlas, and exposing the vertebral artery between the axis and atlas. Bone wax or other hemostatic agents can be used to pack and compress this area, or "blind" application of surgical clips deep into the wound may staunch the bleeding.

Because of the anatomic difficulties in vascular control of the vertebral artery, angiographic embolization represents an acceptable alternative. If the injured vertebral artery is discovered in the initial evaluation by angiography, the surgeon has a "road map" in planning the operative approach. Additionally, preoperative angiography allows for selection of patients who may not require ligation, specifically those with vertebral artery narrowing or occlusions. The approach to patients with pseudoaneurysms, dissections, arteriovenous fistulas, or extravasations will depend on the skill and judgment of the trauma surgeon, as well as the availability of experienced neuroradiologists.

Some series (Reid and Weigelt, 1970) noted several cases in which a disrupted artery, as seen operatively, had been diagnosed inaccurately as an occlusion by preoperative angiography. As a result, they recommended neck exploration for all angiographically diagnosed vertebral artery injuries unless deemed minimal. In the recent series from San Francisco (Yee and colleagues, 1995), five of six patients with vertebral artery occlusion were treated by clinical observation, whereas one underwent embolization. No adverse symptoms or neurologic sequelae were seen in these five patients. In addition, three patients with angiographic narrowing were treated by observation without complication, which are findings consistent with those reported by others. In the series reported by Demetriades and colleagues (1996b), 22 patients with vertebral artery injuries were reviewed. Only four patients required an emergency operation. Most of the injuries (13/22) were successfully managed by observation. Five patients were managed by angiographic embolization, which was successful in three. In three patients with an aneurysm and arteriovenous fistula, proximal embolization of the vascular lesion was not adequate and a sub-

occipital craniectomy was required for distal ligation. Neurologic sequela from vertebral embolization is very uncommon (Demetriades and Stewart, 1985). These data support the conclusion that most vertebral artery injuries can safely be managed without an operation or by angiographic embolization (Fig. 11–8). Surgical intervention should be reserved for patients with severe bleeding or in whom embolization has failed (Demetriades and colleagues, 1989).

Venous Injuries

Injuries to the innominate, subclavian, axillary, or internal jugular vein may be the source of severe hemorrhage. All of these veins can be ligated if the destruction is severe. In stable patients, they may be repaired. In a recent series of 49 consecutive patients with cervical and thoracic venous injuries (Nair, Robbs, and Muckart, 2000), the vessels involved were internal jugular in 25, subclavian in 15, brachiocephalic in 6, and superior vena cava in 3. Injured veins were ligated in 25 patients and repaired by lateral suture in 22. No complex repairs were performed. There were eight perioperative deaths and five cases of transient postoperative edema (Makins, 1919). In the case of severe bilateral jugular venous injury, ligation will carry significant clinical consequences. In this setting, reconstruction with autologous conduit is advisable.

SUMMARY

The escalating civilian violence of modern times is contributing to increasing frequency of vascular injuries in the neck. Early deaths are related to airway compromise or exsanguinating hemorrhage. If the patient arrives stable to the hospital, an orderly assessment and diagnosis may be made and the wounds successfully managed. Late deaths are from neurodeficits secondary to cerebral hypoxia. Advances in the management of penetrating vascular injuries on the horizon include noninvasive diagnostic testing and nonoperative radiologic procedures of endovascular

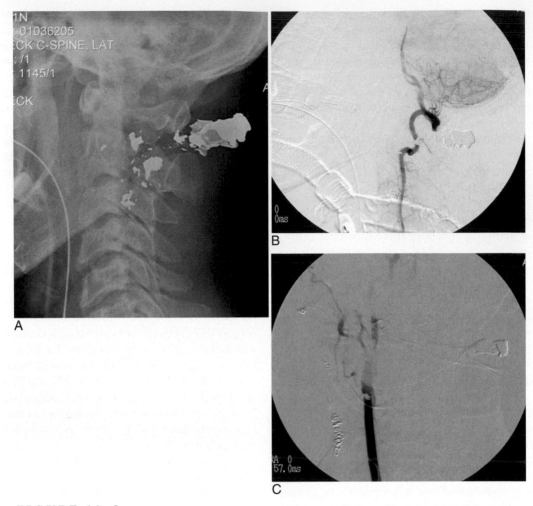

■ **FIGURE 11–8**

A, Lateral view of a patient with a gunshot wound of the neck with active bleeding from the wound. The injury to the cervical vertebra is evident. *B* and *C,* Angiography reveals injury to the vertebral artery. After confirming a complete circle of Willis, this was embolized successfully. (Courtesy T. Marrone and J. Tisnado.) ■

stenting and grafting. All of this progress is directly attributable to the early foundations laid down by the Vietnam Vascular Registry.

REFERENCES

Asensio JA, Chahwan S, et al: Penetrating esophageal injuries: multicenter study of the American Association for the Surgery of Trauma. J Trauma 2001;50(2):289-296.

Asensio JA, Valenziano CP, et al: Management of penetrating neck injuries. The controversy surrounding zone II injuries. Surg Clin North Am 1991;71(2):267-296.

Assali AR, Sdringola S, Moustapha A, et al: Endovascular repair of traumatic pseudoaneurysm by uncovered self-expandable stenting with or without trans stent coiling of the aneurysm cavity. Cathet Cardiovasc Interv 2001;53:253-258.

Azuaje RE, Jacobson LE, Glover J, et al: Reliability of physical examination as a predictor of vascular injury following penetrating neck trauma. Paper presented at the 15th Scientific Assembly of EAST; Orlando; January 15-19, 2002.

Bradley EL: Management of penetrating carotid artery injuries. An alternative approach. J Trauma 1973;13:248-255.

De Bakey ME, Simeone FA: Battle injuries of arteries in World War II: an analysis of 2471 cases. Ann Surg 1946;123:534-579.

Demetriades D, Asensio JA, et al: Complex problems in penetrating neck trauma. Surg Clin North Am 1996a;76:661-683.

Demetriades D, Skakkides J, Fofianos C, et al: Carotid artery injuries (1989): experience with 124 cases. J Trauma 1989;29:91-94.

Demetriades D, Stewart M: Penetrating injuries of the neck. Ann R Coll Surg Engl 1985;67:71-74.

Demetriades D, Theodorou D, et al: Penetrating injuries of the neck in patients in stable condition. Physical examination, angiography, or color flow Doppler imaging. Arch Surg 1995;130:971-975.

Demetriades D, Theodorou D, Asensio J, et al: Management options in vertebral artery injuries. Br J Surg 1996b;83:83-86.

Fields CE, Cassano AD, et al: Indirect carotid-cavernous sinus fistula after shotgun injury. J Trauma 2000;48(2):338-341.

Flemming D. Case of rupture of the carotid artery and wounds of several of its branches treated by tying the common trunk of the carotid itself. Med Chir J Rev 1817;3:2.

Fogelman MJ, Stewart RD: Penetrating wounds of the neck. Am J Surg 1956;91:581.

Friedman D, Flanders A, et al: Vertebral artery injury after acute cervical spine trauma: rate of occurrence as detected by MR angiography and assessment of clinical consequences. AJR Am J Roentgenol 1995;164:443-447.

Fry WR, Dort JA, et al: Duplex scanning replaces arteriography and operative exploration in the diagnosis of potential cervical vascular injury. Am J Surg 1994;168:693-695.

Golueke PJ, Goldstein AS, et al: Routine versus selective exploration of penetrating neck injuries. A randomized, prospective study. J Trauma 1984;24:1010.

Harris JP, Anterasian G, et al: Management of carotid artery transection resulting from a stab wound to the ear. Laryngoscope 1985;95(7, pt 1):782-785.

Hirshberg A, Wall MJ, et al: Transcervical gunshot injuries. Am J Surg 1994;167(3):309-312.

Huhges CW: Arterial repair during the Korean War. Ann Surg 1958;147:555.

Kordestani RK, Counelis GJ, et al: Cerebral arterial spasm after penetrating craniocerebral gunshot wounds: transcranial Doppler and cerebral blood flow findings. Neurosurgery 1997;41:351-359.

Krabbe-Hartkamp MJ, van der Grond J, et al: Circle of Willis: morphologic variation on three-dimensional time-of- flight MR angiograms. Radiology 1998;207:103-111.

Lawrence KB, Sheffts LM, et al: Wounds of the common carotid arteries. Reports of seventeen cases from World War II. Am J Surg 1948;76:29.

LeBlang SD, Nunez DB Jr: Helical CT of cervical spine and soft tissue injuries of the neck. Radiol Clin North Am 1999;37:515-532.

Ledgerwood AM: Neck: vascular injuries. In: Ivatury RR, Cayten CG, eds. The textbook of penetrating trauma. Philadelphia: Williams & Wilkins, 1996.

Ledgerwood AM, Mullins RJ, Lucas CE: Primary repair vs. ligation for carotid artery injuries. Arch Surg 1980;115:488-493.

Liekwig WG Jr, Greenfield LJ: Management of penetrating carotid artery injury. Ann Surg 1978;188:587.

Makins GH: Gunshot injuries to the blood vessels. Bristol: John Wright and Sons, Ltd, 1919.

Marks MW, Argenta LC, et al: Traumatic arteriovenous malformation of the external carotid arterial system. Head Neck Surg 1984;6:1054-1058.

Mittal VK, Paulson TJ, et al: Carotid artery injuries and their management. J Cardiovasc Surg (Torino) 2000;41:423-431.

Monson DO, Saletta JD, et al: Carotid vertebral trauma. J Trauma 1969;9:987-999.

Montalvo BM, LeBlang SD, et al: Color Doppler sonography in penetrating injuries of the neck. AJNR Am J Neuroradiol 1996;17:943-951.

Múnera F, Soto JA, Palacio D, et al: Diagnosis of arterial injuries caused by penetrating trauma to the neck: comparison of helical CT angiography and conventional angiography. Radiology 2000;216:356-362.

Nair R, Robbs JV, Muckart DJ: Management of penetrating cervicomediastinal venous trauma. Eur J Vasc Endovasc Surg 2000;19(1):65-69.

Ofer A, Nitecki SS, Braun J, et al: CT angiography of the carotid arteries in trauma to the neck. Eur J Vasc Endovasc Surg 2001;21:401-407.

Panetta TF, Sales CM, et al: Natural history, duplex characteristics, and histopathologic correlation of arterial injuries in a canine model. J Vasc Surg 1992;16:867-874.

Prabhu VC, Patil AA, et al: Magnetic resonance angiography in the diagnosis of traumatic vertebrobasilar complications: a report of two cases. Surg Neurol 1994;42:245-248.

Puchades-Orts A, Nombela-Gomez M, et al: Variation in form of circle of Willis: some anatomical and embryological considerations. Anat Rec 1976;185:119-123.

Rao PM, Ivatury RR, Sharma P, et al: Cervical vascular injuries: a trauma center experience. Surgery 1993;114(3):527-531.

Reid JD, Weigelt JA: Forty-three cases of vertebral artery trauma. J Trauma 1988;28:1007-1012.

Rich NM, Baugh JH, et al: Acute arterial injuries in Vietnam: 1,000 cases. J Trauma 1970; 10(5):359-369.

Robless P, Okonko D, et al: Vascular surgical society of great Britain and Ireland: platelet function during carotid endarterectomy and the antiplatelet effect of dextran 40. Br J Surg 1999;86(5):709.

Romily RC, Newell DW, Grady MS, et al: Gunshot wounds of the internal carotid artery at the skull base: management with vein bypass grafts and a review of the literature. J Vasc Surg 2001;33:1001-1007.

Sekharan J, Dennis JW, Veldenz H, et al: Continued experience with physical examination alone for evaluation and management of penetrating zone 2 neck injuries: results of 145 cases. J Vasc Surg 2000;32:483.

Thal ER, Snyder WH III, et al: Management of carotid artery injuries. Surgery 1974;76:955-962.

Unger S, Jorgensen J, Hoffman M: Carotid artery trauma. Surgery 1990;87:47740.

Watson WL, Silverstone SM: Ligature of the common carotid artery in cancer of the head and neck. Ann Surg 1939;109:1.

Weaver FA, Yellin AE, et al: The role of arterial reconstruction in penetrating carotid artery injuries. Arch Surg 1988;123:1106-1111.

Yee LF, Olcott EW, Knudson MM, et al: Extraluminal, transluminal, and observational treatment for vertebral artery injuries. J Trauma 1995; 39:480-486.

12

Blunt Cervical Vascular Injury

WALTER L. BIFFL
ERNEST E. MOORE
JON M. BURCH

Blunt cervical vascular injuries (BCVIs), those to the extracranial carotid and vertebral arteries (VAs), have historically been considered rare, yet they are recognized as potentially devastating events. Given the dearth of experience with BCVIs, even in busy trauma centers, there is essentially no class I literature to guide their management. Furthermore, BCVIs present a unique set of challenges because (1) they often occur in the setting of multisystem trauma, particularly head injuries, and symptoms may be masked by depressed consciousness or attributed to intracranial injury; (2) they are typically not diagnosed until after cerebral ischemic injury, making it difficult to achieve a good outcome; (3) they may occur following relatively minor neck "trauma," and so even with a high index of awareness of BCVIs, patients might not be considered at risk until they manifest cerebral ischemia; (4) the only reliable diagnostic test is invasive, resource

241

intensive, and associated with its own risks, and alternative noninvasive diagnostic tests may miss early subtle lesions; (5) the natural history of various injury types is unknown, and thus, it must be presumed that all injuries should be treated; and (6) treatments are potentially risky, there is no consensus on the optimal treatment for various lesions, and efficacy of treatment is largely unproven. In sum, BCVIs present dilemmas in risk assessment, screening, diagnosis, and treatment.

ANATOMIC CONSIDERATIONS

The left common carotid artery (CCA) originates from the aortic arch within the thorax, whereas the right CCA is a terminal branch of the innominate artery behind the sternoclavicular joint. There are no significant arterial branches from the CCA. It generally divides into the internal carotid artery (ICA) and external carotid artery (ECA) at the level of the C3-C4 disc space, corresponding to the superior border of the thyroid cartilage. The ECA does not directly supply circulation to the brain; thus, traumatic injuries to the ECA are usually well tolerated neurologically unless there is preexisting cerebrovascular disease. On the other hand, in the presence of carotid or VA occlusive disease, the ECA branches may provide critical collateral flow. The ICA can be separated anatomically into four segments: cervical, petrous, cavernous, and cerebral (supraclinoid). The cervical portion has no named branches because it ascends ventral to the transverse processes of the C1-C3 vertebral bodies (a relationship that is pivotal in the pathophysiology of many injuries, as described later in this chapter). The petrous segment traverses the carotid canal in the petrous portion of the temporal bone; here, it is at risk of laceration in the setting of a basilar skull fracture. The cavernous portion (also called the *carotid siphon* because of its gentle S shape) is the first part of the ICA within the cranial vault. It is suspended between the layers of the dura matter that form the cavernous sinus. At the anterior clinoid process, the ICA perforates the dura and becomes the supraclinoid, or cerebral, segment. The ICA divides

terminally into the anterior and middle cerebral arteries.

The VAs originate from the subclavian arteries, enter the cervical vertebral foramina at the level of C6, exit the transverse foramen of C2, and merge intradurally to form the basilar artery. There is considerable asymmetry to the point of agenesis (2% of right and 3% of left VAs). The circle of Willis connects the anterior and posterior circulation but is intact and symmetric in just 20% of individuals. The frequency of variations in collateral circulatory routes may explain unusual clinical presentations of arterial injuries and underscores the need to image the entire cerebral circulation in cases of BCVI.

MECHANISMS OF INJURY

There are four fundamental mechanisms of carotid injuries. The most common is associated with hyperextension and rotation of the head and neck. The lateral articular processes and pedicles of the upper three cervical vertebrae (C1-C3) project more anteriorly than those of C4-C7; thus, the overlying distal cervical ICA is prone to stretch injury during cervical hyperextension. Rotation at the atlantoaxial joint may result in anterior movement of the contralateral C1 lateral mass, further exacerbating the stretch (Fig. 12–1). A direct blow to the neck may crush the artery, or it may be compressed between the mandible and the vertebral prominences in acute cervical hyperflexion injuries. Intraoral trauma may injure the ICA, typically seen in children who have fallen with a hard object (such as a pencil) in their mouth. Finally, basilar skull fractures that involve the sphenoid or petrous bones may result in laceration of the artery.

The third segment of the VA, which extends from the level of C2 to the dura, is most commonly injured by blunt trauma because of the increased degree of stretching and compression (Fig. 12–2); the relationship between the VA and the cervical bodies puts the VA at risk when the vertebral body—particularly the foramen transversarium—is fractured.

Of note, numerous case reports in the literature have documented BCVI following

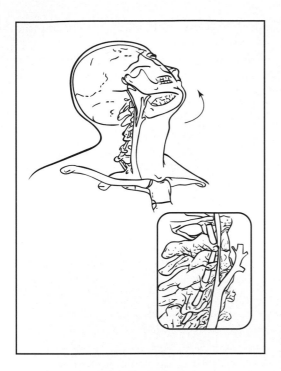

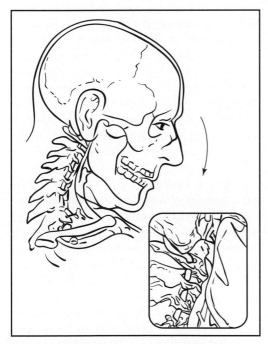

■ **FIGURE 12–1**
Rotation at the atlantoaxial joint may result in anterior movement of the contralateral C1 lateral mass, further exacerbating the stretch. ■

"trivial trauma." These include virtually any athletic endeavor, chiropractic manipulation, visiting the hairdresser, "head banging" to music, "bottoms-up" drinking, rapid head turning, and everyday activities such as coughing, shaving, vomiting, nose blowing, and scolding a child. This is in contradistinction to "spontaneous" carotid dissection, which by definition occurs in the absence of trauma. Reported risk factors for spontaneous dissection include hypertension, Marfan's syndrome, fibromuscular dysplasia, syphilis, arteriopathies, and Erdheim's cystic medial necrosis. It is the contention of some that truly spontaneous dissections are rare, but that such risk factors simply predispose patients to BCVI following trivial trauma. The absence of trauma from an individual's history does not exclude it as an etiology, because patients often consider events too insignificant (or embarrassing) to relate.

PATHOPHYSIOLOGY

Regardless of the underlying mechanism of injury, the final common pathway of BCVI in most cases is intimal disruption. This exposes thrombogenic subendothelial collagen, promoting platelet aggregation with subsequent embolization, partial thrombosis with low flow, or complete thrombosis. In addition, the intimal tear offers a portal of egress for a dissecting column of blood. Dissection may result in progressive luminal narrowing and subsequent occlusion. Whether caused by thromboembolism or occlusion, the end result, particularly in the setting of multisystem trauma with hypotension, is cerebral ischemia. Less commonly, partial or complete transection of the artery occurs, resulting in pseudoaneurysm formation or free rupture. The former may increase in size to compress and occlude the vessel lumen; it may be the source of platelet thromboembolism; or it may rupture. Rupture may result in hemorrhage or arteriovenous fistula formation.

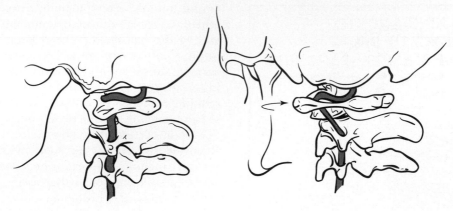

■ FIGURE 12–2
The third segment of the vertebral artery, which extends from the C2 level to the dura, is most commonly injured by blunt trauma because of the increased degree of stretching, which occurs at the atlantoaxial and atlanto-occipital joints during head rotation. ■

CLINICAL PRESENTATION

The clinical manifestations of BCVI depend on the type of injury, the involved artery, and collateral circulation. Premonitory signs and symptoms associated with the vessel injury may suggest the presence of BCVI before manifestations of cerebral ischemia. Pain (neck, ear, face, or periorbital) can be present in up to 60% of patients and is believed to reflect mural hemorrhage or dissection of the vessel wall. Complaints of such pain are often difficult to elicit in the multi-injured patient and may be attributed to other injuries; however, BCVI must be considered in the differential diagnosis of post-traumatic neck pain and headache. Horner's syndrome or oculosympathetic paresis (partial Horner's syndrome) may result from disruption of the periarterial sympathetic plexus. Pupillary asymmetry can have several etiologies in the injured patient. However, if the larger of the pupils is reactive and the smaller pupil is not, carotid injury should be suspected on the side of the smaller pupil.

Systematic neurologic examination will help localize the distribution of cerebral ischemia; however, cerebral ischemic signs or symptoms may be absent in the acute setting, because of (1) the presence of collateral circulatory pathways and (2) a characteristic latent period between the time of injury and the appearance of clinical manifestations. Unless the vessel is immediately occluded, time is required for a platelet plug to form and either limit flow or embolize. In various series, 23% to 50% of patients first developed signs or symptoms of BCVI more than 12 hours after the traumatic event. In our experience, 42% of symptomatic patients manifested more than 18 hours after injury and two exhibited symptoms 7 days later. Delayed recognition may also occur in the face of multisystem trauma, with critical injuries demanding immediate attention, or head injury, which may preclude a meaningful neurologic examination. To make the early diagnosis of BCVI, the surgeon must recognize the signs and symptoms in a trauma patient. These include (1) hemorrhage—from mouth, nose, ears or wound—of potential arterial origin; (2) expanding cervical hematoma; (3) cervical bruit in a patient 50 years old or younger; (4) evidence of cerebral infarction on computed tomographic (CT) scan; or (5) unexplained or incongruous central or lateralizing neurologic deficit, transient ischemic attack (TIA), amaurosis fugax, or Horner's syndrome.

SCREENING AND THE INCIDENCE OF BLUNT CEREBROVASCULAR INJURIES

The incidence of BCVI is difficult to quantify because many remain asymptomatic or symptoms may be attributed to associated brain (or other) injury. However, the incidence of BCVI among blunt trauma victims seems to be increasing. Early multicenter reviews identified an incidence of BCVI of 0.08% to 0.17% among patients admitted to trauma centers following blunt trauma, but more recent series have reported incidences of 0.24% to 0.44%. The argument that the incidence actually is increasing is supported by the fact that nearly all the patients in the series published through 1997 were symptomatic at the time of diagnosis. A number of factors could account for this explosion of BCVI at our center, including (1) higher highway speed limits in Colorado, (2) more widespread use of shoulder restraints and airbags, and (3) our role as a regional trauma center in the Statewide Trauma System, with increasing numbers of individuals being transferred to us following major mechanism injuries. However, without question, screening has identified injuries that would otherwise have been overlooked. In fact, two-thirds of patients diagnosed with BCVI at our center in the 1990s were asymptomatic.

Screening for Blunt Cerebrovascular Injuries

In 1996, Fabian and colleagues suggested that blunt carotid injuries (BCI) were being underdiagnosed. This had been suspected based on the Western Trauma Association multicenter study and demonstrated in a preliminary prospective study of screening at our center. Recognizing the potential to improve neurologic outcome by identifying and treating carotid injuries before occurrence of cerebral ischemia, we instituted an aggressive policy of screening and recently reported an epidemic of BCI. Between January 1990 and June 1996, before screening, our incidence of BCI was 0.1% of blunt trauma admissions—similar to

multicenter reports. During 4.5 years with a formal screening protocol, the incidence of BCVI has approached 1% of all blunt trauma admission to our center. In Memphis, a high index of suspicion and increasingly liberal screening resulted in an incidence of carotid injuries of 0.5%.

Identifying the Patient at Risk

Although the Louisville group has asserted that BCVI cannot be predicted based on clinical grounds, a number of groups have reported higher incidences of BCVI when diagnostic testing is employed for specific injury patterns and mechanisms. We formulated our screening criteria based on a knowledge of injury mechanisms and anatomic considerations. The screening criteria include (1) an injury mechanism compatible with several cervical hyperextension/rotation or hyperflexion, particularly if associated with displaced or complex midface or mandibular fracture, or closed head injury consistent with diffuse axonal injury of the brain; (2) near hanging resulting in cerebral anoxia; (3) seatbelt abrasion or other soft tissue injury of the anterior neck resulting in significant cervical swelling or altered mental status; (4) basilar skull fracture involving the carotid canal: and (5) cervical vertebral body fracture or distraction injury, excluding isolated spinous process fracture. This widespread screening approach requires a tremendous commitment of resources. In an attempt to allocate resources more effectively, we critically evaluated our screening criteria, analyzing the injury mechanisms and patterns of all the patients who underwent arteriography to exclude BCVI over a 9-year period, to identify independent predictors of BCVI. By multivariate analysis, Glasgow Coma Scale score less than 6, petrous bone fracture, diffuse axonal brain injury, and Le Fort II or II fracture were identified as risk factors for carotid injuries. The only independent predictor of VA injury was cervical spine injury. In 4.5 years of screening, we have performed screening cerebral arteriography on 390 patients; of these, 131 (33%) have had BCVI. More than two thirds were asymptomatic at diagnosis. On the other hand, a handful of patients have been transferred from remote facilities who became symptomatic from BCVI following "trivial trauma," who would not have met criteria for screening. We believe these criteria represent a starting point; however, the question of optimal criteria will ultimately require a multicenter collaborative effort.

DIAGNOSTIC EVALUATION

The discovery of signs or symptoms suggestive of BCVI mandates emergent diagnostic evaluation. The gold standard for diagnosis of BCVI is four-vessel biplanar cerebral arteriography. Unfortunately, it is invasive and resource intensive. Its risks include complications related to catheter insertion (1% to 2% hematoma, potential arterial pseudoaneurysm), contrast administration (1% to 2% renal dysfunction, potential allergic reaction), and stroke (<1%). Noninvasive diagnostic alternatives are available for screening asymptomatic patients for BCVI; however, one must recognize that diagnostic sensitivity is compromised in avoiding invasive testing. Duplex ultrasonography is widely considered the modality of choice for imaging the carotid arteries; however, experience in diagnosing BCVI is limited. In the Western Trauma Association multicenter review, duplex scanning had 86% sensitivity for ICA injury. In that series, the lesions missed by duplex were located at the base of the skull. Because most ICA injuries involve the artery at or near the base of the skull, this is a major potential weakness. Furthermore, although duplex scanning can provide indirect evidence of injuries by detecting turbulence and other flow disturbances, these findings are not reliable in the presence of stenoses of less than 60%. Unfortunately, we have witnessed the potential for innocuous-appearing luminal irregularities to cause devastating cerebrovascular accidents and thus do not believe duplex scanning is adequate for BCVI screening. CT angiography (CTA) is attractive because most multisystem trauma patients have indications for CT scanning. However, our experience has shown that CTA has a sensitivity no better than that of duplex ultrasonography. To image the cerebral vessels in their entirety with a slice thickness and pitch adequate for sufficiently sensitive reconstruction is not practical; in addition, bony artifact is in the carotid canal, potentially obscuring injuries. Of all the noninvasive screening modalities, magnetic resonance angiography (MRA) holds the greatest promise to reliably supplant cerebral arteriography. Advantages of MRA include the capability to simultaneously image the remainder of the head and neck and detect cerebral infraction earlier than CT scanning while avoiding contrast administration. Major impediments include a lack of timely availability at many institutions and incompatibility of ventilatory and orthopedic fixation equipment with the magnet. Recent prospective trials have reported suboptimal accuracy of MRA as well as CTA. Until more rigorous evaluation, arteriography remains the gold standard.

INJURY GRADING

Carotid artery and VA injuries are a heterogeneous mix of lesions. Several groups have suggested that different types of injuries might be managed differently; the absence of a formal BCVI grading scale, however, has been a major impediment to formulating sound practice guidelines. We hypothesized that different injury types had distinct implications in terms of response to therapy and ultimate neurologic outcome. Thus, we developed a grading scale based on the literature and our collective experience with 109 carotid injuries (Table 12–1). We reported that stroke incidence increased with injury grade. In contrast, recent analysis of our experience with VA injuries revealed no similar correlation between injury grade and posterior circulation stroke (Table 12–2).

TREATMENT AND OUTCOME

The optimal management of BCVI remains controversial. The three primary choices for

TABLE 12–1

BLUNT CAROTID AND VERTEBRAL ARTERY INJURY GRADING SCALE

			AIS 90	
Injury Grade	Description	ICD-9*	Intracranial	Cervical†
I	Luminal irregularity or dissection with <25% luminal narrowing	900.03	3	3
II	Dissection or intramural hematoma with >25% luminal narrowing, intraluminal thrombus, or raised intimal flap	900.3	3	3
III	Pseudoaneurysm	900.03	3	3
IV	Occlusion	900.03	4	3
V	Transection with free extravasation	900.03	5	4

*Internal carotid artery injury; ICD-9 code for common carotid artery injury is 900.01.
†Add 1 if neurologic deficit (stroke) is not related to head injury.
AIS-90, Abbreviated Injury Scale, 1990 revision; ICD-9, International Classification of Diseases, 9th revision.

TABLE 12–2

STROKE RATE AND MORTALITY OF BLUNT CAROTID AND VERTEBRAL ARTERY INJURIES, STRATIFIED BY INJURY GRADE

	BCAI (%)		BVAI (%)	
Worst Injury Grade	Stroke	Mortality	Stroke	Mortality
I	3	11	19	31
II	11	11	40	0
III	33	11	13	13
IV	44	22	33	11
V	100	100	—	—

BCAI, blunt carotid artery injury; BVAI, blunt vertebral artery injury.

management include observation, surgical therapy, and nonsurgical therapy (e.g., anticoagulation and endovascular techniques). In determining the treatment for an individual, one must consider the location and grade of the injury, as well as symptomatology.

Observation cannot be considered optimal therapy, given the natural history of symptomatic BCVI; early reports established morbidity and mortality rates of 58% and 28%, respectively. Extrapolating from penetrating trauma literature, wherein neurologic morbidity and mortality were better in those undergoing operation, early series recommended surgery in the absence of completed hemiplegic deficits. However, most blunt injuries involve the ICA at or above the base of the

skull. Thus, inaccessibility precludes direct surgical repair. Extracranial-intracranial bypass has been successfully employed in select patients, but this remains a controversial concept.

In 1996, Fabian and colleagues reported a large single-institution experience with carotid artery injuries. Anticoagulation improved neurologic outcome of patients presenting with minor and major neurologic deficits. In fact, logistic regression analysis identified heparin as the only factor independently associated with improved neurologic outcome. We similarly found that symptomatic patients who are anticoagulated showed a trend toward greater neurologic improvement at the time of discharge compared with those who were not anticoagulated (Table 12–3). An important finding of our series was that identification and treatment of carotid injuries before the onset of symptoms appear critical in improving neurologic outcome. In our analysis of outcomes following VA injuries, we again found that heparin improves neurologic outcomes (Table 12–4). Neurologic outcomes were better in the group as a whole, as well as in the subgroup suffering stroke. In addition, anticoagulation resulted in favorable trends including (1) preventing progression of lesions to higher injury grades (Table 12–5); (2) preventing neurologic deterioration from diagnosis to discharge; and (3) preventing stroke.

Obviously, bleeding complications are a concern in patients with multisystem injuries. We have experienced a 10% incidence of bleeding complications with our anticoagulation protocol. Presently, we are exploring an alternative in lower risk patients. Specifically, we are prospectively comparing the safety and efficacy of antiplatelet therapy versus systemic heparinization in the treatment of asymptomatic grade I BCVI (intimal irregularity without luminal stenosis, intraluminal thrombus, or a visible intimal flap).

Deployment of endovascular stents is gaining increasing favor in the treatment of vascular lesions. We deploy stents to treat persistent traumatic pseudoaneurysms (grade III BCVI), in an attempt to tack down the intima and exclude the pseudoaneurysm from the circulation. In addition, we stent grade II stenoses that threaten to occlude the vessel. Given the risk of stroke during manipulation of devices in an acutely injured artery, we recommend waiting 7 days, if possible, before attempting stent placement. Until more data are available, we recommend full anticoagulation after stenting for BCVI. It must be

TABLE 12–3

NEUROLOGIC OUTCOME OF BLUNT CAROTID ARTERY INJURIES, STRATIFIED BY TREATMENT; COMBINED EXPERIENCE FROM DENVER AND MEMPHIS

Outcome	Systemic Heparin (%)	No Systemic Heparin (%)	*P* Value
Neurologic improvement, diagnosis to discharge	49	19	<.05
Neurologic deterioration, diagnosis to discharge	5	24	<.05
Good neurologic outcome	50	30	<.05
Poor neurologic outcome	30	60	<.05

TABLE 12–4

NEUROLOGIC OUTCOME OF BLUNT VERTEBRAL ARTERY INJURIES, STRATIFIED BY TREATMENT

Outcome	Systemic Heparin (%)	No Systemic Heparin (%)	*P* Value
Poor neurologic function (all BVAI patients)	6	60	<.05
Poor neurologic function (stroke victims)	17	100	<.05
Progression of injury grade	25	60	.18
Neurologic deterioration, diagnosis to discharge	19	60	.11
Stroke	14	35	.13

BVAI, blunt vertebral artery injury.

TABLE 12–5
ARTERIOGRAPHIC OUTCOME OF GRADED CAROTID ARTERIAL LESIONS

| Initial Injury Grade | Treatment | Healed (5) | Final Injury Grade (%) | | | |
			I	II	III	IV
I	Heparin	16 (70)	6 (26)	—	1 (4)	—
	No heparin	12 (67)	4 (22)	1 (6)	1 (6)	—
II	Heparin	1 (10)	1 (10)	1 (10)	6 (60)	1 (10)
	No heparin	—	—	—	—	—
III	Heparin	1 (8)	—	—	11 (85)	1 (8)
	No heparin	—	—	—	3 (100)	—
IV	Heparin	—	—	—	—	1 (100)
	No heparin	—	—	—	—	1 (100)

emphasized that these devices are not approved for these indications, and their use should be restricted to research protocols.

Angiographic embolization has been employed widely for maxillofacial arterial injuries, but ICA embolization has not been supported because of concern of brain infarction. Our experience with attempted embolization in the ICA distribution has been confined to grade V injuries; in each instance, embolization has proven futile. On the other hand, angiographic embolization has been promoted as an alternative to surgical ligation in the management of VA injuries. Experience with this technique is still limited. Another alternative to surgical ligation of the VA is endovascular balloon occlusion.

SUMMARY AND GUIDELINES

BCVIs are infrequently diagnosed but may be overlooked in many patients. Symptoms may be masked by central nervous system injuries, but the large majority are asymptomatic at the time of presentation. Early diagnosis and institution of treatment appear to improve outcomes. Thus, the following guidelines have been adopted by our center.

Emergent cerebral arteriography should be performed to exclude BCVI in the presence of the following signs or symptoms: (1) hemorrhage—from mouth, nose, ears, or wounds—of potential arterial origin; (2) expanding cervical hematoma; (3) cervical bruit in a patient younger than 50 years; (4) evidence of cerebral infarction on CT scan; (5) unexplained or incongruous central or lateralizing neurologic deficit, TIA, amaurosis fugax, or Horner's syndrome.

Consideration should be given to screening individuals with injury mechanisms or patterns consistent with BCVI. These include (1) an injury mechanism compatible with severe cervical hyperextension/rotation or hyperflexion, particularly if associated with displaced or complex midface or mandibular fracture, or closed head injury consistent with diffuse axonal injury of the brain; (2) near-hanging resulting in cerebral anoxia; (3) seatbelt abrasion or other soft tissue injury of the anterior neck resulting in significant cervical swelling or altered mental status; (4) basilar skull fracture involving the carotid canal; and (5) cervical vertebral body fracture or distraction injury, excluding isolated spinous process fracture.

Our current diagnostic standard remains four-vessel cervical arteriography. All BCVIs are treated. Surgically accessible grade II, III, IV, and V injuries are repaired. Symptomatic patients with BCVI should receive some form of antithrombotic therapy, unless absolutely contraindicated by central nervous system injury. In asymptomatic patients with cerebral intraparenchymal hemorrhage or fractures in regions with the potential to develop an underlying epidural hematoma, anticoagulation is not initiated until follow-up CT scan in 24 hours excludes a significant change of the lesion. If there has been progression of the brain injury, anticoagulation is held until CT scans are stable at 24-hour intervals. Anticoagulation is not withheld for punctate intraparenchymal, small subarachnoid, or intraventricular hemorrhages. Our anticoagulation protocol is to begin a heparin infusion at 15 U/kg/hr, without an initial bolus dose. The partial thromboplastin time (PTT) is measured 6 hours after therapy is started, and the infusion rate is adjusted to maintain the PTT at 40 to 50 seconds. Follow-up arteriography is performed 7 to 10 days after injury. Healing of the injury allows discontinuation of therapy, whereas persistence warrants 3 months of warfarin (Coumadin) therapy. Progression of the lesion prompts alteration in therapy, including endovascular stent placement or a change in the anticoagulant regimen, as well as additional follow-up imaging. Patients undergo arteriography again after 3 months, to determine the need for further treatment.

REFERENCES

Biffl WL, Moore EE, Ellicott JP, et al: The devastating potential of blunt vertebral arterial injuries. Ann Surg 2000;231:672-681.

Biffl WL, Moore EE, Offner PJ, et al: Optimizing screening for blunt cerebrovascular injuries. Am J Surg 1999;178:517-522.

Biffl WL, Moore EE, Offner PJ, et al: Blunt carotid arterial injuries: Implications of a new grading scale. J Trauma 1999;47:845-853.

Biffl WL, Moore EE, Ryu RK, et al: The unrecognized epidemic of blunt carotid arterial injuries: Early diagnosis improves neurologic outcome. Ann Surg 1998;228:462-470.

Biffl WL, Ray, CE, Moore EE, et al: Noninvasive diagnosis of blunt cerebrovascular injuries: A preliminary report. J Trauma 2002;53:850-856.

Carrillo EH, Osborne DL, Spain DA, et al: Blunt carotid artery injuries: Difficulties with the diagnosis prior to neurologic event. J Trauma 1999;46:1120-1125.

Eachempati SR, Vaslef SN, Sebastian MW, Reed RL II: Blunt vascular injuries of the head and neck: Is heparinization necessary? J Trauma 1998; 45:997-1004.

Fabian TC, Patton JH Jr, Croce MA ,et al: Blunt carotid injury: Importance of early diagnosis and anticoagulant therapy. Ann Surg 1996;223:513-525.

Giacobetti FB, Vaccaro AR, Bos-Giacobetti MA, et al: Vertebral artery occlusion associated with cervical spine trauma: A prospective analysis. Spine 1997;22:188-192.

Miller PR, Fabian TC, Croce MA, et al: Prospective screeing for blunt cerebrovascular injuries: Analysis of diagnostic modalities and outcomes. Ann Surg 2002;236:386-395.

Rogers FB, Baker EF, Osler TM, et al: Computed tomographic angiography as a screening modality for blunt cervical arterial injuries: Preliminary results. J Trauma 1999;46:380-385.

13

Penetrating Thoracic Vascular Injury

SCOTT A. LEMAIRE
LORI D. CONKLIN
MATTHEW J. WALL, JR.

The lethality of penetrating chest wounds has been well recognized throughout history. More than 90% of the penetrating thoracic wounds described in Homer's *Iliad* and Virgil's *Aeneid* were fatal. The first successful repair of a penetrating thoracic vascular injury did not occur until October 1913, when a 30-year-old Russian surgeon named Yustin Djanelidze closed an 8-mm stab wound to the ascending aorta with three interrupted sutures.

Currently, nearly 4% of patients with penetrating chest wounds have an injury involving the thoracic great vessels: the aorta and its brachiocephalic branches, the pulmonary arteries and veins, the superior and intrathoracic inferior venae cavae, and the innominate and azygos veins. The incidence of great vessel injury is substantially higher following gunshot wounds (5%) than after stab wounds (2%).

INITIAL EVALUATION AND MANAGEMENT

Prehospital Management

Patients sustaining penetrating thoracic trauma should be immediately transported to the nearest trauma center capable of managing thoracic vascular injuries. Intravenous access should be avoided in the upper extremities, particularly on the side of injury, because the central venous structures may be transected or thrombosed. Allowing mild hypotension is preferable to aggressive attempts to increase blood pressure with fluid boluses, military antishock trousers (MAST suits), or pressors. Even transient increases in blood pressure may dislodge a soft clot and increase bleeding. In a randomized trial of patients with penetrating truncal trauma, Bickell and colleagues (1994) compared standard fluid resuscitation with no preoperative fluid resuscitation and demonstrated a significant survival advantage in patients who had delayed resuscitation. Similarly, the use of MAST suits in hypotensive patients sustaining penetrating thoracic trauma is associated with increased mortality. These pneumatic compression devices elevate blood pressure by increasing afterload and are equivalent to placing a cross clamp distal to a vascular injury, a clearly counterproductive maneuver.

EMERGENCY CENTER EVALUATION AND MANAGEMENT

Patient presentation can range from minimal symptoms to cardiac arrest necessitating resuscitative thoracotomy. Penetrating vascular injuries may produce intraluminal intimal flaps or thrombosis, arteriovenous fistulas, and pseudoaneurysms. The resulting clinical manifestations include external bleeding, hemothorax, cardiac tamponade, mediastinal hematoma, stroke, and limb ischemia. The diagnosis and treatment of the life-threatening manifestations occur concomitantly during the primary survey and resuscitation phase.

Primary Survey and Resuscitation

HISTORY

The history may provide the first clues suggesting a thoracic vascular injury. Information regarding the length of a knife, the firearm type and number of rounds fired, and the patient's distance from the firearm—though not always reliable—is important to obtain from the patient or accompanying persons. In addition to information involving the mechanism of injury, the emergency transport personnel can provide medical information important in evaluating the potential for a thoracic great vessel injury, such as the amount

of hemorrhage at the accident scene and hemodynamic instability during transport.

INITIAL EXAMINATION

The primary survey addresses the most life-threatening manifestations of intrathoracic vascular injury by including focused attention to airway obstruction, massive hemothorax, and pericardial tamponade. As always, establishing satisfactory airway, breathing, and cervical spine protection are the first concerns. An expanding upper mediastinal hematoma can cause stridor due to airway compression. The subsequent circulation assessment increases the focus on potential thoracic vascular injuries. Hypotension immediately raises the suspicion for a great vessel injury; the critical distinction is whether the hypotension is due to hypovolemia or tamponade from an intrapericardial injury. Tracheal deviation away from the side of injury may indicate mediastinal shift due to a massive hemothorax. Among the classic signs of tamponade (e.g., distended neck veins, pulsus paradoxus exceeding 10 mm Hg, and muffled heart sounds), venous engorgement is an important early sign of pericardial tamponade. Tamponade should be considered in the setting of progressive hypotension without evidence of ongoing blood loss. In many trauma centers, immediate ultrasonography can be performed at the bedside in the emergency department to rapidly determine whether a hemopericardium is present; this is a standard component of the Focused Abdominal Sonography for Trauma examination.

INTRAVENOUS ACCESS AND FLUID ADMINISTRATION

As a general rule, patients with suspected injuries to the major thoracic venous branches should have large-bore intravenous access established in the lower extremities whenever possible. The saphenous vein can be cannulated percutaneously or via saphenous vein cutdown at the ankle or in the groin; when placing the catheter through a cutdown, sterile intravenous extension tubing can be inserted directly in the vein. If an upper extremity or subclavian venous catheter is required in a patient with a potential subclavian vascular injury, the contralateral side should be used for cannulation.

The treatment of severe shock should include blood transfusion. However, in patients with mild hypotension, rapid infusions of either blood or crystalloid should be avoided before operation because they may increase the blood pressure to a point that a protective soft perivascular clot is "blown out" and fatal hemorrhage ensues.

TUBE THORACOSTOMY

By evacuating the initial hemothorax, placement of an appropriately sized chest tube (Table 13–1) restores effective breathing and allows an assessment regarding ongoing hemorrhage. The tube is usually placed in the fourth or fifth intercostal space (near nipple level) at the anterior to mid-axillary line. Intrapleural blood loss that results in hypotension is termed *massive hemothorax*. If a massive hemothorax is suspected, based either on clinical findings or on the chest radiograph findings, a repository that allows autotransfusion can be connected to the chest tube before insertion. Indications for urgent thoracotomy include (1) large initial chest tube output (>1500 mL in adults and >20% of estimated blood volume in children), (2) significant ongoing hemorrhage (>200 to 250 mL per hour in adults and >1 to 2 mL/kg per hour

in children), and (3) a significant increase in bleeding.

PERICARDIOCENTESIS

If hemopericardium is present and the patient is hemodynamically unstable, a subxiphoid pericardial catheter should be placed in the emergency center. Intermittent removal of pericardial blood may prevent sudden hemodynamic deterioration while preparing the patient for surgery. Therefore, after insertion, the catheter is secured in position to allow repeated drainage as needed during transport to the operating room and induction of anesthesia.

EMERGENCY CENTER THORACOTOMY

Emergency center thoracotomy in patients presenting with signs of life and hemodynamic collapse may reveal injuries to major thoracic vessels. In this setting, the thoracotomy allows rapid resuscitation and temporary control of bleeding in preparation for subsequent transfer to the operating room and definitive repair. A pericardiotomy anterior to the phrenic nerve is performed to relieve pericardial tamponade and allow effective cardiac compressions. Bleeding from subclavian vessels can be temporized by tightly packing the thoracic apex or by inserting large balloon catheters through the wounds. Either cross clamping the entire hilum or twisting the lung 180 degrees after releasing the inferior pulmonary ligament can control major hemorrhage from the pulmonary hilum.

TABLE 13–1
APPROPRIATE CHEST TUBE SIZES IN PATIENTS WITH TRAUMATIC HEMOTHORAX

Age	Chest Tube Size
Newborn	12-16 French
Infants	16-18 French
School age children	18-24 French
Adolescents	28-32 French
Adult	36 French

Secondary Survey

The secondary survey includes a search for more subtle signs of vascular injury. Each region of the body is thoroughly examined. All penetrating wounds are noted and marked with radiopaque markers. Substantial external bleeding is more common after stab wounds than gunshot wounds. Because vascular thrombosis or an intimal flap may

TABLE 13–2
CLUES TO PENETRATING THORACIC VASCULAR INJURY

Physical Examination	Chest Radiography
Shock	Large hemothorax
Superior vena cava syndrome	Foreign bodies (bullets or shrapnel) or their trajectories in proximity to the great vessels
Pulse or pressure disparity between right and left upper extremities	A foreign body out of focus with respect to the remaining radiograph, which may indicate its intracardiac location
Pulse or pressure disparity between upper and lower extremities	A trajectory with a confusing course, which may indicate a migrating intravascular bullet
Intrascapular murmur	"Missing" missile in a patient with a gunshot wound to the chest, suggesting distal embolization
Hematoma at base of neck	
Signs of pericardial tamponade:	
Elevated venous pressure	
Muffled heart sounds	
Pulsus paradoxus	

completely occlude an injured vessel, the absence of significant bleeding does not rule out a major vascular injury. Examination of the chest may reveal an expanding hematoma at the thoracic inlet or an intrascapular murmur. Thrills or bruits near the clavicles may indicate the presence of an arteriovenous fistula, which most commonly involves the innominate or subclavian vessels. During assessment of extremity circulation, the presence of a distal pulse does not rule out a proximal injury because blood flow can continue while the surrounding hematoma is contained by perivascular tissue. Loss of an extremity pulse may indicate intravascular embolization of a bullet from an aortic injury. Unequal blood pressures or pulses in the upper extremities suggest an innominate or subclavian artery injury. An injury involving the descending thoracic aorta may cause pseudocoarctation syndrome with upper extremity hypertension and diminished lower extremity pulses and pressures. Clinical signs indicative of penetrating thoracic great vessel injuries are summarized in Table 13–2.

As part of the secondary survey, a supine anteroposterior chest radiograph is performed in the emergency center after placing radiopaque markers on all entrance and exit wounds; findings that suggest an intrathoracic vascular injury are listed in Table 13–2. In many cases, the radiographic findings are suf-ficient to warrant immediate arteriography or direct transport to the operating room.

DIAGNOSTIC STUDIES

Unlike penetrating abdominal vascular trauma, the operative approach to intrathoracic vascular injuries varies substantially and depends on the location of the injury (Table 13–3). Therefore, imaging studies play a critical role in diagnosing and localizing the injury so that the optimal approach can be planned.

Catheter Arteriography

In stable patients with penetrating thoracic trauma, catheter angiography is indicated for suspected innominate, carotid, or subclavian arterial injuries. Different thoracic incisions are required for proximal and distal control of each the brachiocephalic vessels. Arteriography, therefore, is essential for localizing the injury and planning the appropriate incision. Proximity of a missile trajectory to the brachiocephalic vessels, even without any physical findings of vascular injury, is an indication for arteriography.

Although aortography may also be useful in hemodynamically stable patients with

TABLE 13–3
RECOMMENDED INCISIONS FOR THORACIC VASCULAR INJURIES

Injured Vessel	Incision
Uncertain injury (hemodynamically unstable)	Left anterolateral thoracotomy ± transverse sternotomy ± right anterolateral thoracotomy (clamshell)
Ascending aorta	Median sternotomy
Transverse aortic arch	Median sternotomy ± neck extension
Descending thoracic aorta	Left posterolateral thoracotomy (fourth intercostal space)
Innominate artery	Median sternotomy with right cervical extension
Right subclavian artery or vein	Median sternotomy with right cervical extension
Left common carotid artery	Median sternotomy with left cervical extension
Left subclavian artery or vein	Left anterolateral thoracotomy (third or fourth intercostal space) with separate left supraclavicular incision ± connecting vertical sternotomy ("book" thoracotomy)
Pulmonary artery	
Main/intrapericardial	Median sternotomy
Right or left hilar	Ipsilateral posterolateral thoracotomy
Pulmonary vein	Ipsilateral posterolateral thoracotomy
Innominate vein	Median sternotomy
Intrathoracic vena cava	Median sternotomy

suspected penetrating aortic injuries, its limitations in this setting must be recognized. If the laceration has temporarily "sealed off," or if the column of aortic contrast overlies a small area of extravasation, the resulting "negative" aortogram may foster a false sense of security. To maximize sensitivity, therefore, an effort must be made to obtain views that are tangential to possible injuries (Figs. 13–1 and 13–2).

Computed Tomography

Until recently, conventional computed tomography (CT) had a limited role in evaluating vascular injuries. Although CT could demonstrate hemomediastinum and other suggestive signs, it did not provide the diagnostic capability of standard aortography. However, newer helical CT equipment is much faster, uses advanced computer analysis, and performs techniques different from first- or second-generation CT scanners. Not only is the resolution much greater than in former models, but the current machines also allow for computerized anatomic reconstruction, which was not available earlier. Compared to

catheter arteriography, CT angiography (CTA) is faster and less expensive, and it eliminates complications related to arterial catheterization. Data regarding its reliability in evaluating acute injuries, however, are limited and few trauma centers are equipped for its routine use. Although prospective trials will be required to verify its accuracy, CTA with three-dimensional reconstruction is rapidly evolving and may replace catheter arteriography as the study of choice in the future. Although magnetic resonance angiography can generate similarly detailed information, its application in these potentially unstable trauma patients is not currently practical.

TREATMENT OPTIONS

Endovascular Stenting

Evolving techniques in endovascular stenting are providing new options for the treatment of vascular trauma. Endovascular grafts can seal vascular lacerations from within the lumen without compromising blood flow. In

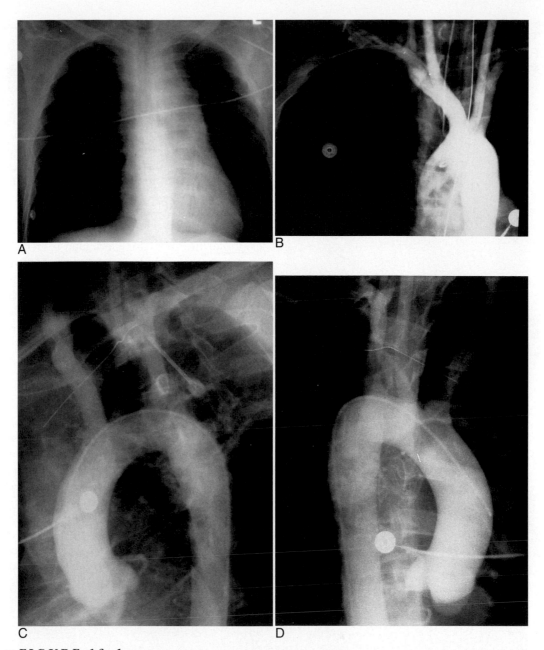

■ **FIGURE 13–1**

Missed injury by aortography. Chest radiograph *(A)* of a patient with a tiny puncture wound from a Philips screwdriver in the left second intercostal space at the sternal border. The patient arrived in the emergency room 30 minutes after being wounded and had stable vital signs for the following 48 hours. Anteroposterior *(B)*, left anterior oblique *(C)*, and near-lateral *(D)* projections of the aortogram were each interpreted by staff radiologist as showing no injury. Subtraction aortography in the lateral projection *(E)* demonstrates tiny outpouching of the thoracic aorta anteriorly at the base of the innominate artery and posteriorly on the undersurface of the transverse aortic arch. Penetrating injury of the transverse aortic arch was confirmed intraoperatively. (From Mattox KL: Approaches to trauma involving the major vessels of the thorax. Surg Clin North Am 1989;69:83.) ■

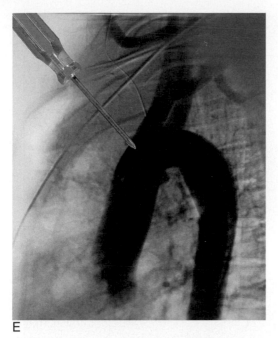

E

■ **FIGURE 13–1, cont'd**

principle, several aspects of vascular trauma make it well suited for transcatheter repair. These injuries occur predominately in relatively young patients without peripheral vascular occlusive disease. Furthermore, remote access can minimize the morbidity and technical difficulty often associated with direct surgical repair, particularly when the traumatic lesion occurs in the presence of a large hematoma, pseudoaneurysm, or arteriovenous fistula. Although direct vascular repair is generally successful, the wide surgical exposure that is often required can cause persistent pain and various degrees of disability. For example, the need for clavicular resection increases the morbidity of subclavian vascular repairs. Despite the advantages of a less invasive approach, many trauma patients, such as those who are hemodynamically unstable or those with heavily contaminated wounds, will not be suitable candidates for endovascular repairs.

Despite these caveats, endovascular techniques are being successfully applied with increasing frequency. Parodi and colleagues (1999) reported a series of 29 patients who

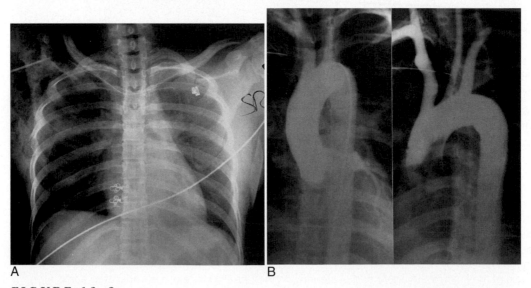

A   B

■ **FIGURE 13–2**
Plain chest radiograph *(A)* of a patient with a penetrating chest wound. *B,* The aortogram demonstrates no apparent injury in the anteroposterior projection but reveals a defect in the anterior aortic wall on the left anterior oblique projection. (From Mattox KL, Wall MJ Jr, LeMaire SA: Injury to the thoracic great vessels. In: Mattox KL, Feliciano DV, Moore EE, eds, Trauma, 4th ed. New York: McGraw-Hill, 2000.) ■

underwent endovascular stent placement for post-traumatic false aneurysms (10 patients) and arteriovenous fistulas (19 patients). Twenty-two of these injuries were located in thoracic or neck vessels, that is, the subclavian artery (9 injuries), axillary artery (3 injuries), aorta (2 injuries), common carotid artery (5 injuries), and internal carotid artery (3 injuries). The false aneurysms or arteriovenous fistulas were closed completely by one or more stent-graft devices in 28 of 29 patients. One patient died 1 month after the stent-graft false aneurysm closure. Twenty-three of twenty-nine patients continued to demonstrate stent-graft patency and remained asymptomatic after 24 months mean follow-up. Event-free survival at 3 years was 83%. In 2000, du Toit and colleagues published a series of 10 patients who qualified for stent-graft placement. The vessels involved were subclavian artery (in 7 patients), carotid artery (2 patients), and axillary artery (1 patients). Seven had arteriovenous fistulas and three presented with pseudoaneurysms. On average follow-up of 7 months, no complications were encountered.

Surgical Repair

Whenever possible, imaging studies are used to establish the diagnosis and plan the surgical approach. Clinical deterioration before obtaining these studies requires immediate transfer to the operating room for thoracotomy; indications for urgent operation include hemodynamic instability, hemopericardium, major hemorrhage from chest tubes, and radiographic evidence of a rapidly expanding mediastinal hematoma.

PREOPERATIVE CONSIDERATIONS

It is important to inform patients and their families of the potential for neurologic complications, such as paraplegia, stroke, and brachial plexus injuries, following surgical reconstruction of the thoracic great vessels. Careful documentation of preoperative neurologic status is critical. With any suspicion of vascular injury, prophylactic antibiotics are administered preoperatively. In hemodynamically stable patients, fluid administration is limited until vascular control is achieved in the operating room. An autotransfusion device should be prepared. During the induction of anesthesia, wide swings in blood pressure are avoided; although profound hypotension is clearly undesirable, hypertensive episodes can have equally devastating consequences.

The operative approach to great vessel injury varies depending on both the overall patient assessment and the specific injury. The initial steps of patient positioning and incision selection (see Table 13–2) are particularly important in surgery for thoracic vascular injuries, as adequate exposure is mandatory for proximal and distal control. Preparing and draping the patient should provide access from the neck to the knees to allow management of all contingencies. For the hypotensive patient with an undiagnosed injury, the mainstay of thoracic trauma surgery is the left anterolateral thoracotomy with the patient in the supine position. In stable patients, preoperative arteriography may dictate an operative approach by another incision.

Appropriate graft materials should be available. Although an infected prosthetic graft may form a pseudoaneurysm, a saphenous vein graft is a devitalized collagen tube susceptible to bacterial collagenase, which can cause graft dissolution leading to acute rupture and uncontrolled hemorrhage. Therefore, for vessels larger than 5 mm, prosthetic graft material is the conduit of choice, especially in potentially contaminated wounds. However, because of patency considerations, a saphenous vein graft may need to be used when smaller grafts are required. For soft vessels, such as the subclavian artery and the aorta in young people, a soft knitted Dacron graft is useful. Antibiotic irrigation of the graft material may help prevent subsequent infection.

DAMAGE CONTROL

Patients with severely compromised physiologic reserve, including those in extremis and those with massive or multiple complex thoracic injuries, often require damage control injury management to achieve survival. The two approaches to thoracic damage control are (1) definitive repair of injuries using quick and simple techniques that restore survivable physiology during a single operation and (2) abbreviated thoracotomy that restores survivable physiology and requires a planned subsequent operation for definitive repairs. Performing a pneumonectomy using stapling devices can quickly control severe hilar vascular injuries. Temporary vessel ligation or placement of intravascular shunts can control bleeding until subsequent correction of acidosis, hypothermia, and coagulopathy allows the patient to be returned to the operating room. En mass closure of a thoracotomy with a continuous heavy suture is more hemostatic than towel-clip closure. A plastic "Bogota bag" can be used as a temporary closure of a median sternotomy in cases with associated cardiac dysfunction.

SPECIFIC INJURIES

Thoracic Inlet

SUBCLAVIAN ARTERY AND VEIN

Penetrating trauma to the periclavicular region with injury to the innominate, sub-

clavian, and axillary vessels continues to pose a challenging problem for the surgeon because of the significant morbidity and mortality that occurs following damage to these vessels. The subclavian vessels are the most commonly injured great thoracic vessels: 21% of thoracic great vessel injuries involve the subclavian arteries and 13% involve the subclavian veins. Venous injuries have a significantly higher mortality than arterial injuries; in a series of 228 penetrating subclavian vessel injuries reported by Demetriades (1987), the overall mortality was 82% and 60%, respectively ($P < .01$). Approximately 61% of patients sustaining injuries to the subclavian vessels are dead on arrival to the emergency center. Of those who reach the hospital alive, most require operative intervention, with an operative mortality of up to 16% and substantial surgical morbidity. External or intrathoracic bleeding from the subclavian vessels may be difficult to control with direct pressure given their anatomic position behind the clavicle. In the presence of a supraclavicular wound, balloon tamponade using one or two Foley catheters placed through the wound may control bleeding until the patient arrives in the operating room (Fig. 13–3).

Patients with injury to the subclavian vessels may present with hard signs of vascular injury, such as absent distal pulses, expanding or pulsatile hematomas, or massive external hemorrhage. However, a subset of patients will not

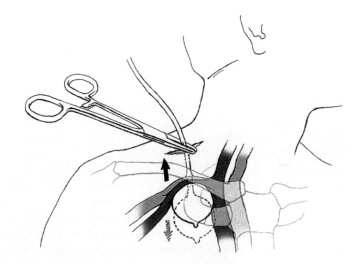

■ **FIGURE 13–3**
Balloon tamponade of subclavian vascular bleeding. A Foley catheter is inserted into the supraclavicular wound and is advanced as far as it can go. The balloon is then inflated and firm traction is applied to the catheter. The balloon compresses the subclavian vessels against the clavicle and the first rib. If there is persistent external bleeding, a second catheter is inserted and the balloon is inflated inside the wound tract, superficial to the first balloon. (Modifed from Demetriades D. Penetrating injuries to the thoracic great vessels. J Card Surg 1997;12:173-180.) ■

exhibit any of these findings, and their injury may be found on angiograms obtained solely on the basis of location of injury or chest radiograph findings.

One pitfall in subclavian injuries is failure to anticipate the exposure necessary for proximal control. When approaching the subclavian artery via a supraclavicular incision without proximal control, exsanguination may occur. A median sternotomy with a cervical extension is employed for exposure of right-sided subclavian injuries. For left subclavian artery injuries, proximal control is obtained through an anterolateral thoracotomy (above the nipple, third or fourth intercostal space), while a separate supraclavicular incision provides distal control. In the extremely difficult left-sided subclavian artery injury, a formal "book" thoracotomy incision may be required. This approach is associated with a high incidence of postoperative "causalgia" type of neurologic complications; therefore, its use should be limited. Although this carries significant morbidity, resection of the clavicle may also aid in obtaining proximal control. Alternatively, for distal injuries, a combination of supraclavicular and infraclavicular incisions may be used to avoid the morbidity of clavicular resection. In obtaining exposure, it is important to avoid injuring the phrenic nerve, which is located anterior to the scalenus anticus muscle, and the brachial plexus. Many patients with subclavian injuries will present with associated brachial plexus injuries, so careful documentation of preoperative neurologic status is important.

In most instances, repair of the subclavian artery requires either lateral arteriorrhaphy or graft interposition. A primary end-to-end anastomosis is usually not possible because of the fragility of the artery and limited mobilization. Associated injuries to the lung should be managed with stapled wedge resection or pulmonary tractotomy.

Achievement of adequate surgical exposure can be difficult and may be associated with postoperative neurologic complications; therefore, certain patients sustaining penetrating injuries to the subclavian vessels may benefit from stent-graft treatment. The success of stent-graft treatment for traumatic lesions depends largely on patient selection. Patients must be hemodynamically stable, and it must be possible to traverse the damaged segment with a guidewire. To avoid endoleaks with this technique, the proximal-distal lumen discrepancy must not be too large, and in the case of injuries to the subclavian artery, all side-branches, which potentially participate in the lesion, must be embolized before stent deployment (Fig. 13–4).

INNOMINATE ARTERY AND VEIN

The innominate artery is injured in approximately 9% of patients sustaining penetrating thoracic vascular trauma. Injuries to the left innominate vein are three times more common than those to the shorter right innominate vein. These injuries are approached through a median sternotomy with a right- or left-sided extension into the neck. Isolated venous injuries can be managed with primary repair or ligation. Division or ligation of the innominate vein can also be used to enhance exposure of the underlying artery.

In selected patients with only partial tears, the innominate artery may be primarily repaired using 4-0 polypropylene suture. More often, injuries to this vessel require repair via the bypass exclusion technique, which does not require cardiopulmonary bypass, hypothermia, systemic anticoagulation, or shunting. Bypass grafting is performed from the ascending aorta to the distal innominate artery using a Dacron tube graft (usually a 10-mm graft in adults). The area of injury is carefully avoided until the bypass is completed. The proximal anastomosis connects the graft to the ascending aorta away from the innominate artery origin; this is accomplished using a partial occluding, "side-biting" clamp on the ascending aorta. The distal anastomosis requires proximal and distal control of the innominate artery. If the proximal portion of the artery is injured, a partial occluding clamp can be placed across the adjacent aorta. For distal control, a vascular clamp is placed proximal to the bifurcation of the innominate artery to allow collateral flow from the right subclavian artery

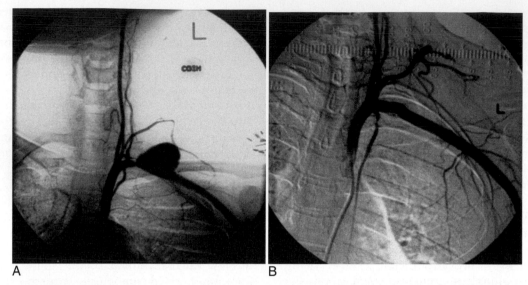

A   B

■ **FIGURE 13–4**
Treatment of a pseudoaneurysm of the left subclavian artery. *A,* Selective left subclavian artery arteriogram demonstrating the pseudoaneurysm; *B,* complete exclusion of the lesion after stent-graft deployment. (From du Toit DF, Strauss DC, Blaszczyk M: Endovascular treatment of penetrating thoracic outlet arterial injuries. Eur J Vasc Endovasc Surg 2000;19:489-495.) ■

to perfuse the right carotid artery. After the bypass is completed, the aorta is controlled with a partial occluding clamp and is oversewn. If concomitantly injured or previously divided, the innominate vein may be ligated with impunity. Alternatively, in stable patients, the vein can be reanastomosed. If the vein remains intact, a pedicled pericardial flap can be positioned between the vein and overlying graft to prevent erosion. With the bypass principle, reconstruction of innominate vascular injury carries an extremely low mortality rate and minimal morbidity, except in patients with preoperative neurologic injury or complex associated injuries.

LEFT COMMON CAROTID ARTERY

Injuries to the left common carotid artery are relatively uncommon when compared with other sites, especially since penetrating thoracic outlet injuries account for less than 5% of all civilian vascular trauma. The early management of these patients is critical and cannot be overemphasized. Immediate airway control is a priority because more

than 50% of these patients require urgent or semiurgent intubation because of the expanding hematoma. Tracheostomy is avoided because it may disrupt an underlying hematoma and cause severe bleeding. A baseline neurologic examination should be documented. Intraoperative endoscopy should be considered to rule out associated tracheal or esophageal injuries. The operative approach for injuries of the left carotid artery mirrors that used for an innominate artery injury: a median sternotomy with a left cervical extension added when necessary. As with other great vessel injuries, the use of shunts or pumps is unnecessary. If the artery is transected near its origin, repair with the bypass principle is preferred over a primary end-to-end anastomosis.

Thoracic Aorta

ASCENDING AORTA

Although penetrating injuries involving the ascending aorta (see Fig. 13–2) are uncommon, they do occur more often than blunt ascending aortic injuries. Survival rates approach 50% for patients having stable vital signs on arrival at a trauma center.

Although primary repair of anterior lacerations can be accomplished without adjuncts, cardiopulmonary bypass may be required if there is an additional posterior injury. The possibility of a peripheral bullet embolus must always be considered in these patients.

TRANSVERSE AORTIC ARCH

Penetrating aortic arch injuries are increasing in frequency because of the escalating use of firearms; however, the overall incidence of these injuries remains small, perhaps because of its short length and restricted location. The dominant clinical presentation is a penetrating thoracic wound with intrathoracic hemorrhage and shock.

When approaching an injury to the transverse aortic arch, extension of the median sternotomy to the neck is important to obtain complete exposure of the arch and brachiocephalic branches. If necessary, exposure can be further enhanced by division of the innominate vein. When hemorrhage limits exposure, the use of balloon tamponade is useful as a temporary measure. Simple lacerations may be repaired by lateral aortorrhaphy. With difficult lesions, such as posterior lacerations or those with concomitant pulmonary artery injuries, cardiopulmonary bypass is recommended. As with injuries to the ascending thoracic aorta, survival rates approaching 50% are possible.

DESCENDING THORACIC AORTA

Penetrating injury to the descending thoracic aorta occurs in 21% of patients presenting with wounds to the thoracic vasculature and is often accompanied by other organ injuries, such as the esophagus and heart. Patients may present to the emergency center with exsanguination, enlarging hemothorax, or bullet embolism to the lower extremity.

Injuries to the descending thoracic aorta are ideally approached via a posterolateral thoracotomy through the fourth intercostal space.

However, these are often found during emergent exploration via anterolateral thoracotomy. Although lateral aortorrhaphy is usually possible, the surgeon must also be prepared to perform patch graft aortoplasty or interposition grafting.

While gaining proximal control at the upper descending thoracic aorta, care must be taken to avoid injuring the left recurrent laryngeal nerve. If it is suspected that the injury extends to the aortic arch or ascending aorta, cardiopulmonary bypass should be available in the operating room. If the patient has had previous coronary artery bypass surgery with use of the left internal mammary artery as a conduit, repair may require profound hypothermic circulatory arrest.

The most feared complication of descending thoracic aortic injury is paraplegia, which has been associated with perioperative hypotension, injury or ligation of the intercostal arteries, and the complexity of the injury. We have advocated simple clamp and repair for injuries to the descending thoracic aorta (without the use of systemic anticoagulation or shunts), a technique that continues to be used with excellent results.

Other Major Intrathoracic Vessels

PULMONARY ARTERY AND VEIN

The pulmonary artery is damaged in 16% of patients presenting to the emergency center with penetrating trauma to the thoracic vessels, while the pulmonary veins are injured in 9%. These injuries are associated with mortality rates that approach 70%. The most common presenting manifestation of pulmonary artery injuries is hypotension or shock in association with either massive hemothorax or hemoptysis.

Distal pulmonary artery injuries are ideally approached through an ipsilateral posterolateral thoracotomy. These injuries are often identified during an emergent exploration via anterolateral thoracotomy. If a major injury to the hilum is present, rapid pneumonectomy may be a lifesaving maneuver. The use of a large balloon catheter may control exsanguinating hemorrhage. The intrapericardial pulmonary arteries are approached via median sternotomy. When this approach is used, minimal dissection is needed to expose the main and proximal left pulmonary arteries. Exposure of the intrapericardial right pulmonary artery is achieved by dissecting between the superior vena cava and ascending aorta. Although anterior injuries can be repaired primarily without adjuncts, repair of a posterior injury usually requires cardiopulmonary bypass. If ligation of the right or left pulmonary artery is required, a pneumonectomy is performed.

Injury to the pulmonary veins is difficult to manage through an anterior incision. With major hemorrhage, temporary occlusion of the entire hilum may be necessary. If a pulmonary vein must be ligated, the appropriate lobe needs to be resected. Pulmonary vein injuries are often associated with concomitant injuries to the heart, pulmonary artery, aorta, and esophagus.

THORACIC VENA CAVA

Isolated injury to the suprahepatic or superior vena cava is infrequently reported. Injury at either location has a high incidence of associated organ trauma and carries a mortality rate greater than 60%. Intrathoracic inferior vena cava injury produces hemopericardium and cardiac tamponade. Exposure of the posterior thoracic inferior vena cava is extremely difficult unless the patient is placed on total cardiopulmonary bypass with the inferior cannula inserted via the groin to the abdominal inferior vena cava. Repair is accomplished by a right atriotomy and intracaval balloon occlusion to prevent air entering the venous cannula and limit blood return to the heart. The injury is repaired from inside the cava via the right atrium. Superior vena cava injuries are repaired by lateral venorrhaphy. At times, an intracaval shunt is necessary. For complex injuries patch angioplasty or an interposition tube graft (Dacron or ringed polytetrafluoroethylene) can be used safely and is more expedient than the time-consuming construction of saphenous vein panel grafts.

AZYGOS VEIN

The azygos vein is not usually classified as a thoracic great vessel, but because of its size and high flow, azygos vein injuries must be considered potentially fatal. Penetrating wounds of the chest can produce combinations of injuries involving the azygos vein, innominate artery, trachea or bronchus, and superior vena cava. These complex injuries have a very high mortality rate and are particularly difficult to control if approached through an anterior incision. Combined incisions and approaches are often needed for successful repair. When injured, the azygous vein is best managed by suture ligature on both sides of the injury. Concomitant injury to the esophagus and bronchus should be considered and ruled out with a combination of direct exploration, esophagoscopy, and bronchoscopy before the patient leaves the operating room.

INTERNAL THORACIC AND INTERCOSTAL ARTERIES

Injury to the internal thoracic (i.e., the internal mammary) artery in a young patient can produce extensive hemothorax or even pericardial tamponade, simulating a cardiac injury. Such injuries are usually serendipitously discovered at the time of thoracotomy for suspected great vessel or heart injury. Persistent hemothorax can be caused by simple lacerations of the intercostal arteries. Because of difficulty in exposure, precise ligature can be difficult. Rapid control is best achieved by circumferential ligatures around the rib on either side of the intercostal vessel injury. These injuries are often missed during the initial operation because of arterial spasm; bleeding ensues later when the spasm resolves.

SPECIAL PROBLEMS

Mediastinal Traverse Injuries

Because penetrating injuries that traverse the mediastinum are classically felt to have a high probability of injury to the thoracic great vessels and other critical structures, mandatory exploration remains a justifiable approach. The evaluation of stable patients using less invasive means, such as combined aortography, bronchoscopy, echocardiography, and esophagoscopy, is gaining proponents. Thoracoscopic evaluation of the mediastinal structures is another potential alternative that warrants investigation.

Thoracic Duct Injury

Injuries to the thoracic great vessels may be complicated by concomitant thoracic duct injury, which if unrecognized may produce devastating morbidity because of marked nutritional depletion. Diagnosed by chylous material draining from the chest tube, this condition is usually treated medically. Continued chest tube drainage, coupled with a diet devoid of long-chain fatty acids, usually results in spontaneous closure in less than 1 month. Prolonged hyperalimentation beyond 3 weeks has not consistently resulted in spontaneous closure of thoracic duct fistula. If thoracotomy is required, a heavy fatty meal to increase the chylous flow and facilitate identification of the fistula is given to the patient a few hours before surgery. The fistula is simply ligated.

Systemic Air Embolism

A fistula between a pulmonary vein and bronchiole due to a penetrating lung injury may result in a systemic air embolism (Fig. 13–5). The fistula allows air bubbles to enter the left heart and embolize to the systemic circulation, including the coronary and cerebral arteries. Intrabronchial pressure of more than 60 mm Hg increases the incidence of this complication. Manifestations include seizures and cardiac arrest. Resuscitation requires thoracotomy, clamping of the pulmonary hilum to prevent further air embolization, and aspiration of air from the left ventricle and ascending aorta. Cardiopulmonary bypass can be considered, but very few survivors have been reported.

Foreign Body Embolism

Because of their central location, the thoracic great vessels may serve as both an entry site and a final resting place for intravascular bullet emboli. These migratory foreign bodies present a diagnostic and therapeutic dilemma. As the result of intravascular embolization, bullets may produce infection, ischemia, or injury to organs distant from the site of trauma.

Bullets and catheters can embolize to the pulmonary vasculature; 25% of migratory bullets finally lodge in the pulmonary arteries. Although small fragments, such as those the size of a BB, can probably be left in place without causing problems, larger bullet emboli should be removed to prevent pulmonary thrombosis, sepsis, or other complications. Nonoperative management of foreign bodies located in the left side of the heart should be performed only in selected asymptomatic patients, such as those presenting long after the initial injury and in whom imaging studies confirm that the foreign body is encapsulated by fibrous tissue. Percutaneous retrieval of the foreign body using transvenous catheters and fluoroscopic guidance may obviate the need for thoracotomy. Intraoperative imaging is necessary to rule out unsuspected migration of the foreign body during patient positioning.

POSTOPERATIVE MANAGEMENT

A significant portion of the in-hospital mortality associated with great vessel injury is secondary to the nature of the multisystem trauma in this group of patients. The operating surgeon is best qualified to direct postoperative management. Careful hemodynamic monitoring, with avoidance of both hypertension and hypotension, is critical. Although urinary output is a generally a good indicator of cardiac function, for the patient with massive injuries, Swan-Ganz monitoring is often necessary to optimize hemodynamic parameters and manage fluids, pressors, and vasodilators.

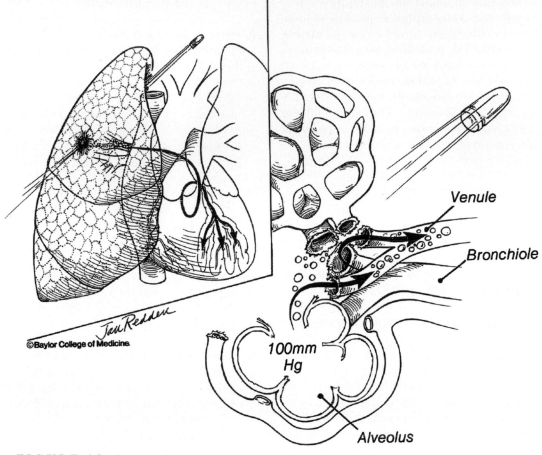

■ **FIGURE 13–5**
Drawing depicting the mechanism of systemic air embolism following a penetrating lung injury. (From Baylor College of Medicine, Houston, Texas.) ■

Various pulmonary problems, including atelectasis, respiratory insufficiency, pneumonia, and acute respiratory distress syndrome, represent the primary postoperative complications in this group of patients, necessitating careful fluid administration. Associated pulmonary contusions also contribute to respiratory problems. Positive end-expiratory pressure can be provided to hemodynamically stable intubated patients, to minimize atelectasis. Patient mobility is important, and adequate medication for pain relief results in fewer pulmonary complications. For the management of pain related to a thoracotomy or multiple rib fractures, postoperative thoracic epidural anesthesia should be considered in stable patients without spinal injuries; alternatively, intercostal nerve blocks can be performed intraoperatively and repeated in the intensive care unit.

Postoperative hemorrhage may be due to a technical problem but is often the result of coagulopathy related to hypothermia, acidosis, and massive blood transfusion. Coagulation studies must be carefully monitored and corrected with administration of appropriate blood products. Blood draining via chest tubes can be collected and autotransfused.

The presence of a prosthetic vascular graft requires special attention aimed at avoiding bacteremia. During the initial resuscitation of these critically injured patients, various intravascular lines are often rapidly placed at the expense of strict sterile technique; such lines should be replaced after the patient has stabilized in the intensive care unit.

Antibiotic therapy should be continued into the postoperative period until potential sources of infection are eliminated. Patients are counseled regarding the necessity of antibiotic prophylaxis during invasive procedures, including dental manipulations.

Most late complications are related to infections or sequelae from other injuries. Long-term complications specifically related to the vascular repair, including stenosis, thrombosis, arteriovenous fistula, graft infection, and pseudoaneurysm formation, are uncommon.

REFERENCES

Bickell WH, Wall MJ Jr, Pepe PE, et al: Immediate versus delayed fluid resuscitation for hypotensive patients with penetrating torso injuries. N Engl J Med 1994;331:1105-1109.

Demetriades D: Penetrating injuries to the thoracic great vessels. J Card Surg 1997;12:173-180.

du Toit DF, Strauss DC, Blaszcyk M, et al: Endovascular treatment of penetrating thoracic outlet arterial injuries. Eur J Endovasc Surg 2000; 19:489-495.

Demetriades D, Rabinowitc B, Pezikis A, et al: Subclavian vascular injuries. Br J Surg 1987;74: 1001-1003.

Feliciano DV: Trauma to the aorta and major vessels. Chest Surg Clin North Am 1997;7(2):305-323.

Mattox KL, Wall MJ: Trauma of the chest: newer diagnostic measures and emergency management. Chest Surg Clin North Am 1997;7(2):213-226.

Parodi JC, Schonholz C, Ferreira LM, Bergan J: Endovascular stent-graft treatment of traumatic arterial lesions. Ann Vasc Surg 1999;13(2):121-129.

Richardson JD, Miller FB, Carrillo EH, Spain DA: Complex thoracic injuries. Surg Clin North Am 1996;76(4):725-748.

Wall MJ, Granchi T, Liscum KR, Mattox KL: Penetrating thoracic vascular injuries. Surg Clin North Am 1996;76(4):749-761.

14

Blunt Thoracic Vascular Injury

AURELIO RODRIGUEZ
DAVID C. ELLIOTT

BLUNT THORACIC VASCULAR TRAUMA

A 30-year-old man is ejected from his pickup truck after falling asleep at the wheel and striking an embankment. Brought rapidly by helicopter to a level I trauma center, he is found by expeditious evaluation to have sustained a mild closed head injury, a stable pelvic fracture, and multiple rib fractures. Of more concern, his diagnostic peritoneal lavage returns grossly positive and his supine chest radiograph reveals a widened mediastinum with distortion of the aortic knob.

How will the diagnostic evaluation proceed from here? Will aortography precede or follow laparotomy? If a ruptured thoracic aorta is found, will a Gott shunt, a Bio-Medicus pump, or a "clamp-and-sew" strategy be pursued? Will you perform a primary repair of the injured aorta or place a synthetic graft? What perioperative measures can you employ to minimize postoperative complications such as paraplegia? These are a few of the often controversial questions surrounding evaluation and treatment of the patient with traumatic rupture of the thoracic aorta, which we attempt to address in this chapter. In addition, the less commonly seen blunt injuries to other thoracic vascular structures are also reviewed.

Blunt thoracic aortic injury (BTAI) is a major cause of morbidity and mortality in the United States, with one fifth of motor vehicle accident deaths attributable thereto. Despite advances in surgical technique and postoperative care, survival has not changed much since 1958, when Parmley and colleagues from the Armed Forces Institute of Pathology and Walter Reed U.S. Army Hospital provided the classic pathophysiologic and epidemiologic description of BTAI. In their series of 275 patients, 86% died at the scene. Of those who initially survived, only 26% were alive at 2 weeks. More recent series report comparable figures for death at the scene, whereas for those who survived transport to a trauma center, survival to discharge rates of 50% to 75% are reported. Except those presenting to the emergency department *in extremis* or who have obviously ruptured, injured patients with BTAI who are stable enough to undergo thoracotomy and repair have a chance of survival of 85%.

DEMOGRAPHICS AND PATTERN OF INJURY

BTAI classically occurs at the aortic isthmus 1 cm distal to the left subclavian artery (at the site of the ligamentum arteriosum). In the series by Parmley and colleagues (1958), 45% of all aortic injuries and 63% of those in early survivors were at this site, which agrees well with results from more recent autopsy series. Other sites of injury, such as ascending, descending, and abdominal aorta, are less common and are often associated with spine fractures. Injury to other great vessels in the chest, such as the innominate artery and the subclavian artery and vein, comprises 5% or less of all blunt thoracic vascular trauma.

One prospective study of 1500 patients sustaining significant blunt chest trauma found that using multivariate logistic regression analysis, BTAI was associated with high-speed collisions (>60 miles per hour) and higher Injury Severity Scores (ISSs), but not direction of impact, ejection from the vehicle, sudden deceleration, or other fatalities in the vehicle. A second recent study assessing direction of impact found that half of BTAI victims (48 of 97) sustained lateral impact collisions, and 83% of these were wearing restraints. As in motor vehicle collisions, BTAI has also been found to be a common cause of death among pedestrians struck by motor vehicles, responsible in one series for 13% of pedestrian deaths, with a mortality rate of 93% overall. In the single largest prospective, multi-institutional study of BTAI (274 patients), the mean ISS was 42, the Glasgow Coma Scale (GCS) score was 12, 93% of injuries were at the aortic isthmus, and 46 patients (17%) arrived to the hospital *in extremis* or exsanguinated from free rupture soon thereafter. Multiple injuries were commonplace and included head injury (51%), rib fractures (46%), pelvic and long bone fractures (34%), and abdominal injuries (22%). Traumatic rupture of the aorta rarely (<30% of all cases)

TABLE 14–1
ASSOCIATED INJURIES TRAUMATIC RUPTURE OF THE AORTA

Study	Patients (n)	Closed Head Injury (%)	Abdominal Injury (%)	Pulmonary Contusion (%)	Pelvic Fracture (%)
Duhaylongsod, Glower, and Wolfe (1992)	67	31	37	45	27
Hilgenberg and colleagues (1992)	51	40	29	39	25
Hunt and colleagues (1996)	144	37	25	16	26
Kieny and Charpentier (1991)	73	62	18		25
Fabian and colleagues (1998)	274	51	22	38	31
Szwerc and colleagues (1999)	30	37	53	40	33

Associated injuries recorded as percent of patients afflicted.

occurs without significant associated injuries. Table 14–1 lists nine recent series of patients with BTAI and commonly associated injuries. In four series, the ISS was calculated, and the average excluding the aortic component was 18.

Although free rupture of the aorta is immediately lethal, the circumferential extent of contained tears is not clearly associated with increased mortality. In the Parmley and colleagues (1958) series, 24% of early survivors had complete circumferential tears. Again, this finding has been reproduced in more recent series. Patients with partial-thickness tears who survive without surgical repair develop a fibrous pseudoaneurysm. These may be discovered incidentally on routine chest x-ray films years after the inciting injury. Alternatively, these pseudoaneurysms may become symptomatic or result in delayed rupture in one third of patients. Therefore, it is recommended that pseudoaneurysms of the thoracic aorta are repaired whenever found. Death from BTAI appears to follow a bimodal distribution, with early deaths (<4 hours) being due to free rupture of the aorta and exsanguination and late deaths uncommonly due to bleeding, but due to associated injuries and resultant multiorgan failure.

PRESENTATION

Despite the dire nature of the injury, the diagnosis of BTAI is often subtle because history and physical examination after blunt thoracic trauma are neither sensitive nor specific for aortic injury. Certain clues should, however, raise the index of suspicion: appropriately severe mechanism (high-speed motor vehicle collision, pedestrian struck, or a fall from great height); dyspnea; dysphagia; interscapular pain; significant chest wall trauma (multiple rib fractures or steering-wheel imprint); new cardiac or interscapular murmur; left-sided hemothorax; left supraclavicular hematoma; and pseudocoarctation (relative upper extremity hypertension). In particular, left-sided hemothorax greater than 500 mL, left supraclavicular hematoma, and pseudocoarctation may be signs of imminent free rupture.

DIAGNOSIS

Aortogram

The gold standard for the diagnosis of BTAI has been the aortogram. Not only is conventional aortography highly sensitive and specific for aortic injury, but it also provides precise anatomic localization of the injury, which may help guide surgical repair (Fig. 14–1). Conversely, aortography is expensive, invasive, and time and resource intensive, requires patient transport away from the trauma bay, and has a morbidity rate of up to 10%, making it unsuitable as a general screening examination. Digital subtraction angiography may

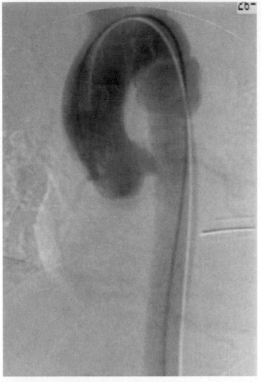

■ FIGURE 14–1
Digital subtraction aortogram demonstrating a pseudoaneurysm of the proximal descending thoracic aorta. (Courtesy S. Mirvis.) ■

improve diagnostic accuracy while decreasing contrast loads.

Chest X-ray

Because of the limitations of aortography and the lack of sensitivity and/or specificity of the clinical presentation, all patients with blunt trauma should undergo an initial supine anteroposterior chest x-ray. The purpose of this study is to detect indirect evidence of BTAI such as mediastinal hemorrhage or bony fractures indicating high-energy transfer. Frequently cited signs suggestive of BTAI are listed in Box 14–1.

Many of the signs listed in Box 14-1 are technique dependent and repeated evaluation in the upright position or standard posteroanterior projection is advocated if there is no clinical contraindication (Fig. 14–2). Using the presence of any of the aforementioned signs as a trigger for further evaluation, some aortic injuries will still be missed. In a review of the radiologic literature, Woodring and Dillon (1984) found that of 656 cases of BTAI, 7.3%

BOX 14–1
CHEST X-RAY SIGNS SUGGESTIVE OF AORTIC RUPTURE

Mediastinal widening > 8 cm
Mediastinal-to-chest width ratio > 0.25
Abnormal aortic contour
Loss of the aorticopulmonary window
Shift of the trachea to the right
Shift of the orogastric/nasogastric tube to the right
Left apical cap
Widening of the paraspinal lines
Depression of the left mainstem bronchus
Left pleural effusion
Scapular fracture
Sternal fracture
Thoracic spine fracture
First or second rib fracture
Multiple rib fractures

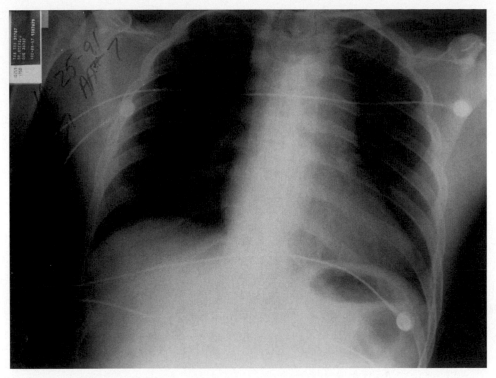

■ **FIGURE 14–2**
Anteroposterior "true erect" chest radiograph showing a widened mediastinum, loss of aortic contour, tracheal deviation, loss of the aorticopulmonary window, and a widened left paraspinal line. The patient sustained an aortic rupture. (Courtesy S. Mirvis). ■

had none of the standard radiologic criteria for mediastinal hemorrhage. Other recent series also report a significant incidence of normal chest x-ray film among patients with BTAI. Select patients, with compelling mechanism of injury, should therefore undergo further evaluation despite a normal screening chest x-ray film (Fig. 14–3).

Computed Tomography

The role of computed tomography (CT) in the evaluation of blunt thoracic trauma is contested: Does it supplement or possibly replace the role of chest x-ray and aortography, or is it merely a waste of time and resources? Over the last 10 years, CT has evolved from an adjunct to an inadequate or equivocal chest radiograph to an all-purpose screening and diagnostic tool, potentially supplanting both chest x-ray and aortography. Many earlier series have documented that standard chest CT with intravenous contrast can consistently

document mediastinal hemorrhage associated with BTAI, reporting a zero false-negative rate and conclude that chest CT can safely decrease the need for aortography by greater than 50%.

The latest generation of spiral and helical CT scanners have greatly increased the accuracy of making a diagnosis of BTAI through noninvasive means. Used with a dynamic bolus of contrast and three-dimensional reconstruction algorithms, CT aortography can perhaps obviate the need for most conventional aortograms. A recent series by Gavant and colleagues applied this technique to 1518 patients with blunt chest trauma over an 11-month period. Of these, 127 patients had abnormal CT scans and subsequently underwent conventional aortography. CT sensitivity for BTAI was 100% versus 94% for conventional aortography, and specificity was 82% for the CT versus 96% for conventional aortography. A follow-up study with 38 thoracic aortic and great-vessel injuries demonstrated that CT aortography can not only accurately diagnose BTAI but also provide

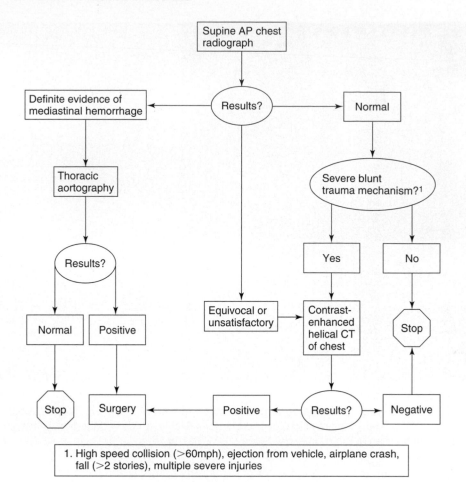

■ **FIGURE 14–3**
Suggested algorithm for radiographic evaluation of patients sustaining significant blunt thoracic trauma. ■

sufficient anatomic detail (previously only available through conventional aortography) to guide management. In our hands, CT was superior to angiography in the diagnosis of BTAI. Mirvis and colleagues have also documented the steady progress made with thoracic CT in the diagnosis of BTAI, in an earlier series showing that nonhelical CT can reliably (100% sensitivity and negative predictive value) pick up the presence of mediastinal hematoma, but in the latest series showing the same reliability and accuracy with helical CT in demonstrating the actual aortic injury, precluding the need for aortography. Three prospective series similarly add to the growing body of evidence that helical CT is equal or superior to aortography in the diagnosis of BTAI, that this technology represents a significant improvement over previous non-

helical CT, and that up to 95% of angiography scans can be obviated through use of CT (Fig. 14–4).

The preceding discussions on the merits of CT and aortography in the diagnosis of BTAI must be viewed in light of their major drawback: Both require transport away from the trauma bay and therefore are only useful in a hemodynamically stable patient. Fabian and colleagues point out that CT has the advantage in this regard; compared to aortography, helical CT is faster, easier, more available, and less invasive. Nonetheless, like any other technologic imaging innovation, results depend on user experience. The near-perfect diagnostic accuracy cited may not be universally reproducible at facilities where the volume of trauma patients is insufficient to allow adequate experience with this technique to

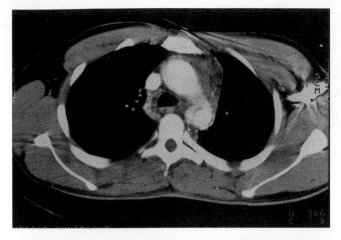

■ **FIGURE 14-4**
Axial dynamic thoracic computed tomogram revealing a mediastinal hematoma anteriorly and an aortic intimal flap. The patient had sustained an aortic rupture. (Courtesy S. Mirvis). ■

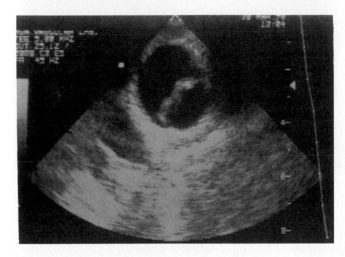

■ **FIGURE 14-5**
Transesophageal echocardiogram revealing an intimal flap of disrupted descending thoracic aorta. (From Brooks SW, Young JC, Cmolik B, et al: J Trauma 1992;32:761-766.) ■

accrue. In such situations, the time-tested modality of aortography may represent the diagnostic test of choice.

Transesophageal Echocardiography

Since its introduction in the early 1980s, transesophageal echocardiography (TEE) has become the study of choice for various cardiac diseases and is increasingly used for the evaluation of the thoracic aorta. TEE is well suited for this role because of the close anatomic proximity between the esophagus and the thoracic aorta.

In a representative study by Smith and colleagues (1995), TEE was attempted in 101 blunt trauma patients but only completed in 93. TEE diagnosis of BTAI was corroborated with aortography and surgery and/or autopsy. Overall, TEE sensitivity was 100% and specificity was 98% with one false-positive result. In these and other authors' hands, TEE is both sensitive and specific in the diagnosis of BTAI. Also, TEE provides precise anatomic localization of the site of injury and does not require patient transport, making it better suited for the unstable patient (Fig. 14-5). On the negative side, TEE cannot be used in all trauma patients (7% in this study) because of patient combativeness, cervical spinal or maxillofacial injury, and airway difficulty. In addition, results are operator dependent, and other authors have not been able to reliably reproduce such excellent results, with sensitivity for BTAI only 57% in one series. In analyzing 10 series totaling 407 patients undergoing TEE to diagnose BTAI, Ben-Menachem (1997) found this test's sensitivity for BTAI to be 86% and inferior to that of aortography. To summarize, the diagnostic accuracy of TEE is open to question, it possesses "blind spots" to include the ascending aorta, the aortic arch, and its branches, and certain patients cannot tolerate the procedure. However, it possesses a few advantages over other techniques, including portability, rapidity, and its safety profile. Until incontrovertible documentation of superior accuracy, TEE might best be reserved for the following circumstances:

- Evaluation of unstable patients who are poor risks for transport to the CT scanner or the angiography suit

- Evaluation of patients in the operating room during emergent laparotomy for intra-abdominal hemorrhage

- Evaluation of the morbidly obese patient whose weight may exceed table limits of the CT scanner or angiography suite

PREOPERATIVE MANAGEMENT

Multisystem injuries are common in patients with BTAI; thus, keeping the entire clinical scenario in perspective is important when discussing management. It has been noted that hypotension in patients with BTAI is generally not due to the aortic injury because bleeding from the aorta is rapidly fatal. Therefore, as in all trauma patients, it is imperative to discover and address the etiology of hypotension. Primary and secondary surveys will reveal sites of external hemorrhage and sites of possible occult blood loss such as pelvic and long bone fractures. Chest x-ray and/or tube thoracostomy will expose significant intrapleural hemorrhage. Intra-abdominal hemorrhage is best evaluated in this situation by diagnostic peritoneal lavage (DPL), CT, or abdominal ultrasonography. The advantages of DPL and ultrasonography reside in their ability to be performed quickly, in both unstable and stable patients. The use of abdominal CT takes longer and requires a stable patient but gives more information and can be performed coincident to CT of the chest, if already planned. In cases of combined thoracic and abdominal injury, laparotomy should follow thoracotomy when

signs of imminent BTAI rupture exist such as left hemothorax, pseudocoarctation, or supraclavicular hematoma. Otherwise, laparotomy should generally precede aortography and/or thoracotomy.

A subset of patients with BTAI and severe associated injuries are poor candidates for immediate aortic repair. Initial nonoperative management can allow sufficient physiologic recovery for delayed aortic repair. Akins and colleagues (1981) suggest the following criteria for delayed repair:

- Major intracranial injury
- Extensive burns
- Severe respiratory failure
- Extensively contaminated wound
- Sepsis

Similarly, some authors have advocated nonoperative therapy for patients with minimal aortic injury (e.g., aortic intimal irregularity without extravasation of contrast). These patients should be followed with serial angiography or TEE to document resolution of their aortic injury. Afterload reduction and β-blockade are useful medical adjuncts, temporizing patients with delayed operative and primary nonoperative management by minimizing aortic wall stress.

Increasing experience with delayed operative management of BTAI is resulting in an overall paradigm shift and change in management strategy for this injury. There is now substantial evidence supporting that excepting BTAI patients presenting *in extremis,* in-hospital rupture can be effectively prevented by keeping the systolic blood pressure below 140 mm Hg. Most of these data have been accrued through retrospective analysis of prospective medical protocols using a combination of esmolol, labetalol, and sodium nitroprusside, and although outcomes were simply compared to historical controls, virtually no deaths resulting from in-hospital rupture of BTAI have occurred in these series when adequate medical control of blood pressure is ensured. This allows for a planned, considered, and prepared approach to the repair of this problematic injury, ensuring optimal patient physiologic condition and optimal hospital resource support, rather than the sense of hurry and panic that can be engendered from the perceived need to thwart a potential intrathoracic "time bomb."

It is further recommended that adequate sedation be used at the time of endotracheal intubation, should this be required, and that fluid resuscitation be particularly judicious, to minimize wall stress on the attenuated aorta. Pneumatic antishock garments (PASGs), a once common appliance of patients with multiple trauma brought to trauma centers, are more clearly detrimental. No benefit to these devices has been demonstrated clinically in the management of BTAI and in a porcine model of aortic injury, 100% of pigs with and 0% of pigs without PASG died of their injury.

Approximately one half of patients with BTAI will also have a closed head injury (see Table 14–1). Optimally, a head CT scan should be obtained before BTAI repair so craniotomy can be planned if needed. Head CT findings will also bear on surgical technique; for example, systemic heparinization is contraindicated in the presence of intracranial hemorrhage.

SURGICAL TECHNIQUE

Most patients with blunt thoracic vascular injury are best served by repair via a left posterolateral thoracotomy, because this approach gives the best exposure to the aortic isthmus where most injuries occur. There are two main technical variables in the surgical repair of a classic (aortic isthmus) BTAI (Fig. 14–6), as follows:

- "Clamp-and-sew" technique *versus* shunt and
- Interposition graft versus primary repair

The clamp-and-sew technique is less complex and more expedient than shunting. Proponents of this technique argue that it is superior to shunting in all cases of BTAI because it does not require systemic heparinization, does not have adjunct-associated complications (e.g., insertion site hemorrhage or aortic dissection), and does not require special equipment. Arguably, morbidity and mortality rates are similar between clamp-and-sew and shunt techniques. In short, the key technical points in the clamp-and-sew technique are as follows:

SURGICAL MODALITIES

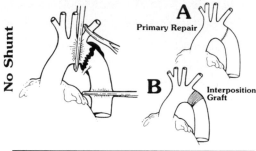
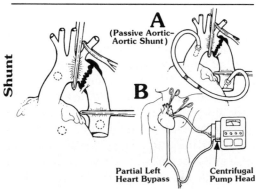

■ **FIGURE 14–6**
Options in operative repair techniques for rupture of the descending thoracic aorta. *A,* Primary or direct repair. *B,* Graft interposition without a mechanical adjunct (clamp and sew). Use of a mechanical adjunct in aortic repair: *A,* Aortoaortic (Gott's) shunt. *B,* Left atrial femoral artery bypass with a Bio-Medicus centrifugal flow pump. ■

1. Position the patient in the right lateral decubitus position and create a standard left posterolateral thoracotomy.
2. Identify left vagus and phrenic nerves; retract left vagus.
3. Circumferentially dissect left subclavian artery and secure with an umbilical tape.
4. Perform sharp and blunt dissection between the left subclavian and left common carotid arteries and place umbilical tape around the proximal aorta.
5. Circumferentially dissect descending aorta below hematoma and secure with an umbilical tape.
6. Ligate and/or control intervening intercostal arteries.
7. Administer intravenous mannitol
8. First cross-clamp aortic arch, followed by descending aorta and subclavian artery.

9. Open hematoma and control back-bleeding.

10. Débride devitalized aortic wall.

11. Anastomose aorta with or without intervening prosthetic graft.

12. Back-bleed and vent aorta before securing suture line.

13. Notify anesthesiologist, then release subclavian and descending aorta clamps, followed by aortic arch clamp.

Shunt techniques of BTAI repair are similar to "clamp and sew" with the exception that a conduit is inserted proximal and distal to the aortic injury. Benefits of this arrangement include afterload reduction of the left ventricle and preserved systemic perfusion during aortic cross-clamp. The least complicated of these techniques involve passive conduits such as the heparin-bonded Gott shunt. This is typically inserted into the left ventricle or ascending aorta proximally and the femoral artery distally. Passive conduits such as the Gott shunt rely on cardiac output and therefore may not provide adequate distal perfusion if cardiac performance is impaired. Active shunts employing centrifugal or roller pumps are cardiac output independent but are at the risk of stealing perfusion from the cerebral and coronary circulation. In a trauma setting, centrifugal pumps have the advantage over roller pumps of not requiring systemic heparinization. Like passive conduits, the distal insertion of these shunts is usually in the femoral artery and the proximal insertion is in the left atrial appendage. Shunts may decrease the incidence of ischemic spinal cord injury, systemic acidosis, and renal injury, and although the evidence in the trauma literature on this subject has in the past been divided, more recent series support that the incidence of postoperative paraplegia is lower at centers that use partial left heart bypass with a centrifugal flow pump. A recent prospective nationwide survey of trauma centers performing BTAI repair found that although mortality was no different between the two groups, the incidence of postoperative paraplegia was 16.4% among the 73 patients treated with the clamp-and-sew technique, versus 2.9% among the 69 patients treated using centrifugal pump bypass ($P < .004$). Citing similar results, another recent study showed by multivariate regression analysis that the factors independently predicting postoperative paraplegia included older age, operative technique (clamp and sew), clamp time greater than 30 minutes, and the occurrence of intraoperative hypotension.

Choice of primary repair versus use of prosthetic graft is largely dictated by the physical characteristics of the native aorta and the extent of aortic disruption. The advantages of primary repair include shorter cross-clamp times, decreased risk of infection, and less intercostal artery sacrifice (possibly contributing to ischemic spinal cord injury). In the pediatric population, primary repair abates the need for reoperation to upsize an outgrown aortic prosthesis. Generally, prosthetic grafts are better suited for instances when the edges of the torn aorta are widely distracted making a tension-free anastomosis impossible. One prominent series, however, reports 32 consecutive aortic injuries repaired primarily despite up to 5-cm separation of the torn aortic edges. Another recent series wherein primary repair was the preferential mode of therapy for BTAI reports mortality and paraplegia rates comparable to that those reported with use of the centrifugal pump bypass. Use of both Dacron and polytetrafluoroethylene (PTFE) have been described in the literature, and both provide similarly good results.

Still in its infancy, endovascular repair of BTAI appears to be a promising area for study. One published series of nine patients sustaining BTAI reports TEE-guided endoluminal stent repair from 1 to 8 months after injury with excellent results: no mortality, no rupture, no occlusions, and no need for revision after the initial procedure.

BLUNT INJURY TO OTHER THORACIC VESSELS

Innominate Artery

Innominate and proximal carotid artery injury is rare, comprising less than 5% of all blunt thoracic vascular trauma, although the innominate artery is probably the most common thoracic vessel injured by blunt trauma after the thoracic aorta. Focal neurologic deficits may be present with this injury, but most injuries are picked up through screening chest radiography, CT, and aortography.

Optimal exposure is via median sternotomy, plus or minus right neck extension, and repair is advocated over ligation because of the concern for cerebral ischemia and resultant neurologic injury. Because most blunt innominate injuries occur at its aortic insertion and native tissue at that location may be compromised, anastomosis at this location should be avoided. Rather, the preferred approach involves the construction of a Dacron or PTFE bypass graft proximal to the injury by anastomosis to the aorta using a partial-occlusion clamp. No heparin, shunt, or cardiopulmonary bypass is generally employed. The bypass graft is sutured distally to uninjured vessel or vessels, and the aorta at the site of the innominate insertion is oversewn with pledgeted sutures. Outcome is generally excellent, and mortality should be 0% to 10%, based on hemodynamic condition on admission and concomitant injuries (which are common). Of note, endoluminal stent repair has also been performed successfully for blunt innominate artery injury.

Subclavian Artery

Approximately 1% to 5% of blunt thoracic vascular trauma involves the subclavian artery. In contrast to BTAI, shoulder harness seat belts have been implicated in the pathogenesis of this injury. Signs concerning for subclavian injury include supraclavicular hematoma, pulse deficit, brachial plexus injury, clavicular fracture, and bruit (although none are particularly sensitive or specific). Pulse deficit is most characteristic but may be absent because of extensive collateral flow often present about the shoulder. Diagnosis of subclavian artery injury, as in BTAI, is best made with aortography. Optimal surgical exposure is debated (see Table 14–2), although most favor median sternotomy for right subclavian and proximal left subclavian lesions, and left supraclavicular incision for mid-subclavian to distal subclavian injuries of the left side. Reconstruction is generally done with prosthetic graft. Concomitant subclavian vein injury occurs in up to 20% of patients and can often be treated with simple ligation. If collateral venous return is compromised, reconstruction of the subclavian vein is recommended and can be performed with a saphenous vein interposition graft or an end-to-end subclavian jugular vein bypass.

One variant of blunt subclavian vessel injury occurs in the syndrome of scapulothoracic

TABLE 14–2
OPTIMAL AND ALTERNATIVE EXPOSURE FOR THORACIC VASCULAR INJURIES

Injured Vessel	Optimal Exposure	Alternate Exposure
Ascending aorta	MS	
Right subclavian	**P**: MS with supraclavicular ext.	**D**: R. supraclavicular
Innominate	MS	
Proximal common carotid	MS	
Left subclavian	**D**: L. supraclavicular	**P**: L. anterolateral thoracotomy
Aortic arch	MS	
Aortic isthmus	L. posterolateral thoracotomy	
Descending aorta	L. posterolateral thoracotomy	
SVC	MS	
Suprahepatic IVC	Thoracoabdominal	

D, distal; IVC, inferior vena cava; L, left; MS, median sternotomy; P, proximal; R, right; SVC, superior vena cava.

dissociation. In this devastating injury, a strong torsion or rotational force is applied to the shoulder joint, shearing the scapula and shoulder girdle from the chest wall, resulting in extensive complex fractures of the upper extremity and avulsion of the brachial plexus and subclavian vessels as they emerge from the thoracic cavity. Patients present in shock with massive swelling of the ipsilateral chest and neurovascular deficiency of the arm. For survival, treatment requires early recognition, control of bleeding, reversal of shock, and usually, substantial amputation of the involved extremity.

Vena Cava

Blunt injury to the thoracic vena cava, though less common than BTAI, has similar mortality. This difference in incidence between arterial and venous injuries is most likely due to differences in vessel wall plasticity. Surgical approach to the vena cava, and in particular the suprahepatic vena cava, is problematic and may require heroic measures such as total hepatic vascular occlusion and atriocaval shunting. When feasible, primary repair with lateral venorrhaphy is preferred even though this may result in vessel narrowing.

Pulmonary Artery and Vein

Blunt trauma to the pulmonary artery and vein is rare. Patients with these injuries present in shock from hemorrhage and/or cardiac tamponade. The treatment of choice for these injuries is lateral repair, but if the tear in the vessel wall is not amenable to this, pneumonectomy is an option.

SUMMARY

BTAI is a common and often lethal injury. For those who survive the initial insult, patients with this injury are best served by expeditious evaluation and prompt repair. A high index of suspicion, based on mechanism of injury, will ensure that few of these injuries are missed. Chest helical CT is increasingly becoming both the screening and the diagnostic test of choice in centers that serve significant numbers of blunt trauma patients; however, chest radiography and aortography remain gold standards in the diagnostic algorithm.

Attentive medical management, based around the use of intravenous β-blockers to keep systolic blood pressure below 140 mm Hg, should be employed early in patients with probable BTAI and may prevent in-hospital rupture. Technique of operative repair is controversial, and no single nationwide standard of care has emerged for definitive operative strategy. However, the preponderance of medical evidence increasingly points to decreased incidence of paraplegia after BTAI repair when heparin-less centrifugal pump bypass is employed.

Because of the common occurrence of BTAI, the proclivity of its presence and repair to result in mortality or morbidity, and the wide diversity of management options that have been used for care, it is strongly recommended that each trauma center that deals with this injury consider the use of a clinical practice guideline for BTAI that would encourage a single safe standard for the diagnosis and management of this injury. An excellent example of such a practice guideline has been developed and published by the Eastern Association for the Surgery of Trauma.

REFERENCES

Albrink MH, Rodriguez E, England GJ, et al: Importance of designated thoracic trauma surgeons in the management of traumatic aortic transection. Southern Med J 1994;87:497-501.

Akins CW, Buckley MJ, Daggett W, et al: Acute traumatic disruption of the thoracic aorta: A 10-year experience. Ann Thorac Surg 1981;31:305-309.

Ali J, Vanderby B, Purcell C: The effect of the pneumatic antishock garment (PASG) on hemodynamics, hemorrhage, and survival in penetrating thoracic aortic injury. J Trauma 1991;31:846-851.

Attar S, Cardarelli MG, Downing SW, et al: Traumatic aortic rupture: Recent outcome with regard to neurologic deficit. Ann Thorac Surg 1999;67:959-965.

Axisa BM, Loftus IM, Fishwick G, et al: Endovascular repair of an innominate artery false aneurysm following blunt trauma. J Endovasc Ther 2000;7:245-250.

Baker SP, O'Neill B, Haddon W, et al: The Injury Severity Score: A method for describing patients with multiple injuries and evaluating emergency care. J Trauma 1974;14:187-196.

Ben-Menachem Y: Rupture of the thoracic aorta by broadside impacts in road traffic and other collisions: Further angiographic observations and preliminary autopsy findings. J Trauma 1993;35:363-367.

Ben-Menachem Y: Assessment of blunt aortic-brachiocephalic trauma: Should angiography be supplanted by transesophageal echocardiography? J Trauma 1997;42:969-972.

Borman KR, Aurbakken CM, Weigelt JA: Treatment priorities in combined blunt abdominal and aortic trauma. Am J Surg 1982;144:728-732.

Brundage SI, Haruff R, Jurkovich GJ, et al: The epidemiology of thoracic aortic injuries in pedestrians. J Trauma 1998;45:1010-1014.

Buckmaster MJ, Kearney PA, Johnson SB, et al: Further experience with transesophageal echocardiography in the evaluation of thoracic aortic injury. J Trauma 1994;37:989-995.

Buscaglia LC, Walsh JC, Wilson JD, et al: Surgical management of subclavian artery injury. Am J Surg 1987;154:88-90.

Clark DE, Zieger MA, Wallace KL, et al: Blunt aortic trauma: Signs of high risk. J Trauma 1990;30:701-705.

Cohn SM, Burns GA, Jaffe C, et al: Exclusion of aortic tear in the unstable trauma patient: The utility of transesophageal echocardiography. J Trauma 1995;39:1087-1090.

Cooper C, Rodriguez A, Omert L: Blunt vascular trauma. Curr Probl Surg 1992;29:291-357.

Cox CS, Allen GS, Fischer RP, et al: Blunt versus penetrating subclavian artery injury: Presentation, injury pattern, and outcome. J Trauma 1999;46:445-449.

Demetriades D, Gomez H, Velmahos GC, et al: Routine helical computed tomographic evaluation of the mediastinum in high-risk blunt trauma patients. Arch Surg 1998;133:1084-1088.

Duhaylongsod FG, Glower DD, Wolfe WG: Acute traumatic aortic aneurysm: The Duke experience from 1970 to 1990. J Vasc Surg 1992;15:331-343.

Dyer AD, Moore EE, Ilke DN, et al: Thoracic aortic injury: How predictive is mechanism and is chest computed tomography a reliable screening tool?

A prospective study of 1561 patients. J Trauma 2000;48:673-682.

Ebraheim NA, An HS, Jackson WT, et al: Scapulothoracic dissociation. J Bone Joint Surg 1988; 70:428-432.

Fabian TC, Davis KA, Gavant ML, et al: Prospective study of blunt aortic injury: Helical CT is diagnostic and antihypertensive therapy reduces rupture. Ann Surg 1998;227:666-676.

Fabian TC, Richardson JD, Croce MA, et al: Prospective study of blunt aortic injury: Multicenter trial of the American Association for the Surgery of Trauma. J Trauma 1997;42:374-380.

Feczko JD, Lynch L, Pless JE, et al: An autopsy case review of 142 nonpenetrating (blunt) injuries of the aorta. J Trauma 1992;33:846-849.

Fenner MN, Fisher KS, Sergel NL, et al: Evaluation of possible traumatic aortic injury using aortography and CT, Am Surg 1990;56:497-499.

Finkelmeier BA, Mentzer RM, Kaiser DL, et al: Chronic traumatic thoracic aneurysm. Influence of operative treatment on natural history: An analysis of reported cases, 1950-1980. J Thorac Cardiovasc Surg 1982;84:257-266.

Fisher RG, Oria RA, Mattox KL, et al: Conservative management of aortic lacerations due to blunt trauma. J Trauma 1990;30:1562-1566.

Forbes AD, Asbaugh DG: Mechanical circulatory support during repair of thoracic aortic injuries improves morbidity and prevents spinal cord injury. Arch Surg 1994;129:494-497.

Gavant JL, Flick P, Menke P, et al: CT aortography of thoracic aortic rupture. AJR Am J Roentgenol 1996;166:955-961.

Gavant ML, Menke PG, Fabian T, et al: Blunt traumatic aortic rupture: Detection with helical CT of the chest. Radiology 1995;197:125-133.

Hajarizadeh H, Rohrer MJ, Cutler BS: Surgical exposure of the left subclavian artery by median sternotomy and left supraclavicular extension. J Trauma 1996;41:136-139.

Hilgenberg AD, Logan DL, Akins CW, et al: Blunt injuries of the thoracic aorta. Ann Thorac Surg 1992;53:233-239.

Hoff SJ, Reilly MK, Merrill WH, et al: Analysis of blunt and penetrating injury of the innominate and subclavian arteries. Am Surg 1994;60:151-154.

Hunick MGM, Bos JJ: Triage of patients to angiography for detection of aortic rupture after blunt chest trauma: Cost-effectiveness analysis of using CT. AJR Am J Roentgenol 1995;165:27-36.

Hunt JP, Baker CC, Lentz CW, et al: Thoracic aorta injuries: Management and outcome of 144 patients. J Trauma 1996;40:547-556.

Johansen K, Sangeorzan B, Copass MK: Traumatic scapulothoracic dissociation: Case report. J Trauma 1991;31:147-149.

Johnston RH, Wall MJ, Mattox KL: Innominate artery trauma: A thirty-year experience. J Vasc Surg 1993;17:134-140.

Katyal D, McLellan BA, Brenneman FD, et al: Lateral impact motor vehicle collisions: Significant cause of blunt traumatic rupture of the thoracic aorta. J Trauma 1997;42:769-772.

Kearney PA, Smith DW, Johnson SB, et al: Use of transesophageal echocardiography in the evaluation of traumatic aortic injury. J Trauma 1993; 34:696-701.

Kieny R, Charpentier A: Traumatic lesions of the thoracic aorta: A report of 73 cases. J Cardiovasc Surg 1991;32:613-619.

Kram HB, Wohlmuth DA, Appel PL, et al: Clinical and radiographic indications for aortography in blunt chest trauma. J Vasc Surg 1987;6:168-176.

Kudsk KA, Bongard F, Lim RC: Determinants of survival after vena caval injury: Analysis of a 14-year experience. Arch Surg 1984;119:1009-1012.

Madayag MA, Kirshenbaum KJ, Nadimpalli SR, et al: Thoracic aortic trauma: Role of dynamic CT. Radiology 1991;179:853-855.

Mattox KL: Symposium: New approach in vascular trauma. J Vasc Surg 1988;7:725-729.

Mattox KL, Feliciano DV, Burch J, et al: Five thousand seven hundred sixty cardiovascular injuries in 4459 patients: Epidemiologic evolution 1958 to 1987. Ann Surg 1989;209:698-707.

Mattox KL, Holzman M, Pickard LR, et al: Clamp/repair: A safe technique for treatment of blunt injury to the descending thoracic aorta. Ann Thorac Surg 1985;40:456-463.

McCroskey BL, Moore EE, Moore FA, et al: A unified approach to the torn thoracic aorta. Am J Surg 1991;162:473-476.

Minard G, Schurr MJ, Croce MA, et al: A prospective analysis of transesophageal echocardiography in the diagnosis of traumatic disruption of the aorta. J Trauma 1996;40:225-230.

Mirvis SE, Pais So, Gens DR: Thoracic aortic rupture: Advantages of intraarterial digital subtraction angiography. AJR Am J Roentgenol 1986; 146:987-991.

Mirvis SE, Shanmuganathan K, Buell J, et al: Use of spiral computed tomography for the assess-ment of blunt trauma patients with potential aortic injury. J Trauma 1998;45:922-930.

Mirvis SE, Shanmuganathan K, Miller BH, et al: Traumatic aortic injury: Diagnosis with contrast-enhanced thoracic CT. Five-year experience at a major trauma center. Radiology 1996;200:413-422.

Morgan PW, Goodman LR, Aprahamian C, et al: Evaluation of traumatic aortic injury: Does dynamic contrast-enhanced CT play a role? Radiology 1992;182:661-666.

Myers SI, Harward TRS, Cagle L: Isolated subclavian artery dissection after blunt trauma. Surgery 1991;109:336-338.

Nagy K, Fabian T, Rodman G, et al: Guidelines for the Diagnosis and Management of Blunt Aortic Injury. Eastern Association for the Surgery of Trauma: Available at http://www.east.org. 2000.

Omert L, Rodriguez A, Simon B, et al: Blunt vascular torso trauma: A review of 310 cases. Panam J Trauma 1991;2:102-111.

Parmley LF, Mattingly TW, Manion WC, et al: Non-penetrating traumatic injury of the aorta. Circulation 1958;17:1086-1101.

Pate JW, Fabian TC, Walker W: Traumatic rupture of the aortic isthmus: An emergency? World J Surg 1995;19:119-126.

Pate JW, Gavant ML, Weiman DS, et al: Traumatic rupture of the aortic isthmus: Program of selective management. World J Surg 1999;23:59-63.

Pre'tre R, Chilcott M, Murith N, et al: Blunt injury to the supra-aortic vessels. Br J Surg 1997;84:603-609.

Ramadan F, Rutledge R, Oller D, et al: Carotid artery trauma: A review of contemporary trauma center experiences. J Vasc Surg 1995;21:46-56.

Raptopoulos V: Chest CT for aortic injury: Maybe not for everyone. AJR Am J Roentgenol 1994; 162:1053-1055.

Razzouk AJ, Gundry SR, Wang N, et al: Repair of traumatic aortic rupture: A 25-year experience. Arch Surg 2000;135:913-918.

Read RA, Moore EE, Moore FA, et al: Partial left heart bypass for thoracic aorta repair: Survival without paraplegia. Arch Surg 1993;128:746-752.

Richardson P, Mirvis SE, Scorpio R, et al: Value of CT in determining the need for angiography when findings of mediastinal hemorrhage on chest radiographs are equivocal. AJR Am J Roentgenol 1991;156:273-279.

Richardson JD, Smith JM III, Grover FL: Management of subclavian and innominate artery disruption due to blunt trauma. Am J Surg 1977;134:780.

Richardson JD, Wilson ME, Miller FB: The widened mediastinum: Diagnostic and therapeutic priorities. Ann Surg 1990;211:731-737.

Rodriguez A, Elliott D: Blunt traumatic rupture of the thoracic aorta. In Maull et al. (eds): Advances in Trauma and Critical Care. St. Louis, Mosby, 1993;8:145-181.

Rousseau H, Soula P, Perreault P, et al: Delayed treatment of traumatic rupture of the thoracic aorta with endoluminal covered stent. Circulation 1999;99:498-504.

Saletta S, Lederman E, Fein S, et al: Transesophageal echocardiography for the initial evaluation of the widened mediastinum in trauma patients. J Trauma 1995;39:137-142.

Schmidt CA, Smith DC: Traumatic avulsion of arch vessels in a child: Primary repair using hypothermic circulatory arrest (case report). J Trauma 1989;29:248-250.

Schmidt CA, Wood MN, Razzouk AJ, et al: Primary repair of traumatic aortic rupture: A preferred approach. J Trauma 1992;32:588-592.

Sharma S, Reddy V, Ott G, et al: Surgical management of traumatic aortic disruption. Am J Surg 1997;173:416-418.

Smith MD, Cassidy JM, Souther S, et al: Transesophageal echocardiography in the diagnosis of traumatic rupture of the aorta. New Engl J Med 1995;332(6):356-362.

Sweeney MS, Young DJ, Frazier OH, et al: Traumatic aortic transections: Eight-year experience with the "Clamp-Sew" technique. Ann Thorac Surg 1997;64:384-389.

Szwerc MG, Benckart DH, Lin JC, et al: Recent clinical experience with left heart bypass using a centrifugal pump for repair of traumatic aortic transection. Ann Surg 1999;230:484-492.

Townsend RN, Colella JJ, Diamond DL: Traumatic rupture of the aorta critical decisions for trauma surgeons. J Trauma 1990;30:1169-1174.

Turney SZ, Rodriguez A: Injuries to the great thoracic vessels. In Turney SZ, Rodriguez A, Cowley RA (eds): Management of Cardiothoracic Trauma. Baltimore, Williams & Wilkins, 1990: 229-260.

Vignon P, Gueret P, Vedrinne JM, et al: Role of transesophageal echocardiography in the diagnosis and management of traumatic aortic disruption. Circulation 1995;92:2959-2968.

Von Oppell UO, Dunne TT, De Groot KM, et al: Spinal cord protection in the absence of collateral circulation: Metaanalysis of mortality and paraplegia. J Card Surg 1994;9:685-691.

Wahl WL, Michaels AJ, Wang SC, et al: Blunt thoracic aortic injury: Delayed or early repair? J Trauma 1999;47:254-259.

Walls JT, Boley TM, Curtis JJ et al: Experience with four surgical techniques to repair traumatic aortic pseudoaneurysm. J Thorac Cardiovasc Surg 1993;106:283-287.

Weiman DS, McCoy DW, Haan CK, et al: Blunt injuries of the brachiocephalic artery. Am Surg 1998;64:383-387.

Williams JS, Graff JA, Uku JM, et al: Aortic injury in vehicular trauma. Ann Thorac Surg 1994; 57:726-730.

Woodring JH, Dillon ML: Radiographic manifestations of mediastinal hemorrhage from blunt chest trauma. Ann Thorac Surg 1984;37:171-178.

Zeiger MA, Clark DE, Morton JR: Reappraisal of surgical treatment of traumatic transection of the thoracic aorta. J Cardiovasc Surg 1990;31:607-610.

15

Wounds of the Heart

MATTHEW J. WALL, JR.
DAVID RICE
ERNESTO SOLTERO

HISTORY

The heart has always been regarded as the sustainer of life, and its wounds have been approached through the ages with awe and apprehension. Homer provided antique literature with many references to heart wounds. Their fatality was clear.

285

The insulting victor with disdain bestrode
The prostrate prince and on his bosom trod;
Then drew the weapon from his panting heart,
The reeking fibers clinging to the dart;
From the wide wound gushed out a stream of
*   blood*
And the soul issues in the purple flood.
*   Beall, Gasior, and Brickeret (1971)*

Attempts to treat wounds of the heart have been recorded as early as the first century AD, when Galen described therapy based on anatomic and experimental study through surgery of the pericardium. Ambroise Paré tried to dispel the general belief that cardiac injuries were usually fatal in his sixteenth century reports. Yet even in 1709, Boerhaave wrote that all heart wounds resulted in death.

Larrey is often credited with the first successful decompression of the pericardium in 1810 during the Napoleon wars, but it is only in the last 100 years that treatment of heart wounds has been repeatedly beneficial to the patient. Until 1896, pericardiocentesis, either alone or combined with phlebotomy, was the only method of surgical treatment for heart wounds. Those treated were usually small penetrating wounds of the pericardium. In 1896, however, Cappelen attempted to repair a heart by suturing a myocardial laceration. Although this operation failed, in the same year Rehn, in Frankfurt, was successful in relieving a cardiac tamponade and in suturing a knife wound of the heart. Rehn's accomplishment is generally regarded as the first actual repair of a heart wound, although in 1908, Matas reported that Farina had performed a similar operation, also in 1896. On September 14, 1902, Dr. Hill of Montgomery, Alabama, became the first American physician to successfully repair a cardiac injury.

Thus it is interesting that H.M. Sherman in 1902 noted, "The road to the heart is only 2 to 3 cm in a direct line, but it has taken surgery nearly 2400 years to travel it," Considerable controversy continued regarding the best approach in managing penetrating cardiac trauma. In 1943, Blalock and Ravitch still advocated pericardiocentesis as a form of definitive treatment for cardiac tamponade secondary to penetrating wounds of the heart.

While originally recommending pericardiocentesis, Beall, in 1961, advocated aggressive use of thoracotomy and direct repair even in the emergency center (EC). Currently, this is the most common approach, with pericardiocentesis being used only rarely for temporary decompression of cardiac tamponade, if indicated, before direct cardiac repair.

INCIDENCE

In 1908, Matas noted that there had been 160 reported cases of heart wounds after the operations of 1896. Recent reports show an increasing incidence of recognized cardiac trauma. The greater number of gunshot wounds in many urban centers is associated with the rise in cases of penetrating heart wounds, and true blunt cardiac trauma is associated with high-speed transportation.

Parmley, Mattingly, and Manion (1958) evaluated 456 postmortem cases of penetrating wounds of the heart and aorta but stressed that the true incidence of cardiac trauma had not been established. Assessing numbers is complicated by the high early mortality rate of patients with these injuries. Isaacs (1959) reported, for instance, that from 1937 to 1959, more than 50% of the 133 patients were dead on arrival at Johns Hopkins Hospital. Only 86 of the 459 patients analyzed by Sugg (1968) arrived alive in the EC of Parkland Hospital in Dallas.

Other reports of note were those of Griswold and Drye (1954), who found 108 cardiac wounds at Louisville General Hospital in 20 years (1933 to 1953); Naclerio (1964), who recorded 249 penetrating wounds in 13 years (1950 to 1963); Wilson and Bassett (1966), who saw 200 patients and 205 wounds in 16.5 years (1949 to 1965); and Beall and colleagues (1972) who had 269 patients with penetrating cardiac injuries in Houston within 20 years (1951 to 1971). Similarly, in Atlanta, Symbas, Harlaftis, and Waldo (1976) treated 102 patients with penetrating cardiac heart wounds, between 1964 and 1974. In 1997, Wall and Mattox reported 711 heart injuries over a 30-year period in Houston, of which 60 were complex.

The true incidence of cardiac trauma in the military experience is difficult to ascertain. On the battlefield, many cardiac wounds are immediately fatal. This is emphasized by one of the typical case reports from World War I. Dixon and McEwan (1916) reported one wounded heart in a series of 123 wounds of the thorax. These authors proclaimed, "probably nearly all cardiac wounds produced death from hemorrhage too quickly to allow the patients being removed alive even to a short distance from the battlefield." Interest in wounds of the heart increased greatly during World War II. Harken (1946) reported a unique experience in removing foreign bodies from the heart and adjacent major vessels in 134 patients.

There was one major report of injuries to the heart during the Korean conflict. Valle (1955) reported an incidence of 4.2% of injuries to the heart and mediastinum: 117 injuries in a group of 2811 chest casualties treated at Tokyo Army Hospital from August 1950 to March 1953. In this group, however, there were only 19 cases of foreign bodies in the heart and 42 pericardial effusions. The remainder of the injuries were to the mediastinum and structures adjacent to the heart.

Cardiac trauma during the Vietnam War has not been completely documented. Gielchinsky and McNamara (1970) reported 10 heart injuries at the 24th Evacuation Hospital, an incidence of 2.8%. The records of nearly 120 patients with cardiac wounds in Vietnam are included in the long-term follow-up effort in the Vietnam Vascular Registry. Specifically, details of 96 cardiac injuries were evaluated by Geer and Rich (1972). Most of these injuries occurred between 1968 and 1970. At least 21 different surgical facilities participated in the care of patients with cardiac injuries (Table 15–1).

CLINICAL PATHOLOGY

Penetrating wounds of the pericardium and/or the myocardium caused by sharp instruments or low-velocity missiles are the most frequent types of injuries reported. Recent reports emphasize the vulnerability of the right

TABLE 15–1
ETIOLOGY OF CARDIAC TRAUMA IN VIETNAM

Wounding Agent	No. of Patients	%	Deaths
Fragment	71	74.0	7
Gunshot	11	11.5	1
Fléchette	3	3.1	0
Stab	3	3.1	0
Unknown	8	8.3	2
Total	96	100	10

From T.M. Geer and N.M. Rich, Vietnam Vascular Registry, unpublished data, 1972.

ventricle because of its anterior location. Our service found that the site of injury among patients with penetrating wounds of the pericardium was the right ventricle in 40% of patients, the left ventricle in 40% of patients, the right atrium in 24%, and the left atrium in 3% (multiple injuries included) (Fig. 15–1).

The World War II combat experience as described by Samson (1948) varies somewhat in that the left ventricle was involved more often than the right ventricle. This is the exception, however, because the location of cardiac wounds in the Vietnam experience again emphasizes the predominance of wounds of the right ventricle (Table 15–2). As alluded to earlier, most of these wounds are penetrating wounds.

True blunt cardiac trauma usually results in diffuse contusion of the myocardium. However, the extent of cardiac injuries secondary to blunt trauma to the chest may range

TABLE 15–2
CARDIAC TRAUMA IN VIETNAM: LOCATION OF WOUNDS

Site	No.	%
Right ventricle	40	44.9
Left ventricle	22	24.7
Right atrium	7	7.9
Left atrium	5	5.6
Unknown	15	16.9
Total	89	100

From T.M. Geer and N.M. Rich, Vietnam Vascular Registry, unpublished data, 1972.

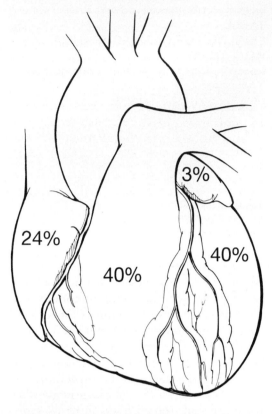

© Baylor College of Medicine 1997

■ **FIGURE 15–1**
Distribution of injuries to the four chambers of
the heart (multiple injuries included). The
posterior nature of the relatively protected left
atrium probably accounts for its low incidence
of injury. ■

from minor subepicardial or subendocardial
hemorrhage to actual rupture of the
myocardium. When there is sufficient force
involved in a nonpenetrating injury to cause
actual cardiac laceration, a fatal outcome frequently occurs. Patients who have had blunt
trauma to the chest with cardiac trauma of
varying degrees may have electrocardiographic changes, dysrhythmias, cardiac failure,
cardiac tamponade, or hemothorax. Cardiac
injuries from blunt trauma to the chest wall
may or may not be associated with rib fractures or obvious chest wall deformity. When
Parmley and colleagues (1958) reviewed 546
autopsies in patients who had nonpenetrating traumatic cardiac injuries, they found that
353 of the 546 patients died of rupture of the

heart. Of these 353 patients, 106 had multiple chamber ruptures.

In addition to the injuries of the myocardial surface, other more unusual types of
injuries can be seen to the valves, the interventricular or interatrial septum, the coronary
vessels, and the conduction system of the
heart. Representative case reports of these
unusual injuries include the removal of a wire
lodged in the interventricular septum by
Kleinsasser (1961); two patients with penetrating wounds of cardiac valves, one with
mitral insufficiency and the other with tricuspid insufficiency (Pate and Richardson,
1969); three patients with intracardiac lesions
including an aortic right ventricular fistula
(Hardy and Timmis, 1969); and coronary arterial injuries (Tector and colleagues, 1973).
Patients have developed left ventricular
aneurysms after penetrating wounds, as
reported in the civilian experience by Kakos
and colleagues (1971) and in the military
experience by Aronstam and colleagues
(1970). There have been, in addition, more
recent series by Demetriades (1990),
Thandroyen (1981), and Wall (1997). In the
later, 60 patients had complex heart wounds
out of a total of 711 into the hemothorax.

Associated pathology frequently accompanies cardiac wounds. This is emphasized by
the report of Ricks and colleagues, who found
that concomitant organ injury was associated
with a striking rise in the mortality from 12%
when there was injury of one associated organ
to 69% with two or more associated organ
injuries in their 31 patients with gunshot
wounds of the heart. All but 1 of the 31 patients
had one or both lungs injured together with
the associated cardiac wound. Sugg and colleagues found that 30 survivors of penetrating heart wounds had no associated injuries.
However, 33 patients who survived penetrating wounds of the heart had a total of 84 associated injuries.

PATHOPHYSIOLOGY

Injuries to the heart can be divided into
simple and complex. Simple injuries to the
myocardium that result in bleeding from

an injured chamber can present two ways. If the injury through the pericardium is so small that the bleeding is contained, tamponade physiology results. The pericardium does not distend acutely and can prevent the passive filling of the heart. Thus the patient essentially has an empty beating heart. If the injury through the pericardium is large, the patient may exsanguinate either externally or into the hemithorax. How much blood is in the left pleural cavity is often helpful to note during an empiric exploration for cardiac injury because the approach may be altered based on whether exsanguination or tamponade physiology is present. Most cardiac injuries are simple lacerations and can be managed with direct repair. However, complex cardiac injuries that involve the coronary arteries, cardiac valves, subvalvular apparatus, or the cardiac septum, though rare, present a different challenge. Injuries to the coronary arteries can result in an area of ischemic myocardium. Treatment options are based on the distribution and amount of ischemic myocardium at risk. Injuries to the atrioventricular valves often result in regurgitation, which is commonly diagnosed postoperatively when a new murmur is noticed. Significant injury to the aortic valve is not well tolerated in the acutely hypotensive patient, and most of these patients die before arrival at the hospital, so they are rarely seen. Cardiac septal injuries from penetrating trauma often initially are small and diagnosed postoperatively as a new murmur. Thus the common scenario is that many of the valvular and septal injuries are detected postoperatively after the acutely bleeding cardiac injury is controlled and are repaired subacutely at a later operation.

PREHOSPITAL MANAGEMENT

These patients most commonly present with a pattern of injury of penetrating trauma with proximity to the heart with either hypovolemia or tamponade physiology. Early consideration of the possibility of a cardiac injury with appropriate transport to a center that can manage it may be lifesaving. If the patient has a sys-

tolic blood pressure more than 80 mm Hg and is awake, ancillary measures to artificially elevate the blood pressure may not be helpful. Thus time should not be wasted on large-volume crystalloid resuscitation or the placement of pneumatic antishock trousers. In a patient in extremis, endotracheal intubation to control ventilation and maximally oxygenate the remaining circulating blood may be one of the few efficacious prehospital maneuvers.

EMERGENCY CENTER

The diagnosis of a cardiac injury in the EC is based on a high index of suspicion. A penetrating injury in the area of the middle third of the chest between the nipples laterally and from the xiphoid to the sternal notch vertically is a common presentation. The patients often present in extremis and the cardiac injury is diagnosed on empiric exploration during EC thoracotomy. Low-energy mechanisms such as stab wounds can be problematic because tamponade physiology may not immediately develop. Awake patients usually have a profound anxiety. There are also reports of tamponade manifesting 2 to 3 days after the injury. Muffled heart sounds, distended neck veins, and hypotension are classically described. However, distended neck veins and an elevated central venous pressure are common in the anxious patient, and muffled heart sounds are difficult to detect in the noisy EC. Few diagnostic studies are usually needed and only delay transfer to the operating room for definitive therapy. The problematic patients are the ones who present hemodynamically stable with no signs of tamponade that are being investigated for proximity. These patients most benefit from monitoring and further investigation.

Chest radiographs are commonly obtained. This is often unhelpful for the diagnosis of cardiac injury because these patients usually have a normal mediastinum. Their primary efficacy is to detect a pneumothorax or hemothorax. Wound clips marking entrance and exit wounds can be helpful, although missiles often do not follow straight lines between these clips. Unexplained missile trajectories can be problematic and may represent either a missile bouncing off bony structures or an intravascular missile that has embolized.

One diagnostic procedure that has had a significant impact on the diagnosis of cardiac injury has been ultrasound in the EC by the surgical team. Blood around the heart may be readily seen and diagnosed before the hemodynamic affects of tamponade. In skilled hands and the appropriate body habitus, the use of ultrasound has probably superseded other diagnostic entities such as central venous pressure monitoring and subxiphoid pericardial window. Formal echocardiography (either transthoracic or transesophageal) has little use in the hypotensive patient and only delays therapy. Their primary use may be as a second study or as a follow-up study after operative repair of a cardiac injury to document wall motion, septal integrity, and valvular function.

EMERGENCY CENTER PROCEDURES

A patient with a penetrating wound to the chest often requires a tube thoracostomy for a concomitant hemothorax or pneumothorax. In the hypotensive patient with a suspected cardiac wound, an empiric tube thoracostomy may be used to rule out a tension pneumothorax, which can present in a similar manner. Chest tubes should be placed no lower than the nipple level (to avoid the diaphragm) in the midaxillary line directing the tube posteriorly. After developing a tunnel and dividing intercostal muscles, the pleural space should be entered bluntly with the finger to avoid injuring the lung or the heart. During tube thoracostomy, the lung, diaphragm, and pericardium should be palpated. This is often referred to as a digital thoracotomy. Before the wide use of ultrasound, balloting the pericardium could be used to detect a tamponade and provide an indication for operation. In a patient with suspected stab wounds to the heart, the tube thoracostomy incision is often placed slightly more anterior so the apex of the heart can

be more readily palpated. Balloting the heart to detect tamponade is a subtle maneuver and should be done during each tube thoracostomy.

Pericardiocentesis is often recommended in some resuscitation courses to temporize tamponade. Unfortunately, it is an unreliable procedure that often results in significant iatrogenic injuries. Even when a catheter is successfully placed, the clotted blood is unreliably removed and may result in a false sense of security. Thus with the availability of ultrasound, the use of pericardiocentesis as a diagnostic maneuver has practically disappeared. At best, it may be a temporizing maneuver en route to the operating room.

EC thoracotomy is one of the original damage control procedures in surgery. Many patients with cardiac injuries are often premorbid on arrival and will not survive the trip to the operating room. Using EC thoracotomy to bring techniques of definitive care to the EC has resulted in survivors. The primary thrust of EC thoracotomy for cardiac injuries is accessing the heart, relieving the tamponade, and controlling bleeding. Once this is accomplished, the patient can be moved to the operating room for completion of the procedure.

The EC thoracotomy is performed with the patient supine after abducting the left arm. The incision is made immediately below the nipple in the male patient or beneath the breast tracking up to the fourth intercostal space in the female patient. The incision is made from the sternum to the posterior axillary line following the rib. Intercostal muscles are divided entering the chest in one area and the intercostal incision extended with the scissors. The rib retractor is placed with the rack toward the table and the retractor widely opened. The pleural cavity is inspected for the amount of blood to determine exsanguination versus tamponade and the pericardium inspected. If tamponade is present and the heart is still beating, the pericardium is grasped between clamps anterior to the phrenic nerve and the pericardium is opened with the scissors. This is extended superiorly and inferiorly evacuating the clot and may result in a return of cardiac output. The heart is brought into the left side of the chest and inspected for injuries. For injuries to the right side of the heart, the incision may need to be extended across the chest with a Gigli saw, Lebsche knife, or sternal saw. If relief of tamponade does not result in return of perfusion, the aorta is cross clamped with an aortic clamp just distal to the left subclavian artery, being careful to avoid the esophagus.

Immediate control of the injury is obtained with the surgeon's finger. A 4-0 polypropylene suture on a large needle is then used to rapidly close the laceration in a gentle running fashion. The suture may be tied by an assistant while the surgeon continues to hold the heart. Because the incidence of needle stick during EC cardiorrhaphy approaches more than 30%, the skin stapler has often been used to achieve rapid vascular control and minimize the incidence of injury to the surgical team (Fig. 15–2). After repair, warm saline is poured on the heart and the patient is rapidly transferred to the operating room for definitive repair. Pitfalls during the EC thoracotomy involve taking too long to perform it, not making a large enough incision initially, injuring the heart and lung while opening the chest, and injuring segmental vessels or the esophagus during aortic cross clamping. The outcomes of EC thoracotomy hinge on patient selection. A significant number of patients who have signs of life after an isolated stab wound to the heart can be salvaged. Recent data by Moore suggest that if a sustainable blood pressure is not obtained in the EC, further efforts in the operating room may be futile.

OPERATIVE MANAGEMENT OF CARDIAC INJURIES

Incisions

For abdominal trauma, the midline laparotomy offers almost universal exposure. However, there are multiple incisions that can be made to manage chest trauma. The two most common incisions employed to manage cardiac injuries are left anterolateral thoracotomy with possible extension across the sternum or median sternotomy. Each incision has advantages and disadvantages. The

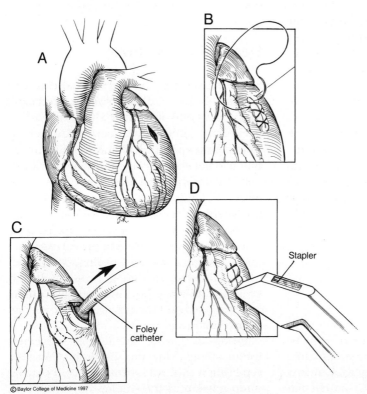

© Baylor College of Medicine 1997

■ **FIGURE 15–2**
Acute management of cardiac injuries. *A,* Laceration of the left ventricle. *B,* Continuous fine polypropylene suture placed for both repair and hemostasis. *C,* A Foley balloon catheter can be useful to achieve hemostasis in the beating heart before placement of sutures. *D,* Because of the high incidence of needle stick during cardiorrhaphy, the skin stapler may be useful acutely in the emergency center for initial control. ■

median sternotomy, the standard elective cardiac incision, is a midline incision that is relatively bloodless. Though easy to perform, it has the disadvantage of being difficult to clamp the aorta for resuscitation. In addition, efforts to retract the heart to repair a posterior injury may result in intractable ventricular fibrillation in the cold, irritable injured heart. In many centers the left anterolateral thoracotomy is the incision of choice for cardiac trauma. It is easily made with a minimal number of instruments and offers excellent exposure of the heart and descending thoracic aorta. In most cases the patient is positioned supine with the arms out so they are available to the anesthesia service. For right-sided injuries, a transsternal extension into the opposite chest is helpful. Left anterolateral thoracotomy has the additional advantage in that injuries to the posterior heart can be more readily visualized from this viewpoint with less retraction and manipulation.

Aortic Occlusion

Occlusion of the descending thoracic aorta may be helpful as a resuscitative maneuver. The aorta is cross clamped just distal to the left subclavian origin, being careful to avoid injury to the esophagus. It is useful to dissect anterior and posterior to the aorta and actually encircle it with a finger before applying the clamp to ensure accurate positioning. This ensures that blood is preferentially diverted to the brain and heart. As the patient is resuscitated, the aortic cross clamp can be gradually weaned and removed. It is extremely common after hemorrhage is controlled for patients to be over-resuscitated and the heart may become distended. One technique to decompress the heart is to remove the aortic cross clamp and vent the heart into the systemic circulation momentarily.

Cardiac Manipulation

The cold, empty injured heart can be extremely irritable. Even minor manipulation can cause significant dysrhythmias. Unfortunately, in the cold patient, ventricular fibrillation is often refractory. Thus all manipulations of the heart should be gentle and retraction minimized.

It has been learned from elective cardiac surgery that significant retraction of the heart can be performed if done slowly and in such a manner that the heart can fill. Because the filling of the heart is passive, it is important not to compress the cardiac chambers as it is retracted. Gentle manipulation with a dragging motion can often allow one to completely invert the heart out of the chest and still maintain cardiac output while allowing access to the posterior aspect of the left atrium. If the heart is not beating in an organized rhythm, manual cardiac compression may be required. This is best performed with a two-handed technique gently alternating between allowing the heart to fill and compressing it from apex to base. Cardiac compressions often are performed with one hand by some doctors. Unfortunately, the distended right ventricle can be extremely thin walled and may be injured by the thumb or fingers. In the bradycardic heart, manual compression may serve to prevent it from becoming distended by manually emptying the chambers. Sutured temporary epicardial leads can be helpful also.

Hemorrhage Control

Some injuries may be extremely difficult to manage because of massive hemorrhage. These may often be managed by cardiac inflow occlusion to empty the heart before repair. The superior and inferior vena cava can be pinched between the fingers or clamped with vascular clamps and the heart allowed to empty. The injury can then be visualized and the repair performed. If after a left-sided injury is repaired there is concern about intracardiac air, the patient should be placed in a head-down position and the ascending aorta vented while a cardiac rhythm is restored. Inflow occlusion allows a short interval of an empty beating heart and the repair must be accomplished before its arrest.

Inflow occlusion can also be extremely useful in repairing the distending heart or repairing a thin soft aorta. To avoid placing undo tension as the stitches are tied down, inflow occlusion can be accomplished to temporarily decrease the blood pressure while tying down the repair.

The right atrium is a commonly injured cardiac structure. Upon diagnosis of a right atrial injury, it is helpful to extend the incision across the sternum for better visualization. Initially, the injury is controlled with the finger. Other adjuncts that may be useful are a partial occluding clamp or a Foley catheter placed through the injury for temporary control (Fig. 15–2). A 4-0 polypropylene or 5-0 polypropylene suture is then used in a simple continuous manner to close the injury and effect repair. The repair of atrial injuries close to the superior vena cava–right atrial appendage junction may involve the sinoatrial node and result in dysrhythmias.

Injuries to the left atrium can be difficult to manage. The heart is gently and slowly retracted while avoiding compression and permitting passive filling of the heart. All instruments and sutures should be prepared before retracting the heart, and sutures can often be placed in a back-hand manner. It may be helpful for the surgeon to retract with one hand and sew with the other so the cardiac performance can be monitored and the heart returned to the chest before arrest. It may take multiple episodes of suturing to close these injuries. As described earlier, inflow occlusion can decrease bleeding through a posterior injury so it can be more readily visualized. Repairs in the empty heart should raise the surgeon's suspicion of intracardiac air, and the patient can be placed head down and the aorta vented before restitution of inflow.

Whereas the left ventricle is a thick muscular structure, the anterior wall of the right ventricle is only approximately 5 mm thick. Repair of the right ventricle can be initially managed with digital pressure, followed by repair with a fine suture. Pledgeted sutures are not routinely needed though may be used if the repair fails or the heart distends. Avoiding over-resuscitation and inflow occlusion may be helpful adjuncts in these repairs. Injuries to the left ventricle are performed in a similar manner, although these are often on the posterior surface and require some measure of retraction. If possible, the ventricle should be carefully inspected to identify injury to adjacent coronary arteries. It should be remembered that the heart is a relatively soft muscle and a gentle technique with a fine suture often gets better results. Again, initial control with a finger or a Foley balloon catheter to arrest hemorrhage is often helpful. With no intravenous access available, the Foley catheter can be connected to an intravenous catheter for direct infusion. It is our preference not to aggressively resuscitate the heart before repair because the empty bradycardic heart is ideal for the placement of sutures. Overzealous crystalloid resuscitation results in an overdistended heart that not only fails to hold stitches but also fails to beat well after repair. Administration of pressor drugs before repair results in a rapidly beating empty heart that is extremely difficult to sew. Multiple injuries and complex lacerations portend a poorer prognosis.

Complex Injuries

Anterior stab wounds often occur immediately adjacent to the left anterior descending coronary artery. If the coronary artery is uninjured, it is important to repair the laceration without compromising the coronary artery. Deep mattress sutures beneath the coronary artery will permit repair while avoiding the coronary artery. When a coronary artery is injured, decision making is guided by its location and the amount of myocardium at risk. Small secondary branches of the coronary arteries can usually be ligated. The patient can then be observed for dysrhythmias or the development of an akinetic area of the heart. If there is any concern, many will place a horizontal mattress suture and use a snare tourniquet and observe the heart before tying the suture down. If a significant area of the heart becomes akinetic and fails, then coronary artery bypass may be indicated. If a small area of the heart becomes akinetic and cardiac function is borderline after ligation, the placement of an intra-aortic balloon pump may temporize the injury and the patient may be treated similar to those having had a small myocardial infarction. Though uncommon, most coronary artery injuries that require emergent bypass are proximal injuries of the

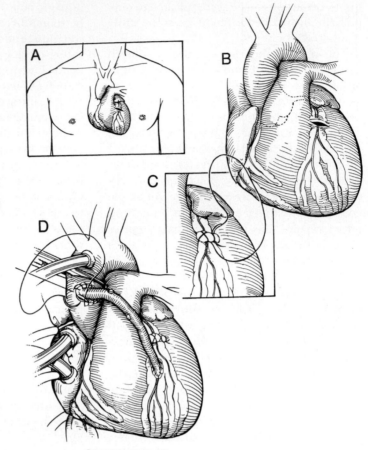

■ **FIGURE 15–3**
Coronary artery bypass grafting for injury involving the left anterior descending coronary artery. *A,* Anterior stab wound to the chest. *B,* Injury involves the proximal left anterior descending coronary artery, resulting in a large area of ischemic myocardium. *C,* Hemostasis is initially obtained with continuous suture of the laceration. *D,* Coronary artery bypass from the ascending aorta to the distal left anterior ascending coronary artery using cardiopulmonary bypass. Fortunately, this is seldom needed in most patients. ■

© Baylor College of Medicine 1997

primary branches such as the left anterior descending or the right coronary artery (Fig. 15–3). Although off-pump methods would seem attractive, these patients often require cardiopulmonary bypass to support the failing heart. Because this is an emergent lifesaving activity, the saphenous vein is most commonly used as the conduit.

Cardiac Septal Injuries

The most common presentation for cardiac septal injuries is when a new murmur is noted postoperatively in the intensive care unit. Most patients who survive cardiac repair who have a septal injury often have small injuries that may not be hemodynamically significant. The diagnosis is confirmed with echocardiography. A saturation run during catheterization of the right side of the heart may be diagnostic and can be used to calculate shunt fraction. If indicated, most of these patients undergo cardiopulmonary bypass in a subacute fashion often weeks after the initial injury. A shunt fraction of more than 2:1 is often used as an indication for surgery. Smaller injuries with smaller shunt fractions may be observed. The patient however should be counseled about the risk of endocarditis if they undergo other invasive procedures.

These injuries are repaired using cardiopulmonary bypass usually via a median sternotomy. For anterior stab wounds resulting in ventricular septal defects, the injury may be repaired through the previous myocardial repair. Although ventriculotomy is avoided in elective cardiac surgery, this area is often scarred from the initial injury and offers excellent exposure of the septal injury (Fig. 15–4).

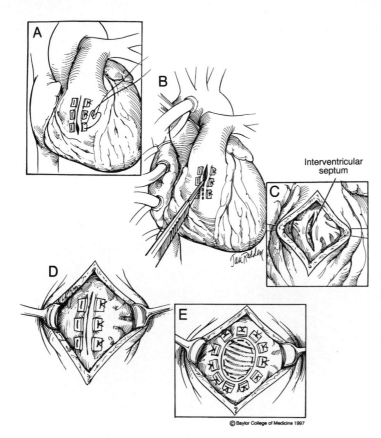

Interventricular
septum

© Baylor College of Medicine 1997

■ **FIGURE 15–4**
Repair of traumatic ventricular septal defect. *A,* The acute management of the injury to the surface of the heart is with either continuous or pledgeted sutures controlling the hemorrhage. Later in the intensive care unit, a murmur is detected and the ventricular septal defect is diagnosed. *B,* These injuries are most commonly repaired subacutely often weeks after the initial injury. Because of the scarring from the initial injury, ventriculotomy can be performed through the original scar. *C,* This results in good visualization of the septal wound. These can be repaired with either *(D)* interrupted pledgeted sutures or *(E)* larger defects closed with a Dacron patch. ■

Knowledge of the conduction system of the heart and counseling the patient preoperatively about the risk of conduction defects is helpful. Smaller defects can be closed primarily, but often the use of a prosthetic material such as Dacron may be required. Small ventricular septal defects located near the apex of the heart can be extremely difficult to localize and repair. Atrial septal defects can be approached via the standard incision in the right atrium. Again, knowledge of the path of the conduction system can help avoid iatrogenic injuries.

Cardiac Valvular Injury

Similar in presentation to septal injuries, most cardiac valvular injuries in survivors are detected as a new murmur postoperatively in the intensive care unit. They are usually injuries of the mitral or tricuspid valve and are evaluated with echocardiography. Trans-

esophageal echocardiography may be helpful to adequately visualize the subvalvular apparatus of the mitral valve. The injuries may involve the leaflets of the valve or the subvalvular apparatus. Although it is often hoped that a simple repair can be performed, upon exploration, the valve often is found to be totally destroyed and in need of being replaced. Replacement is performed via median sternotomy and the standard approach using cardiopulmonary bypass. Injury to the right-sided heart valves is not common. The indications for operation are the same as those for elective cases. Choice of technique and prosthesis depends on the pathology encountered at exploration.

Intrapericardial Inferior Vena Cava Injury

One injury that requires acute cardiopulmonary bypass is a posterior injury to the

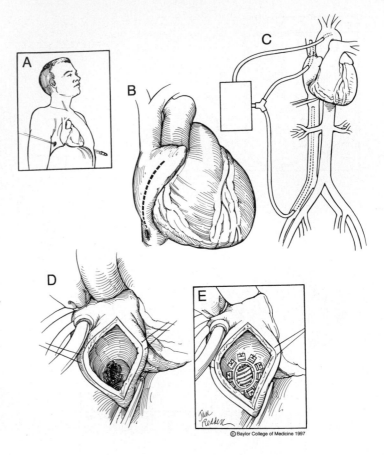

© Baylor College of Medicine 1997

■ **FIGURE 15–5**
Unusual injury of posterior intrapericardial inferior vena cava. *A,* These are often from transaxial gunshot wounds. *B,* The injury is extremely difficult to visualize and access. *C,* Cardiopulmonary bypass is instituted with cannulation of the superior vena cava directly and the inferior vena cava via the groin for venous drainage. *D,* Total cardiopulmonary bypass allows the right atrium to be opened and the injury repaired from within. *E,* Larger injuries may require the use of a Dacron or pericardial patch. ■

intrapericardial inferior vena cava. This area is extremely difficult to access, is a short vessel, and difficult to visualize posteriorly. One technique available to address it is to cannulate the groin for cardiopulmonary bypass and place a superior vena caval cannula for total cardiopulmonary bypass. The superior vena cava is snared around the cannula and the inferior vena cava is clamped immediately above the liver. The injury is accessed by opening the right atrium and repairing it from inside. Though extremely uncommon, this is one of the few areas in which cardiopulmonary bypass may assist in managing cardiac injuries acutely (Fig. 15–5).

SUMMARY

Injuries to the heart have fascinated trauma surgeons for ages. As with many other injuries,

a repair that was originally thought to be futile, with advances in technique, has resulted in significant salvage. Cardiac injuries can present as either tamponade or exsanguination and can be classified as either simple or complex. Simple injuries primarily involve the myocardium, and complex injuries involve the coronary arteries, cardiac septa, and cardiac valves. The EC thoracotomy is one of the original damage-control procedures and has resulted in a significant salvage rate for patients with low-energy penetrating injuries to the heart. Ultrasound has significantly aided in the diagnostic accuracy of patients who present hemodynamically stable. Cardiac injuries are managed in the operating room via left anterolateral thoracotomy with extension across the sternum. Cross clamping of the descending thoracic aorta could be a significant adjunct and various maneuvers such as digital compression, Foley catheter occlusion, stapling, and a partial occluding clamp may provide initial hemostasis. The avoidance of resuscitation until repair is complete, the avoidance of cyclic hyper-resuscitation and the avoidance of overdistention of the heart can result in improved outcomes. It is important to evaluate the patient postoperatively with physical examination and echocardiography to document wall motion and assess the patient for occult septal and valvular injuries. Most cardiac injuries can be managed by the trauma surgeon without any specialized cardiac technique. The need for cardiopulmonary bypass is extremely rare and is seen in fewer than 1% of these patients.

REFERENCES

Surgical approach and initial management of patients with cardiac injuries

Asensio JA, Stewart BM, Murray J, et al: Penetrating cardiac injuries. Surg Clin North Am 1996;76:685.

Beall AC Jr, Ochsner JL, Morris GC, et al: Penetrating wounds of the heart. J Trauma 1961;1:195.

Ivatury RR, Shah PM, Ito K, et al: Emergency room thoracotomy for the resuscitation of patients with "fatal" penetrating injuries of the heart. Ann Thorac Surg 1981;32:377.

Mattox KL, Beall AC, Jordan GL, et al: Cardiorrhaphy in the emergency center. J Thorac Cardiovasc Surg 1974;68:886.

Diagnosis and management of complex cardiac injuries to the coronary arteries, septa, and valves

Demetriades D, Charalambides C, Sareli P, Pantanowitz D: Late sequelae of penetrating cardiac injuries. Br J Surg 1990;77:813-814.

Fallahnejad M, Kutty ACK, Wallace HW: Secondary lesions of penetrating cardiac injuries: A frequent complication. Ann Surg 1980; 191:228-233.

Symbas PN, DiOrio DA, Tyras DH, et al: Penetrating cardiac wounds: Significant residual and delayed sequelae. J Thorac Cardiovasc Surg 1973;66:526-532.

Wall MJ, Mattox KL, Chen C-D, Baldwin JC: Acute management of complex cardiac injuries. J Trauma 1997;42(5):905-912.

Management of intracardiac injuries

Asfaw I, Thoms NW, Arbulu A: Interventricular septal defects from penetrating injuries of the heart: A report of 12 cases and review of the literature. J Thorac Cardiovasc Surg 1975;69:450-457.

Espada R, Whisennand HH, Mattox KL, Beall AC Jr: Surgical management of penetrating injuries to the coronary arteries. Surgery 1975;78:755-760.

Thandroyen FT, Matisonn RE: Penetrating thoracic trauma producing cardiac shunts. J Thorac Cardiovasc Surg 1981;81:569-573.

Whisennand HH, Van Pelt SA, Beall AC Jr, et al: Surgical management of traumatic intracardiac injuries. Ann Thorac Surg 1979;28:530-536.

Ventricular aneurysms after cardiac injury

Aronstam EM, Strader LD, Geiger JP, Gomez AC: Traumatic left ventricular aneurysms. J Thorac Cardiovasc Surg 1970;59:239-242.

Morales RA, Garcia F, Grover FL, Trinkle JK: Aneurysm of the left ventricle after repair of a penetrating injury. J Thorac Cardiovasc Surg 1973;66:632-635.

Injury to Abdominal Aorta and Visceral Arteries

DAVID V. FELICIANO

GENERAL

Incidence

The incidence of injuries to the abdominal aorta, celiac trunk or major branches, superior mesenteric artery, and renal artery is surprisingly high in urban trauma centers in the United States. This is a reflection of rapid transport by prehospital emergency medical services and the large number of patients who are treated for penetrating wounds, particularly those caused by low-velocity civilian handguns.

In one recently published review from the Grady Memorial Hospital in Atlanta, Georgia, 300 patients with 205 abdominal arterial and 284 abdominal venous injuries were treated at laparotomy during a 10-year period. Of interest, the mechanism of injury was a penetrating wound in 86.7% of patients, with abdominal gunshot wounds (78%) accounting for the majority. The group of patients with abdominal arterial injuries included 77 (37.5%) with injuries to the abdominal aorta, 18 (8.8%) with injuries to the renal artery, 16 (7.8%) with injuries to the superior mesenteric artery, and 16 with injuries to the celiac trunk or major branches. This group therefore accounted for 62% of all abdominal arterial injuries treated.

Another recently published review from the Los Angeles County Hospital described 302 patients with 238 abdominal arterial and 266 abdominal venous injuries that were treated at laparotomy during a 6-year period. Of interest, the mechanism of injury was a penetrating wound in 88% of patients, with abdominal gunshot wounds (81%) accounting for the majority. Patients with injuries to the aorta, celiac trunk or major branches, superior mesenteric artery, and renal artery accounted for 57% of all abdominal arterial injuries treated.

In contrast to the aforementioned reports, injuries to all abdominal vessels have been uncommon in reviews of military conflicts. This low incidence reflects the greater wounding power of high-velocity military weapons and the longer delays to definitive operation that occur in all war zones. In the report by DeBakey and Simeone of 2471 arterial injuries during World War II, only 49 (2%) occurred in the abdomen. In similar fashion, the report by Hughes of 304 arterial injuries from the Korean War included only 7 (2.3%) that occurred in the abdomen. Finally, the report by Rich and colleagues of 1000 arterial injuries treated in the Vietnam conflict described only 29 (2.9%) involving abdominal vessels.

Pathophysiology

Penetrating injuries to the abdominal aorta or visceral branches most commonly cause lateral wall defects with intraperitoneal bleeding or expanding pulsatile retroperitoneal or mesenteric hematomas. A less common injury is complete transection of a visceral artery with secondary bleeding, an expanding hematoma, or complete thrombosis of both ends of the vessel. On occasion, the track of a missile may be in proximity to a visceral vessel and cause a thrombosis because of disruption of the intima from a blast effect. The rarest injury related to a penetrating wound is the creation of an upper abdominal arteriovenous fistula involving the hepatic artery and portal vein, the superior mesenteric vessels, or the renal vessels.

Blunt injuries to the abdominal aorta or visceral branches are most commonly caused by deceleration, a direct anterior crushing mechanism (lap-type seatbelt), or a posterior blow to the spine. Deceleration or direct anterior blows have most commonly caused either thrombosis of the infrarenal abdominal aorta, superior mesenteric artery, or renal artery or lateral wall defects in the superior mesenteric artery at the base of the mesentery. Posterior blows to the spine have most commonly caused an intimal flap and secondary thrombosis of the infrarenal abdominal aorta.

Clinical Presentation

In patients with either a penetrating or a blunt mechanism of injury, the clinical presentation will depend on several factors. The first of these is the type of aortic or visceral arterial injury. In patients with defects in the lateral wall, hemorrhage will occur and lead to hypotension with or without peritonitis. With complete transection of a visceral vessel and hemorrhage, the presentations will be the same. Should transection lead to thrombosis of both ends of the visceral vessel, a rare event in my experience, only abdominal pain (superior mesenteric artery) or hematuria (renal artery) may be present. The same presentations along with ischemia of both lower extremities (abdominal aorta) would occur if blunt trauma, an intimal flap, and secondary arterial thrombosis were present.

Clinical presentation is affected by the presence or absence of retroperitoneal or mesenteric tamponade, as well. In patients with defects in the lateral wall of the abdominal aorta or visceral arteries, retroperitoneal or mesenteric tamponade is the most common finding at a subsequent laparotomy. All patients who have arterial injuries and tamponade are still hypotensive at some point in the preoperative period—in the field, in the emergency center, or in the operating room as general anesthesia is initiated. In contrast to patients with abdominal venous injuries and tamponade, any improvement in blood pressure secondary to the infusion of crystalloid solutions and blood is transient. If retroperitoneal or mesenteric tamponade does not occur and there is active hemorrhage into the peritoneal cavity, a confused or moribund patient with profound hypotension, clear-cut peritonitis, and a tight abdomen is the presentation.

Areas of Abdominal Vascular Injuries

As has been discussed in numerous other texts, it is often helpful to describe the approaches to abdominal vascular injuries in a "geographic zone" fashion. Zone 1 includes the midline retroperitoneum and base of the mesentery, zone 2 is the upper lateral retroperitoneum (renal vessels), and zone 3 is the pelvic retroperitoneum (iliac vessels). Because they are uncommon, injuries to the vessels in the porta hepatis or retrohepatic area are usually described separately, as well.

Zone 1, the topic of discussion in this chapter, is best divided into *supramesocolic* and *inframesocolic* areas, because the operative approach is different for each, as is described. A midline supramesocolic area of hematoma or hemorrhage is likely to contain an injury to the suprarenal abdominal aorta, celiac trunk, proximal superior mesenteric artery, proximal renal artery, superior mesenteric vein, or obviously the pancreas. A midline inframesocolic area of hematoma or hemorrhage is likely to contain an injury to the infrarenal abdominal aorta, left renal vein, or inferior vena cava.

As a general rule, all hematomas in zone 1 (either supramesocolic or inframesocolic) from either penetrating or blunt trauma are opened by the surgeon using techniques to be described. Hematomas from penetrating wounds in zones 2, 3, and in the porta hepatis are opened, as well. In contrast, hematomas from blunt trauma that are located in zones 2 and 3 or in the retrohepatic area are opened only if they are pulsatile, expanding rapidly, or have already ruptured.

OPERATION

Supramesocolic Area of Zone 1

SUPRARENAL ABDOMINAL AORTA

The presence of a hematoma in the midline supramesocolic area will usually give the surgeon time to obtain proximal control of the supraceliac abdominal aorta. Such a hematoma is more likely to be present when the injury to the abdominal aorta is in the *diaphragmatic aorta* (in the aortic hiatus, itself) rather than in the *visceral aorta* (origins of visceral arteries) (Fig. 16–1).

The left-sided medial mobilization maneuver is the preferred operative approach. This maneuver includes division of the retroperitoneal attachments and reflection of the left colon, left kidney, spleen, tail of the pancreas, and fundus of the stomach to the midline (Fig. 16–2). The advantage of this technique is that it allows visualization of the entire abdominal aorta from the aortic hiatus of the diaphragm

Divisions of Suprarenal Aorta

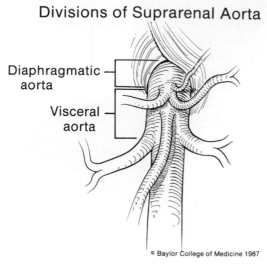

Diaphragmatic —
aorta

Visceral —
aorta

© Baylor College of Medicine 1987

■ **FIGURE 16–1**
Penetrating wounds of the diaphragmatic abdominal aorta may be tamponaded by muscle fibers of the aortic hiatus, and wounds of the visceral abdominal aorta are obviously more complex. (From Baylor College of Medicine, 1987.) ■

to the aortic bifurcation (Fig. 16–3). Disadvantages include the time required to complete the maneuver (4 to 5 minutes in inexperienced hands); risk of damage to the spleen, left kidney, or posterior left renal artery

Plane of Dissection

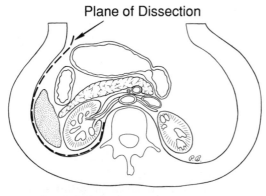

■ **FIGURE 16–2**
Left medial mobilization maneuver is initiated by dividing lateral retroperitoneal attachments of left colon, left kidney, spleen, tail of pancreas, and fundus of stomach. (From Feliciano DV: Truncal vascular trauma. In Callow AD, Ernst CB [eds]: Vascular Surgery. Theory and Practice. Stamford, Conn, Appleton & Lange, 1995, pp 1059-1085.) ■

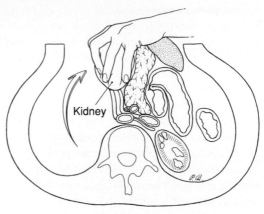

Kidney

■ **FIGURE 16–3**
Completion of left medial mobilization maneuver with all left-sided intra-abdominal viscera elevated to the midline. ■

during the maneuver; and anatomic distortion that results when the left kidney is rotated anteriorly. One alternative is to leave the left kidney in its fossa, thereby eliminating potential damage to or distortion resulting from rotation of this structure.

There are three significant obstacles to completing the maneuver once the viscera are mobilized. These include the length of the hiatal muscle fibers surrounding the diaphragmatic aorta, the dense nature of the celiac plexus of nerves connecting the right and left celiac ganglia, and the thickened lymphatic tissue around the aorta at this level. Although it is possible to peel the hiatal muscle fibers away and dissect through the celiac plexus of nerves and lymphatics, these maneuvers may be too time consuming in profoundly hypotensive patients (Fig. 16–4). It is much easier to transect the left crus of the aortic hiatus of the diaphragm at the 2-o'clock position to allow for exposure of the distal descending thoracic aorta above the hiatus. With the distal descending thoracic aorta or abdominal aorta in the hiatus exposed, the supraceliac aortic clamp can be applied without difficulty.

An alternative approach in the patient with a supramesocolic hematoma is to perform an extensive Kocher maneuver, elevate the *C*loop of the duodenum and the head of the pancreas to the left, and incise the retroperitoneal tissue to the left of the inferior vena cava. This

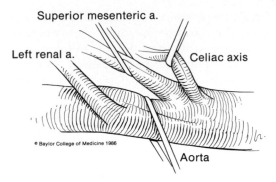

■ **FIGURE 16–4**
View of suprarenal abdominal aorta and major branches after left-sided medial mobilization maneuver and removal of all neural and lymphatic tissue. Note the fold in the visceral abdominal aorta created by mobilization of the left kidney and renal artery. (From Baylor College of Medicine, 1986.) ■

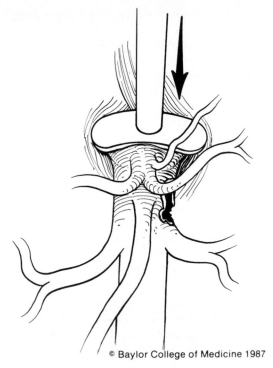

© Baylor College of Medicine 1987

■ **FIGURE 16–5**
Aortic compression device applied to supraceliac abdominal aorta for temporary proximal control superior to wound in visceral abdominal aorta. (From Baylor College of Medicine, 1987.) ■

will expose the suprarenal abdominal aorta between the celiac axis and the superior mesenteric artery. The disadvantage of this approach is that the exposure obtained is below the level of any wounds to the supraceliac aorta in the hiatus.

If active hemorrhage is coming from the supramesocolic area of the abdominal aorta, the surgeon may obtain temporary control manually or with one of the aortic compression devices (Fig. 16–5). If this compression prevents exposure and repair of the aortic injury, the next maneuver is to divide the lesser omentum manually, retract the stomach and esophagus to the left, and digitally separate the muscle fibers of the crura from the supraceliac aorta to obtain the same exposure as described for the left-sided medial mobilization maneuver, but anteriorly and more quickly. Distal control of the aorta in this location is awkward because of the presence of the visceral vessels. In young patients with injury confined to the supraceliac aorta, the celiac axis should be ligated and divided to allow for more space for the distal aortic clamp and subsequent vascular repair.

With small perforating wounds to the aorta at this level, lateral aortorrhaphy with 3-0 or 4-0 polypropylene suture is preferred. If two small perforations are adjacent to one another,

they should be connected and the defect closed in a transverse fashion with the polypropylene suture. When closure of the perforation(s) results in significant narrowing or if a portion of the aortic wall is missing, patch aortoplasty with polytetrafluoroethylene (PTFE) is indicated in the patient who is hemodynamically stable without hypothermia, significant acidosis, or an intraoperative coagulopathy. The other option is to resect a short segment of the injured aorta and perform an end-to-end anastomosis. This is difficult because of the limited mobility of both ends of the aorta at this level.

On rare occasions, patients with extensive injuries to the diaphragmatic or supraceliac aorta will require insertion of a synthetic vascular conduit or spiral graft after resection of the area of injury. Many of these patients have associated gastric, enteric, or colonic injuries. Therefore, much concern has been expressed about placing a synthetic conduit, such as a

12-, 14-, or 16-mm woven Dacron, albumin-coated Dacron, or PTFE prosthesis, in the aorta. The data in the American literature describing young patients with injuries to nondiseased abdominal aortas do not support the concern about infection occurring in Dacron interposition grafts, and there are few data relating to the use of PTFE grafts in penetrating trauma to the abdominal aorta. Despite the available data, some authors continue to recommend an extra-anatomic bypass when injury to the abdominal aorta would require replacement with a conduit in the presence of gastrointestinal contamination.

To lower the risk of infection in a prosthetic patch or graft inserted into the abdominal aorta at any level, one should not perform repairs of the intestine and the aorta simultaneously. Once the perforated bowel with occlusion clamps applied has been packed away and the surgeon has changed gloves, the aortic prosthesis is sewn in place with 3-0 or 4-0 polypropylene suture. After appropriate flushing of both ends of the aorta and removal of the distal aortic clamp to flush air out from the graft, the proximal aortic clamp should be removed very slowly as the anesthesiologist rapidly infuses fluids. If a long aortic clamp time has been necessary, the prophylactic administration of intravenous bicarbonate is indicated to reverse the "washout" acidosis from the previously ischemic lower extremities. The retroperitoneum is then copiously irrigated with an antibiotic solution and closed in a watertight fashion with an absorbable suture. At this point, the injuries to the gastrointestinal tract are repaired.

The survival rate of patients with injuries to the suprarenal abdominal aorta is approximately 30% (Table 16–1). Combined injuries to the suprarenal aorta and inferior vena cava had a 100% mortality rate in the large series from the Ben Taub General Hospital in 1987.

CELIAC TRUNK

When branches of the *celiac trunk* are injured, they are often difficult to repair because of the surrounding dense neural and lymphatic tissue and the small size of the vessels in a patient in shock with secondary vasoconstriction. Therefore major injuries to either the left gastric or the proximal splenic artery should be ligated. The common hepatic artery may have a larger diameter than the other two vessels, and an injury to this vessel may occasionally be amenable to lateral arteriorrhaphy, end-to-end anastomosis, or the insertion of a saphenous vein or prosthetic graft. In general, one should not worry about ligating the common hepatic artery proximal

---

TABLE 16–1
SURVIVAL WITH INJURIES TO THE SUPRARENAL ABDOMINAL AORTA

Reference	No. Patients	No. Survivors	% Survival
Arch Surg 109:706, 1974	17	5	29.4
Am J Surg 128:823, 1974	28	10	35.7
Ann Surg 42:1, 1976	5	4	80.0
J Trauma 22:481, 1982	3	3	100.0
J Trauma 22:672,1982	9	4	44.4
Surg Gynecol Obstet 160:313, 1985	15	7	46.6
Am J Surg 154:613, 1987	74	21	28.4
Am Surg 58:622, 1992	4	0	0.0
J Trauma 50:1020, 2001			
Diaphragmatic	9	1	11.1
Visceral	9	1	11.1
Suprarenal	13	0	0.0
Pararenal	5	1	20.0
Overall	191	57	29.8

to the origin of the gastroduodenal artery, because the extensive collateral flow from the inferior pancreaticoduodenal artery in the midgut will maintain the viability of the liver. If the entire celiac trunk is injured, it is best to ligate all three vessels and make no attempt at repair. Ligation of the celiac trunk has never caused any short-term morbidity or mortality in properly resuscitated patients.

SUPERIOR MESENTERIC ARTERY

Injuries to the *superior mesenteric artery* may occur at several levels. In 1972 Fullen and colleagues described an anatomic classification of injuries to the superior mesenteric artery that has been used only infrequently by subsequent authors in the trauma literature. If the injury to the superior mesenteric artery is beneath the pancreas (Fullen zone I), the pancreas may on rare occasions have to be transected between Glassman or Dennis intestinal clamps to control the bleeding point. Because the superior mesenteric artery has few branches at this level, proximal and distal vascular control is relatively easy to obtain once the overlying pancreas has been divided. Another option is to perform medial rotation of the left-sided intra-abdominal viscera, as previously described, and apply a clamp from the left side of the aorta directly to the proximal superior mesenteric artery at its origin. In this instance the left kidney may be left in the retroperitoneum as the medial rotation is performed.

Injuries to the superior mesenteric artery also occur beyond the pancreas at the base of the transverse mesocolon (Fullen zone II, between the pancreaticoduodenal and middle colic branches of the artery). Although there is certainly more space in which to work in this area, the proximity of the pancreas and the potential for pancreatic leaks near the arterial repair make injuries in this location almost as difficult to handle as the more proximal injuries. If the superior mesenteric artery has to be ligated at its origin from the aorta or beyond the pancreas (Fullen zone I or II), collateral flow from both the foregut and the hindgut should theoretically maintain the viability of the midgut in the distribution of this

vessel. Exsanguinating hemorrhage from injuries in this area, however, often leads to profound shock with intense vasoconstriction of the distal superior mesenteric artery. For this reason, collateral flow is often inadequate to maintain viability of the distal midgut, especially the cecum and ascending colon. In the hemodynamically unstable patient with hypothermia, acidosis and a coagulopathy, the insertion of a temporary intraluminal shunt into the débrided ends of the superior mesenteric artery is a better choice than ligation and fits the definition of *damage control*. If replacement of the proximal superior mesenteric artery is to be performed at a first operation or at a reoperation after *damage control,* it is safest to place a saphenous vein or prosthetic graft on the distal infrarenal aorta, away from the injury to the pancreas and other upper abdominal organs (Fig. 16–6). A graft in this location should be tailored so that it will pass through the posterior aspect of the mesentery of the small bowel and then be sutured to the mid or distal superior mesenteric artery in an end-to-side or end-to-end fashion without significant tension. It is mandatory to cover the proximal suture line on the infrarenal aorta with retroperitoneal fat or a viable omental pedicle to avoid an aortoenteric fistula at a later time. Injuries to the more distal superior mesenteric artery beyond the transverse mesocolon (Fullen zone III, beyond the middle colic branch) should be repaired if at all possible to avoid ischemia of the distal midgut. Injuries to the segmental branches (Fullen zone IV) are usually ligated and followed by resection of portions of the midgut as needed.

The survival rate among patients with penetrating injuries to the superior mesenteric artery during the 1970s and 1980s was approximately 58%, and this is still true (Table 16–1). This decreases to 20% to 25% when any form of repair more complex than lateral arteriorrhaphy is necessary. In three more recent series in which 84 patients with injuries to the superior mesenteric artery were described (Asensio and colleagues, 2000; Davis and colleagues, 2001; Tyburski and colleagues, 2001), survival was approximately 49% (Table 16–2).

A large multi-institutional review of such injuries was reported in 2001 by Asensio and

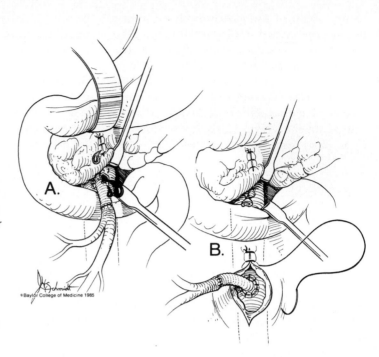

■ **FIGURE 16-6**
It may be dangerous to place the proximal suture line of a graft in Fullen zone I or II of the superior mesenteric artery near an associated pancreatic injury. The proximal suture line should be on the lower aorta, away from the upper abdominal injuries, and covered with retroperitoneal tissue. (From Baylor College of Medicine, 1985.) ■

colleagues. There were 250 patients with injuries to the superior mesenteric artery (52% penetrating; 48% blunt) treated in 34 trauma centers over a 10-year period. Data were available on operative management in 244 patients including 175 (72%) with ligation, 53 (22%) with suture repair, and 16 (6%) with insertion of an autogenous (no. 10) or PTFE (no. 6) graft. Overall survival was 61% and ranged from 23.5% for patients with Fullen zone I injuries to 76.9% for those with Fullen zone IV injuries. Finally, logistic regression analysis was used to identify independent risk factors for mortality. These risk factors

TABLE 16–2
SURVIVAL WITH INJURIES TO THE SUPERIOR MESENTERIC ARTERY

Reference	No. Patients	No. Survivors	% Survival
J Trauma 12:656, 1972	8	5	62.5
Surgery 84:835, 1978	45	27	60.6
Ann Surg 193:30, 1981	15	10	66.7
J Trauma 22:672,1982	6	4	66.7
J Trauma 23:372, 1983	20	14	70.0
J Trauma 26:313, 1986	22	7	31.8
Am J Surg 180:528, 2000	28	13	46.4
Am Surg 67:565, 2001*	15	8	53.3
J Trauma 50:1020, 2001	41	20	48.8
J Am Coll Surg 193:354, 2001 (multi-institutional)	250	153	61.2
Overall	450	261	58.0

*Excludes patients with exsanguination before repair or ligation.

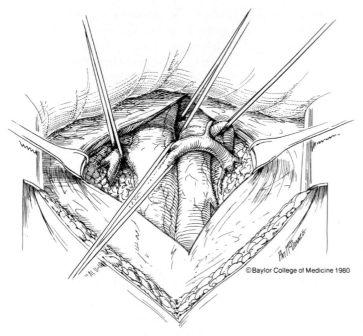

©Baylor College of Medicine 1980

■ **FIGURE 16-7**
Vessel loops or umbilical tapes
are placed around the proximal
renal vessels before perirenal
hematomas are entered. (From
Baylor College of Medicine,
1980.) ■

included the following: transfusion of more
than 10 units of packed red blood cells; intraoperative acidosis; dysrhythmias; injury in
Fullen zone I or II; or the development of
multisystem organ failure.

RENAL ARTERY

Injuries to the *proximal renal arteries* may also
present with a supramesocolic hematoma or
with hemorrhage in this area. With an injury
to the proximal renal artery, supraceliac
control of the abdominal aorta by either of
the methods previously described will be necessary. A tamponaded injury closer to the renal
hilum allows for proximal control of the renal
artery in the midline retroperitoneum (Fig.
16–7). The transverse mesocolon is retracted
superiorly, and the small bowel is eviscerated
to the right. The ligament of Treitz is then
divided as the inferior mesenteric vein is
retracted to the left. With extensive mobilization of the duodenojejunal junction, the
left renal vein crossing over the juxtarenal
abdominal aorta is exposed and mobilized,
as needed, by ligation and division of the left
adrenal, gonadal, and renal lumbar veins.
Such extensive mobilization will allow this vein

to be retracted 6 to 7 cm in a superior direction. The origin of the left renal artery at the
4-o'clock position on the juxtarenal abdominal aorta is readily identified by dissection of
the surrounding retroperitoneal tissue of
modest density. A vessel loop is then passed
around the proximal left renal artery. To
expose the origin of the right renal artery at
the 7-o'clock position on the juxtarenal
abdominal aorta, the surgeon may need to
retract the adjacent infrarenal inferior vena
cava to the right with a vein retractor. The right
renal vein cannot be looped until an extensive Kocher maneuver is performed to expose
the juxtarenal inferior vena cava. Options for
repair of either the proximal or the distal renal
artery are described later in this chapter.

Inframesocolic Area of Zone 1

INFRARENAL ABDOMINAL AORTA

The second major area of hematoma or
hemorrhage in the midline retroperitoneum
is the inframesocolic area. Patients with
injuries to the *infrarenal (or suprarenal) abdominal aorta* and signs of life upon arrival in the
operating room always have a massive midline

hematoma in the retroperitoneum. The size of this hematoma is often intimidating to the inexperienced trauma surgeon, but one simple rule should be kept in mind: The hole in the aorta is under the highest point of the hematoma. Therefore, an injury just below the base of the mesocolon is likely to involve the juxtarenal abdominal aorta and demands proximal aortic control in the upper abdomen by using the previously described techniques. A midline hematoma over the lower lumbar area is likely to be over an injury to the infrarenal abdominal aorta, and exposure and control will be easier. With either a true inframesocolic hematoma or an area of hemorrhage, proximal aortic control is obtained as described previously for exposure of the proximal renal arteries. The transverse mesocolon is elevated superiorly, the small bowel is eviscerated to the right, and the ligament of Treitz is divided to allow for application of an aortic cross clamp in the infrarenal position (Fig. 16–8). Exposure to allow for application of the distal vascular clamp is obtained

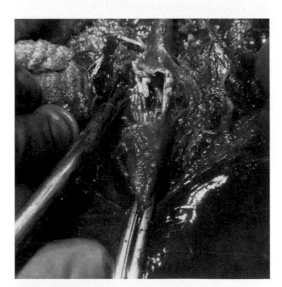

■ **FIGURE 16–8**
Gunshot wound of infrarenal abdominal aorta viewed through standard inframesocolic exposure (head of patient is toward the proximal clamp). (From Feliciano DV, Burch JM, Graham JM: Abdominal vascular injury. In Mattox KL, Moore EE, Feliciano DV [eds]: Trauma, 1st ed. Stamford, Conn, Appleton & Lange, 1988, pp 519-536.) ■

by dividing the midline retroperitoneum down to the aortic bifurcation, carefully avoiding the left-sided origin of the inferior mesenteric artery; however, this vessel may be sacrificed whenever necessary for exposure in young trauma patients.

As with injuries to the suprarenal aorta, injuries in the infrarenal abdominal aorta are repaired in a transverse fashion with 3-0 or 4-0 polypropylene suture or by patch aortoplasty, end-to-end anastomosis, or insertion of a woven Dacron graft, an albumin-coated Dacron graft, or a PTFE graft, none of which requires preclotting. Because of the small size of the aorta in young trauma patients, it is unusual to be able to place a tube graft larger than 12, 14, or 16 mm in diameter if one is required, as previously noted. The principles of completing the suture lines and flushing are exactly the same as those for aortic repairs in the suprarenal area. Because the retroperitoneal tissue is often thin in young patients, it may be worthwhile to cover an extensive aortic repair or the suture lines of a prosthesis with mobilized omentum before closure of the retroperitoneum. One option is to divide the gastrocolic omentum, flip the omentum superiorly into the lesser sac, and make a window in the left side of the transverse mesocolon. The mobilized pedicle is passed through the window and placed over the aortic repair or graft. The other option is to mobilize the gastrocolic omentum away from the right side of the transverse colon. This mobilized pedicle is then placed lateral to the ligament of Treitz and over the aortic repair or graft. With either technique, 2-0 or 3-0 absorbable sutures are used to attach the omental pedicle to the opened retroperitoneal edges around the area of repair in the infrarenal abdominal aorta.

The survival rate among patients with penetrating injuries to the infrarenal abdominal aorta during the 1970s, 1980s, and early 1990s was approximately 46% (Table 16–3). In a more recent series with 35 patients, the survival rate was 34.3% (Tyburski and colleagues, 2001). In three other recent series (Coimbra and colleagues, 1996; Asensio and colleagues, 2000; Davis and colleagues, 2001) in which 140 patients with injuries to the abdominal "aorta" (not specified as to whether the loca-

TABLE 16–3
SURVIVAL WITH INJURIES TO THE INFRARENAL ABDOMINAL AORTA

Reference	No. Patients	No. Survivors	% Survival
Arch Surg 109:706, 1974	15	7	46.7
Am Surg 41:755, 1975*	40 (aortoiliac)	17	42.5
J Trauma 22:672, 1982	9	4	44.4
J Trauma 22:481, 1982	12	7	58.3
Surg Gynecol Obstet 160:313, 1985	10	4	40.0
Am Surg 58:622, 1992	7	4	57.1
J Trauma 50:1020, 2001	35	12	34.3
Overall	88	38	43.2

*Not included in overall figures.

tion was suprarenal or infrarenal) were treated, the survival was 42.8% (12/28), 20.6% (13/63), and 39.1% (25/64, excluding 13 patients who exsanguinated before repair) (Table 16–4). The overall survival of approximately 32% for all aortic injuries in these recent reviews, a decrease of approximately 6% of all the aortic injuries before 1993 (Tables 16–1 and 16–3) are included, is quite interesting. The recent survival figures may reflect shorter scene times in urban environments, which would bring more exsanguinated patients to the trauma center, or this change may be a manifestation of more patients with multiple penetrating wounds and/or injuries.

There is one interesting report by Soldano and colleagues (1988) of the long-term follow-up of 11 survivors of penetrating wounds to the abdominal aorta (9 infrarenal injuries and 5 suprarenal injuries in the 11 patients) from

the Vietnam War. Ankle-to-brachial pressure ratios were decreased in five (one only with exercise), and all had calcification of the area of repair on abdominal computed tomography (CT).

Zone 2 or Upper Lateral Retroperitoneum

RENAL ARTERY

If a hematoma or hemorrhage is present in the lateral perirenal area, injury to either the *distal renal artery*, the *renal vein*, or *both* or the *kidney* should be suspected. In hemodynamically stable patients who have suffered blunt abdominal trauma and have normal preoperative IVP, renal arteriogram, or CT of the kidneys, there is no justification for exploring the kidney through its perirenal

TABLE 16–4
RECENT SURVIVAL WITH INJURIES TO THE ABDOMINAL AORTA (NOT OTHERWISE SPECIFIED)

Reference	No. Patients	No. Survivors	% Survival
Am J Surg 172:541, 1996	28	12	42.8
Am J Surg 180:528, 2000			
Isolated injury	46	10	21.7
With other arterial injury	17	3	17.6
Am Surg 67:565, 2001*	64	25	39.1
Overall	155	50	32.3

*Excludes patients with exsanguination before repair.

hematoma at a laparotomy performed for other injuries. As previously noted, the perirenal hematoma should be opened if it is pulsatile, expanding rapidly, or has already ruptured partially.

In highly selected and hemodynamically stable patients with penetrating wounds to the flank, CT has been used to document an isolated minor renal injury and operation has been avoided. All other patients found to have a perirenal hematoma at the time of exploration for a penetrating abdominal wound should have unroofing of the hematoma and exploration of the underlying kidney ("Huey Long rule").

If the hematoma is not rapidly expanding and there is no free intra-abdominal bleeding, most surgeons will loop the ipsilateral renal artery with a vascular tape in the midline at the base of the mesocolon as previously described. It should be noted that there is little consensus on the value of preliminary arterial control at the midline in stable patients.

If there is active bleeding from the kidney through Gerota's fascia or from the retroperitoneum overlying the renal vessels, no central renovascular control is necessary. The surgeon should simply open the retroperitoneum lateral to the injured kidney, divide Gerota's fascia, and manually elevate the kidney directly into the wound. A large vascular clamp can be applied proximal to the hilum or just lateral to the inferior vena cava on the right to control any further bleeding.

Renovascular injuries from penetrating trauma are difficult to manage, especially when the renal artery is involved. It is an extraordinarily small vessel that is deeply embedded in the retroperitoneum. Occasionally, small perforations of the artery from penetrating wounds can be repaired by lateral arteriorrhaphy or resection with an end-to-end anastomosis. Interposition grafting using either a saphenous vein or a PTFE graft or use of borrowed arteries, such as the splenic artery to replace the left renal artery and the hepatic artery to replace the right renal artery, is indicated only when the renal artery to the patient's only kidney is injured. In other patients with multiple intra-abdominal injuries or a long preoperative period of ischemia, nephrectomy is a better choice, as long as

intraoperative palpation has confirmed a normal contralateral kidney. The survival rate for patients with injuries to the renal arteries from penetrating trauma in two older series (1980; 1990) was approximately 87%, with renal salvage in only 30% to 40%.

Controversy continues to surround the role of renal revascularization after the delayed diagnosis of thrombosis of the renal artery from blunt trauma. Intimal tears in the renal arteries may result from deceleration in motor vehicle crashes, automobile-pedestrian crashes, and falls from heights. These usually lead to secondary thrombosis of the vessel and complaints of upper abdominal and flank pain. One literature review in 1980 noted that only 30% of patients with intimal tears in the renal arteries had gross hematuria, 43% had microscopic hematuria, and 27% had no blood in the urine. A more recent report in 1998 documented that seven of eight patients in whom a urinalysis was performed had hematuria. Therefore, the diagnosis may be missed, because an IVP or CT may not be performed in stable patients with normal abdominal examinations and no hematuria or microhematuria, only, after blunt trauma.

Lack of enhancement of a kidney with intravenous contrast on an abdominal CT is pathognomonic of blunt thrombosis of the ipsilateral renal artery. As the intimal tear is always 2 to 4 cm from the abdominal aorta, the value of a follow-up renal arteriogram to confirm the diagnosis is questionable (Fig. 16–9).

The operative technique when renal revascularization is attempted is straightforward. Resection of the area of the intimal tear and an end-to-end anastomosis, insertion of an aortorenal artery bypass graft, or ex vivo perfusion of the ischemic kidney followed by autotransplantation into the pelvis can all be performed by an experienced vascular or transplantation surgery team. The value of external cooling of the ischemic kidney or infusing a cold renal perfusion solution before a revascularization procedure after the artery is opened is unclear. The same can be said for the value of decapsulation of the previously ischemic kidney to prevent a post-revascularization "kidney compartment syndrome."

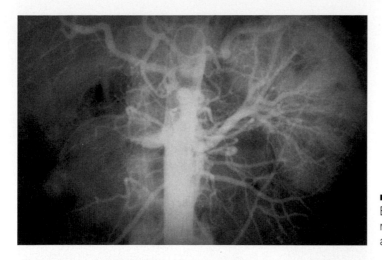

■ **FIGURE 16-9**
Blunt occlusion of the right
renal artery on an abdominal
aortogram. ■

The controversy regarding revascularization is related to the poor results that have been reported. The time from injury to revascularization appears to be critical, as would be expected when dealing with one kidney that receives 12.5% of the cardiac output each minute. In one review in 1978, some renal function was restored in 80% of patients undergoing renal revascularization within 12 hours of occlusion. This figure decreased to 57% if revascularization did not occur for 18 hours. A more recent report of 12 patients with blunt thrombosis of the renal artery (one bilateral) by Haas and colleagues in 1998 is even more discouraging. In the group of five patients who underwent attempted revascularization of the renal artery at a median warm ischemia time of 5 hours (4.5 to 36 hours), four were felt to be "technically successful." Immediate nephrectomy was performed in another, with an unsuccessful attempt at revascularization. The outcomes for the four patients with successful revascularization were as follows: nephrectomy at 1 day (no function on postoperative renal scan) in one; death on hemodialysis at 2 months in another; nephrectomy at 6 months because of delayed hypertension in a third; and minimal function (9% differential) at 1 month on a renal scan in the fourth. In the same series, seven patients with blunt thrombosis of the renal artery did not undergo revascularization. A delayed nephrectomy was required at a mean time of 5 months in three patients (43%) who developed hypertension, and four were normotensive at a mean

time of 11 months from injury. Based on the historical and recent data, it is difficult to recommend revascularization of one renal artery in a patient with a functioning contralateral kidney after sustaining blunt trauma. This is especially true if the patient has other serious injuries and time to revascularization would exceed 6 hours from injury. This conclusion, of course, would not be acceptable to the authors of case reports or reviews documenting successful late renal revascularization (one or both kidneys) after *bilateral* thrombosis of the renal arteries. Such successful repairs have been performed at 12, 15, 18, and 19 hours, as reported by Greenholz and colleagues (1986). Patients *not* undergoing revascularization of one thrombosed renal artery need to be monitored for 6 to 12 months after injury to allow for early detection of delayed hypertension.

There are isolated case reports in which patients with failure of bilateral renal revascularization *and* no revascularization because of biopsy-proven renal necrosis had return of renal function starting at 4 to 8 weeks after injury. This phenomenon is presumably related to maintenance of some renal viability via collateral flow to renal capsular vessels and to recanalization of the thromboses in the renal arteries. If patients with bilateral thrombosis with or without attempts at renal revascularization remain dependent on hemodialysis, they should be put on a waiting list for renal transplantation.

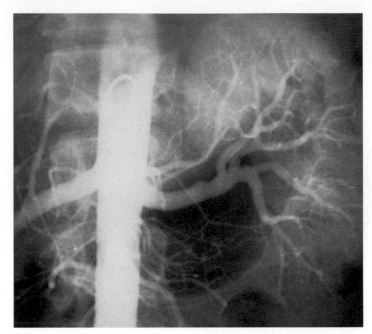

■ **FIGURE 16–10**
Blunt intimal tear in the left renal artery demonstrated on a "pullout" abdominal aortogram. (From Feliciano DV, Burch JM, Graham JM: Vascular injuries of the chest and abdomen. In Rutherford RB, et al [eds]: Vascular Surgery, 3rd ed. Philadelphia, WB Saunders, 1989, pp 588-603.) ■

There are patients with blunt trauma who undergo "pullout" abdominal aortograms after evaluation of the thoracic aorta or preliminary abdominal aortography before pelvic arteriography who are found to have intimal tears in the renal artery without thrombosis (Fig. 16–10). When there is no extravasation of contrast at the site of injury, observation and follow-up arteriography within the first week after injury are appropriate. The role of anticoagulation is problematic because so many of these patients have associated injuries. In the absence of serious associated injuries, anticoagulation would seem appropriate, recognizing the absence of meaningful data. An intimal or wall defect that was the presumed source of embolic infarctions in the ipsilateral kidney has been treated successfully by insertion of an endovascular stent in one recent report by Villas and colleagues (1999).

Complications

The complications of repairs of the abdominal aorta or visceral arteries include distal embolization, thrombosis, dehiscence of a suture line, and infection. Occlusion is not uncommon when small vasoconstricted vessels, such as the superior mesenteric artery or renal artery, undergo lateral arteriorrhaphy. In such patients, it may be valuable to perform a second-look operation within 12 to 24 hours after the patient's blood pressure, temperature, and coagulation abnormalities have returned to normal. When this is done, correction of a vascular thrombosis may be successful.

As previously noted, dehiscence of vascular suture lines in the superior mesenteric artery near a pancreatic injury may occur if a small pancreatic leak occurs in the postoperative period. For this reason the proximal anastomosis of such a graft should be on the infrarenal aorta far away from the pancreas as described.

In addition, the postoperative development of vascular enteric fistulas occurs most commonly in patients who have anterior aortic repairs, aortic grafts, or grafts to the superior mesenteric artery from the aorta. Again, this problem can be avoided by proper coverage of suture lines on the aorta with retroperitoneal tissue or a viable omental pedicle and on the recipient vessel with mesentery.

REFERENCES

Asensio JA, Britt LD, Borzotta A, et al: Multiinstitutional experience with the management of superior mesenteric artery injuries. J Am Coll Surg 2001;193:354-366.

Asensio JA, Chahwan S, Hanpeter D, et al: Operative management and outcome of 302 abdominal vascular injuries. Am J Surg 2000;180:528-534.

Asensio JA, Forno W, Roldan G, et al: Abdominal vascular injuries: Injuries to the aorta. Surg Clin North Am 2001 Dec;81(6):1395-1416, xiii-xiv. Review.

Coimbra R, Hoyt D, Winchell R, et al: The ongoing challenge of retroperitoneal vascular injuries. Am J Surg 1996;172:541-545.

Davis TP, Feliciano DV, Rozycki GS, et al: Results with abdominal vascular trauma in the modern era. Am Surg 2001;67:565-571.

Feliciano DV: Management of traumatic retroperitoneal hematoma. Ann Surg 1990;211:109-123.

Feliciano DV, Burch JM, Graham JM: Abdominal vascular injury. In Mattox KL, Feliciano DV, Moore EE (eds): Trauma, 4th ed. New York, McGraw-Hill, 2000, pp 783-805.

Fry WR, Fry RE, Fry WJ: Operative exposure of the abdominal arteries for trauma. Arch Surg 1991;126:289-291.

Haas CA, Dinchman KH, Nasrallah PF, Spirnak JP: Traumatic renal artery occlusion: A 15-year review. J Trauma 1998;45:557-561.

Meghoo CA, Gonzalez EA, Tyroch AH, Wohltmann CD: Complete occlusion after blunt injury to the abdominal aorta. J Trauma 2003 Oct;55(4):795-799.

Roth SM, Wheeler JR, Gregory RT, et al: Blunt injury of the abdominal aorta: A review. J Trauma 1997;42:748-755.

Tyburski JG, Wilson RF, Dente C, et al: Factors affecting mortality rates in patients with abdominal vascular injuries. J Trauma 2001;50:1020-1026.

Injuries of the Inferior Vena Cava and Portal Venous System

ROBERT F. BUCKMAN, JR.
ABHIJIT S. PATHAK
KEVIN M. BRADLEY

Venous injury in the upper abdomen most often involve the inferior vena cava (IVC) and the portal venous system. Often such injuries occur simultaneously. The literature on these injuries is usually presented separately; therefore, these injuries are presented in two sections of this chapter.

INJURIES OF THE INFERIOR VENA CAVA

The IVC, though deeply protected against the accidents of nature, is by no means immune to wounding. It has been estimated that 10% to 15% of cases of abdominal penetration result in an injury to a major vein and that 1 of every 50 gunshot wounds to the abdomen strikes the IVC (Starzl and colleagues, 1962; Wiencek and Wilson, 1986). Although penetrating mechanisms cause most caval injuries and can involve any portion of the IVC, the retrohepatic and intrapericardial sections are the only portions of the vessel that are injured by blunt trauma.

Whether caused by blunt or penetrating mechanisms, caval wounds are highly lethal. As many as 50% of patients with such injuries die before reaching the hospital and the mortality among patients who arrive at a trauma center with signs of life has ranged between 20% and 57% (Duke, Jones, and Shires, 1965; Quast and colleagues, 1965; Weichert and Hewitt, 1970; Burns and Sherman, 1972; Graham and colleagues, 1978; Kudsk, Sheldon, and Lim, 1982; Feliciano and colleagues, 1984; Wiencek and Wilson, 1986; Klein, Baumgartner, and Bongard, 1994; Burch and colleagues, 1998; Asensio and colleagues, 2001). The three factors that are most important in the prognosis for survival are the hemodynamic condition of the patient on arrival, the occurrence of spontaneous tamponade of the caval injury, and to a lesser degree, the location of the caval laceration (Weichert and Hewitt, 1970; Graham and colleagues, 1978; Kashuk and colleagues, 1982; Kudsk, Sheldon, and Lim, 1982; Wiencek and Wilson, 1986; Klein, Baumgartner, and Bongard, 1994; Burch and colleagues, 1998). Patients who arrive in shock and fail to respond to initial resuscitative measures, those who are still actively bleeding at the time of laparotomy, and those with wounds of the retrohepatic vena cava have a low probability of survival. Death is most commonly due to intraoperative exsanguination (Nakamura and Tzuzuki, 1981; Wiencek and Wilson, 1986; Burch and colleagues, 1998).

Surgical Anatomy

The IVC originates by the confluence of the common iliac veins just anterior to the body of the fifth lumbar vertebra and posterior to the right common iliac artery. As it ascends along the right side of the lumbar vertebral bodies, the cava receives numerous tributaries including four or five pairs of lumbar (sometimes called "segmental") veins, the right gonadal vein, the renal veins, the right adrenal vein, and finally the hepatic and phrenic veins. It then traverses the mid-diaphragm to reach the right atrium. The IVC is a relatively delicate and thin-walled vessel, 1.5 inches in diameter, valveless throughout its length, with a high flow at an intraluminal pressure of about 5 cm H_2O.

The intra-abdominal vena cava may be divided into five sections, each of which has anatomic peculiarities that affect the exposure and control of injuries that section (Weichert and Hewitt, 1970). The lowest section is the bifurcation. Above this are the infrarenal, the perirenal, the suprarenal/subhepatic, and the retrohepatic sections. The management of injuries in each of these segments is discussed separately.

An important anatomic feature of both the bifurcation and the infrarenal sections of the IVC is an abundant collateral circulation, of which the lumbar veins constitute the principal elements. These paired veins are connected with one another, with the common iliac, hypogastric, iliolumbar, and renal veins and with the azygos and hemiazygos system through bilateral ascending lumbar veins. This extensive network is capable of bypassing any obstruction of the bifurcation or of the infrarenal segment of the vena cava, but the very richness of the collateral circulation also confounds efforts to achieve proximal and distal control of injuries in these zones (Fig. 17–1).

The perirenal area extends about 1 inch above and below the renal veins and lies posterior to the pancreas and duodenum. The high flow from the renal veins requires that these vessels and the IVC itself be occluded to control bleeding from wounds in this section of the cava (Wiencek and Wilson, 1986; Burch and colleagues, 1998).

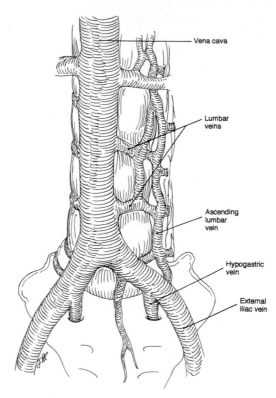

■ **FIGURE 17–1**
The abundant collaterals of the infrarenal vena cava. Lumbar veins communicate with ascending veins that drain into the azygos and hemiazygos systems. (From Buckman RF Jr, Pathak AS, Badellino MM, Bradley KM: Injuries of the inferior vena cava. Surg Clin North Am 2001;81[6]:1433.) ■

Between the perirenal segment and the beginning of the retrohepatic segment is a short, suprarenal-subhepatic region of the IVC. Injuries in this segment are difficult to control because of the renal vessels below and the proximity of the liver above, with the passage of the cava underneath the liver into the retrohepatic zone. The portal vein lies immediately anterior to this short segment of the IVC.

The segment of the IVC that has the most unique anatomic features is the retrohepatic section, lying above the right adrenal vein and below the phrenic veins. This portion of the cava, 7 to 10 cm in length, lies in a groove or tunnel on the posterior aspect of the liver within its "bare" area (Nakamura and Tzuzuki, 1981). This area, completely circumscribed by the hepatic suspensory ligaments with the diaphragm behind and the liver in front, has the ability to confine or contain bleeding associated with retrohepatic caval injuries, provided that the diaphragm, the posterocentral liver, or hepatic ligaments are not themselves severely disrupted by the traumatic event or by surgical intervention (Buckman, Miraliakbari, and Badellino, 2000). The retrohepatic vena cava is joined by two or three major hepatic veins shortly before it traverses the diaphragm and below this by seven or more accessory hepatic veins of varying sizes. These numerous tributaries bind the cava to the liver, making its circumferential mobilization dangerous. The exposure of caval injuries in the retrohepatic zone is exceptionally difficult and is usually unnecessary if spontaneous containment of hemorrhage has been achieved by the suspensory ligaments, the liver, and the diaphragm.

Patterns of Injury

With the exception of the retrohepatic and intrapericardial vena cava, which may be injured by blunt or penetrating trauma, virtually all other IVC injuries are caused by penetrating mechanisms. Gunshot wounds are much more likely than stab wounds to lacerate the IVC and generate far more destructive wounding patterns. Although stab wounds cause linear lacerations of the vena cava, which often spontaneously tamponade, gunshot wounds, especially the high-energy wounds of the current era, produce large tangential avulsions involving varying amounts of the circumference or actual transection of the vessel.

Almost every patient with a penetrating wound of the vena cava has injuries to other viscera, other major vessels, or both (Bricker and Wukasch, 1970; Bricker and colleagues, 1971; Mattox and colleagues, 1974, 1975). Injuries of the liver, duodenum, pancreas, bowel, and colon are common. Approximately 10% of the patients wounded in the IVC have a second major vascular injury, most commonly involving the aorta or portal vein (Mattox and colleagues, 1975; Linker and colleagues, 1982). In rare instances, the combined penetration of the vena cava with the aorta leads to the development of an aortocaval fistula. Acute traumatic fistulas may also occur between the cava and the renal arteries or the cava and the duodenum.

Blunt injuries to the IVC are generally caused by shearing forces in violent deceleration accidents and may take the form of avulsion of the atriocaval junction or tearing of hepatic veins from the retrohepatic vena cava. Intraparenchymal lacerations of the hepatic veins or the anterior surface of the retrohepatic cava may occur in severe blunt fractures of the posterocentral liver caused by crushing injuries.

For a caval or other venous injury to bleed freely, there must exist, in addition to the venous wound itself, a major breach of surrounding tissues normally capable of confining or containing low-pressure hemorrhage. The capacity for self-tamponade is characteristic of caval injuries because it is of all venous injuries and has important clinical implications. Among patients with IVC injuries, more than half will spontaneously contain the site of injury with cessation of bleeding (Ochsner, Crawford, and DeBakey, 1961; Starzl and colleagues, 1962; Duke, Jones, and Shires, 1965; Weichert and Hewitt, 1970; Burch and colleagues, 1998). This phenomenon is more likely to occur with oblique, crossing, low-velocity gunshot wounds and with stab wounds than with straight, front-to-back, high-powered gunshot wounds or massive hepatic fractures. A beveled or slit-like retroperitoneal track favors containment and tamponade. Spontaneous tamponade is also likely to occur in wounds of the cava that are behind the pancreas, duodenum, or liver, provided that the overlying viscera are not extensively disrupted. In such instances of a tamponaded injury, profuse iatrogenic rebleeding occurs at the time of surgical exposure.

Numerous authors have observed that the retroperitoneal hematoma associated with a caval injury may not be large, and that there may be minimal free intraperitoneal blood if the tamponade occurs early. Although survival is far more likely in patients with spontaneous cessation of bleeding (Starzl and colleagues,

1962; Duke, Jones, and Shires, 1965; Weichert and Hewitt, 1970; Mattox and colleagues, 1974), not all patients who have tamponaded will survive. Up to 40% of them may die of exsanguination after the tamponade is surgically decompressed unless the hemorrhage from the cava and associated vascular injuries can be completely and quickly controlled (Duke, Jones, and Shires, 1965).

Initial Assessment and Management

Approximately half of patients with wounds of the IVC will present with some degree of hypotension, often with profound hemodynamic compromise (Ochsner, Crawford, and DeBakey, 1961; Wiencek and Wilson, 1986; Beal, 1990; Klein, Baumgartner, and Bongard, 1994). Of these, most will show temporary improvement with the institution of appropriate intravenous fluid resuscitation (Feliciano and colleagues, 1984). The failure of the hypotensive patient to respond to initial volume repletion correlates with the presence of continued active bleeding, that is, a failure of spontaneous tamponade, and portends a poor prognosis. At the other extreme, patients with IVC injuries who have achieved early spontaneous containment of their bleeding are often normotensive on arrival. Rare presentations of caval injury include acute cavalduodenal fistula with hypotension and copious emesis of dark blood or acute aortocaval fistula characterized by a wide pulse pressure, abdominal bruit, and hematuria (Linker and colleagues, 1982).

Patients whose wound trajectories or clinical presentations suggest the possibility of major intraabdominal vascular wounding should have supradiaphragmatic intravenous access and be taken directly the operating room. Those with the most extreme degrees of cardiovascular collapse, who fail to respond to initial appropriate resuscitative measures, may require resuscitative thoracotomy, performed in the emergency department. Most patients, however, will show a dramatic hemodynamic improvement with volume repletion and can be transported for operation.

Exposure and Control

Injuries of the IVC most often present at operation as stable hematomas of the central retroperitoneum (Ochsner, Crawford, and DeBakey, 1961; Starzl and colleagues, 1962; Duke, Jones, and Shires, 1965; Burch and colleagues, 1998). Varying amounts of free intraperitoneal blood may be present, although active hemorrhage from the cava often has ceased. When active bleeding is occurring, the initial operative maneuver should be the manual tamponade of the bleeding point with a tightly rolled gauze pack. Aortic compression may be indicated in severely compromised patients until the hemodynamic condition improves.

In most patients, tamponade having been achieved either spontaneously or by the assistance of the surgeon, some circumspection is possible before exploration of the hematoma. It is often feasible, on the basis of the location of the points of retroperitoneal penetration to deduce the path of the wounding agent relative to major retroperitoneal structures.

Recalling that the vast majority of patients who die from IVC injuries succumb to intraoperative exsanguination (Ochsner, Crawford, and DeBakey, 1961; Duke, Jones, and Shires, 1965; Weichert and Hewitt, 1970) and that many of these patients have spontaneously tamponaded the wound before exploration, the first question that the surgeon must ask is whether the hematoma surrounding the suspected caval injury truly requires exploration. Early writers on the subject of caval injury and many experienced surgeons subsequently have urged restraint in the exploration of stable, nonpulsating retroperitoneal hematomas, especially those behind the liver, unless an injury to the pancreas, duodenum, colon, kidney, or ureter or an associated arterial injury is strongly suspected and demands exposure (Ochsner, Crawford, and DeBakey, 1961; Starzl and colleagues, 1962; Duke, Jones, and Shires, 1965; Graham and colleagues, 1978; Burch and colleagues, 1998; Buckman, Miraliakbari, and Badellino, 2000).

Nonpulsatile hematomas accompanying presumed injuries to the retrohepatic (or the immediately subhepatic) vena cava that have spontaneously tamponaded or that can be induced to tamponade by manual compression or gauze packing are not often associated with other retroperitoneal injuries and are probably better left unexplored. Decompression of such hematomas by radical hepatic mobilization is often associated with massive, sometimes lethal, hemorrhage that cannot any longer be controlled by packing after the natural containment structures have been surgically destroyed. Although rebleeding following spontaneous or assisted tamponade of presumed caval injuries is rare, an estimated 10% to 40% of patients with originally stable hematomas bleed to death following operative exposure of a caval wound (Ochsner, Crawford, and DeBakey, 1961; Duke, Jones, and Shires, 1965; Weichert and Hewitt, 1970; Burch and colleagues, 1998). Most hematomas below the level of the immediate subhepatic segment of vena cava require exploration not just to fix a possible caval wound, but because of the risk of injuries to other retroperitoneal visceral or vascular structures (Duke, Jones, and Shires, 1965).

Having reached whatever conclusions are possible regarding the probable location and nature of the vascular injury in a central hematoma, and having determined that either active hemorrhage or the risk of associated injuries outweighs the dangers of caval exploration, preparations to enter the hematoma should include an adequate supply of blood, an autotransfuser, vascular instruments, skilled assistance, large-bore venous access above the diaphragm, rolled packs, stick sponges, adequate suction, intravascular balloon occlusion catheters, and 4-0 vascular suture on large needles. Preliminary aortic control is obtained if a major arterial injury is suspected and the patient should be placed in a slight, reverse Trendelenburg position to obviate venous air embolism (Bricker and colleagues, 1971). As the hematoma is opened, massive hemorrhage should be expected. When encountered, it must be immediately tamponaded with a tightly rolled pack held by an assistant, until more definitive control is established with clamps or occlusion catheters. In most wounds of the IVC, attempts to obtain remote proximal and distal control, before entering the

area of caval wounding, are not valuable because of the abundant collateral circulation.

Wide exposure of the caval wound and any associated injury is of the utmost importance. Wounds of the vena cava from the immediate subhepatic segment to the bifurcation are best exposed by a mobilization of the duodenum, the head of the pancreas, the right colon, and the base of the mesentery from the cecum to the duodenojejunal flexure (Fig. 17–2). This combined rotational maneuver provides exposure, not only of the entire vena cava below the liver but also of any associated aortic or renovascular injury below the origin of the superior mesenteric artery (Cattell and Braasch, 1960; Hunt and colleagues, 1971; Mattox and colleagues, 1975; Feliciano, 1988). In the course of this wide exposure, if a major bleeding source is encountered, the mobilization maneuvers are interrupted while a tamponading pack is placed and held by an assistant over the source of hemorrhage. Full mobilization is then completed. It has been observed that in most cases of caval injury, shock is not maximal at the onset of the operation but during that portion of the procedure when the hematoma is opened and caval hemorrhage and caval compression occur. The anesthesiologist should be forewarned of this possibility (Weichert and Hewitt, 1970; Burch and colleagues, 1998).

Three sections of the intra-abdominal IVC, the perirenal, the bifurcation, and the retrohepatic areas, may require special exposure maneuvers beyond those listed earlier. The posterior elements of wounds of the perirenal area may require medial rotation of one kidney or division of the renal vein between clamps to visualize the back of the cava at its junction with a renal vein.

Full exposure of the caval bifurcation zone is best achieved by division of the right common iliac artery between clamps with subsequent arterial reanastomosis (Salam and Stewart, 1985). This maneuver is more likely to be necessary if repair of the IVC is desired rather than simple caval ligation.

Active hemorrhage from the retrohepatic cava, *which cannot be controlled by any form of tamponade,* may rarely require caval exposure to attempt hemostasis. Exposure of the retrohepatic or immediate subhepatic cava

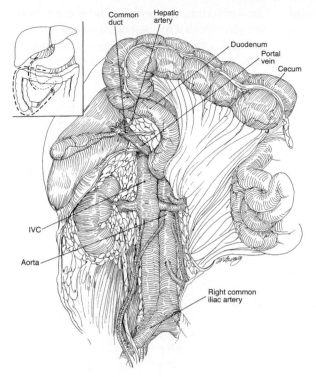

Common duct
Hepatic artery
Duodenum
Portal vein
Cecum
IVC
Aorta
Right common iliac artery

■ **FIGURE 17–2**
Exposure of the inferior vena cava from the liver to the bifurcation is best achieved by a medial rotation of the duodenum and pancreas together with the right colon and mesenteric base. (From Buckman RF Jr, Pathak AS, Badellino MM, Bradley KM: Injuries of the inferior vena cava. Surg Clin North Am 2001;81[6]:1438.) ■

necessitates extensive mobilization of the right triangular ligament, including its caval crossing point at the level of the right adrenal vein (Mattox and colleagues, 1974). For left-sided injuries, full incision of the left triangular ligament is necessary. Because the anterior surface of the retrohepatic cava is bound to the liver by numerous tributaries, it cannot be exposed except by dividing the liver along the interlobar plane. Although some have used resection of the left lateral segment of liver to gain access to the left anterior aspect of the retrohepatic vena cava (Klein, Baumgartner, and Bongard, 1994) and Schrock, Blaisdell, and Mathewson (1968) have actually suggested division of the liver along the interlobar plane to expose the entire retrohepatic cava, such maneuvers cannot be recommended unless they constitute mere completions of massive traumatic fractures along these planes. A right thoracoabdominal incision or preferably a median sternotomy often is required, in addition to the extensive division of hepatic suspensory ligaments to expose the retrohepatic cava (Klein, Baumgartner, and Bongard, 1994). It cannot be too strongly emphasized that *radical hepatic*

mobilization and *exposure of retrohepatic vena cava injuries* is associated with an extremely high mortality and is not advisable unless active bleeding is present and cannot be contained by perihepatic packing (Beal and Ward, 1989; Beal, 1990; Cue and colleagues, 1990; Buckman, Miraliakbari, and Badellino, 2000).

CONTROL OF HEMORRHAGE: INFRAHEPATIC INFERIOR VENA CAVA

Most wounds of the infrahepatic vena cava can be controlled by manual or pack pressure until proximal and distal dissection is carried out or a partial occlusion clamp applied. Care must be taken to avoid avulsion of lumbar veins during these attempts to gain clamp control of the caval wound (Graham and colleagues, 1978).

The abundant lumbar collateral circulation makes satisfactory proximal and distal control of the infrarenal cava or confluence difficult. In areas where there is a problem achieving control with clamps, intraluminal balloon catheters may permit bleeding control with minimal dissection (Ravikumar and Stahl, 1985; Buckman, Miraliakbari, and Badellino, 2000). Both urinary catheters and Fogarty vascular catheters have been used for this purpose. The widely recommended proximal and distal compression of the IVC with stick sponges is rapid but cumbersome and difficult to maintain during repair of the vein (Graham and colleagues, 1978; Feliciano, 1988).

The method for control of caval wounds used by the authors of this chapter consists of the immediate tamponade of the wound with a tightly rolled pack, followed by the slow rolling of the pack down the wound from one end, exposing small portions of the injury while the remainder of the injury is still compressed. As the opalescent venous intima is visualized, revealing the location of the wound edges, Babcock clamps are applied sequentially to each exposed portion until the entire wound has been coapted (Fig. 17–3). The clamps are applied vertically in most wounds but can be applied transversely to produce less caval narrowing in suitable injuries.

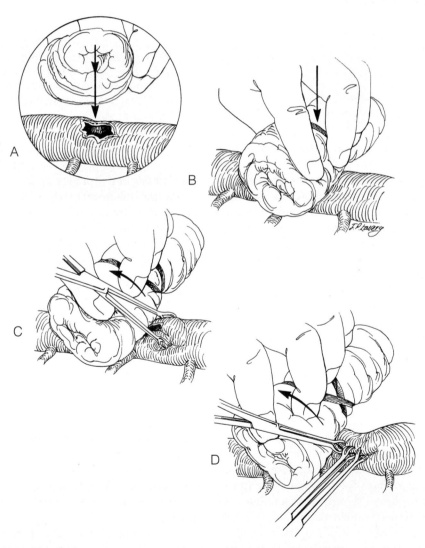

■ **FIGURE 17-3**
Method of control of the inferior vena cava wound using tightly-rolled pack and Babcock clamps. (From Buckman RF Jr, Pathak AS, Badellino MM, Bradley KM: Injuries of the inferior vena cava. Surg Clin North Am 2001;81[6]:1440.) ■

Once the hemorrhage has been controlled by this method, the injury can be secondarily underclamped with a partial occlusion clamp or with Crafoord or "bulldog" clamps from each end, to permit exact suturing or patching of the defect (Fig. 17–4). Alternatively, the Babcock clamps themselves can be simply under-run with suture from end to end, with this suture line constituting the final repair.

Once the anterior and lateral aspects of the wound have been controlled, lumbar veins can be divided between ligatures and, if necessary, the cava can be rotated to repair the posterior parts of the wounds. The best "control" for caval hemorrhage is with a rapid repair, which can then be revised if improvement of the initial closure is deemed necessary.

CONTROL OF HEMORRHAGE: RETROHEPATIC INFERIOR VENA CAVA

The extreme dangers associated with exposure of the retrohepatic vena cava have been previously described. The most dire problems with the initial control of caval hemorrhage are those that occur following wide hepatic mobilization and decompression of retrohepatic caval wounds (Carmona, Peck, and Lim, 1984; Beal and Ward, 1989; Buechter and colleagues, 1989; Beal, 1990; Cue and colleagues, 1990; Burch and colleagues, 1998).

This disaster is best avoided by *reinforcing* the structures capable of tamponading a retrohepatic bleeding site rather than *destroying* them by mobilizing the liver (Weichert and Hewitt, 1970; Sharp and Locicero, 1992).

In cases of transparenchymal hepatic venous or caval hemorrhage, containment may be restored by omental packing, deep liver sutures, and perihepatic gauze packing (Weichert and Hewitt, 1970; Stone and Lamb, 1975; Carmona, Peck, and Lim, 1984; Beal, 1990; Cue and colleagues, 1990; Fabian and colleagues, 1991). Intracaval shunts generally do not constitute a method of initial hemorrhage control (Shrock, Blaisdell, and Mathewson, 1968; Beal and Ward, 1989; Burch and colleagues, 1998). In order to place the shunt, if its use is deemed indispensable, bleeding control should be achieved by tamponade *before* the insertion of the shunt (Bricker and colleagues, 1971; Wiencek and Wilson, 1986; Rovito, 1987; Beal and Ward, 1989; Burch and colleagues, 1998). However, if bleeding can be stopped by packing, the use of the atriocaval shunt is required only to attempt a direct suture repair of the suspected caval or hepatic vein injury (Shrock, Blaisdell, and Mathewson, 1968). There is no evidence supporting the need for venous repair in this area of the cava, and strategies that seek such repairs are associated with mortality rates of 70% to 90%. (Kudsk, Sheldon, and Lim, 1982; Moore, Moore, and Seagraves, 1985; Beal and

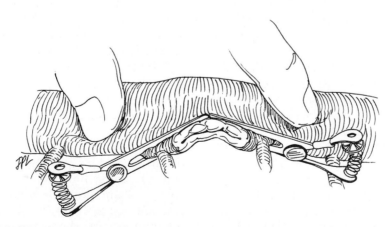

■ **FIGURE 17–4**
Technique of controlling caval wound by partially underclamping the wound from each end to control lumbar inflow. (From Buckman RF Jr, Pathak AS, Badellino MM, Bradley KM: Injuries of the inferior vena cava. Surg Clin North Am 2001;81[6]:1441.) ■

Ward, 1989; Burch and colleagues, 1998; Cogbill and colleagues, 1998).

Direct clamping of the suprahepatic and infrahepatic vena cava, together with the application of portal inflow occlusion by a Pringle maneuver, has also been advocated by some as a method to limit retrohepatic bleeding in pursuit of the strategy of direct repair of the retrohepatic vena cava (Yellin, Chaffee, and Donovan, 1971; Klein, Baumgartner, and Bongard, 1994). Vascular isolation by this technique carries the danger of triggering a cardiac arrest in a severely hypovolemic patient (Weichert and Hewitt, 1970; Klein, Baumgartner, and Bongard, 1994). Like all methods used to approach and suture retrohepatic vena caval injuries, its use is associated with an extremely high likelihood of death and cannot be recommended in any case in which retrohepatic hemorrhage has ceased spontaneously or can be contained by perihepatic packing.

Venovenous bypass (Baumgartner and colleagues, 1995) and hypothermic circulatory arrest (Shrock, Blaisdell, and Mathewson, 1968; Carmona, Peck, and Lim, 1984) have also been reported to permit vascular isolation and repair of the retrohepatic vena cava in rare cases. These are not hemorrhage control tactics but are practicable only when prior control of the caval injury by manual or pack tamponade has gained sufficient time to institute the bypass procedure. As is true for the techniques of atriocaval shunting and clamp vascular isolation of the liver, their sole value is in pursuing the highly dubious goal of direct suture repair of the retrohepatic cava.

Nearly all successful repairs of retrohepatic vena caval injuries, in case reports describing actual clinical events, have occurred in patients who had stable hematomas at the time of operation (Bricker and Wukash, 1970; Burns and Sherman, 1972; Fullen and colleagues, 1974; DePinto, Mucha, and Powers, 1976; Mullin, Lucas, and Ledgerwood, 1980; Misra, Wagner, and Boneval, 1983; Rovito, 1987; Hartman and colleagues, 1991; Baumgartner and colleagues, 1995; Feldman, 1996). These hematomas, having been disrupted by hepatic mobilization, released a massive hemorrhage that was then, in the *fortunate* patients, stopped by manual tamponade. Control by tamponade allowed time for the insertion of an intracaval shunt or for the institution of venovenous bypass in pursuit of direct suture repair of the caval injury. This sequence permitted, in a few lucky patients, successful repair of the injuries. Aside from case reports such as those described earlier, it is doubtful whether there are any successful applications of these techniques. Despite the occasional technical feasibility of carrying it out, there is *no* evidence that injuries of the retrohepatic or immediate subhepatic vena cava, associated with spontaneously contained hematomas, *require* repair to prevent recurrent hemorrhage or thromboembolic complications. All strategies and techniques designed to effect such repairs, at the cost of disrupting a stable hematoma, are ill founded and are less likely to produce survival than methods that produce tamponade or reinforce the spontaneously occurring containment of retrohepatic hemorrhage (Buckman, Miraliakbari, and Badellino, 2000).

Inferior Vena Cava Repair

At the outset of the discussion of definitive caval repair, it is necessary to emphasize three important facts: First, patients who do not die of uncontrolled intraoperative hemorrhage or the consequences of prolonged shock tend to be long-term survivors regardless of the method of managing the caval injury (Weichert and Hewitt, 1970; Bricker and colleagues, 1971; Graham and colleagues, 1978; Wiencek and Wilson, 1986; Burch and colleagues, 1998). Second, complications of caval repairs or of the expectant management of spontaneously tamponaded caval injuries are very uncommon (Beal, 1990). Third, the long-term outcome for ligation of the infrarenal IVC is about the same as that for repair (Duck, Jones, and Shires, 1965; Quast and colleagues, 1965; Weichert and Hewitt, 1970; Graham and colleagues, 1978; Burch and colleagues, 1998). It follows that minimization of the shock period and rapid control of active caval hemorrhage are the principal goals to be pursued in the definitive operative management of wounds of the intra-abdominal IVC. Sometimes, as indicated earlier in this chapter, these goals can be met without exposing or suturing the caval wound.

Caval wounds that have demanded exposure can be rapidly repaired, in most cases, using a lateral suture technique with 4-0 cardiovascular suture material (Fullen and colleagues, 1974; Burch and colleagues, 1998). The posterior portion of a wound may be accessed by extension of the anterior wound or by rotation of the cava. This type of repair, in a patient with severe or multiple injuries and shock, is preferable to struggling with fine suture material on a tiny needle or attempting elegant caval reconstruction in locations, such as the bifurcation or the infrarenal vena cava, where precise repair has no provable impact on outcome. After lateral repair, if the narrowing of the cava is deemed unacceptable and the patient is stable, revision by patch angioplasty or graft replacement to restore luminal diameter can be considered. However, the need for revision is not common.

Because retrohepatic caval injuries are best managed expectantly or by tamponade, and because there is no credible evidence that caval narrowing or even ligation (Mullins, Lucas, and Ledgerwood, 1980; Burch and colleagues, 1998) below the renal veins affects long-term outcome, the issue regarding complex reconstruction of the vena cava really devolves down to injuries of the suprarenal and perirenal segments. In these sections, it is not known how much narrowing of the vena cava can be tolerated, although caval ligation above the renal veins is claimed to be incompatible with survival. A reduction of up to 75% of the luminal cross section probably would be tolerated, but this cannot be stated with certainty (Burch and colleagues, 1998). In the absence of certainty, it is advisable that unless the patient is exsanguinating, a lumen of at least 25% or more should be preserved during repair of the suprarenal or perirenal IVC. After the initial repair, if the lumen is believed to be less than this and the hemodynamic condition of the patient permits, patch angioplasty, using vein or polytetrafluoroethylene (PTFE) can be done (Klein, Baumgartner, and Bongard, 1994). Very rarely the replacement of a damaged segment of the perirenal or suprarenal IVC with panel grafts of vein or externally supported PTFE may be justified (Fig. 17–5).

Revision of narrowed repairs of the infrarenal vena cava cannot be easily justified because there is no evidence that the long-term outcome is better with patent than with thrombosed repairs or with *any* repair rather than ligation. In severe caval wounds, especially with profound shock and multiple vascular injuries, ligation of the infrarenal vena cava or bifurcation, with separate ligation or clipping of any lumbar veins entering the wounded segment, is an acceptable method of management (Duke, Jones, and Shires, 1965; Agarwal and colleagues, 1982; Moore, Moore, and Seagraves, 1985; Burch and colleagues, 1998). All evidence suggests that rapid enlargement of existing abundant lumbar collaterals and the ascending lumbar veins will allow the continuation of caval flow around the area of ligation. It has been reported that even suprarenal caval ligation can be safely carried out, if the pressure in the vena cava below the ligature does not rise above 30 cm of saline and if indigo carmine excretion by the kidney, following intravenous administration, is demonstrated (Caplan, Halasz, and Bloomer, 1964). The same network of collaterals to the azygous and hemiazygous systems that permits infrarenal ligation may also prove adequate in the case of suprarenal ligation. The evidence on this subject is not sufficient for a definite conclusion to be drawn.

For an exposed but irreparable injury of the suprarenal IVC in a patient unable to withstand complex reconstruction, an alternative to ligation might be placement of a temporary heparin-bonded shunt. In an experimental model, caval shunts have maintained their patency for up to 24 hours (Aldridge, Buckman, and Badellino, 1997). Clinical experience with this desperate expedient is limited (Burch and colleagues, 1998).

Postoperative Management

Regardless of whether the IVC is repaired or ligated or managed by tamponade, stagnation

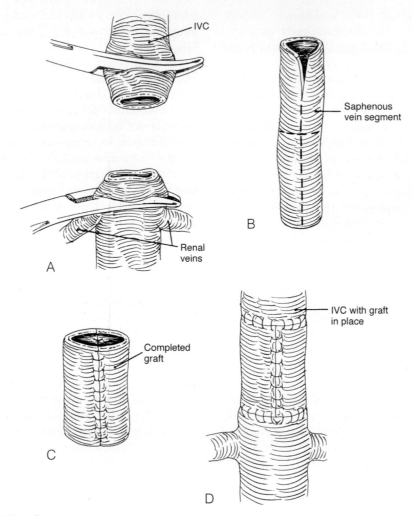

■ **FIGURE 17–5**
A–D, Reconstruction of a destroyed suprarenal segment of the inferior vena cava using a panel graft of saphenous vein. (From Buckman RF Jr, Pathak AS, Badellino MM, Bradley KM: Injuries of the inferior vena cava. Surg Clin North Am 2001;81[6]:1444.) ■

of blood in the lower extremities is undesirable. Leg elevation, elastic bandage wrapping, and sequential compression devices promote venous flow and may reduce thromboembolic complications at and below the caval repair. Whether the use of anticoagulants improves the outcome of narrowed IVC repairs is not known, but a postoperative infusion of dextran for 24 hours is empirically used by many surgeons. Edema of the lower extremities may occur in the early postoperative period following caval repair or ligation, but it is almost never a long-lasting or severe problem

(Mullins, Lucas, and Ledgerwood, 1980; Burch and colleagues, 1998).

Sudden death due to pulmonary embolism has been reported to occasionally occur following IVC repair, especially in patients older than 50 years (Burch and colleagues, 1998). Use of vena cava filters, placed above the repair, may be considered in this subgroup. The actual incidence of subclinical thrombotic complications following caval repair or ligation has not been determined by systematic investigation.

Summary

Injuries of the IVC, whether caused by blunt or penetrating mechanisms, are highly lethal. Patients who arrive in shock and fail to respond to initial resuscitative measures, those who are still actively bleeding at the time of laparotomy, and those with wounds of the retrohepatic vena cava have a low probability of survival. Death is most commonly due to intraoperative exsanguination. Knowledge of the anatomy and exposure techniques for the five segments of the intraabdominal vena cava is very important to the trauma surgeon. Although some wounds of the vena cava are best left unexplored, especially those of the retrohepatic vena cava, most injuries below this level can be exposed and repaired by lateral suture technique. Preservation of a lumen of at least 25% of normal is probably important in the suprarenal vena cava but is of no provable value below the renal veins. There is no evidence supporting the need to expose and repair wounds of the vena cava that have spontaneously stopped bleeding. Such wounds, especially in the retrohepatic area, may be managed expectantly provided there is no strong suspicion of an associated injury to a major artery or hollow viscus.

PORTAL VEIN INJURIES

Wounds of the portal vein, though uncommon, represent one of the most highly lethal of all vascular injuries. The reported case-fatality rate among patients with such wounds who reach the hospital alive has been 39% to 71% in most series (Chisholm and Lenio, 1972; Mattox, Espada, and Beall, 1974; Bostwick and Stone, 1975; Graham, Mattox, and Beall, 1978; Peterson, Sheldon, and Lim, 1979; Busuttil and colleagues, 1980; Stone, Fabian, and Turkelson, 1982; Sheldon and colleagues, 1985; Dawson, Johansen, and Jurkovich, 1991; Jurkovich and colleagues, 1995). This high death rate is due mainly to intraoperative exsanguination during attempts to control the injured vessel (Mattox, Espada, and Beall, 1974; Bostwick and Stone,

1975). Portal vein injuries are caused in 90% of cases by penetrating trauma (Mattox, Espada, and Beall, 1974; Bostwick and Stone, 1975; Graham, Mattox, and Beall, 1978; Peterson, Sheldon, and Lim, 1979; Busuttil and colleagues, 1980), with gunshot wounds more commonly the cause of the injury and far more lethal than stab wounds. Not only has there been no decrease in mortality from this form of trauma over the last 20 years, but the case-fatality rate may actually be increasing, despite all the advances in prehospital and hospital care, because of the increased frequency of gunshot as the wounding mechanism and the greater destructive power of wounding weapons.

Surgical Anatomy

The portal system drains the splanchnic territories supplied by the celiac and mesenteric arteries. Collecting effluent from the unpaired abdominal viscera, the portal vein delivers this blood, rich in oxygen and nutrients, to the liver, accounting for nearly 80% of total hepatic blood flow. Despite its high flow, portal pressure is normally less than 6 mm Hg.

PORTAL VEIN

The portal vein forms by the confluence of the superior mesenteric vein and the slightly smaller splenic vein behind the upper third of the neck of the pancreas (Fig. 17–6). This confluence is located just to the right of the body of the second lumbar vertebra and immediately anterior to the left border of the vena cava. The inferior mesenteric vein, the third major tributary contributing its flow to the portal vein, joins either the splenic or the superior mesenteric vein in the immediate vicinity of the major confluence. In as many as 30% of patients, the inferior mesenteric vein enters at the angle of the major confluence itself (Ivatory and colleagues, 1987). The retropancreatic confluence zone is not intimately related to the superior mesenteric artery, the bile duct, or the hepatic artery. A sound knowledge of the anatomy of the portal confluence

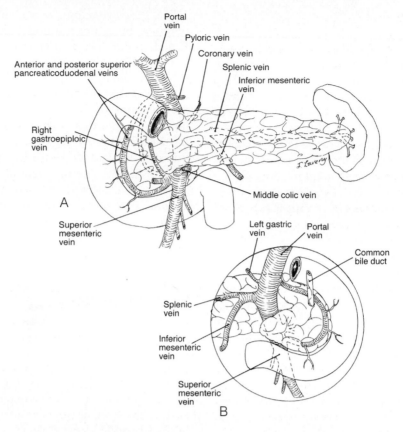

Portal
vein

Pyloric vein

Coronary vein

Anterior and posterior superior
pancreaticoduodenal veins

Splenic vein

Inferior mesenteric
vein

Right
gastroepiploic
vein

A

Middle colic vein

Superior
mesenteric
vein

Left gastric
vein

Portal
vein

Common
bile duct

Splenic
vein

Inferior
mesenteric
vein

Superior
mesenteric
vein

B

■ **FIGURE 17–6**
Anterior *(A)* and posterior *(B)* views of the portal vein and its major tributaries in relation to the
pancreas. Wounds of the retropancreatic confluence zone are the most difficult portal injuries to
control and repair. (From Buckman RF Jr, Pathak AS, Badellino MM, Bradley KM: Portal vein injuries.
Surg Clin North Am 2001;81[6]:1450.) ■

(and potential anomalies) is of utmost importance to the trauma surgeon attempting to manage injuries in this dangerous and unfamiliar area.

From its origin, the valveless portal vein passes cephalad, inclining slightly rightward over its course of 3 to 4 inches, to reach the hilum of the liver, where it divides extrahepatically into right and left branches. During its course, it passes, in succession, behind the upper pancreatic neck, and the first portion of the duodenum. Then, upon entering the hepatoduodenal ligament, it comes into relationship with the hepatic artery and bile duct, lying behind these structures and forming the anterior border of the foramen of Winslow. Throughout its length, the portal vein lies immediately anterior to the suprarenal segment of the IVC.

In addition to its main tributaries, the portal vein receives the pyloric vein from the pancreas and duodenum, the coronary (left gastric) vein, and the superior pancreaticoduodenal vein (see Fig. 17–6). A cystic vein, if present, also drains into the portal vein. These veins represent major potential collaterals in cases of portal vein obstruction.

SUPERIOR MESENTERIC AND SPLENIC VEIN

In addition to the anatomy of the portal vein itself, certain features of its major tributaries are important to the trauma surgeon. The superior mesenteric vein, representing the confluence of all the tributaries that correspond to the branches of the superior mesenteric artery, is formed in the mesentery as numerous intestinal veins. The ileocolic, right colic, and middle colic veins join the main venous trunk. The mesenteric vein also receives the right gastroepiploic vein, the inferior pancreaticoduodenal vein, and in some cases, the inferior mesenteric vein. In addition, a number of small unnamed veins drain into the right lateral aspect of the superior mesenteric vein from the head of the pancreas.

The main trunk of the superior mesenteric vein passes anterior to the third portion of the duodenum and in front of the uncinate process. Then, it courses behind the neck of the pancreas to enter confluence zone where it converges with the splenic vein to form the main portal vein. The proximal portion of the superior mesenteric vein is located in a groove of the pancreas behind the neck and may be completely encircled by the pancreatic tissue. The numerous tributaries entering the superior mesenteric vein all along its course provide abundant collateral pathways in the event of obstruction of this vein. Of particular importance are the gastroepiploic vein and the inferior pancreaticoduodenal vein, which join the superior mesenteric just before its confluence with the splenic vein, and communicate with the portal vein above the confluence.

The most important distinctions regarding the superior mesenteric vein, from the trauma surgical standpoint, are first that a part of the superior mesenteric vein is retropancreatic and difficult to expose, while most of it is infrapancreatic and easily accessible; and second, that it has abundant collaterals.

The splenic vein, as it courses along the dorsum of the pancreas, receives many small pancreatic branches and often receives the inferior mesenteric vein just prior to the confluence of the splenic vein with the superior mesenteric vein. In addition to the splenic and pancreaticoduodenal veins, a large accessory pancreatic vein may be present and may enter the portal vein directly.

COLLATERALS IN PORTAL OBSTRUCTION

It is obvious from the regional vascular anatomy that in the event of portal obstruction in the hepatic hilum, there would be virtually no way for antegrade portal flow to be reconstituted. In such a case, the portosystemic collaterals would expand to drain the effluent of the portal circulation. However, it is equally evident that the closer any of the major veins (i.e., portal, mesenteric, or splenic) is obstructed to the confluence of these veins, the more abundant are the potential major collateral veins that could reconstitute portal flow. The regional vascular anatomy makes it apparent that *any retropancreatic injury of the portal vein and its main tributaries could be ligated, with probable preservation, not only of adequate splanchnic drainage, but also, with the expectation of collateral antegrade portal flow.*

Patterns of Injury

ASSOCIATED INJURIES

Because of the dense crowding of major vessels and viscera in the upper midabdomen, penetrating portal venous injuries are almost always associated with injury to the liver, biliary tract, pancreas, duodenum, or bowel. Of far greater concern, however, than these visceral injuries, are major vascular wounds of the IVC, aorta, superior mesenteric artery, or renal vessels, which accompany portal vein wounds in 70% to 90% of patients (Mattox, Espada, and Beall, 1974; Bostwick and Stone, 1975; Graham, Mattox, and Beall, 1978; Perterson, Sheldon, and Lim, 1979; Stone, Fabian, and Turkelson, 1982; Jurkovich and colleagues, 1995). The suprarenal vena cava, which lies just behind the entire course of the portal vein, is the most common vessel to be injured in association with the portal vein, as might be expected. In rare cases, the simultaneous wounding of a major artery and the portal vein may lead to an arteriovenous fistula (Smith and Northrop, 1976; Dingledin, Proctor, and Jaques, 1977; Robb and Costa, 1984; Epstein and colleagues, 1987;

Deitrick and colleagues, 1990; Lumsden and colleagues, 1993).

Associated major vascular injuries are nearly always posterior to the plane of the portal vein itself and may be multiple, involving both arteries and veins and tending, together with the portal venous wound, to produce massive and chaotic retropancreatic hemorrhage, which is extremely difficult to control.

Portal venous wounds have been reported to involve the supraduodenal and retropancreatic zones of the vein with similar frequency (Peterson, Sheldon, and Lim, 1979; Sheldon and colleagues, 1985; Dawson, Johansen, and Jurkovich, 1991; Jurkovich and colleagues, 1995). Hilar wounds are more rare. Whereas stab wounds tend to produce limited portal lacerations or clean transections, high-energy gunshot wounds striking the portal vein produce extensive avulsions or transection of the impacted vessel and may disrupt important potential collateral pathways, as well as the main trunk of the portal vein. Damage to other viscera and vessels is also more severe with gunshot wounds. Wounds of this type, involving the retropancreatic portal confluence zone, are almost uniformly fatal due to rapid transpancreatic exsanguination (Stone, Fabian, and Turkelson, 1982).

Initial Assessment and Management

Most patients with portal venous injuries arrive at the hospital in hemorrhagic shock, with many in advanced circulatory collapse (Mattox, Espada, and Beall, 1974; Bostwick and Stone, 1975). Approximately one half of such patients will respond to initial fluid resuscitation, and these will usually be found at operation to have achieved some degree of spontaneous tamponade of their vascular wounds. The remaining patients have active hemorrhage and require immediate operation as an indispensable element of their resuscitation. In patients with the most dire degrees of hemodynamic collapse, resuscitative thoracotomy and aortic cross clamping may be required in the emergency department. Few such patients will survive. More commonly, immediate transport to the operating room for emergency laparotomy is required.

Exposure and Initial Vascular Control

Even when accompanied by other vascular wounds, especially to the IVC, portal injuries may present at operation as stable hematomas of the upper central retroperitoneum, hepatoduodenal ligament, or mesenteric root. In perhaps one half of patients, active intraperitoneal bleeding is continuing at the time of laparotomy. This bleeding may have its origin from the portal vein injury itself or from an associated vascular wound.

STABLE HEMATOMA

If there is a stable hematoma, determination of the location of the points of retroperitoneal penetration and consideration of the probable wound tract may allow a deduction to be reached concerning the vessels most likely to be wounded. Before opening the hematoma, it is prudent to prepare the equipment that may be necessary to control multiple vascular injuries. Vascular instruments, balloon occlusion catheters, stick sponges, tightly rolled laparotomy pads, and an adequate supply of blood for transfusion must be at hand. If an autotransfusion apparatus is available, it should be prepared for use. When a major arterial injury is suspected, preliminary control of the aorta is desirable. It is also wise to place the patient in a mild reverse Trendelenburg position to obviate the possibility of venous air embolism if a caval injury is disclosed.

In penetration of the region of the portal vein, *multiple* vascular injuries are the *rule,* and an apparently minor hematoma with modest free hemoperitoneum may harbor major wounds of both the portal vein and the vena cava, which will bleed most impressively once unroofed. The vast majority of patients who die from portal vein injuries exsanguinate intraoperatively, after exposure of their vascular wounds. This misfortune may befall even those who were stable preoperatively. Because the prevention of this type of death is the major problem in the management of injuries of the portal vein, the issue of vascular control assumes the highest importance.

The initial procedure upon entry into the abdomen of a severely shocked patient with active transpancreatic hemorrhage is to manually compress the aorta at its hiatus and then to locate and manually compress the site of bleeding. As these things are done, volume repletion and the transfusion of blood may be performed, to remove the patient from the immediate danger of cardiac arrest.

Some reduction in flow in the portal vein and other vessels in the region may be obtained by double clamping the aorta, both above the celiac axis and below the renal

vessels. This maneuver will reduce, but not abolish, flow through the celiac and superior mesenteric arteries, aorta, vena cava, and renal vessels and will indirectly decrease portal vein flow.

SUPRAPANCREATIC EXPOSURE

In patients with suspected injury to the portal vein or its major tributaries, wide exposure to locate and immediately control the sources of hemorrhage is crucial. Wounds of the suprapancreatic portal vein can be exposed by a wide Kocher maneuver with rotation of the hepatic flexure of the colon as needed (Fig. 17–7). If a major source of hemorrhage is

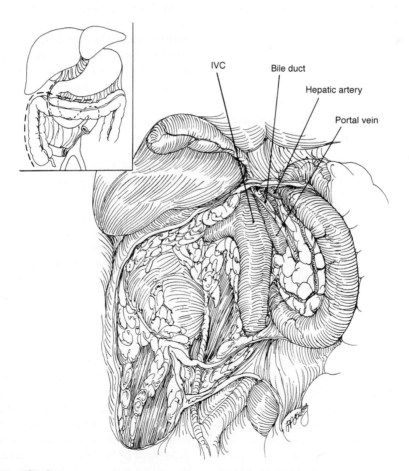

■ **FIGURE 17–7**
Exposure of the retropancreatic portal vein and vena cava by a combined medial rotation of the pancreas, duodenum, and hepatic flexure. (From Buckman RF Jr, Pathak AS, Badellino MM, Bradley KM: Portal vein injuries. Surg Clin North Am 2001;81[6]:1455.) ■

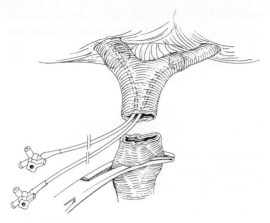

■ FIGURE 17–8
Control of a suprapancreatic portal vein injury
using intraluminal catheters for control of the
bifurcation and a clamp proximally. A wound of
this type may require an interposition vein graft.
(From Buckman RF Jr, Pathak AS, Badellino
MM, Bradley KM: Portal vein injuries. Surg Clin
North Am 2001;81[6]:1456.) ■

encountered, it must be immediately controlled with a pack held by an assistant. Following preliminary hepatic inflow occlusion
and the division of the cystic duct to facilitate
exposure, the suprapancreatic portal vein may
be dissected to obtain distal control with a vascular clamp or occlusion catheter (Peterson,
Sheldon, and Lim, 1979) (Fig. 17–8).

RETROPANCREATIC EXPOSURE

Retropancreatic wounds involving the portal
confluence or its major tributaries and suprapancreatic wounds with suspected additional
injury of the IVC or other vessels are exposed
by a combination of the Kocher maneuver and
mobilization of the entire right colon and
mesenteric base, from the cecum to the duodenojejunal flexure (Cattell and Braasch,
1960; Peterson, Sheldon, and Lim, 1979).
When combined with leftward mobilization
of the hepatic flexure, this maneuver provides
access to the entire portal vein and the proximal portions of its major tributaries. It also
exposes the entire infrahepatic vena cava and
the aorta up to the origin of the superior

mesenteric artery. Rarely, left medial rotation
of the spleen and the tail of the pancreas may
be necessary to expose the left lateral aspect
of the portal vein confluence (Fish, 1966).

PANCREATIC DIVISION

Surgical transection of the neck of the pancreas has been occasionally used as a method
of exposing portal injuries (Stone, Fabian, and
Turkelson, 1982). This maneuver takes time
and (in the opinion of the authors) is rarely
of value in controlling retropancreatic hemorrhage. Visualization of the anterior aspect
of a portal or superior mesenteric vein injury
is the *only* advantage gained by dividing the
pancreas, and the maneuver has generally
been performed in pursuit of precise lateral
repair of a portal or superior mesenteric
vein injury. It is not clear that this maneuver
is justified unless it represents the mere completion of a traumatic pancreatic fracture,
which would itself have necessitated proximal
or distal pancreatectomy. It is *not* a good
emergency maneuver for hemorrhage
control.

CONTROL OF MULTIPLE
VASCULAR INJURIES

Once the retroperitoneal hematoma has been
entered, the surgeon must be prepared to
immediately control *two or more* major vascular injuries. Clamp control of the portal injury
is often of secondary concern. Great vessel
lacerations deep to the plane of the portal vein
must usually be managed first while the
fingers of an assistant compress the portal
venous injury, behind or above the mobilized
pancreas. Rotation of the duodenum and
pancreatic head during a Kocher maneuver
provides an opportunity for broad manual
compression of the retropancreatic portal vein
and its major tributaries in a plane anterior
to the great vessels of the retroperitoneum.
This *must* provide immediate portal hemorrhage control while deeper and more desperate associated vascular injuries are
addressed.

Definitive Repair

SUPRAPANCREATIC WOUNDS

In the suprapancreatic or hilar portions of the portal vein, precise lateral repair, with or without vein patching, or even vein graft interposition, may be used after proximal and distal control has been obtained. In cases of combined hepatic artery and portal vein wounding, repair of the portal vein, following ligation of the hepatic artery, is generally recommended (Fuller and Anderson, 1978). Reconstruction of a divided bile duct may also be necessary in this location (Sheldon and colleagues, 1985). End-to-end anastomosis of the portal vein in the suprapancreatic zone is generally not feasible because, as has been described by Stone, Fabian, and Turkelson (1982), there is a loss of exposure as the two ends of the vein are brought together. For this reason, interposition saphenous vein grafting may be a wiser choice for the management of a divided suprapancreatic portal in which reconstruction is necessary. Ligation of the portal vein in this location is compatible with survival, provided that the hepatic artery is intact (Fish, 1966; Pachter and colleagues, 1979).

RETROPANCREATIC WOUNDS

Wounds of the retropancreatic confluence zone of the portal vein offer fewer and more difficult options for repair. Although the suprapancreatic portal vein can be fully mobilized and exposed for precise repair, except perhaps in the hilum itself, the situation in the retropancreatic zone is far more challenging. Because of the relatively medial location of the vein, and its fixation to the pancreas by its numerous tributaries, only the posterior aspect of the vein can be visualized by the standard rotation maneuvers. Visualization of the anterior portion of the vein requires transection of the pancreas or full mobilization of the confluence from the numerous, laterally inserting tributaries. Because of these hardships, as well as the near inevitability of major hemorrhage, and the

difficulties of obtaining proximal and distal control in a vessel with so many tributaries, the opportunities for repair are severely limited in wounds of the retropancreatic zone (Stone, Fabian, and Turkelson, 1982). Many authors who have reported lateral "repairs" in this zone have likely often oversewn the vein in a way that amounted to complete or near-complete obliteration of the lumen, not only of the portal vein itself but also of its major tributaries. No major complications have been reported from the use of this approach.

PORTAL VEIN LIGATION

A second approach to devastating wounds in the retropancreatic zone, and an approach that has been found to be life saving by experienced surgeons, is the deliberate and immediate ligation of any portal injury that cannot be easily repaired by lateral suture. Despite the reports from some experienced surgeons that ligation has, in their hands, been associated with a higher mortality than lateral repair (Mattox, Espada, and Beall, 1974; Graham, Mattox, and Beall, 1978; Peterson, Sheldon, and Lim, 1979; Busuttil and colleagues, 1980; Sheldon and colleagues, 1985; Jurkovich and colleagues, 1995), the reported experience does not permit a conclusion that all or any of their purported repairs remained patent, or that any form of repair offered a survival advantage compared to ligation. The best evidence on this subject comes from a large series reported by Stone, Fabian, and Turkelson (1982), in which survival was achieved in 17 of 20 patients in whom immediate portal ligation was carried out "whenever lateral repair was impossible or impractical."

Because the cause of most deaths in portal injury is uncontrolled hemorrhage, the method that provides the quickest definitive control should be preferred. Portal vein repair is desirable, but prolonged efforts to carry out complex venous repair, in the face of continuing blood loss and shock, to avoid ligation, cannot be justified by the existing evidence. In fact, prolonged reconstructive efforts, followed by ligation as a desperation maneuver, may explain why ligation has had a high mortality in some series in which it was rarely employed (Mattox, Espada, and Beall, 1974; Graham, Mattox, and Beall, 1978; Busuttil and colleagues, 1980; Sheldon and colleagues, 1985; Jurkovich and colleagues, 1995), but not in other series in which ligation was done quickly (Stone, Fabian, and Turkelson, 1982).

Although a preponderance of evidence casts doubt on the wisdom of undertaking technically difficult and time-consuming reconstruction of most portal venous injuries, special circumstances make repair of the portal vein necessary. The first is the destruction of the hepatic artery, as alluded to earlier in this chapter. When both of the hepatic inflow vessels are divided, one of them must be repaired to permit survival (Fuller and Anderson, 1978; Sheldon and colleagues, 1985; Jurkovich and colleagues, 1995). Most authors have recommended that the portal vein be reconstructed in this situation. The second circumstance in which portal vein reconstruction might be unavoidable would be an extensive destruction of the potential collateral pathways, in association with transection of the portal vein itself. Under these rare conditions, regardless of difficulty, the portal vein may require reconstruction. Interposition grafting using saphenous vein (Symbas, Foster, and Scott, 1961; Stone, Fabian, and Turkelson, 1982), a segment of transposed splenic vein (Busuttil and colleagues, 1980), or externally supported PTFE to bridge a gap in the portal vein may be technically feasible. Alternatively, the distal end of the splenic vein may be anastomosed to the proximal stump of the superior mesenteric vein (Busuttil and colleagues, 1980) (Fig. 17–9).

Portocaval or mesocaval shunting has been used to provide effluent flow from the intestines following portal vein ligation. Experience with this method has been uniformly unfavorable, with nearly all patients becoming encephalopathic. It should not be considered an acceptable approach to the management of portal or mesenteric vein injuries (Fish, 1966; Stone, Fabian, and Turkelson, 1982).

Postoperative Management

The postoperative care of patients who have undergone portal vein reconstruction or ligation is similar to that of any patient who has suffered abdominal wounding with major vascular injury and hemorrhagic shock. However, certain additional considerations apply to patients who have undergone either portal ligation or a repair of the portal vein in which venous narrowing has led to the threat of repair site thrombosis.

Acute occlusion of the portal vein causes certain predictable effects, which were described by Child and colleagues (1952) in a classic series of experiments carried out a half-century ago and by Milnes and Child (1949). There is a major but transient decrease in systemic blood pressure caused by pooling of blood in the splanchnic viscera, accompanied by a marked elevation of the portal pressure below the ligature or thrombosis. Massive bowel edema is common. The hypotensive effect of portal occlusion can be ameliorated by intravenous volume repletion in an amount sufficient to compensate for blood trapped in the splanchnic veins. The effects of splanchnic venous hypertension resolve as collateral pathways enlarge over a period of days to weeks. Chronic portal hypertension appears to be rare (Pachter and colleagues, 1979).

Any patient who has undergone portal vein ligation or a venous repair that has markedly constricted the portal vein may be expected to have extraordinary fluid requirements in the immediate postoperative period. Replacement of this volume may be best guided with a pulmonary artery catheter. Most will also develop marked bowel edema with some small risk of venous intestinal infarction (Bostwick and Stone, 1975; Pachter and colleagues, 1979; Peterson, Sheldon, and Lim, 1979; Sheldon and colleagues, 1985). In the anticipation of these consequences of portal vein ligation or the acute thrombosis of a repair, consideration may given to skin-only suture of the abdominal wall at the conclusion of the procedure or even the placement of a temporary abdominal wall prosthesis to avoid abdominal compartment syndrome when the bowel edema becomes maximal over the first 24 to

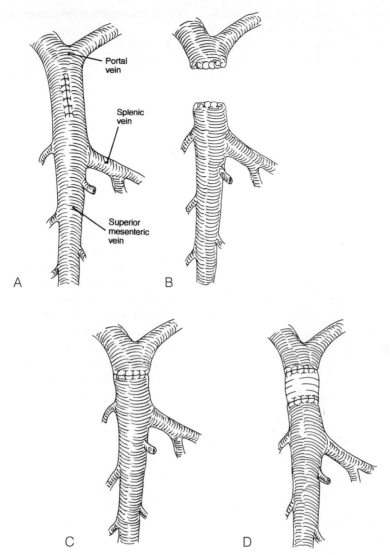

Portal vein

Splenic vein

Superior mesenteric vein

A   B

C   D

■ **FIGURE 17–9**
Four methods of managing portal vein injuries. Of these, only lateral repair *(A)* and ligation *(B)* have been commonly used. End-to-end anastomosis *(C)* and graft *(D)*. (From Buckman RF Jr, Pathak AS, Badellino MM, Bradley KM: Portal vein injuries. Surg Clin North Am 2001;81[6]:1460.) ■

48 hours. The use of a "second-look" procedure to inspect the bowels for viability has been recommended by some (Pachter and colleagues, 1979; Peterson, Sheldon, and Lim, 1979).

Administration of anticoagulants to prevent mesenteric thrombosis is not justified by existing evidence. Follow-up of the portal vein repair using abdominal ultrasound has been recommended (Milnes and Child, 1949).

Summary

Wounds of the portal vein are caused most commonly by penetrating trauma and have a very high mortality. Most deaths are due to exsanguination, occurring intraoperatively as the surgeon struggles to control the hemorrhage from the portal vein and associated vascular injuries. A thorough knowledge of the anatomy of the area and the likely patterns of wounding is important. At operation, the surgeon must be prepared to deal with multiple vessel wounding. Although most authors have advocated lateral repair of the portal vein when it can be accomplished, portal ligation appears to be a safe alternative. Complex repairs are justified only when a contraindication to ligation exists. Postoperative care must recognize the need for extraordinary fluid replacement and the small risk of postoperative bowel infarction following repair or ligation of the portal vein.

REFERENCES

Agarwal N, Shah PM, Clauss RH, et al: Experience with 115 civilian venous injuries. J Trauma 1982;22:827-832.

Aldridge SA, Buckman RF, Badellino MM: Extended patency of intravascular shunts in an experimental model of vascular injury. J Cardiovasc Surg 1997;38:183-186.

Asensio JA, Chahwan S, Hanpeter D, et al: Operative management and outcome of 302 abdominal vascular injuries. Am J Surg 2001;180:528-534.

Baumgartner F, Scudamore C, Nair C, et al: Venovenous bypass for major hepatic and caval trauma. J Trauma 1995;39:671-673.

Beal SL: Fatal hepatic hemorrhage: an unresolved problem in the management of complex liver injuries. J Trauma 1990;30:163-169.

Beal SL, Ward RE: Successful atrial caval shunting in the management of retro-hepatic venous injuries. Am J Surg 1989;158:409-413.

Bostwick J, Stone HH: Trauma to the portal venous system. South Med J 1975;68(11):1369-1372.

Bricker DL, Morton JR, Okies JE, et al: Surgical management of injuries to the vena cava: Changing patterns of injury and newer techniques of repair. J Trauma 1971;11:725-735.

Bricker DL, Wukasch DC: Successful management of an injury to the supra-renal inferior vena cava using an internal vena caval shunt. Surg Clin North Am 1970;50:999-1002.

Buckman RF, Miraliakbari R, Badellino MM: Juxtahepatic venous injuries: A critical review of reported management strategies. J Trauma 2000;48:978-983.

Buckman RF, Pathak AS, Badellino MM, Bradley KM: Injuries of the inferior vena cava. Surg Clin North Am 2001;81(6):1431-1447.

Buechter KJ, Sereda D, Gomez G, Zeppa R: Retrohepatic vein injuries: Experience with 20 cases. J Trauma 1989;29:1698-1704.

Burch JM, Feliciano DV, Mattox KL, Edelman M: Injuries of the inferior vena cava. Am J Surg 1998;156:548-552.

Burns GR, Sherman RT: Trauma of the abdominal aorta and inferior vena cava. Am Surg 1972; 38:303-306.

Busuttil RW, Kitahama A, Cerise E, et al: Management of blunt and penetrating injuries to the porta hepatis. Ann Surg 1980;191(3):641-648.

Caplan BB, Halasz NA, Bloomer WE: Resection and ligation of the supra renal inferior vena cava. J Urol 1964;92:25-29.

Carmona RH, Peck DZ, Lim RC Jr: The role of packing and planned re-operation in severe hepatic trauma. J Trauma 1984;24:779-784.

Cattell RB, Braasch JW: A technique for exposure of the third and fourth portions of the duodenum. Surg Gynecol Obstet 1960;113:379-380.

Child CG III, Holswade GR, McClure RD Jr, et al: Pancreaticoduodenectomy with resection of the portal vein in the Macaca mulatta monkey and in man. Surg Gynecol Obstet 1952;94:31-45.

Chisholm TP, Lenio PT: Traumatic injuries of the portal vein. Am J Surg 1972;124:770-773.

Cogbill TH, Moore EE, Jurkovich GL, et al: Severe hepatic trauma: A multicenter experience with 1335 liver injuries. J Trauma 1998;28:1433-1438.

Cue JL, Cryer HG, Miller FB, et al: Packing and Planned re-exploration for hepatic and retroperitoneal hemorrhage: Critical refinements of a useful technique. J Trauma 1990;30:1007-1013.

Dawson DL, Johansen KH, Jurkovich GJ. Injuries to the portal triad. Am J Surg 1991;161:545-551.

Deitrick J, McNeill P, Posner MP, et al: Traumatic superior mesenteric artery—portal vein fistula. Ann Vasc Surg 1990;4:72-76.

DePinto DJ, Mucha SJ, Powers PC: Major hepatic vein ligation necessitated by blunt abdominal trauma. Ann Surg 1976;183:243-246.

Dingledin GP, Proctor HJ, Jaques PF: Traumatic aorto–caval–portal–duodenal fistula: Case Report. J Trauma 1977;17:474-476.

Douglas BE, Baggenstoss AH, Hollinshead WH: The anatomy of the portal vein and its tributaries. Surg Gynecol Obstet 1950;91:562-576.

Duke JH Jr, Jones RC, Shires GT: Management of injuries to the inferior vena cava. Am J Surg 1965;110:759-763.

Epstein BM, Bocchiola FC, Andrews JC, Bester L: Case report: Traumatic arterio-venous fistula involving the portal venous system. Clin Radiol 1987;38:91-93.

Fabian TC, Croce MA, Stanford GG, et al: Factors affecting morbidity following hepatic trauma: A prospective analysis of 482 injuries. Ann Surg 1991;21:540-548.

Feldman EA: Injury to the hepatic vein. Am J Surg 1996;111:244-246.

Feliciano DV: Approach to major abdominal vascular injury. J Vasc Surg 1988;7:730-735.

Feliciano DV, Bitondo CG, Mattox KL, et al: Civilian trauma in the 1980s. A one-year experience with 456 vascular and cardiac injuries. Ann Surg 1984;199:717-724.

Fish JC: Reconstruction of the portal vein: Case reports and literature review. Am Surgeon 1966;32(7):472-478.

Fullen WD, McDonough JJ, Popp MJ, Altemeier WA: Sternal splitting approach for major hepatic or retrohepatic vena cava injury. J Trauma 1974;14:903-911.

Fuller JW, Anderson PH: Operative management of combined injuries to the portal vein and hepatic artery. South Med J 1978;71:423-424.

Graham JM, Mattox KL, Beall AC: Portal venous system injuries. J Trauma 1978;18:419-422.

Graham JM, Mattox KL, Beall AC Jr, Debakey MD: Traumatic injuries of the inferior vena cava. Arch Surg 1978;113:413-418.

Hartman AR, Yunis J, Frei L, et al: Profound hypothermic circulatory arrest for the management of penetrating retrohepatic venous injury: Case report. J Trauma 1991;31:1310-1311.

Hunt TX, Leeds FH, Wanebo HJ, Blaisdell FW: Arteriovenous fistulas of major vessels in the abdomen. J Trauma 1971;11:483-493.

Ivatury RR, Nallathambi M, Lankin DH, et al: Portal vein injuries. Ann Surg 1987;206(6):733-737.

Jurkovich GJ, Hoyt DB, Moore FA, et al: Portal triad injuries. J Trauma 1995;39(3):426-433.

Kashuk JL, Moore EE, Millikan JS, Moore JB: Major abdominal vascular trauma—A unified approach. J Trauma 1982;22:672-679.

Klein SR, Baumgartner FJ, Bongard FA: Contemporary management strategy for major inferior vena caval injuries. J Trauma 1994;37:35-42.

Kudsk KA, Sheldon GF, Lim RC Jr: Arterial-caval shunting (ACS) after trauma. J Trauma 1982;22:81-85.

Linker RW, Crawford FA Jr, Rittenbury MS, Barton M: Traumatic aorto-cava fistula. J Trauma 1982;22:81-85.

Lumsden AB, Allen RC, Sreeram S, et al: Hepatic arterioportal fistula. Am Surg 1993;59:722-726.

Mattox KL, Espada R, Beall AC: Traumatic injury to the portal vein. Ann Surg 1974;181(5):519-522.

Mattox KL, McCollum WM, Jordon GL, et al: Management of upper abdominal vascular trauma. Am J Surg 1974;128:823-828.

Mattox KL, Whisennand HH, Espada R, Beall AC Jr: Management of acute combined injuries to the aorta and inferior vena cava. Am J Surg 1975;130:720-725.

Milnes RF, Child CG III: Acute occlusion by ligature of the portal vein in the macacus rhesus monkey. Proc Soc Exp Biol Med 1947;70:332-333.

Misra B, Wagner R, Boneval H: Injuries of hepatic veins and retrohepatic vena cava. Am Surg 1983;49:55-60.

Moore FA, Moore EE, Seagraves A: Non-resectional management of major hepatic trauma: An evolving concept. Am J Surg 1985;150:725-729.

Mullins RJ, Lucas CE, Ledgerwood AM: The natural history following venous ligation for civilian injuries. J Trauma 1980;20:737-743.

Nakamura S, Tzuzuki T: Surgical anatomy of the hepatic veins and inferior vena cava. Surg Gynecol Obstet 1981;152:43-50.

Ochsner JL, Crawford ES, Debakey ME: Injuries of the vena cava caused by external trauma. Surgery 1961;49:397-405.

Pachter HL, Drager S, Godfrey N, et al: Traumatic injuries of the portal vein: The role of acute ligation. Ann Surg 1979;189(4):383-385.

Pachter HL, Spencer FC, Hofstetter SR, et al: The management of juxtahepatic venous injuries without an atriocaval shunt: Preliminary clinical observation. Surgery 1986;99:569-575.

Peterson SR, Sheldon GF, Lim RC: Management of portal vein injuries. J Trauma 1979;19(8):616-620.

Quast DC, Shirkey AL, Fitzgerald JB, et al: Surgical correction of injuries of the vena cava: An analysis of sixty-one cases. J Trauma 1965;5:1-10.

Ravikumar S, Stahl WM: Intra-luminal balloon catheter occlusion for major vena cava injuries. J Trauma 1985;25:458-460.

Robb JV, Costa M: Injuries to the great veins of the abdomen. South Afr J Surg 1984;22(4):223-228.

Rovito PF: Atrial caval shunting in blunt hepatic vascular injury. Ann Surg 1987;205:318-321.

Salam A, Stewart MT: New approach to wounds of the aortic bifurcation and inferior vena cava. Surgery 1985;98:105-108.

Sharp KW, Locicero RJ: Abdominal packing for surgically uncontrollable hemorrhage. Ann Surg 1992;215:467-474.

Sheldon GF, Lim RC, Yee ES, et al: Management of injuries to the porta hepatis. Ann Surg 1985;202(5):539-545.

Shrock T, Blaisdell W, Mathewson C Jr: Management of blunt trauma to the liver and hepatic veins. Arch Surg 1968;96:698-704.

Smith CR, Northrop CH: Stab wound causing mesenteric-portal arteriovenous fistula: An unusual case with a spontaneous closure. J Trauma 1976;16:408-410.

Starzl TH, Kaupp HA, Beheler EM, et al: The treatment of penetrating wounds of the inferior vena cava. Surgery 1962;51:195-204.

Stone HH, Fabian TC, Turkelson ML: Wounds of the portal venous system. World J Surg 1982;6:335-341.

Stone HH, Lamb JM: Use of pedicled omentum as an autogenous pack for control hemorrhage in major injuries to the liver. Surg Gynecol Obstet 1975;141:92-94.

Symbas PN, Foster JH, Scott HW: Experimental vein grafting in the portal venous system. Surgery 1961;50:97-106.

Weichert RF, Hewitt RL: Injuries to the inferior vena cava: report of 35 cases. J Trauma 1970;10:649-657.

Wiencek RG, Wilson RF: Abdominal venous injuries. J Trauma 1986;26:771-778.

Yellin AE, Chaffee CB, Donovan AJ: Vascular isolation in the treatment of juxtahepatic venous injuries. Arch Surg 1971;102:566-573.

18

Iliac Vessel Injuries

DEMETRIOS DEMETRIADES
JAMES A. MURRAY
JUAN A. ASENSIO

INTRODUCTION

Iliac vessel injuries are among some of the most lethal injuries sustained by trauma patients. Their complex anatomy and the often associated injuries, particularly to the gastrointestinal and genitourinary structures, may challenge the skills of even the most experienced trauma surgeons. Rapid transport to

339

a trauma center, prompt recognition of the injury, good knowledge of the local anatomy, and sound surgical judgment remain the cornerstone for survival.

ANATOMY

The abdominal aorta bifurcates at approximately the level of the fourth and fifth lumbar vertebra into two common iliac arteries. The level of the bifurcation corresponds roughly to the level of the umbilicus. The common iliac arteries course inferiorly and laterally through the pelvis and divide at the level of the sacroiliac joint into the internal and external iliac arteries. The ureter crosses over the bifurcation of the common iliac artery. The external iliac artery courses along the pelvis, exiting anteriorly beneath the inguinal ligament to become the common femoral artery. The internal iliac artery provides blood supply to the pelvic viscera. It divides at the level of the sciatic notch into anterior and posterior divisions. The anterior division includes the vesicular, obturator, pudendal, and inferior gluteal branches. The main posterior division includes the iliolumbar, superior gluteal, and lateral sacral branches.

The common iliac veins join at the level of the fifth lumbar vertebra to form the inferior vena cava. The confluence of the two veins occurs below the level of the aortic bifurcation and behind the right common iliac artery (Fig. 18–1). The left common iliac vein courses behind and medial to the left common iliac artery. The right common iliac vein passes inferiorly behind the junction of the right external iliac and the right internal iliac artery. This anatomic arrangement makes combined arterial venous injuries common and complicates the exposure of the right common iliac vein.

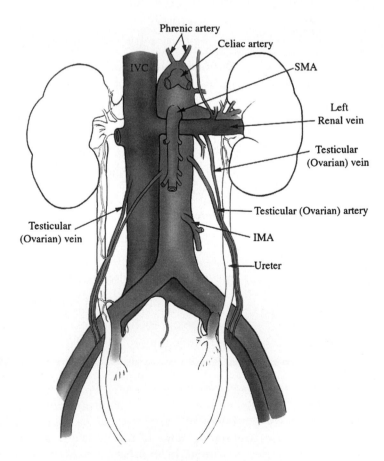

■ **FIGURE 18–1**
Anatomy of the iliac vessels. Note the confluence of the two common iliac veins behind the right iliac artery and the relationship of the ureter with the bifurcation of the common iliac artery. ■

TABLE 18–1

INCIDENCE OF ILIAC VESSEL INJURIES IN PATIENTS UNDERGOING LAPAROTOMY FOR TRAUMA

Mech-anism of Injury	No. of Laparotomies	Patients with Iliac Vessel Injuries (%)	Patients with Iliac Artery Injuries (%)	Patients with Iliac Vein Injuries (%)	Combined Artery-Vein Injuries (%)
Gunshot wound	1310	131 (10)	64 (5)	67 (5)	35 (2.7)
Stab wound	638	12 (2)	6 (1)	6 (1)	2 (0.3)
Blunt trauma	633	33 (5.5)	30 (5)	3 (0.5)	1 (0.2)

From USC Trauma Center, 1993-2000. Unpublished trauma registry data.

Each common iliac vein is formed by the junction of an internal and external iliac vein. The external iliac vein accompanies the external iliac artery, and the internal iliac vein is formed by numerous small and delicate tributaries.

INCIDENCE AND EPIDEMIOLOGY

Though uncommon, iliac vessel injuries are not necessarily rare in busy urban trauma centers. The incidence of iliac artery injury varies depending on the setting. During World War II DeBakey and Simeone (1946) reported 43 iliac arterial injuries in 2471 patients for an incidence of 1.7%. Both Hughes (1958) during the Korean conflict and Rich, Baugh, and Hughes (1970) during the Vietnam conflict reported incidences of 2.3% and 2.6%, respectively.

Iliac vessel injuries are reported with greater frequency from the civilian arena. The incidence of iliac vascular injuries in patients undergoing laparotomy for trauma at the University of Southern California trauma center is shown in Table 18–1. Overall, the incidence of iliac vessel injuries is 10% for gunshot wounds, 2% for stab wounds, and 5.5% in blunt trauma. In a recent survey at an urban level I trauma center, Bongard (1990) reported that iliac arterial injuries represented only 10% of abdominal vascular injuries and less than 2% of all vascular trauma. Mattox and col-

leagues (1989), in a series of 5760 cardiovascular injuries in 4459 patients, reported 232 iliac artery and 289 iliac venous injuries, for an overall incidence of 12% of patients or 9% of cardiovascular injuries. In a series of 504 abdominal vascular injuries from the Los Angeles County and University of Southern California trauma center, there were 112 iliac vessel injuries (22% of all abdominal vascular injuries).

Burch and colleagues (1990) in a series of 233 patients sustaining iliac vessel injuries reported that the common iliac artery was the most frequently injured vessel, with an incidence of 40%, and both external and internal iliac arteries accounted for 30% of these injuries. In the venous system, the common iliac vein was the most frequently injured vessel (48%), the external iliac vein was injured in 32% of the patients, and the internal iliac vein accounted for 20% of the venous injuries. In this series, Burch and colleagues (1990) reported a 70% incidence of combined arteriovenous injuries.

In contrast to penetrating injuries, blunt trauma usually involves the internal iliac vessels and their branches. Injury to the common or external iliac artery following blunt trauma is not common, although there are several case reports. The usual mechanism is stretching of the vessel over the pelvic wall, resulting in intimal tear and possibly thrombosis (Fig. 18–2). In addition, direct laceration of a vessel may occur from a bone fragment.

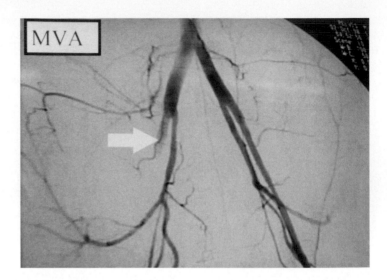

■ FIGURE 18–2
Blunt trauma with pelvic fracture. The patient had an absent femoral pulse. Angiography shows occlusion of the right common iliac artery. ■

CLINICAL PRESENTATION

Penetrating injuries to the lower abdomen, hips, or buttock, especially in the presence of shock, should prompt suspicion of an associated iliac vessel injury. Some of the signs and symptoms associated with these injuries include hemorrhagic shock, abdominal distention, and absent or diminished femoral pulse. Additional evidence of injury to the pelvic viscera such as gross hematuria or evidence of rectal injuries should heighten concerns for the presence of iliac vascular injury. In most cases the diagnosis of vascular injury is made intraoperatively.

Blunt injuries to the iliac arteries are typically but not always associated with pelvic fractures. Absent or diminished femoral pulse is highly suggestive of injury to the common or external iliac arteries. Hemorrhage is typically due to injury to the branches of the internal iliac vessels. These patients may demonstrate signs and symptoms of severe hemorrhagic shock upon initial presentation requiring aggressive resuscitation. Other patients may present with gradual and persistent bleeding. Both these scenarios require exclusion of intraperitoneal hemorrhage. In the absence of intraperitoneal hemorrhage or peritonitis, these patients should undergo immediate angiographic evaluation and possibly embolization. In rare occasions with blunt trauma, an arterial intimal tear may remain undetected during the initial hospitalization, only to manifest at a later stage with signs of leg ischemia due to secondary thrombosis.

In patients with suspected pelvic fractures, a thorough physical examination can determine the stability of the pelvis by examining the anterior, lateral, and posterior components of the pelvic ring. Injudicious and repeated examinations can exacerbate bleeding and lead to life-threatening hemorrhage. Therefore once a patient has been noted to have an unstable pelvis by one examiner, further examinations by other physicians are contraindicated. Radiographic examination of the pelvis to confirm the clinical diagnosis should follow expeditiously and measures to stabilize the pelvis should be promptly instituted. Early application of a pelvic binder or external pelvic fixation may contain the expansion of the pelvic hematoma and reduce bleeding (Fig. 18–3).

DIAGNOSTIC INVESTIGATIONS

Radiographic Studies

Radiographic evaluation of penetrating injuries to the abdomen should be performed only if the patient is hemodynamically fairly stable. These investigations may include a

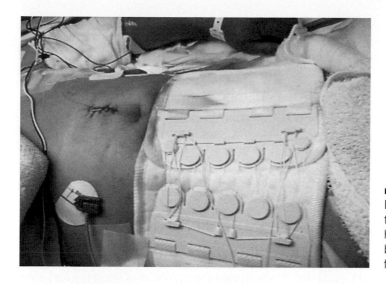

■ **FIGURE 18–3**
Pelvic binder may contain
the expansion of a pelvic
hematoma and reduce
bleeding from a pelvic
fracture. ■

plain radiograph of the abdomen and pelvis. The presence of missiles or fragments in the pelvis, especially in the presence of hypotension, should prompt the physician to suspect injury to the iliac vessels (Fig. 18–4). In blunt trauma, radiographic findings from the pelvis known to be associated with increased risk of bleeding from the internal iliac vessels include the presence of symphysis pubis diastasis of greater than 2.5 cm, sacroiliac joint disruption, and the presence of superior and inferior rami fractures bilaterally ("butterfly fracture"). In our center these patients undergo early angiographic embolization before hemodynamic decompensation and massive transfusions are required.

COMPUTED TOMOGRAPHY

Computed tomography continues to play a major role in the evaluation of hemodynamically stable blunt trauma patients. The presence of a significant pelvic hematoma is suggestive of an injury to the internal iliac vessels or their branches. Extravasation of intravenous contrast is diagnostic of arterial bleeding or false aneurysm and requires

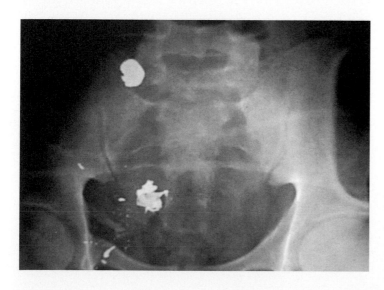

■ **FIGURE 18–4**
Missiles in the pelvis on
radiographs, especially in the
presence of shock, are
suggestive of iliac vessel
injury. ■

prompt angiographic evaluation and possibly embolization. Lack of contrast opacifying the lumen of the major iliac vessels is consistent with thrombosis and should be investigated further with angiography to confirm the diagnosis, provided the extremity does not appear threatened by ischemia. If the extremity appears compromised, prompt surgical exploration should be performed.

ANGIOGRAPHY

Angiography has dramatically improved the management of patients with hemorrhage from pelvic fractures secondary to blunt trauma. It should be considered early in patients with clinical evidence of severe bleeding from the pelvis (low hematocrit or hypotension) as soon as intraperitoneal bleeding or peritonitis has been ruled out. Similarly, the presence of extravasation of intravenous contrast on computed tomographic scan or certain radiographic findings on plain pelvic films (pubis diastasis >2.5 cm, major sacroiliac joint disruption, and "butterfly" fracture) should prompt the surgeon to seek an early angiogram. It is critical that during angiography the patient is closely monitored and resuscitated continuously under the supervision of a senior member of the trauma team.

Angiography is able to identify the site and severity of bleeding and control bleeding with embolization. Additionally, it may identify occlusions or major intimal tears of the common or external iliac arteries that require operative intervention. If massive hemorrhage from a major artery is identified at the time of angiographic evaluation, temporary control of the bleeding may be achieved with an intraluminal balloon while the patient is transported to the operating room (Fig. 18–5).

OPERATIVE MANAGEMENT

The operative findings depend on the mechanism of injury, associated injuries, and the nature of vascular injury. In blunt trauma the usual finding is a zone 3 retroperitoneal hematoma, which may or may not be pulsatile or expanding. However, in some cases with intimal tear and thrombosis, often there is a small or even no local hematoma and the injury may be missed. A zone 3 retroperitoneal hematoma resulting from blunt trauma should not be explored routinely. Exploration is indicated only if there is a suspicion of iliac artery injury—that is, absent or diminished femoral pulse.

In penetrating iliac vessel injuries upon entering the abdominal cavity, the surgeon may encounter free intraperitoneal bleeding, a zone 3 hematoma, or a combination of both. It is an important surgical principle that all

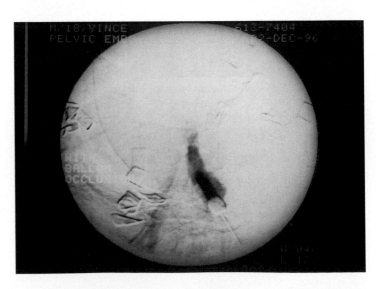

■ **FIGURE 18–5**
Motor vehicle accident with severe pelvic fracture. Angiography showed massive bleeding from the left common iliac artery. Balloon occlusion of the injured artery achieved temporary control of the bleeding and the patient was taken to the operating room. ■

zone 3 hematomas caused by penetrating trauma be explored.

Arterial Injuries

Any active bleeding is controlled initially by direct compression and subsequently by proximal and distal vascular control. The iliac vessels may be exposed by direct dissection of the peritoneum over the vessels or by dissection of the paracolic peritoneum and medial rotation of the right or left colon. Care should be taken to avoid injury to the ureter, which crosses over the bifurcation of the common iliac artery.

The anatomic level of proximal control depends on the site of bleeding and the site and size of the hematoma. For suspected iliac artery injuries near the bifurcation of the aorta, proximal arterial control may be achieved with aortic cross clamping above the bifurcation. In more distal external iliac artery injuries, proximal control can be achieved by applying a vessel tape around the common iliac artery. During the dissection, care should be taken to avoid accidental injury to the underlying vein, especially the right common iliac vein. Isolation and control of the internal iliac artery is essential because the bleeding may continue despite proximal and distal control. The identification and isolation of the internal iliac artery can be facilitated by retracting the vascular tapes proximally and distally and dissecting toward the middle until the vessel is identified. A similar technique of gradual dissection of the vessel and progressive movement of the vascular clamps toward the injury can be used in cases with active bleeding or large hematoma, in which a direct approach to the injured site may be difficult. If the exposure of the distal iliac vessels is difficult, especially in men with a narrow pelvis, extending the midline incision by adding a transverse lower abdominal incision may be necessary. In some cases with bleeding from the vessels near the groin or in the presence of a large hematoma, distal control can be facilitated by a longitudinal incision over the groin and division of the inguinal ligament.

Small common or external iliac artery injuries can be managed by primary repair, using a 4-0 or 5-0 vascular suture and taking care to avoid significant stenosis. In the appropriate cases a venous or PTFE patch may be necessary to avoid stenosis at the repair site. This patch should not be excessive in size in order to avoid aneurysmal dilation. In more extensive injuries, especially in gunshot wounds or blunt trauma in which débridement is always necessary, an end-to-end anastomosis with or without a prosthetic graft (size 6 or 8 PTFE) may be required. It is strongly recommended that all vascular repairs are performed under loupe magnification. Local heparin (20 to 30 mL of solution of 100 units of heparin per 100 mL) should be administered to prevent thrombosis during the vascular repair. A balloon-tipped catheter should always be passed in the distal arterial tree to remove any clots.

More complex procedures, such as extra-anatomic femorofemoral bypass or mobilization and use of the internal iliac artery to replace the external iliac artery, are time consuming and often technically difficult. Extra-anatomic bypasses may be necessary in patients with severe purulent peritonitis. Burch performed six extra-anatomic bypasses with poor results, including three deaths, three amputations, three compartment syndrome, and two graft thrombosis. The existing evidence suggests that the presence of enteric contamination is not a contraindication for an end-to-end repair or a PTFE interposition graft. In a study of 358 penetrating iliac vascular injuries, Burch reported that in general associated gastrointestinal or urologic injuries did not influence the management of vascular injuries. However, many surgeons still suggest that in the presence of significant enteric contamination, an extra-anatomic bypass should be performed. Any enteric spillage should be controlled first and the peritoneum cleaned meticulously before any vascular repair is performed. The peritoneum should be closed over the graft whenever possible.

Ligation of the common or external iliac artery should never be considered, even in the most critically injured patients. Ligation is poorly tolerated and in most cases results

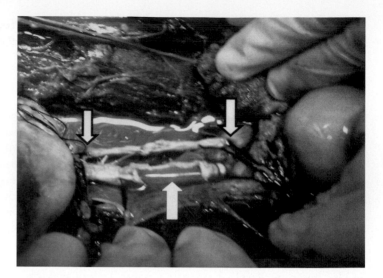

■ **FIGURE 18–6**
Injuries to the right iliac artery and vein. Because of the critical condition of the patient, the vein was ligated *(white and black arrows)* and the artery was shunted with a catheter *(white arrow).* Definitive arterial reconstruction was performed 24 hours later. ■

in ischemia of the leg and in about 50% of patients limb loss. The ischemia may aggravate the general condition of the patient by release of toxic metabolites into the systemic circulation. Subsequent attempts to re-establish blood flow may be even more dangerous because of reperfusion injury. In the critically ill, hypothermic, and coagulopathic patient, a temporary intraluminal shunt with semielective reconstruction of the artery at a later stage should be considered (Fig. 18–6). The fastest and cheapest way to construct a shunt is from a sterile intravenous or nasogastric tube. The shunt is secured in place with proximal and distal ligatures. The incidence of thrombosis of the shunt is high, and the peripheral pulses and perfusion should be monitored closely. Systemic anticoagulation prophylaxis is usually contraindicated because of associated coagulopathy.

Venous Injuries

Iliac venous injuries may be technically more challenging than arterial injuries because of the more difficult surgical exposure and the risk of air embolism. The anatomic location of the right common iliac vein and the confluence of the two common iliac veins behind the right common iliac

artery may make exposure a challenging task, especially in elderly patients with atherosclerosis and adhesions between the artery and vein. These difficulties have led some authors to recommend transection of the overlying iliac artery. We believe that such a drastic approach is excessive and should rarely be considered. As a rule, satisfactory surgical exposure of the vein can be achieved by meticulous and adequate mobilization and retraction of the artery with vessel tapes. Ligation and division of the internal iliac artery may also facilitate exposure.

Repair of iliac venous injuries should always be considered in cases in which it can be performed by lateral venorrhaphy without producing major stenosis. This is usually possible in more than 50% of cases. The management of complex venous injuries, which cannot be repaired by lateral venorrhaphy, is a controversial issue. Burch, in a study that included 192 iliac venous injuries, performed only one PTFE reconstruction on a patient with external iliac vein injury. Repair associated with severe stenosis may result in thrombosis and possibly pulmonary embolism. In these cases, ligation of the vein may be preferable to repair. Burch reported two cases with fatal embolism in a group of 82 patients with common or external iliac vein injuries treated with repair but none in 43 patients treated with ligation.

Although theoretically a caval filter may prevent pulmonary embolism, there is no published clinical experience. The proponents of ligation argue that complex repair with spiral graft or other methods is time consuming and increases blood loss, and that there is no evidence of any improved outcome. Ligation is usually tolerated very well by almost all patients. Most patients develop transient leg edema, which responds well to elevation and elastic bandage wrapping. However, in some cases ligation results in massive edema and extremity compartment syndrome. In some extreme cases with massive leg and scrotal edema, we had to re-operate and re-establish the continuity of the vein with a prosthetic graft.

The management of complex iliac vein injuries becomes even more controversial in patients with associated iliac artery injuries. Some surgeons have suggested that venous repair may protect the arterial repair by avoiding venous hypertension. However, many others challenge this concept and advocate ligation. These major injuries are usually associated with severe blood loss, and any complex procedures prolonging the operation may increase mortality. We believe that the decision to repair or ligate the vein should be individualized according to the condition of the patient and the nature of the venous injury.

Adjunct Measures for Bleeding Control

In some cases bleeding may persist even after repair or ligation of the iliac vessels. The source of bleeding is usually from deep vascular branches to the pelvic wall or the sacrum. Opening of the presacral fascia is ill-advised and often aggravates the bleeding. Damage control by packing, followed by postoperative angiographic embolization, should be considered at an early stage. Carillo and colleagues (1998) reported significantly reduced mortality in patients with iliac vascular injuries undergoing abbreviated laparotomy and damage control.

Bleeding from a gunshot wound involving the bony pelvis can be troublesome and difficult to control. In these cases we have successfully used Foley catheter balloon tamponade. The balloon is inflated in the bone defect and the distal end of the catheter is brought outside the abdominal cavity through a small skin incision (Fig. 18–7). A gentle traction on the catheter is maintained by a clamp applied to the catheter just above the skin. The clamp is removed and the balloon is deflated 2 or 3 days postoperatively, and if no bleeding occurs through the catheter, the Foley catheter is pulled out.

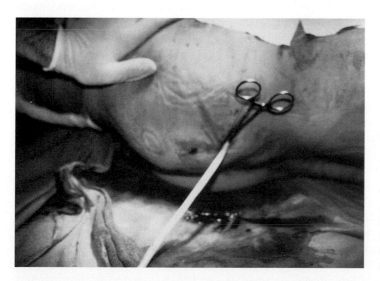

■ **FIGURE 18–7**
Foley catheter balloon tamponade of persistent bleeding from the posterior wall of the pelvis following a gunshot wound. The catheter is exiting through the left buttock. The balloon was removed 4 days later without any recurrent bleeding. ■

Fasciotomy

Therapeutic leg fasciotomy in patients with extremity compartment syndrome should be performed without any delay, even before reconstruction or shunting of any arterial injury. However, the role of liberal prophylactic fasciotomy is controversial. Although some authors advocate prophylactic fasciotomies in all patients with delayed arterial reconstruction or venous ligation, especially in combined arteriovenous injuries, many others practice a policy of "fasciotomy on demand." These authors suggest that fasciotomy is a procedure associated with significant complications and inferior cosmetic results and should be performed only for therapeutic purposes. In a study of 94 patients with fasciotomies for trauma, Velmahos and colleagues (1997) reported local complications in 42% of patients with prophylactic fasciotomies. In 57% of these patients, primary closure of the wounds was not possible and there was a need of skin grafting. If an expectant policy is selected, the patient should be monitored very closely with frequent clinical examinations and measurements of compartment pressures in the appropriate cases. Fasciotomy should be performed with the first signs of compartment syndrome.

PERIOPERATIVE MANAGEMENT

To avoid reperfusion injury following revascularization of the extremity, the surgeon must maintain good hydration and diuresis during the operation and the first few hours postoperatively. In hemodynamically stable patients, administration of mannitol (0.5 g/kg of body weight over 20 minutes) has many beneficial effects because of its oxygen free radical scavenger, rheologic, and osmotic properties. There is evidence that early administration of mannitol blunts the effects of reperfusion injury, reduces the risk of extremity compartment syndrome and the need for fasciotomy, and improves the microcirculation of tissues. It is our practice to administer a second dose 4 to 6 hours after injury.

Mannitol is contraindicated in hypotensive patients because its diuretic effect may aggravate the hypotension. There is also concern that the vasodilating and rheologic properties of mannitol may increase bleeding in patients with active uncontrolled hemorrhage.

The role of postoperative anticoagulation in uncomplicated vascular repairs or in venous ligations is not clear. Some authors use low-molecular-weight heparin prophylaxis for the first few days, followed by aspirin for the next few weeks. In patients with venous thrombosis after repair, oral anticoagulation should be given for at least 3 months.

In venous injuries treated by ligation, it is important to elevate the leg, apply early compression elastic bandages, and monitor closely for extremity compartment syndrome.

Role of Interventional Radiology

Diagnostic angiography has a limited role in the preoperative evaluation of penetrating abdominal trauma. However, it may play a useful therapeutic role postoperatively in patients with incomplete hemostasis from deep iliac artery branches. In blunt trauma angiography may play a major diagnostic and therapeutic role. It remains the most useful investigation for the diagnosis of iliac artery thrombosis or bleeding following blunt trauma to the abdomen or pelvis. Bleeding from peripheral branches may be effectively controlled by embolization in most patients (Fig. 18–8). In cases with major bleeding from the iliac artery, the interventional radiologist may be able to achieve temporary control by inflating an intraluminal balloon at the site of injury until surgical control is achieved in the operating room (Fig. 18–5).

Angiographically placed stents have an important role in selected cases with iliac artery injuries. Patients with false aneurysms, arteriovenous fistulas, or significant intimal tears may benefit from this procedure. Stenting should not be attempted during the acute stage in patients with a thrombosed iliac artery, because of the risk of clot dislodgement and major hemorrhage in cases with a transected vessel. However, angiographic stenting may

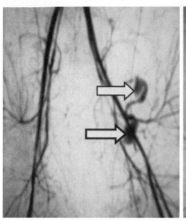
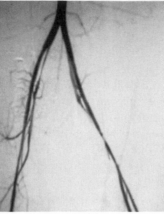

■ FIGURE 18-8
Patient with severe pelvic fracture and major blood loss. Angiography shows two areas of significant bleeding *(arrows)*, which were successfully controlled by embolization *(right frame)*. ■

be a good option in patients with late iliac artery thrombosis. In most cases a skillful interventional radiologist may be able to pass a guidewire through the clot and deploy a stent (Fig. 18–9).

Complications

Complications directly related to the vascular injuries may appear early during the initial hospitalization or late. The overall incidence of early vascular complications in patients surviving for more than 24 hours is about 15% for arterial injuries and 12% for venous injuries.

Thrombosis of the repaired artery remains the most common early arterial complication. The most important factors for early thrombosis are the technique and the use of prosthetic grafts. Burch reported no thrombosis in 25 patients with lateral suturing of the iliac artery. On the other hand, 25% of 16 PTFE grafts and 33% of 6 extra-anatomic bypasses thrombosed. Good surgical techniques, Fogarty balloon exploration and extraction of any clots from the peripheral arteries, intraoperative local heparinization, and liberal use of on-table angiography may reduce the incidence of early failure of the arterial repair. Postoperatively, the peripheral pulses and perfusion should always be monitored closely and

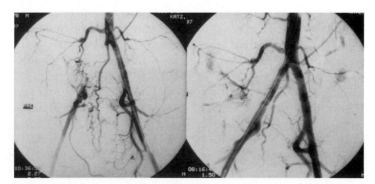

■ FIGURE 18-9
An 18-year-old patient presenting with intermittent claudication many months after a major car accident for which he required a splenectomy and small bowel resection. Angiography revealed occlusion of the right common iliac artery *(left frame)*. The occlusion was successfully stented by interventional radiology *(right frame)*. ■

emergency reoperation should be considered in patients with evidence of arterial thrombosis.

Early postoperative bleeding is another fairly common problem. Bleeding during the first few hours after the operation may be due to a technical problem with the suture line, missed bleeding from a small vessel, or medical bleeding resulting from coagulopathy. Depending on the rate of bleeding and the coagulation status of the patient, reoperation may be necessary. Delayed bleeding a few days after the initial procedure, especially in the presence of other signs of infection, such as fever or leucocytosis, may be due to local sepsis and is an ominous sign. Infection of the repaired vessel, especially in the presence of a prosthetic graft, is a life-threatening complication. The controversies regarding the role of prosthetic grafts in a grossly contaminated field have already been discussed. Early recognition of the infection and aggressive antibiotic treatment may salvage the graft. However, in advanced sepsis, especially in the presence of bleeding, reoperation with removal of the graft and ligation of the vessel combined with an extra-anatomic bypass remain the only option.

The overall incidence and nature of early venous complications following iliac vein injury depend on the extent of venous injury and method of management. Generally, lateral repairs are associated with a lower incidence of venous complications than venous ligations (5% vs. 25% in the series by Burch). Transient leg edema following ligation of the common or external iliac vein is by far the most common complication. The edema can be avoided or minimized by elevation and elastic wraps of the leg. Occasionally, the swelling is so severe that it results in extremity compartment syndrome, requiring fasciotomy.

Deep venous thrombosis may occur in patients treated by ligation of the iliac vein or in cases with thrombosis of the repaired vein. The real incidence of early deep venous thrombosis is not known because no study has ever evaluated systematically all patients with iliac venous injuries. It has been suggested that anticoagulation prophylaxis and elastic wrap on the leg should be used in all patients with venous injuries.

The most dangerous complication following iliac venous injury is pulmonary embolism. Patients with repair producing major venous stenosis are at risk of pulmonary embolism. Earlier military experience suggested that venous repairs may be associated with a high incidence of pulmonary embolism, especially if the lumen is narrowed more than 50%. More recent civilian experience reported an incidence of about 2% of fatal pulmonary embolism in patients treated with venous repair. The role of prophylactic inferior vena cava filters and long-term anticoagulation has not been studied. It might be appropriate to use these modalities in cases with major stenosis of the vein.

The incidence of late complications following iliac vascular trauma is not known. All existing studies are retrospective and lack systematic late follow-up. Late iliac artery complications include false aneurysm and arterial stenosis associated with intermittent claudication or a threatened limb. The method of treatment of these complications, such as open surgery or angiographically placed stents, should be individualized according to the age of the victim, the nature of the arterial pathology, and the experience of the trauma center.

Late venous complications may include chronic venous insufficiency with leg edema and skin ulcers. The incidence of this complication is not known, and the reported figures from existing retrospective studies may be misleading, because those patients returning for late follow-up are usually the symptomatic ones. There is evidence that late venous complications are more likely to occur in patients treated with iliac vein ligation than in patients with lateral repair. Mullins suggested that iliac vein ligation does not often result in chronic venous complications, especially if elevation of the leg is instituted immediately after surgery. The rationale for this practice is that elevation may interrupt the cascade of events, which lead the vascular damage during the critical postinjury period. It certainly makes sense to elevate the leg and apply elastic wraps in these cases, but there is no proven evidence of any benefit.

Mortality

The mortality of iliac vascular injuries is high and depends on the type of vascular trauma (contained or free bleeding), the presence of other associated injuries, the clinical condition of the patient on admission, and the experience of the trauma team.

The mortality of patients undergoing emergency department thoracotomy is almost 100%, with only very few survivors reported. The reported overall mortality varies from 30% to 50% in arterial injuries and 25% to 40% in venous injuries. In isolated vascular injuries, the mortality is about 20% for arterial injuries and about 10% for venous injuries.

REFERENCES

Asensio JA, Chahwan S, Hanpeter D, et al: Operative management and outcome of 302 abdominal vascular injuries. Am J Surg 2000;180: 528-534.

Asensio JA, Lejarraga M: Abdominal vascular injuries. In Demetriades D, Asensio JA (eds): Trauma Management. Georgetown, Tex, Landes BioScience, 2000, pp 356-362.

Asensio JA, Petrone P, Roldan G, et al: Analysis of 185 iliac vessel injuries: Risk factors and predictors of outcome. Arch Surg 2003;138(11): 1187-1193.

Bongard FS, Dubrow T, Klein SR: Vascular injuries in the urban battleground: Experience at a metropolitan trauma center. Ann Vasc Surg 1990;4:415-418.

Burch JM, Richardson RJ, Martin RR, Mattox KL: Penetrating iliac vascular injuries: Recent experience with 233 consenting patients. J Trauma 1990;30:1450.

Carillo EH, WohPtmann CD, Spain DA, et al: Common and external iliac artery injuries associated with pelvic fractures. J Orthop Trauma 1999;13:351-355.

Carillo EH, Spain DA, Wilson MA, et al: Alternatives in the management of penetrating injuries to the iliac vessels. J Trauma 1998;44:1024-1030.

DeBakey ME, Simeone FA: Battle injuries of the arteries in World War II: An analysis of 2,471 cases. Ann Surg 1946;123:534-579.

Degiannis E, Velmahos G, Levy R, et al: Penetrating injuries of the iliac arteries: A South Africa experience. Surgery 1996;119:146-150.

Feliciano DV, Mattox KL, Graham JM, Bitondo CA: Five-year experience with PTFE grafts in vascular wounds. J Trauma 1985;25:75.

Haan J, Rodriguez A, Chiu W: Operative management and outcome of iliac vessel injury: A ten-year experience. Am Surg 2003;69(7):581-586.

Hughes CW: Arterial repair during the Korean War. Ann Surg 1958;147:555-561.

Rich NM, Baugh JH, Hughes CW. Acute arterial injuries in Vietnam: 1,000 cases. J Trauma, 1970:359-369.

Mattox KL: Penetrating injuries to the iliac arteries. Am J Surg 1978;135:663.

Mattox KL, Feliciano DV, Burch J, et al: Five thousand seven hundred and sixty cardiovascular injuries in 4,459 patients. Epidemiologic evolution. Ann Surg 1989;209(6):698-707.

Rogers FB, Cipolle MD, Velmahos G, et al: Practice management guidelines for the prevention of venous thromboembolism in trauma patients: The EAST practice management guidelines work group. J Trauma 2002;53(1):142-164.

Velmahos GC, Theodorou D, Demetriades D, et al: Complications and nonclosure rates of fasciotomy for trauma and related risk factors. World J Surg 1997;21:247-253.

Extremity Vascular Trauma

MICHAEL J. SISE
STEVEN R. SHACKFORD

OVERVIEW OF EXTREMITY VASCULAR TRAUMA

Vascular trauma of the extremities is a highly morbid injury that is becoming more common. Improved prehospital management and regionalization of trauma care with rapid transport have increased the number of these injuries seen at trauma centers in the last 3 decades. Patients who previously died in the field or in transit because of severe isolated peripheral vascular injuries or multiple injuries with associated vascular trauma are now presenting alive.

Successful management of extremity vascular trauma is based on early diagnosis and prompt treatment. The severity of injury and the length of time until restoration of perfusion are the major determinants of outcome. The management strategy must focus on minimizing the duration of ischemia to maximize the chance of successful recovery and rehabilitation. The often insidious nature of extremity vascular trauma significantly increases the opportunity for errors in management. Clinically relevant and practical protocols for both diagnosis and treatment are the best tools for avoiding these errors and ensuring the best possible outcome.

Clinical Presentation

Extremity vascular trauma may be immediately apparent on presentation because of external hemorrhage, hematoma, or obvious limb ischemia. A history of penetrating trauma associated with hypotension, pulsatile bleeding, or a large quantity of blood at the scene suggests potential vascular injury. Blunt trauma is also capable of causing significant vascular injury that can be overlooked when serious head, chest, or abdominal injuries are present (Fig. 19–1).

Peripheral neurologic deficit should alert the examining physician to a possible vascular injury. The deficit may be due to direct injury of a nerve in close anatomic proximity to an artery, or it may be the result of advanced ischemia.

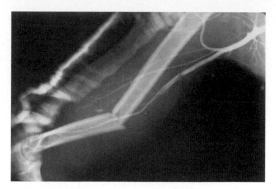

■ **FIGURE 19–1**
Brachial artery occlusion secondary to distal shaft of humerus fracture in patient with multiple injuries. Shown are *(arrows)* collateral flow filling distal brachial artery. Absent pulse and low forearm systolic pressure prompted arteriography. A saphenous vein interposition graft was required to repair this lacerated and contused artery. ■

Diagnosis

A thorough history and careful physical examination of the extremities for signs of vascular injury are the first and most important steps in making the diagnosis of extremity vascular trauma. Careful inspection of the injured sites, examination of wounds, sensory and motor assessment, and pulse examination must be part of the extremity physical examination. The presence of a hematoma, bruit, or thrill must be noted. If distal pulses are diminished or absent, ankle or wrist systolic blood pressure should be determined with a continuous-wave Doppler device and compared with the normal side. A significant difference in systolic blood pressure (>10 mm Hg) between extremities may be an indication of vascular injury. Duplex scanning of the extremities has no role in the acute evaluation of extremity vascular trauma.

Patients with "hard signs" of vascular injury (Table 19–1) should be taken directly to the operating room. In less straightforward cases, arteriography may be indicated to rule out the need for operation. Arteriography is limited to suspected extremity vascular trauma when no clear indication for immediate operative therapy is present or when evidence of peripheral ischemia and multiple sites of

TABLE 19–1
"HARD" AND "SOFT" SIGNS OF VASCULAR INJURY

Hard	Indicate need for operative intervention
	Pulsatile bleeding
	Expanding hematoma
	Palpable thrill
	Audible bruit
	Evidence of regional ischemia
	Pallor
	Paresthesia
	Paralysis
	Pain
	Pulselessness
	Poikilothermia
Soft	Suggest need for further evaluation
	History of moderate hemorrhage
	Injury (fracture, dislocation, or penetrating wound)
	Diminished but palpable pulse
	Peripheral nerve deficit

injury in an extremity exist (e.g., a shotgun injury with multiple pellet wounds) (Fig. 19–2). Arteriography is both sensitive and specific in the diagnosis of extremity vascular injuries. However, arteriography is time consuming, and successful management of these injuries requires prompt control of hemorrhage and a timely restoration of adequate blood flow.

Spiral computed tomographic angiography with the latest generation scanners might prove an acceptable alternative to formal arteriography. Although this imaging technique requires contrast infusion, it does not require arterial catheterization, is easily performed, and is extremely rapid. Its use in the diagnosis of peripheral vascular injury has not yet been systematically evaluated.

Nonoperative Management

The widespread application of arteriography in the evaluation of injured extremities results in the detection of clinically insignificant lesions. Intimal irregularity, focal spasm with minimal narrowing, and small pseudoaneurysms are often asymptomatic and do not progress. Considerable evidence suggests that nonoperative therapy of many asymptomatic lesions is safe and effective. However, successful nonoperative therapy requires continuous surveillance for subsequent occlusion or hemorrhage. Operative therapy is required for thrombosis, symptoms of chronic ischemia, and failure of small pseudoaneurysms to resolve.

A limited role exists for interventional radiologic techniques in the management of extremity vascular injuries. This modality requires special training, expertise, and an established interventional radiology program. Only an experienced interventionalist can successfully manage an extremity vascular injury. A multidisciplinary approach in anticipation of injuries amenable to endovascular therapy is best led by a trauma surgeon skilled in the

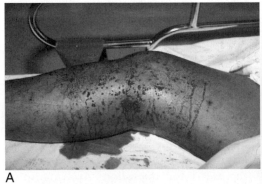
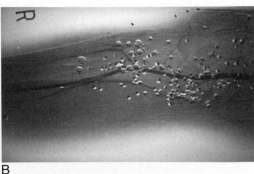

A   B

■ **FIGURE 19–2**
Close-range shotgun injury to right medial knee. Pedal pulses were palpable but diminished. Formal arteriography demonstrated patent popliteal artery and peroneal and posterior tibial arteries. This patient was successfully treated nonoperatively. ■

management of extremity vascular trauma. The indications for endovascular techniques in the extremities are limited to hemorrhage from branch vessels that may be occluded without producing ischemia, acute pseudo-aneurysms with a small lateral wall arterial injury, intimal flap without significant underlying thrombosis, and acute arteriovenous fistulas. Endovascular techniques are not effective in acute arterial occlusion from trauma. Endovascular placement of stents and stent grafts for noniatrogenic vascular trauma remains experimental and should be performed only in the most carefully selected cases (Fig. 19–3). Long-term results are not yet available and their application remains limited to specialized centers.

Operative Management

The operative management of extremity vascular injuries must be carefully orchestrated with the overall care of the patient. Intravenous broad-spectrum antibiotics should be administered preoperatively. Systemic heparin may be given preoperatively to patients with isolated extremity injury (e.g., in whom cavitary hemorrhage has been excluded) to prevent propagation of thrombus. However, heparin should be avoided in multi-injured patients, especially those with central nervous system trauma.

A generous sterile field should be prepared to allow for adequate exposure of vessels, to obtain proximal and distal control. This includes the chest and abdomen in proximal injuries of the upper and lower extremities. An uninjured leg should be prepared for harvesting of autologous venous conduit.

An orthopedic surgeon has an essential role in the surgical management of extremity vascular trauma associated with skeletal injury and should be involved before the surgical procedure begins. Restoration of blood flow is imperative and can be achieved by an initial

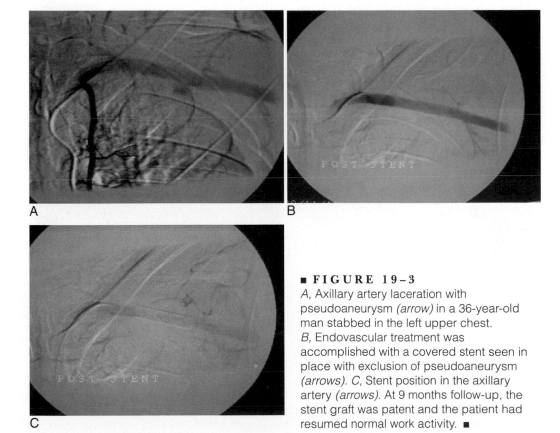

A

B

C

■ FIGURE 19–3
A, Axillary artery laceration with pseudoaneurysm *(arrow)* in a 36-year-old man stabbed in the left upper chest. *B,* Endovascular treatment was accomplished with a covered stent seen in place with exclusion of pseudoaneurysm *(arrows). C,* Stent position in the axillary artery *(arrows).* At 9 months follow-up, the stent graft was patent and the patient had resumed normal work activity. ■

vascular repair or insertion of a vascular shunt. The vascular surgeon's role does not end after perfusion is restored. Careful surveillance must be maintained to ensure that orthopedic appliances do not obstruct the shunt or disrupt the arterial repair. The early involvement of a plastic and reconstructive surgeon is essential for the successful management of vascular injuries associated with large soft tissue defects.

The appropriate treatment of extremity arterial and venous injuries consists of débridement of the damaged vessel, a tension-free repair, use of saphenous interposition grafting when primary repair is not possible, and adequate coverage with healthy vascularized tissue.

A limited role for primary amputation exists in the management of complex extremity vascular injuries. Patients with extensive soft tissue loss, neurologic deficit, extensive fractures, and vascular injuries should be evaluated collaboratively with orthopedic and plastic surgery colleagues to determine whether primary amputation is the best initial management. These mangled extremities can be objectively evaluated using a rating system that accounts for the age of the patient, the type of injury and the severity of the injury (Fig. 19–4; see also Table 19–1). However, the use of this scoring system is for general assessment and should never be a substitute for thoughtful clinical judgment using the skills of orthopedic and plastic surgery consultants.

Fasciotomy, particularly in the setting of prolonged ischemia, remains an important adjunct in the management of extremity vascular injury. Elevated compartment pressure is a sufficient indication to proceed with fasciotomy, even before arterial repair. If normal pressures are obtained, eventual reperfusion edema and subsequent swelling may occur with delayed compartment syndrome. Thus, continuous or intermittent compartment pressure monitoring may be necessary in the postoperative period. Lack of a timely fasciotomy remains the most common error leading to preventable limb loss following vascular trauma.

Frequent postoperative physical examinations of the extremity with vascular repair are essential. Any deterioration in the examination must be investigated. Loss of a palpable pulse is an absolute indication for re-exploration. Early and prompt return to the operating room when thrombosis is

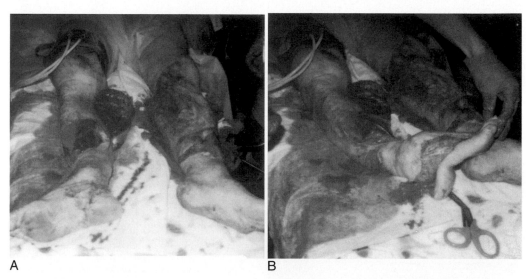

A   B

■ **FIGURE 19–4**

Extensive tissue destruction of the lower extremity in a man struck and rolled over by a bus. *A,* Right leg neurovascular disruption was complete and there were fractures at multiple levels. *B,* The left leg was similarly fractured but neurovascular function was normal. The right leg was amputated right below the knee and external fixation device was placed immediately. Recovery was rapid and functional outcome was acceptable. ■

suspected is the best way to ensure successful limb salvage.

The initial evaluation and management of peripheral vascular trauma is summarized in Table 19–2.

TABLE 19–2
SUMMARY OF THE MANAGEMENT OF PERIPHERAL VASCULAR TRAUMA

1. Perform thorough clinical evaluation; formal arteriography (uncommon).
2. Administer preoperative broad-spectrum antibiotics.
3. Consider systemic heparinization for an isolated vascular injury without any possibility of cavitary hemorrhage.
4. Prepare and drape to allow harvesting of autologous conduit.
5. Achieve proximal and distal control before direct investigation of the injury.
6. Perform proximal and distal catheter thrombectomy; proximal and distal infusion of heparin.
7. Achieve complete débridement of damaged vessel.
8. Cover vascular anastomoses with viable tissue.
9. Consider fasciotomy for elevated compartment pressures or prolonged ischemia.
10. Monitor frequently during the postoperative period.

SUBCLAVIAN ARTERY INJURIES

Surgical Anatomy

The *right* subclavian artery originates from the innominate artery and passes through the base of the neck behind the sternoclavicular joint. The *left* arises from the aortic arch and follows a similar course (Fig. 19–5). Anomalies of the subclavian arteries are rare. The most common anomaly is a *right* subclavian originating from the descending aorta as the most distal branch of the aortic arch and passing *posterior* to the esophagus. This is thought to occur in approximately 1% of the population.

The subclavian artery has three parts based on its relationship to the anterior scalene muscle (Fig. 19–6); first or proximal (proximal to the muscle), second or middle (posterior to the muscle), and third or distal (from the lateral border of the muscle to the lateral border of the first rib).

The first or proximal part gives off three branches (vertebral, internal mammary, and thyrocervical trunk) close to its termination near the anterior scalene muscle. The proximal part of the first portion is free of branches for 1 to 3 cm. Several important structures are

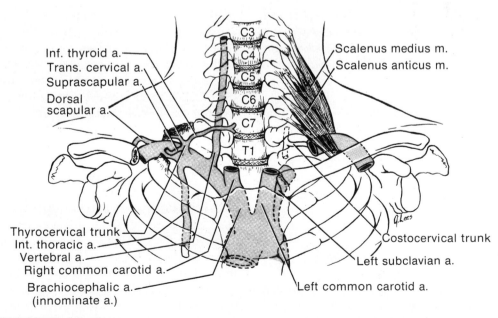

■ **FIGURE 19–5**
Anterior view of subclavian artery with branches of the subclavian artery arising from the right side. ■

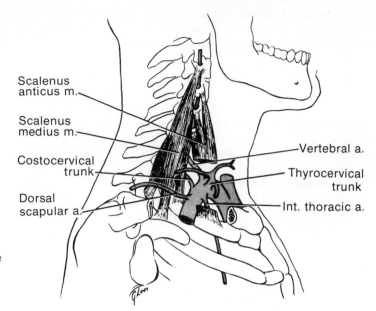

Scalenus anticus m.

Scalenus medius m.

Costocervical trunk

Dorsal scapular a.

Vertebral a.

Thyrocervical trunk

Int. thoracic a.

■ **FIGURE 19–6**
The right lateral view of the subclavian artery illustrating the branches of the subclavian artery with potential collateral anastomoses. ■

related to the first portion: The phrenic and vagus nerves cross anteriorly, the internal jugular-subclavian vein confluence passes anteriorly, and the cervical dome of the pleura is located inferiorly. On *both* sides, the venous confluence will contain the termination of lymphatic channels, which are often multiple. On the left, the thoracic duct is easily injured during retraction.

The second portion usually contains one or two branches (costocervical trunk and dorsal scapular) and is related closely to the brachial plexus. The third portion contains no branches and is closely related to the plexus.

The branches of the subclavian artery provide such a rich collateral network that interruption of flow at any of the three parts rarely produces limb-threatening ischemia (Fig. 19–7). However, adjacent soft tissue destruction can disrupt these collaterals and threaten limb viability in the presence of subclavian artery thrombosis.

Epidemiology and Etiology

Subclavian artery injuries are uncommon and represent fewer than 5% of all arterial injuries noted in most civilian and military series (Rich and Spencer, 1978). This is

because the subclavian artery is relatively short, is well protected by the sternum, clavicle, and first rib, and when partially lacerated, can produce rapid exsanguination and death in the field before patients receive medical attention.

A blunt mechanism of injury can produce several types of subclavian artery injury: avulsion of branches (producing significant hemorrhage); contusion with intimal disruption and prolapse (producing thrombosis); puncture or laceration from shards of bone from either the clavicle or first rib (producing hemorrhage); or severe stretching producing complete separation of intima and media with adventitia intact or disrupted (producing hemorrhage, thrombosis, or pseudoaneurysm). Recent civilian series document a blunt mechanism of injury as high as 45%.

Clinical Features and Diagnosis

Approximately 50% of patients with subclavian artery injuries present to the hospital in shock. The classic signs of advanced ischemia (pulselessness, pallor, paresthesias, poikilothermia, and paralysis) may be present but are not common because of the substantial collateral circulation available. Associated

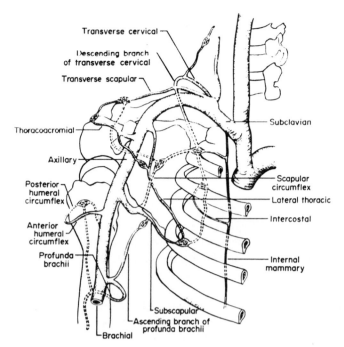

Labels in figure:
Transverse cervical
Descending branch of transverse cervical
Transverse scapular
Thoracoacromial
Axillary
Posterior humeral circumflex
Anterior humeral circumflex
Profunda brachii
Brachial
Ascending branch of profunda brachii
Subscapular
Subclavian
Scapular circumflex
Lateral thoracic
Intercostal
Internal mammary

■ **FIGURE 19–7**

Collateral circulation in the shoulder region. Important collateral vessels are the thoracoacromial, lateral thoracic, subscapular, and anterior and posterior humeral circumflex arteries. (From Levin PM, Rich NM, Hutton JE Jr: Collateral circulation in arterial injuries. Arch Surg 1971;102:392-399.) ■

injuries to the chest wall, lung, and brachial plexus are common.

The diagnosis may be obvious when a patient presents with a penetrating wound at the base of the neck or in the supraclavicular fossa combined with loss of the ipsilateral pulse. If these patients are in shock that is unresponsive to volume resuscitation, they must be taken to the operating room for control of hemorrhage. However, if patients are stable or stabilize with resuscitation, arteriography is extremely useful to plan the operative approach. The arteriogram can elucidate the portion of the artery that has been injured and allow the surgeon to determine the safest exposure for obtaining proximal control. A chest roentgenogram is also useful. In penetrating injuries, the entrance and exit wounds should be marked with radiopaque material before obtaining an x-ray film. In blunt injuries, the chest x-ray film can provide information about the mediastinum and unsuspected fractures of the ribs or clavicle.

Surgical Treatment

Surgical exposure of a subclavian artery injury can be quite difficult because the clavicle and sternum obstruct a direct route to the artery. In addition, the area of the subclavian contains many important anatomic structures that can be injured in the haste to obtain control. Surgical management of the injury is difficult because the subclavian is not a muscular or thick-walled artery and is intolerant of heavy-handed traction or imprecise suturing.

The second and third portions of the subclavian artery can be exposed through a supraclavicular incision. On the *right*, the first portion is best exposed through a median sternotomy. On the *left*, the first portion can be exposed through either a median sternotomy or a left anterolateral thoracotomy. For the first portion on the *left*, we recommend the thoracotomy approach because it is much easier.

The location of the injury, the condition of the wound, and the condition of the patient determine the best approach. For patients in shock or those with a massive hematoma of the neck or chest wall, proximal control of the first portion of the subclavian is the safest approach (even if the injury is in the third portion). Thoracotomy or sternotomy in an uninjured field allows rapid proximal control and can be lifesaving. For patients with an injury to the third portion who are stable, the artery can be approached through a supraclavicular incision. If uncontrollable bleeding is encountered, the wound should be packed and control should be obtained as discussed earlier. If it appears that the bleeding or the wound is directly behind the clavicle, the clavicle can be resected (completely or in part) without significant long-term morbidity. For all of these reasons, we recommend preparing and draping a wide field to include the neck to the mastoid process superiorly, along the trapezius to the deltoid, the entire ipsilateral arm (extended on a board), and the entire chest. The arm should be supported on a board but be mobile. The draping should allow space for one operator to be positioned cephalad to the arm support and one operator to be positioned caudad to the arm support.

The operation follows general guidelines specified previously and elsewhere (Shackford and Rich, 2001). Following débridement, catheter thrombectomy, and regional heparinization, the subclavian should be carefully inspected. Mobilization of the ends to attempt an end-to-end anastomosis is reasonable if no major branches are divided to achieve the mobilization. We recommend interposition grafting rather than attempting an end-to-end anastomosis with *any* tension. If tension exists, the anastomosis may tear

because the artery, by nature, is thin and nonmuscular. Although experience with prosthetic material for interposition grafting of the subclavian is extensive, the first choice for a conduit should be autologous proximal saphenous vein. We have found the size match of the proximal to be reasonable for short segment bypasses in both males and females. Prosthetic material is certainly acceptable when either no available suitable vein exists or the patient's condition is such that prolongation of the operation to harvest a conduit may jeopardize outcome.

Recent series have documented that most injuries are treated with primary repair (42%), followed by interposition grafting with autologous vein (Table 19–3). Another alternative, when the patient is unstable, is ligation. As previously described, the collateral circulation around the shoulder and neck is extensive and ligation of the subclavian artery is rarely associated with limb loss.

Results

Many reports document experience with subclavian artery injuries, but only a precious few document immediate, short-term, or long-term outcome. When outcome is reported, it is usually immediate or short term and focuses either on survival, on the patency

---

TABLE 19–3

SURGICAL TECHNIQUES USED FOR MANAGEMENT OF UPPER EXTREMITY VASCULAR INJURY: SELECTED REVIEW OF THE RECENT LITERATURE*

Artery	Series[†]	Years[‡]	N[§]	None (%)[∥]	Primary (%)[¶]	ASV (%)[**]	Prosthetic (%)[††]	Ligate (%)[‡‡]
Subclavian	6	1988-2000	378	32 (8.5)	160 (42.3)	128 (33.8)	47 (12.4)	11 (3)
Axillary	7	1982-1998	126	0	59 (46.8)	42 (33.3)	20 (15.8)	5 (4.1)
Brachial	5	1984-1994	223	5 (2.2)	121 (54.3)	87 (39)	0	3 (4.5)
Radial/ulnar	5	1984-1994	251	3 (1.1)	161 (64.2)	30 (11.9)	0	57 (22.8)

*References available on request.
[†]Number of published articles reviewed.
[‡]Years covered by the aggregated publications.
[§]Number of patients.
[∥]No repair or exploration undertaken.
[¶]Either vein patch, end to end anastomosis or arteriography.
[**]Saphenous vein interposition.
[††]Prosthetic graft interposition.
[‡‡]Ligation, no repair.

of the repair, or on limb salvage. Unfortunately, these outcome measures lack relevance because survival is rarely dependent solely on repair of the subclavian artery injury and thrombosis of the arterial repair rarely results in amputation of the upper extremity because of its abundant collateral circulation. Rather, long-term outcome is determined primarily by the neurologic function and secondarily by the orthopedic outcome (Hardin and colleagues, 1985).

Mortality rates are highly variable after subclavian artery injury because when death occurs, it is usually because of associated injuries. However, rare cases of death resulting from uncontrolled hemorrhage from subclavian arterial lacerations that either go unnoticed or undergo attempted repair without proximal control have been reported.

Amputation is rare following subclavian injuries and is usually a result of devastating soft tissue loss, multiple arterial injuries, infection (primarily intractable osteomyelitis), or severe neurologic injury with "flail arm" (see "Scapulothoracic Dissociation," later in this chapter). Graft infection (either of prosthetic material or vein) is uncommon and can be treated by ligation and extra-anatomic bypass (either carotid-subclavian or axilloaxillary) if either claudication or limb-threatening ischemia develops.

Complete resolution of infection, swelling, pain, and neurologic deficit and complete healing of all wounds define a good outcome following upper extremity vascular injury (Hardin and colleagues, 1985). When patients with scapulothoracic dissociation are included, the long-term outcome following subclavian artery injury is dismal, and only 30% of patients have a good outcome (Table 19–4). Excluding those with scapulothoracic dissociation improves the good outcome to about 40%, with the balance of patients having persistent disability due to nerve injury, osteomyelitis, or causalgia.

Management of Scapulothoracic Dissociation

Scapulothoracic dissociation is a devastating injury of the upper extremity and shoulder girdle caused by blunt injury. The mechanism is stretch and avulsion of the vascular and neurologic elements of the arm from their more proximal origins in the shoulder and neck regions. Substantial separation and/or fracture of the musculoskeletal attachments of the shoulder girdle can occur. Scapulothoracic dissociation is a rare injury, with only 52 patients reported in the literature (Sampson and colleagues, 1993). On physical examination, there is absence of the radial pulse associated with a significant shoulder or chest wall hematoma and absence of sensory or motor function below the shoulder. Chest radiography will demonstrate a laterally displaced scapula (with acromioclavicular disruption

TABLE 19–4
OUTCOME FOLLOWING REPAIR OF UPPER EXTREMITY VASCULAR INJURY: SELECTED REVIEW OF THE RECENT LITERATURE*

Artery	Series[†]	Years[‡]	N[§]	Die (%)[‖]	AMP (%)[¶]	ABNML (%)[**]	NML (%)[††]
Subclavian	6	1984-1993	103	17 (16.5)	6 (5.8)	45 (43.6)	35 (34.1)
Axillary	4	1982-1990	92	2 (2.2)	1 (1.1)	66 (71.7)	23 (25)
Brachial	4	1984-1994	146	1 (0.6)	5 (3.4)	42 (28.7)	98 (67.3)
Radial/ulnar	4	1984-1994	211	1 (0.5)	7 (3.5)	74 (35)	129 (61)

*References available on request.
[†]Number of published articles reviewed.
[‡]Years covered by the aggregated publications.
[§]Number of patients.
[‖]Death.
[¶]Amputation.
[**]Abnormal function (see text) does not include amputations.
[††]Normal function (see text).

and increased distance between the distal end of the clavicle and the acromion). An associated displaced clavicle fracture or a sternoclavicular disruption is often present (Sampson and colleagues, 1993). Unfortunately, the outcome is uniformly poor because of the neurologic disruption, not the arterial injury. Our experience and that of Sampson and colleagues (1993) suggest that delayed hemorrhage or limb-threatening ischemia is very rare and there are no benefits to revascularization. In the rare patient who is actively bleeding, we recommend ligation. In the infrequent patient with limb-threatening ischemia, primary amputation should be considered.

AXILLARY ARTERY INJURIES

Surgical Anatomy

The axillary artery begins at the lateral margin of the first rib and ends at the lateral margin

of the teres major muscle. Three parts are dependent on their relationship to the pectoralis minor muscle (Fig. 19–8): proximal to the muscle (first) and beneath (second) and distal to the muscle (third). The first part has one branch (superior thoracic), the second has two (thoracoacromial, lateral thoracic), and the third has three (anterior and posterior circumflex, subscapular). These branches provide a rich collateral circulation to this region.

The axillary vein lies anterior and slightly inferior to the axillary artery. Close proximity to the artery provides the anatomic basis for the development of an arteriovenous fistula following relatively minor trauma (e.g., arterial cannulation). A similar close relationship exists to branches of the brachial plexus (Fig. 19–9). Proximally, the plexus is posterior/lateral to the artery. Distally, the three cords of the plexus surround the second and third parts of the artery. This intimate relationship explains the high incidence of concomitant nerve injuries in axillary arterial trauma.

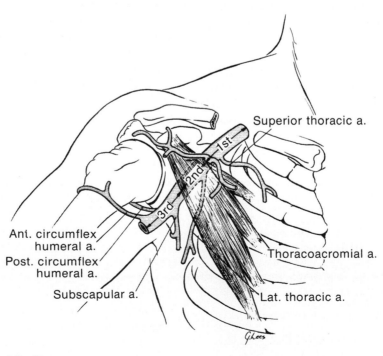

■ **FIGURE 19-8**
Surgical anatomy of the axillary artery with the usual configuration of six branches coming from the three parts of the artery. ■

AXILLARY ARTERIAL INJURIES

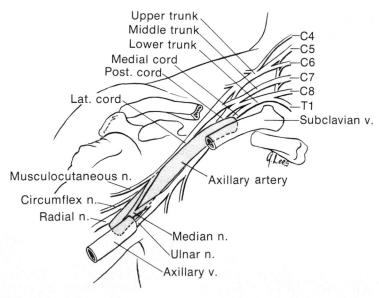

■ **FIGURE 19–9**
The close proximity of the brachial plexus to the cord adjacent to the second part of the axillary artery and the branches surrounding the third part demonstrate why there is a high incidence of concomitant nerve injuries with axillary arterial trauma, as shown above. ■

Epidemiology and Etiology

Axillary artery injuries are only slightly more common than subclavian artery injuries and represent 5% to 10% of all arterial injuries in most military and civilian injuries (Rich and Spencer, 1978). More than 95% of axillary artery injuries are from penetrating trauma. Included in this group are patients with iatrogenic injury following cannulation of the artery for arterial pressure monitoring or contrast studies. Although blunt injuries are rare, two types merit consideration. The first is rupture, contusion, or stretching of the artery following fracture of the proximal humerus or anterior dislocation of the shoulder. Approximately 1% of shoulder dislocations are associated with axillary artery injury (Sparks and colleagues, 2000). The second is thrombosis following chronic repetitive impingement by crutch use.

Clinical Features and Diagnosis

Patients with axillary artery injury commonly present with regional signs and symptoms,
such as a pulse deficit, advanced ischemia, pulsatile bleeding, or an expanding hematoma. Shock solely due to an axillary artery injury is rare. The most common associated injury is vascular (axillary vein) followed very closely by nerve (cords or branches of the brachial plexus).

The diagnosis of an axillary artery injury should be suspected in a patient with a penetrating wound of the axilla, a palpable subclavian pulse (detected by palpation in the supraclavicular fossa), but no distal pulses. If evidence of advanced ischemia is present, the patient should be taken immediately to the operating room.

Occasionally, a patient with a penetrating injury near the axilla will present with a palpable radial pulse and a thrill or bruit in the region of the injury. An arteriovenous fistula should be the primary consideration and formal arteriography should be performed. Formal arteriography can provide needed diagnostic information and, if performed by qualified and experienced angiographers, can afford a potential opportunity for endoluminal treatment (see Chapters 9 and 10).

Surgical Treatment

Anticipate proximal control before entering the site of the injury by preparing the site to include all of the shoulder, ipsilateral neck and supraclavicular fossa (to allow for exposure of the subclavian artery), the arm and hand to the fingertips (to allow intraoperative palpation of the radial pulse), and the contralateral leg (to allow a separate team to harvest) for a conduit (Fig. 19–10). The arm should be supported on a board but be mobile. The draping should allow space for one operator to be positioned cephalad to the arm support and one operator to be positioned caudad to the arm support.

Exposure of the proximal axillary artery is best obtained by an infraclavicular incision, made approximately one fingerbreadth below and parallel to the clavicle. This proximal exposure is recommended for all cases of axillary artery trauma (Graham and colleagues, 1982) because injuries that are more distal are often associated with significant hematoma (Fig. 19–11). Obtaining control of an axillary

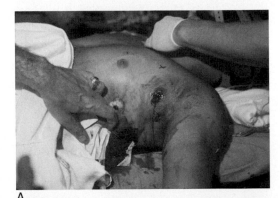

A

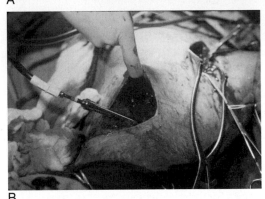

B

■ **FIGURE 19–11**
A, Close range shotgun wound to the anterior axilla. Notice the large hematoma causing significant swelling of the anterior chest wall, axilla, and deltoid region of the arm. *B,* Intraoperative photo from same perspective (patient's head is located toward the right side of this picture) demonstrating the infraclavicular incision and exposure of the injury through a second incision. After proximal control was first obtained through the infraclavicular incision (note the vascular clamp in the wound), the hematoma was opened and evacuated, allowing better visualization of the injury and avoidance of iatrogenic trauma to the brachial plexus. ■

■ **FIGURE 19–10**
Preparing for surgery. Note that the entire arm is being prepared as well as the ipsilateral neck and chest. We prefer to drape the contralateral proximal thigh for a conduit as this allows a second team to harvest the proximal saphenous vein, while the primary team obtains proximal control. The drapes should be placed in such a way as to allow an assistant to stand in the area cephalad to the shoulder and the arm. ■

arterial injury in the midst of a large hematoma is fraught with problems that inevitably lead to increased blood loss and possibly to an iatrogenic brachial plexus injury. The infraclavicular incision can be extended into the axilla and both the pectoralis minor and the major tendons can be divided, if necessary, to obtain distal control.

Conduct of the operation follows general guidelines specified previously and elsewhere (Shackford and Rich, 2001). Clamps should never be blindly placed near the axillary artery because its intimate relationship to the axillary vein and to the brachial plexus mandate precise clamp placement. In the event that uncontrolled bleeding exists, tamponade can be obtained by gentle finger compression or, if the lumen can be visualized, insertion of a balloon tipped catheter followed by careful balloon expansion.

Following débridement, catheter thrombectomy, and regional heparinization, the axillary artery should be carefully inspected. Mobilization of the ends to attempt an end-to-end anastomosis is reasonable if no major branches are divided to achieve the mobilization. Recent series have documented that most injuries are treated with primary repair (47%) followed by interposition grafting with autologous conduit (33%, see Table 19–3). We recommend interposition grafting with autologous proximal saphenous vein rather than attempting an end-to-end anastomosis with *any* tension. Ligation of the axillary artery is acceptable (there is a rich collateral circulation) in patients who are moribund and physiologically unstable, but this is not encouraged. Rather, if both ends of the artery can be visualized, a temporary intravascular shunt can be placed and the wound packed, towel clipped or stapled until the patient has stabilized. These shunts can be left in place several days without systemic anticoagulation (Granchi and colleagues, 2000).

Results

Similar to the literature describing treatment results of subclavian artery injuries, only a few reports document the outcome of axillary artery repair. When outcome is reported, it is usually immediate or short-term and focused on survival, the patency of the repair or limb salvage. Unfortunately, these outcome measures lack relevance because survival is rarely dependent solely on repair of the axillary artery injury and thrombosis of the arterial repair rarely results in amputation of the upper extremity because of the abundant collateral circulation in the shoulder and arm. Rather, long-term outcome is determined primarily by the neurologic function and secondarily by the orthopedic outcome (Hardin and colleagues, 1985).

Mortality and amputation are rare following axillary artery injury (see Table 19–4). A good outcome following axillary repair (as determined by complete resolution of swelling, pain and neurologic deficit) is rare because axillary artery injury is often accompanied by nerve injury, which ultimately leads to long-term neuralgia or causalgia. In four recently published series of axillary artery injuries in which follow-up was documented for 92 patients, only 23 (25%) had a good outcome (see Table 19–4). The other 66 patients had neurologic dysfunction, post-traumatic neuralgia producing disability, or diminished use because of chronic pain associated with osseus or soft tissue injury.

BRACHIAL ARTERY INJURIES

Surgical Anatomy

The brachial artery is a continuation of the axillary artery and begins at the lower border of the teres major muscle. Exiting the axilla, the brachial artery is a relatively superficial structure covered only by skin, subcutaneous tissue, and deep fascia. Proximally, it lies medial to the humerus and is accompanied by the median nerve (superiorly and laterally) and the ulnar and radial nerves (medially). Distally, it lies anterior to the elbow and is crossed by the median nerve, which then lies medial to the artery. Just proximal to the elbow, the ulnar nerve is posterior to the artery as it goes behind the medial epicondyle of the ulna. The brachial artery terminates 1 inch below the elbow skin crease where it divides into the radial and ulnar arteries.

The brachial artery has three main branches (Fig. 19–12). The first (most proximal) is the profunda brachii, which accompanied by the radial nerve passes posteriorly between the medial and long head of the triceps muscle. The profunda brachii provides an important collateral anastomosis with the axillary artery through its posterior circumflex humeral branch. The profunda also has a collateral anastomosis with the radial recurrent artery. The second main branch of the brachial artery is the superior ulnar collateral, which accompanied by the ulnar nerve passes behind the medial epicondyle to provide a collateral anastomosis with the posterior ulnar recurrent. The third (most distal) main branch is the inferior ulnar collateral, which provides a rich anastomotic collateral network around the elbow with the ulnar artery through its anterior recurrent branch.

Epidemiology and Etiology

Brachial artery injury is the most commonly reported arterial injury of the upper extremity. In large military and civilian series, brachial artery injury constitutes 15% to 30% of all peripheral arterial injuries. The reason for this relatively high frequency is that the brachial artery is relatively long, superficial, and exposed as compared to other peripheral

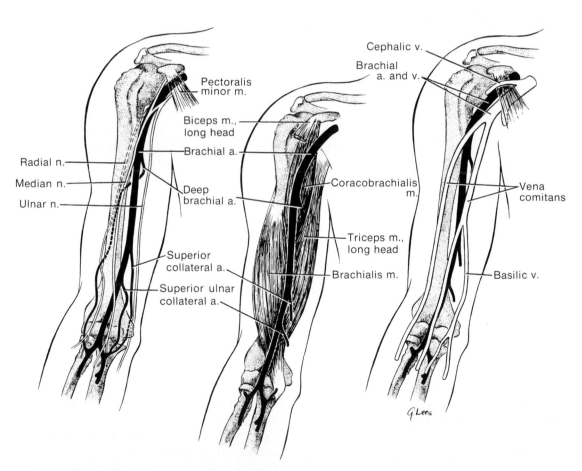

■ **FIGURE 19–12**
The brachial artery is a continuation of the axillary artery at the lower border of the teres major muscle. It terminates approximately 1 inch below the transverse skin crease in the antecubital fossa, where it divides into two branches. Important anatomic relationships include three associated nerves, three associated veins, and three main branches with the brachial artery lying successively on three muscles. ■

arteries. Furthermore, the upper extremity is often used as a lever, hammer, and weapon, as well as a protective or restraining device for the torso, all of which put the brachial artery in harm's way.

Penetrating trauma is the most common cause of brachial artery injury. Recently, the increase in the number of diagnostic cardiac catheterizations has resulted in an increase in the number of brachial artery injuries seen at most tertiary medical centers. Blunt injury of the brachial artery is much less common but deserves emphasis because it can easily be overlooked unless there is a high index of suspicion. Supracondylar fracture of the humerus, particularly with anterior displacement or elbow dislocation (Endean and colleagues, 1992), should alert the clinician to the possibility of a brachial artery injury.

Clinical Features and Diagnosis

Patients with brachial artery injuries classically present with a cool, painful hand, no radial pulse, and diminished sensory and motor function of the forearm and hand. The classic findings, however, are not always present. Patients may have a complete thrombosis of the brachial artery and loss of a palpable radial pulse but have a warm hand without neurologic dysfunction. Conversely, the patient may have a laceration of the brachial artery and have a palpable radial pulse. If symptoms of ischemia associated with "hard" signs are present, the diagnosis is not certain. In patients with a supracondylar fracture or an elbow dislocation where doubt about the diagnosis exists (diminished or absent pulse, but a warm, pink hand), arteriography is indicated. In patients with closed blunt trauma and primarily neurologic signs and symptoms who have a warm pink hand and a palpable radial pulse, plethysmography and segmental pressure determination can avoid a needless arteriogram.

Careful physical examination and comprehensive documentation of the pulses and neurologic findings are essential, particularly in patients who are to undergo operative exploration. This point cannot be overemphasized in patients with brachial artery injuries who have peripheral neurologic deficits before operation. Lack of documentation of the preoperative neurologic status leads to the assumption that the deficits arose out of some operative misadventure.

Surgical Treatment

Bleeding can be controlled by proximal compression against the humerus or by direct pressure over an open wound. Blindly attempting to clamp a bleeding vessel in the arm is never necessary and is fraught with the hazard of significant injury to the median, radial, or ulnar nerve.

For suspected proximal injury, prepare and drape the patient similar to that used to manage an axillary artery injury (see previous discussion). For injuries that are more distal, prepare the arm and hand to the fingertips (to allow intraoperative palpation of the radial pulse) and a leg (to allow a separate team to harvest) for a conduit. The arm should be supported on a board but be mobile. The draping should allow space for one operator to be positioned cephalad to the arm support and one operator to be positioned caudad to the arm support.

Exposure of the brachial artery is best obtained by a longitudinal incision in the palpable groove between the triceps and biceps muscle along the medial aspect of the arm. This incision can be extended distally across the antecubital fossa or proximally across the axilla with an S-shaped curve (Fig. 19–13). No matter where the exposure is obtained (proximally or distally), precise dissection and careful handing of all structures are mandatory. Careless dissection or heavy-handed retraction may result in injury to the associated nerve (particularly the median nerve).

Conduct of the operation follows general guidelines specified previously and elsewhere (Shackford and Rich, 2001). Following débridement, catheter thrombectomy, and regional heparinization, the brachial artery should be carefully inspected. Small lateral injuries, particularly those associated with iatrogenic injuries, may be reapproximated

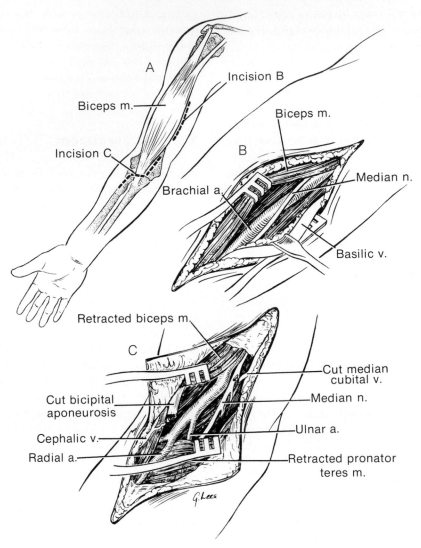

■ **FIGURE 19–13**

Surgical exposure of the brachial artery is rapidly obtained by a longitudinal incision along the course of the artery with an extension as an *S* curve either across the axilla proximally or across the antecubital fossa distally as needed. The median nerve and basilic veins are in close proximity to the artery. ■

with simple interrupted sutures placed in the same axis as the direction of the artery so no luminal compromise occurs. If more than two or three sutures are required, a vein patch is a better alternative because the artery is easily narrowed. Our preference for most injuries is excision of the area of injury and either an end-to-end anastomosis (performed with interrupted sutures and with the ends of the vessel distracted for placement of *all* sutures) or an interposition autologous saphenous vein graft. Recent civilian series support this

approach, with the majority of the repairs being either primary end-to-end or interposition vein grafting (see Table 19–3). If associated orthopedic injuries are present, our preference is to place an indwelling temporary shunt in the artery and let the orthopedic surgeons achieve length and stability of the arm before attempting definitive vascular repair. Ligation should never be a consideration because it carries a significant risk of amputation. If the patient is in extremis from other associated injuries, an indwelling temporary shunt can be placed quickly and left in place for several days without systemic heparinization.

Results

Amputation or death is rare following brachial artery repair. Long-term outcome following brachial artery repair is decidedly better than either subclavian or axillary artery injuries because the incidence of associated nerve injury is much less. In recent civilian series (see Table 19–4), a good outcome (as determined by complete resolution of swelling, pain, and neurologic deficit) was achieved in almost 70% of patients. If patients develop symptoms of arm claudication on follow-up, they should undergo noninvasive vascular testing to include plethysmography, segmental pressure determination, and duplex of the area of injury. If stenosis or occlusion is evident, the patients should have diagnostic arteriography for possible endoluminal or open revision.

RADIAL AND ULNAR ARTERY INJURY

Surgical Anatomy

After the brachial artery crosses through the cubital fossa, it bifurcates into the radial and ulnar artery. The ulnar artery is the larger of the two, but this size discrepancy exists only in the proximal portion of the artery. Two branches immediately arise from the proximal ulnar artery: the anterior and posterior ulnar recurrent arteries that form collateral anastomoses with the brachial artery around the anterior and posterior aspects of the elbow, respectively. The common interosseus also arises from the proximal ulnar artery (Fig. 19–14) and passes laterally and posteriorly toward the interosseus membrane where, at the superior edge of the membrane, it divides into the volar (anterior) and dorsal (posterior) interosseus arteries. The dorsal interosseus gives rise in its proximal portion to the interosseus recurrent, which forms a collateral anastomosis with branches of the brachial artery. The ulnar artery terminates in the superficial or volar palmar arch. In its oblique proximal portion, it is crossed by the pronator teres and by the median nerve. The ulnar nerve joins the artery in its distal third (Fig. 19–15).

The radial artery is unique in that no muscle or nerve crosses it in its relatively direct course to the wrist. The only major branch of the radial artery is the radial recurrent, which passes under the brachioradialis muscle to pass proximally and form a collateral anastomosis with branches of the profunda brachii. The radial artery gives a small branch to the superficial arch but terminates in the deep palmar arch.

Epidemiology and Etiology

Arterial injuries of the forearm are often reported in recent series describing vascular injuries and now make up between 5% and 30% of the total peripheral vascular injuries. Approximately 95% are due to penetrating trauma. A relatively rare form of ulnar artery injury occurs in individuals with a history of repeatedly using their hypothenar eminence as a hammer. It is thought that the repeated trauma can produce aneurysmal dilatation, distal embolization, or thrombosis.

Clinical Features and Diagnosis

Complete interruption of either the radial or the ulnar artery will often have no adverse effect on the circulation of the forearm or hand because of the rich collateral circulation. Signs of advanced ischemia warrant surgical exploration or operating room arteriography. If doubt exists about the integrity of the circulation and the condition of the patient and the condition of the arm permit, formal arteriography with magnification views of the hand are helpful for diagnosis and the planning of operative management.

Puncture wounds of the forearm can be quite insidious because the small skin wound will not allow sufficient egress of venous or

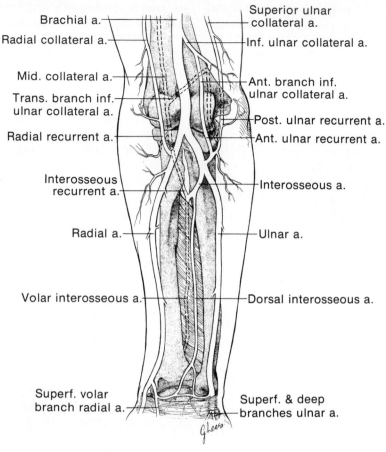

■ **FIGURE 19–14**

As the brachial artery divides into the radial artery (its more direct continuation) and the ulnar artery (the larger of the two branches) in the forearm, there are important collateral branches, which help form the rich anastomosis around the elbow. The common interosseus is also an important branch of the ulnar artery. ■

arterial blood, which can accumulate in significant quantity in the subcutaneous and subfascial planes to produce a forearm compartment syndrome. Physical signs that should alert the examiner to the possibility of an expanding hematoma include marked tension in the dorsal or volar forearm, superficial venous engorgement, paresthesias in the hand, or diminished sensation to light touch in the fingers. Without fasciotomy, these patients are at risk of developing a Volkmann contracture.

Surgical Treatment

Control of hemorrhage from either the radial or the ulnar artery is easily achievable by direct pressure. Tourniquets or blind clamping in an open wound is not warranted. Prepare the arm and hand to the fingertips (to allow intraoperative palpation of the radial pulse) and a leg (to allow a separate team to harvest) for a conduit. The arm should be supported on a board but be mobile. The draping should allow space for one operator to be positioned cephalad to the arm support and one operator to be positioned caudad to the arm support.

Exposure of the proximal portions of both arteries can be accomplished through an *S*-shaped incision in the cubital fossa (Fig. 19–16). The distal arteries can be exposed through longitudinal incisions over the course of the artery just proximal to the hand. Conduct of the operation follows general

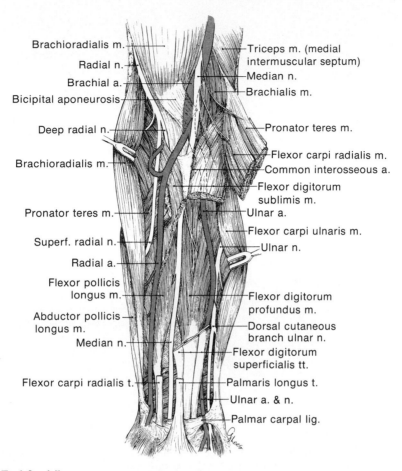

Brachioradialis m.

Radial n.

Brachial a.

Bicipital aponeurosis

Deep radial n.

Brachioradialis m.

Pronator teres m.

Superf. radial n.

Radial a.

Flexor pollicis
longus m.

Abductor pollicis
longus m.

Median n.

Flexor carpi radialis t.

Triceps m. (medial
intermuscular septum)

Median n.

Brachialis m.

Pronator teres m.

Flexor carpi radialis m.

Common interosseous a.

Flexor digitorum
sublimis m.

Ulnar a.

Flexor carpi ulnaris m.

Ulnar n.

Flexor digitorum
profundus m.

Dorsal cutaneous
branch ulnar n.

Flexor digitorum
superficialis tt.

Palmaris longus t.

Ulnar a. & n.

Palmar carpal lig.

■ **FIGURE 19–15**
The relationship of the radial and ulnar arteries to the important nerves, major muscle groups, and tendons. Particularly note the crossing of the proximal ulnar artery by the median nerve and the close approximation of the ulnar nerve to the distal two thirds of the ulnar artery. The cross section through the upper third of the forearm emphasizes the relatively deep location of the ulnar artery compared with the more superficial radial artery. ■

guidelines specified previously and elsewhere (Shackford and Rich, 2001). Following débridement, catheter thrombectomy, and regional heparinization, the area of injury should be carefully inspected. If both arteries are injured, repair of the ulnar is less technically taxing because of its relatively larger size. If only one artery is injured and no sign of ischemia is seen in the hand (as documented by a comprehensive physical examination and confirmed by Doppler signals in the palmar arch and digits), ligation is reasonable (Johnson, Ford and Johansen, 1993). For small "clean" lacerations or puncture wounds, lateral suture repair may suffice. More severe lacerations will require resection and end-to-end anastomosis, which is the most

common technique used in recent series (see Table 19–3). Reversed autologous saphenous vein from the distal leg can be used if significant arterial débridement is required or when an end-to-end anastomosis will create tension on the suture line.

Results

Amputation is rare following radial or ulnar artery injury. When amputation does occur, it is often the result of massive soft tissue destruction (with interruption of both the radial and the ulnar arteries) associated with sepsis or chronic osteomyelitis. Few studies document adequate long-term follow-up.

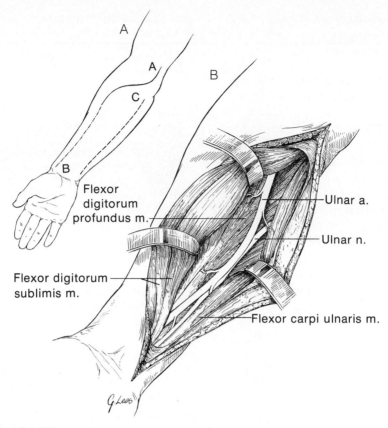

■ **FIGURE 19–16**

Elective incisions that can be used for approach to the radial and ulnar arteries. *A,* An *S*-type incision starting along the course of the distal brachial artery, carried through the antecubital fossa and continued down on the forearm will give excellent exposure of the proximal ulnar and radial arteries, as well as the origin of the common interosseous artery (A). An extension off this incision (B) along the course of the radial artery can be used for exposure to the wrist level. A separate incision can be used over the course of the ulnar artery (C). *B,* This drawing demonstrates exposure of the ulnar neurovascular bundle within the deep muscle layers, which have been split proximally. ■

Recent series with adequate documentation of follow-up demonstrate good results (as determined by complete resolution of swelling, pain, and neurologic deficit) following radial or ulnar repair in 65% of patients (see Table 19–4). Poor results are not related to the vascular repair, but to the associated nerve or tendon injuries. In fact, in one study, patency of the vascular repair when only one artery (either radial or ulnar) was injured was 50% (Johnson, Ford, and Johansen, 1993). Despite the high failure rate of radial or ulnar repairs, no patients had claudication.

VENOUS INJURIES OF THE UPPER EXTREMITY

Injuries to the subclavian or axillary vein should be repaired if the patient's condition permits. In most cases, repair will consist of lateral venorrhaphy or end-to-end anastomosis. After appropriate débridement, when a direct repair cannot be performed because it will result in tension on the suture line or will significantly narrow the vein, repair can be accomplished with autologous vein patch, interposition vein grafting, or a panel or spiral graft made from autologous vein. Early patency of these venous repairs is 50% to 90% (Meyer and colleagues, 1987; Pappas and colleagues, 1997), but long-term patency approaches 100% because it appears that the thrombus recanalizes and provides adequate function (Nypaver and colleagues, 1992; Pappas and colleagues, 1997). If the patient is in extremis, ligation of the subclavian or axillary vein is acceptable with minimal long-term sequelae (Timberlake and Kerstein, 1995). If symptoms of venous claudication or severe swelling develop during rehabilitation or with the return of vigorous arm function, a subclavian venous bypass using autologous vein or a jugular venous "turn down" with temporary distal arteriovenous fistula provides satisfactory relief of symptoms.

COMPARTMENT SYNDROME OF THE UPPER EXTREMITY

A compartment syndrome can develop in either the upper arm (triceps, deltoid, or along the axillary sheath) or the forearm. The forearm compartment syndrome is more common. Increased tissue pressure can follow either blunt or penetrating trauma because of hematoma, post-traumatic transudation of serum into the interstitial space, venous thrombosis, or reperfusion following ischemia (Shackford and Rich, 2001). The possibility of a compartment syndrome must always be a consideration in a patient who has been injured, particularly one with prolonged ischemia before reperfusion.

The diagnosis of compartment syndrome should be suspected in any patient complaining of increasing pain following injury. The physical findings include a tense compartment, pain on passive range of motion, progressive loss of sensation, and weakness. The loss of arterial pulses is a late finding, which usually indicates a poor prognosis. Neurologic signs and symptoms, while helpful, are neither sensitive nor specific in the upper extremity following arterial injury because associated peripheral nerve injury often exists. Early diagnosis must be predicated on measurement of compartment pressures. The

normal tissue compartment pressure ranges from 0 to 9 mm Hg. Much controversy exists about what constitutes a pathologic elevation. Our approach has been to perform fasciotomy when compartment pressure exceeds 30 mm Hg.

Treatment consists of complete fasciotomy of the involved compartment. For the volar compartment, the skin incision begins 1 cm proximal and 2 cm lateral to the medial epicondyle. It is carried obliquely across the skin crease at the antecubital fossa and continued obliquely for the proximal part of the forearm. It is then curved medially, reaching the midline at the junction of the middle and distal third of the forearm, and is continued in a straight line to the wrist crease at a point on the medial side of the palmaris longus tendon. The incision is then curved obliquely across the wrist crease and terminated in the mid palm. This allows routine decompression of the carpal tunnel. A superficial fasciotomy adequately decompresses the volar compartment in most cases. If any doubt exists about adequate decompression, intraoperative measurement of compartment pressures should be performed. For the dorsal compartment, the incision begins 2 cm distal to the lateral epicondyle. It is carried straight distally in the midline for approximately 7 to 10 cm. The skin edges are undermined and the dorsal fascia incised directly in line with the skin incision.

POST-TRAUMATIC CAUSALGIA

Persistent pain following upper extremity vascular injury is common due to associated peripheral nerve injury and resultant traumatic neuralgia. Some patients may have pain that appears to be sympathetically mediated, but not all will have causalgia. Causalgia (complex regional pain syndrome type 2) occurs in about 3% of patients suffering peripheral nerve injuries (Costa and Robbs, 1988) and is often confused with reflex sympathetic dystrophy (complex regional pain syndrome type 1). Several characteristics distinguish causalgia: a burning pain noted within 24 hours of injury of a large mixed nerve with a pain distribution similar to that of the nerve. Onset of reflex sympathetic dystrophy usually occurs weeks to months following the injury, is not always burning in character, and has a distribution that does not follow a specific anatomic distribution of a mixed nerve in the extremity. Causalgia typically presents early and is associated with hypalgesia in the area of the partial denervation followed by constant burning pain that can be increased by nonpainful stimuli (allodynia). Abnormal sympathetic function is evident in the region (e.g., vasomotion or hyperhidrosis) and the pain can be exaggerated by emotional upset.

The diagnosis should be suspected when the aforementioned characteristics are present. It can be confirmed by the relief of symptoms with a sympathetic block (Costa and Robbs, 1988). Some patients may have resolution of the syndrome with a single sympathetic block. For symptom recurrence, surgical sympathectomy is the treatment of choice.

LOWER EXTREMITY VASCULAR INJURIES

Common Femoral and Profunda Femoral Arteries

SURGICAL ANATOMY

The common femoral artery emerges from under the inguinal ligament as a continuation of the external iliac artery at the midpoint between the anterosuperior iliac spine and the pubic tubercle. It is relatively exposed with only subcutaneous fat and lymphatic tissue overlying. Along its course are three to five branches of varying size and location. The most prominent are the superficial circumflex iliac and the superficial epigastric, which arise within 1 cm of the inguinal ligament. Approximately 5 cm below the inguinal ligament, the common femoral artery bifurcates into the superficial femoral and profunda femoral arteries.

The profunda femoral artery usually originates as a single posterolateral branch. However, more than one profunda branch may be present. The lateral femoral circumflex vein crosses the profunda anteriorly and transversely within 3 cm of its origin from the common femoral artery. At this level, the artery usually bifurcates into two large branches, the medial and lateral circumflex arteries. The proximity of the crossing vein demands careful attention when exposing the distal profunda.

Numerous collaterals come from the branches of the hypogastric artery to the profunda femoral artery but are usually not sufficient to sustain adequate blood flow in the presence of an acute occlusion of the common femoral artery. The distal branches of the profunda femoral artery provide collateral flow to the popliteal artery through the lateral superior genicular artery and the descending genicular artery. Following acute occlusion of the superficial femoral artery, these collaterals are not sufficient to sustain adequate blood flow to the lower leg (Fig. 19–17).

The femoral nerve, composed predominantly of the motor fibers of the quadriceps, traverses the femoral region along the lateral aspect of the femoral sheath and can be injured during exposure of the femoral vessels if an inadvertently lateral incision is used or excessive lateral retraction is present.

EPIDEMIOLOGY AND ETIOLOGY

Trauma to the femoral vessels accounts for one third of all vascular injuries in military series and 7% to 35% in civilian series (Rich, Baugh, and Hughes, 1970; Mattox and colleagues, 1989; Humphrey, Nichols, and Silver, 1994; Hafez, Woolgar, and Robbs, 2001). Penetrating injuries are more common than blunt. Low-caliber gunshot wounds are the most common cause of penetrating injuries; knife wounds are less common (Hafez, Woolgar, and Robbs, 2001). Anterior dislocation of the femoral head is a rare cause of blunt injury. Laceration of the common femoral artery can cause severe hemorrhage that can be fatal if not tamponaded or controlled. In survivable injuries, the femoral

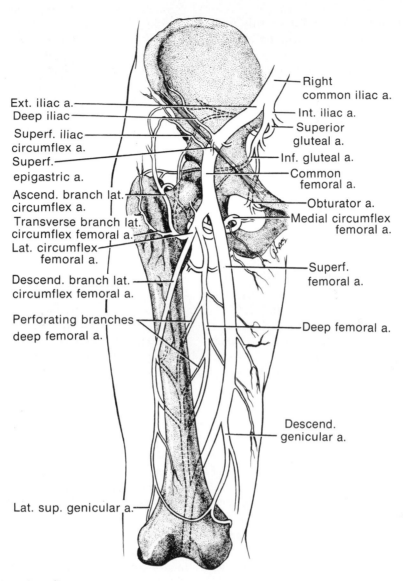

Ext. iliac a.
Deep iliac
Superf. iliac
circumflex a.
Superf.
epigastric a.
Ascend. branch lat.
circumflex a.
Transverse branch lat.
circumflex femoral a.
Lat. circumflex
femoral a.
Descend. branch lat.
circumflex femoral a.
Perforating branches
deep femoral a.

Lat. sup. genicular a.

Right
common iliac a.
Int. iliac a.
Superior
gluteal a.
Inf. gluteal a.
Common
femoral a.
Obturator a.
Medial circumflex
femoral a.
Superf.
femoral a.

Deep femoral a.

Descend.
genicular a.

■ **FIGURE 19–17**
This anatomic drawing traces the course of the superficial femoral artery, the main conduit between
the common femoral and popliteal arteries. In addition to numerous muscular branches, the
supreme genicular (descending genicular) is an important collateral to the rich anastomosis around
the knee. ■

sheath contains the hemorrhage and the
vessel thromboses or forms an acute
pseudoaneurysm.

CLINICAL FEATURES AND DIAGNOSIS

Hemorrhage is the most common presenting
sign. Less commonly, the lacerated or transected common femoral artery thromboses
and distal ischemia results. Associated injury

to the femoral vein is very common in penetrating trauma.

The superficial location of the femoral
bifurcation allows for accurate clinical assessment by inspection and palpation. In patients
with active hemorrhage from the femoral
area, no diagnostic workup is needed; expeditious control of hemorrhage is required.
Arteriography is reserved for patients with
multiple associated injuries and an equivocal
examination. Emergency department arteri-

ogram is usually not helpful in this area because of the difficulty of adequately visualizing the common femoral artery and the femoral bifurcation. If arteriography is required, it should be performed formally in the angiography suite.

SURGICAL TREATMENT

Both groins, the lower abdomen (beginning at the umbilicus), and both lower extremities should be completely prepared and draped. Preparing the lower abdomen allows for proximal extension of the incision and more proximal control if necessary. Having the uninjured groin prepared allows access to an alternative source of inflow. Preparing the uninjured leg provides access to autogenous conduit.

The common femoral artery is best exposed through a longitudinal incision overlying its course from the inguinal ligament inferiorly for 8 to 12 cm (Fig. 19–18). Occasionally, proximal control may require exposure of the external iliac artery. This is best accomplished through an oblique muscle splitting lower quadrant abdominal incision carried down to the retroperitoneum where the artery and vein can be controlled with medial retraction of the peritoneal structures.

The profunda femoral artery is exposed through the same incision used for the common femoral artery. Dissection is carried distal and anterior along the proximal portion of the superficial femoral artery and posterior laterally to identify the origin of the profunda femoral. The proximal 2 cm of the artery is easily exposed. Beyond this point, ligating and dividing the lateral circumflex femoral vein exposes the artery. This vein is broad and short and should be carefully ligated to avoid significant hemorrhage.

Severe hemorrhage usually dictates the initial steps of the surgical procedure. Proximal and distal control prior to exposure of the injury site prevents secondary injury to the vessels. The use of vascular clamps, Silastic vessel loops, optical magnification, and fine monofilament sutures are essential to successful management. There is no role for blind clamp placement. Direct repair, when possible, is preferred. Longitudinal laceration

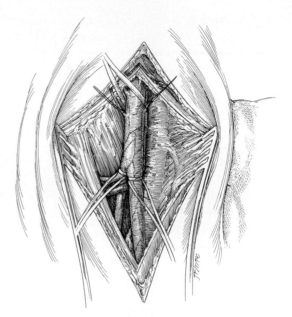

■ FIGURE 19–18
Exposure of the common femoral artery and its branches is best obtained through a longitudinal incision directly over the artery. Silastic loops double passed around the arteries provide control without causing secondary arterial trauma. The profunda femoral artery is exposed by carrying this dissection distally and by ligating the lateral femoral circumflex vein. (From Rutherford RB: Atlas of vascular surgery: Basic techniques and exposures. Philadelphia: WB Saunders, 1993.) ■

or defects may be repaired with a vein patch angioplasty. However, if injury is extensive and débridement results in a significant loss of artery such that there would be tension on the repair, an interposition graft should be placed.

Saphenous vein is the first choice for interposition grafting. However, vein diameter may not be adequate. Although spiral vein graft construction is an alternative, it is time consuming and technically demanding. Dacron or polytetrafluoroethylene (PTFE) interposition grafts are acceptable alternatives. In general, PTFE is preferred because of its relative resistance to infection compared to Dacron. Short-segment synthetic grafts in this area of high flow are durable and have acceptable long-term patency rates (Feliciano and colleagues, 1985, 1988).

Profunda femoral artery injuries should be repaired whenever possible. However, if serious associated injuries are present or the patient is unstable, the vessel should be ligated. Long-term sequelae are uncommon as long as the superficial femoral artery is patent. Proximal injuries to the profunda femoral artery may be managed by placing a short interposition graft or by proximal ligation and reimplantation of the vessel to the proximal superficial femoral artery. The profunda femoral artery should be repaired only if the patient is stable and the repair is relatively easy to accomplish.

RESULTS

Successful repair of the common femoral and profunda femoral arteries is dependent on restoration of adequate arterial lumen diameter and avoiding infection. Once groin wound infection occurs in patients who had an arterial repair, the first priority is to determine whether the graft or suture line is exposed or involved in the infection. If the suture line is involved, immediate graft removal, ligation of the proximal and distal arteries, and extra-anatomic bypass are the only acceptable option to prevent life-threatening hemorrhage and eventual limb loss. If the graft is exposed, but the suture line is not and the graft is patent, the graft may be salvaged by coverage with a proximally based sartorius flap.

Long-term patency rates of successful primary repair and short segment interposition grafts are very good. Acute thrombosis, though uncommon, usually causes limb-threatening ischemia and requires immediate treatment. Early stenosis of vein interposition grafts is uncommon. These patients should have regular follow-up to assess graft patency and the adequacy of limb blood flow. Calf claudication is the first clinical indication of stenosis at the repair site.

Lower extremity function following vascular repair is predominantly determined by the severity of associated musculoskeletal and nerve trauma. The most disabling associated injury is femoral nerve transection. Loss of quadriceps function results in significant gait

problems. Extensive venous injury with venous outflow obstruction at the femoral level causes venous insufficiency with long-term sequelae of venous stasis dermatitis and ulceration.

Amputation rates following femoral artery injury vary from 15% to 35% and are determined by the severity of musculoskeletal and neurologic injury (Mattox and colleagues, 1989; Hafez, Woolgar, and Robbs, 2001). Penetrating injuries are much less likely to result in amputation. In contrast, blunt injuries that cause vascular disruption usually involve force loading sufficient to cause significant neurologic and musculoskeletal injuries with limb-threatening sequelae. The most discouraging outcome is successful revascularization of a limb, which ultimately requires amputation for chronic recurring pressure ulceration and infection because of denervation.

Superficial Femoral Artery

SURGICAL ANATOMY

The superficial femoral artery originates in the femoral triangle and travels from an anterior location to the medial aspect of the thigh at the adductor canal where it transitions to the popliteal artery. It is superficially located in the groin and moves deeper as it traverses the medial thigh beneath the sartorius muscle approaching the adductor magnus muscle. The only significant branch is the descending genicular artery, which forms a collateral anastomosis with the genicular branches of the popliteal artery. The superficial femoral vein travels in close posteromedial proximity to the artery and is frequently duplicated. The saphenous nerve, a cutaneous sensory nerve to the medial calf and foot, lies anterior to the superficial femoral artery for most of its course. The nerve leaves the artery to join the saphenous vein near the adductor hiatus.

EPIDEMIOLOGY AND ETIOLOGY

Penetrating injury of superficial femoral artery is more common than blunt. The presence of a femoral shaft fracture should alert the examining physician of the possibility of a superficial femoral artery injury, but fewer than 5% of fractures will have vascular trauma (Rosental and colleagues, 1975; Romanoff and Goldberg, 1979).

CLINICAL FEATURES AND DIAGNOSIS

Hemorrhage is the predominant feature of penetrating vascular injuries in the thigh, whereas thrombosis is the usual presentation following a blunt mechanism.

High-velocity gunshot wounds of the thigh, though common in the military setting, remain rare in the civilian environment. Contusion and thrombosis of the superficial femoral artery produced by the temporary cavitational effects of high-energy rounds may present as either initial or delayed lower extremity ischemia. The severity of tissue destruction, neurologic deficit, and vascular spasm may make peripheral vascular examination difficult in this setting.

Inspection and palpation with attention to distal pulses is usually accurate in assessing the superficial femoral artery. Frequent re-examination, particularly in patients with midshaft femur fracture, must be performed to avoid missing a delayed arterial thrombosis. Patients with active hemorrhage from penetrating wounds require immediate operation for hemorrhage control and diagnosis. Arteriography is reserved for patients with equivocal signs of arterial injury, palpable but diminished pulses, or the suspicion of pseudoaneurysm or arteriovenous fistula. Emergency department or operating room arteriography is accurate for detecting superficial femoral artery injuries and is time saving in patients with multiple injuries and the need for immediate thoracotomy or celiotomy.

SURGICAL TREATMENT

Both groins and both legs should be prepared and draped. Preparing the contralateral groin provides an alternative source of inflow and the contralateral leg provides a source for autologous conduit. Proximal superficial femoral artery injuries are best exposed through a longitudinal groin incision similar to that used for femoral bifurcation exposure. The middle and distal artery can be approached through an oblique incision in the thigh over the course of the sartorius muscle. The muscle is retracted medially and the artery found immediately below in the adductor (Hunter) canal. Exposure of the distal artery at the superficial femoropopliteal artery junction may require transection of the adductor magnus tendon.

Primary repair is possible for those few wounds that produce a small, clean laceration. Saphenous vein interposition grafting is the best procedure for more severe injuries of the superficial femoral artery. Careful vascular technique, avoiding undue tension in the repair, preserving lumen diameter, and completion angiogram are essential to the successful repair of the superficial femoral artery. A synthetic graft is an acceptable conduit if no vein is available or the patient is too unstable to prolong the procedure to harvest a vein. Long-term patency rates of PTFE and Dacron grafts are significantly lower than that of autologous vein graft.

Primary amputation is rarely indicated in the management of superficial femoral artery injuries. Extensive crush injury with avulsion of the thigh muscles from the femur is one of the few indications for lifesaving above-knee amputation. Refractory hemorrhage into the thigh is striking in these patients and attempts at direct surgical control of hemorrhage are usually futile. High above-knee amputation may be the only way to control life-threatening hemorrhage in this setting.

RESULTS

Superficial femoral artery repair, if done properly, has long-term patency that approaches 100%. Associated neurologic injury is uncommon and femur fractures are usually amenable to successful orthopedic management. Frequent postoperative assessment for graft failure or calf compartment syndrome is necessary to facilitate early reoperation or fasciotomy should these complications occurs. Amputation rates vary from 10% to 30% and depend on the timeliness and success of the vascular repair and the severity of associated injuries (Mattox and colleagues, 1989; Hafez, Woolgar, and Robbs, 2001).

Patients with superficial femoral artery injuries require long-term follow-up. Yearly assessment of distal pulses and, if indicated, segmental lower extremity arterial pressures should be performed. Five percent to twenty percent of patients will require some form of secondary reconstruction for lower extremity arterial insufficiency because of a late failure (stenosis or thrombosis) of the repair.

Popliteal and Tibial Arteries

SURGICAL ANATOMY

The popliteal artery originates at the adductor magnus hiatus as the continuation of the superficial femoral artery. Throughout its course, the popliteal artery is located deep in the popliteal fossa along the posterior aspect of the femur, in proximity to the joint line, and the tibial plateau. The artery is covered proximally by the semimembranous muscle and in its midportion by subcutaneous tissue. The artery continues distally to the upper calf where it terminates at the origin of the anterior tibial artery at the triceps surae formed by the two heads of the gastrocnemius muscle and the soleus muscle. Along its course, the popliteal artery has six to eight small geniculate branches, which are usually paired. These form an anastomotic network around the knee (Fig. 19–19). However, in acute occlusion of the popliteal artery, these branches are not sufficient to provide adequate distal blood flow.

The relationship of the popliteal artery to the muscles of the thigh and calf places it at risk for severe injury in the dislocation of the knee. In full extension of the knee, the popliteal artery is on tension across the back of the knee joint. Knee dislocation stretches the popliteal artery over the posterior edge of the tibial plateau resulting in severe intimal injury or transection.

The three tibial vessels have a variable origin. In 85% to 90% of patients, the popliteal bifurcates into the anterior tibial and tibial peroneal trunk arteries. The posterior tibial

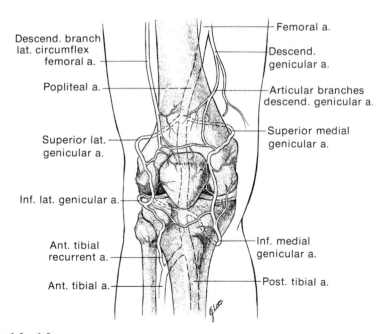

■ FIGURE 19–19
Anterior view of the knee with the popliteal artery and its branches. These collaterals are usually not sufficient to provide adequate distal perfusion in patients with acute traumatic occlusion. ■

and peroneal artery arise 3 to 6 cm distally. In 10% to 15%, variations are seen in the tibial vessel origins from the popliteal artery including an origin of the anterior or posterior tibial arteries at or above the knee joint line. The popliteal and tibial arteries are accompanied in their course by single or paired veins.

The anterior tibial artery traverses the superior edge of the interosseus membrane to enter the anterior compartment of the calf. It courses along the membrane accompanied by the deep peroneal nerve and the anterior tibial vein. This neurovascular bundle lies deep to the extensor muscles. The artery continues across the ankle joint beneath the extensor retinaculum to emerge on the top of the foot at the dorsalis pedis artery. Along its course, the anterior tibial artery gives off numerous muscular branches. The dorsalis pedis terminates in the superficial plantar arch.

The posterior tibial and peroneal arteries originate at the bifurcation of the tibial-peroneal trunk in the upper calf deep to the soleus muscle. The posterior tibial artery continues along the fascia of the deep posterior muscle compartment accompanied by the tibial and paired posterior tibial veins. It traverses the ankle joint posterior to the medial malleolus and terminates in the medial and lateral plantar arteries, which contribute to the deep and superficial plantar arches. Anastomotic connections between the anterior tibial artery and posterior tibial artery allow for adequate foot perfusion as long as one of the vessels remains patent.

The peroneal artery parallels the posterior tibial artery in a lateral course deep to the flexor hallucis longus muscle. It is accompanied by paired veins. Distally it terminates in lateral calcanean branches that anastomose with distal branches of the anterior tibial and posterior tibial arteries. These connections are small and may not be sufficient to supply the foot in acute occlusion of the other tibial vessels. The distal anterior or posterior tibial arteries may be supplied by a large terminal branch of the peroneal artery either as a congenital anomaly or because of collateralization after chronic occlusion of those vessels.

EPIDEMIOLOGY AND ETIOLOGY

Blunt trauma causes most civilian popliteal and tibial arterial injuries. Fracture or dislocation in the area of the knee is the predominate mechanism. In the military experience, penetrating injuries are more common. Occlusion of a single tibial vessel is well tolerated as long as no preexisting occlusion of the other vessels is present.

CLINICAL FEATURES AND DIAGNOSIS

Thrombosis with distal ischemia is the most common presentation of popliteal artery injury. Concomitant venous and neurologic trauma makes these injuries extremely morbid. Most patients with occlusion of the popliteal or more than one tibial artery occlusion have calf and foot ischemia. On the other hand, knee dislocation with spontaneous reduction may be overlooked unless a thorough peripheral vascular examination is performed. In these cases, the dislocation causes a shear effect producing intimal injury and delayed thrombosis.

A thorough peripheral vascular examination in all injured patients is the key to prompt recognition of popliteal and tibial artery injuries. Delays in diagnosis are invariably due to the lack of a physical examination of the pulses augmented with Doppler pressure determination when indicated. Ankle Doppler pressure determination allows rapid assessment of the patient with diminished distal pulses. Absence of Doppler flow sounds, an ankle brachial index of less than 0.8 or a 20 mm Hg decrease compared to the uninjured leg all indicate the need for further evaluation.

Duplex scanning has no role in the assessment of acute arterial trauma, adds nothing to physical examination augmented by Doppler pressure measurement, and is not accurate enough to assist in planning surgical treatment. Even when used by experienced surgeons or technicians, this technology does not obviate the need for arteriography or accurately predict the success of nonoperative therapy.

Arteriography is accurate in the evaluation of patients with suspected popliteal or tibial arterial injury but is time consuming and should be reserved for patients with equivocal physical findings. Emergency department or intraoperative angiography is also accurate and should be considered when formal angiography is not readily available.

SURGICAL TREATMENT

Both groins and both lower extremities should be prepared and draped. Contralateral saphenous vein is the conduit of choice for bypass and should be readily accessible. Popliteal injuries are best approached through a generous medial incision (Fig. 19–20). The simplest landmarks for the incision are the posterior margin of the femur proximally and the posterior margin of the tibia below the knee. During the medial exposure, care should be taken to avoid lacerating the saphenous vein. Post-traumatic deep venous insufficiency is common and this superficial vein may become an important collateral route of venous drainage. The proximal popliteal artery is exposed as it emerges from adductor canal. Exposure of the artery in the area of the knee joint requires division of the medial head of the gastrocnemius, semimembranosus, and semitendinosus muscles. The distal popliteal artery is exposed with an incision along the posterior margin of the tibia (Fig. 19–21).

Tibial vessel exposure requires careful dissection in the upper medial aspect of the calf. The origin of these vessels is exposed by continuing dissection from the distal popliteal artery through the area of the triceps surae. The exposure is facilitated by incising the soleus muscle longitudinally 2 cm posterior to

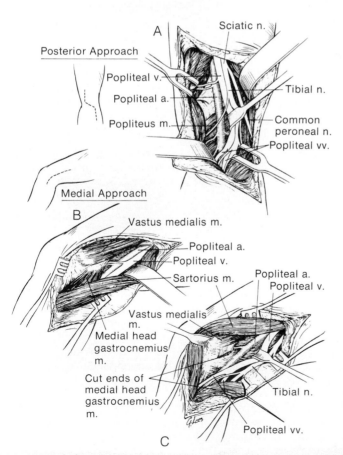

■ **FIGURE 19–20**
The posterior and medial approaches to the popliteal artery. *A,* A modified *S*-shaped incision is used in the posterior approach to avoid contracture across the knee joint. *B,* The medial approach requires a more extensive dissection but provides better access to proximal and distal vessels. *C,* Both approaches can be successfully used in the exposure and repair of the popliteal vessels. ■

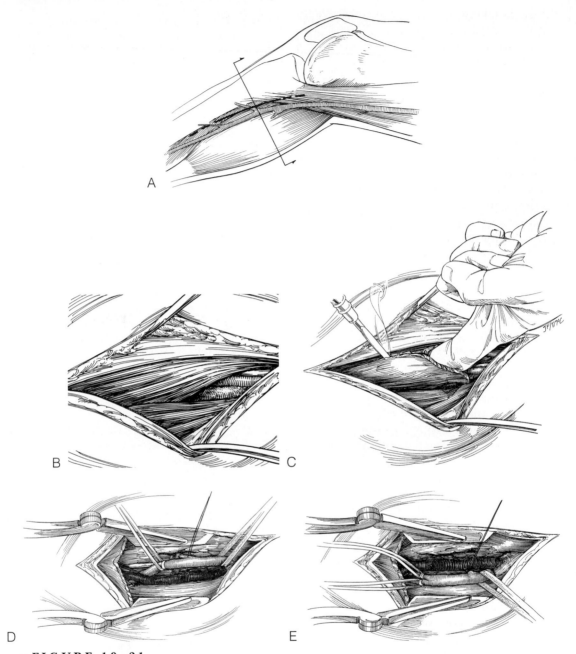

■ FIGURE 19–21

A, Distal popliteal exposure is obtained through an incision posterior to the tibia. *B* and *C,* The soleus muscle is divided longitudinally to expose the neurovascular bundle. *D,* The distal popliteal artery and anterior tibial artery origin is exposed ligating the anterior tibial vein and retracting the popliteal vein posteriorly. *E,* The tibioperoneal trunk and origins of the peroneal and posterior tibial arteries are exposed by retracting the popliteal vein anteriorly. (From Rutherford RB: Atlas of vascular surgery: Basic techniques and exposures. Philadelphia: WB Saunders, 1993.) ■

the tibia, taking care to avoid the soleal plexus of veins adjacent to the tibia. The anterior tibial artery origin is exposed by retracting the popliteal vein posteriorly. The anterior tibial vein should be carefully ligated. This short broad vein is difficult to control if lacerated. Once divided, it allows for exposure of the origin of the anterior tibial artery and the tibial peroneal trunk. The vessels distal to the anterior tibial origin are best exposed by retracting the veins anteriorly. Paired veins with crossing branches envelop the proximal posterior tibial and peroneal arteries. Distal exposure of these vessels is obtained through a medial incision along the posterior margin of the tibia down to the space posterior to the medial malleolus. The anterior tibial artery is exposed through an incision along the middle of the anterior compartment. Dissection is carried deep between the extensor hallucis and extensor digitorum muscles to the level of the interosseus membrane and the artery (Fig. 19–22).

Popliteal and tibial arterial injuries are rarely simple lacerations. Repair usually requires saphenous vein interposition. Primary repair of the popliteal artery is appropriate in lacerations from knife wounds, which result in little arterial disruption. Blunt injuries and gunshot wounds should be treated by careful débridement of all injured vessel wall and tension-free repair with vein interposition grafting (Shah and colleagues, 1985).

Arterial repair at the popliteal and tibial level should always be evaluated with interoperative completion angiography. Any defect in the repair should be immediately addressed with either a catheter thrombectomy or a revision of the anastomosis. Early occlusion with platelet thrombus should be carefully investigated to rule out a technical defect in the repair. If platelet deposition in the area of repair occurs, a continuous infusion of low-molecular-weight dextran should be started. This is a treacherous clinical problem and must be aggressively treated.

Soft tissue coverage of arterial repairs in the region of the knee and calf is essential to successful limb salvage. Infection or exposure of vein interposition grafts always leads to thrombosis or hemorrhage and a high rate of limb loss.

RESULTS

Injury of the popliteal and tibial vessel level is associated with significant long-term disability. The initial outcome is dependent on successful arterial repair and the extent of soft tissue damage and ischemia. Infections of arterial repairs at this level are usually associated with inadequate soft tissue coverage. Long-term results are dependent on the extent of musculoskeletal and neurologic injury. Tibial nerve transection is associated with poor long-term results. Early physical therapy is essential to maximize the recovery of function in all lower extremity vascular injuries.

Lower Extremity Compartment Syndrome

Compartment syndrome may present 12 to 24 hours after reperfusion. If not promptly diagnosed and treated, the risk of limb loss or severe dysfunction is high. Calf compartment syndrome most commonly results from prolonged ischemia or a crush injury. Frequent physical examinations augmented with compartment pressure measurements are necessary to detect this complication in its early stage. The first complaint may be sensory loss in the foot. Thigh compartment syndrome is rare. Thigh muscle swelling and pain out of proportion to the severity of injury are the most common findings.

Mangled Lower Extremity

Every effort must be made to balance the surgical reconstruction of the mangled extremity with the overall status of the patient both immediately following injury and during the rehabilitation phases of care. Primary amputation should be considered in patients with severe soft tissue injury and a dysvascular extremity. Objective rating scales or scoring systems are an adjunct to clinical judgment but not a substitute for careful consideration of what is reasonable and appropriate for the patient's short-term and long-term recovery (Gregory and colleagues, 1985; Johansen

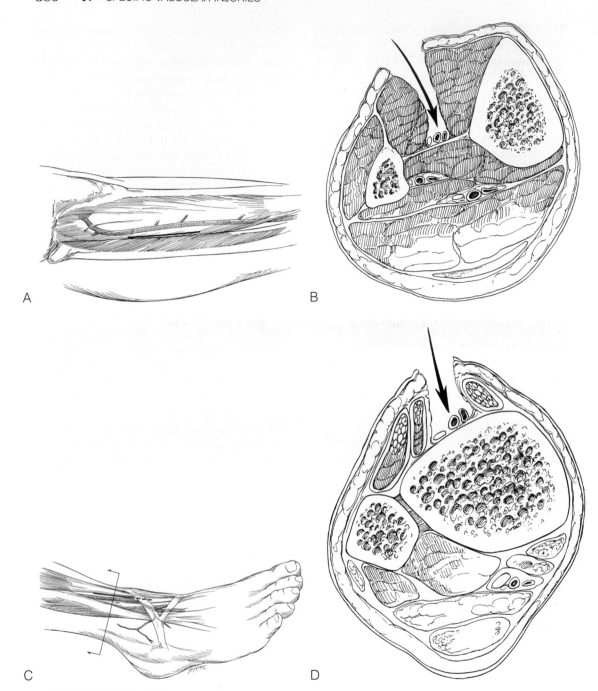

■ FIGURE 19–22

A, Proximal exposure of the anterior tibial artery is obtained through an incision along the anterolateral aspect of the calf. *B,* The extensor muscles are retracted anteriorly and posteriorly to expose the anterior tibial neurovascular bundle on the interosseous membrane. *C,* Distal exposure is obtained through an incision along the extensor digitorum tendon. *D,* The anterior tibial artery lies adjacent to the tibia beneath the flexor tendons and the extensor retinaculum. (From Rutherford RB: Atlas of vascular surgery: Basic techniques and exposures. Philadelphia: WB Saunders, 1993.) ■

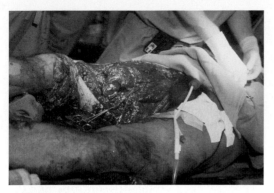

■ **FIGURE 19–23**
Mangled extremity with severe degloving injury
associated with an open femur fracture. This
limb was initially thought to be unsalvageable,
but with appropriate revascularization and
débridement, the extremity was saved and was
functional. ■

and colleagues, 1990; Bonanni, Rhodes, and
Lucke, 1993). Delayed amputation following
initially successful vascular repair remains an
unfortunate possibility in patients with extensive musculoskeletal and neurologic injury.
Most trauma centers pursue an aggressive
approach to young patients with these
complex injuries. Mangled extremities are
often salvaged with a multidisciplinary
approach; however, amputation is eventually
the best choice for a pain-free return to functional status in some patients (Fig. 19–23). This
decision is never easily made and is based on
a strong physician–patient partnership.
Setting reasonable expectations immediately
after injury is the best starting point in
this process. Early involvement of a multidisciplinary approach also allows for a timely
decision about amputation. This remains one
of the most challenging problems for trauma
surgeons.

Venous Injuries of the Lower Extremity

The aggressive approach to arterial injuries
in the extremities has not been matched with
equal enthusiasm for venous repair. Instead,
ligation is frequently performed. However, ligation may result in thrombosis and venous
insufficiency, ultimately leading to significant
chronic disability. A balanced approach that
includes ligation for injuries of minor veins
or for life-threatening injuries in unstable
patients, and repair or reconstruction
whenever possible may be the best strategy
(Nypaver and colleagues, 1992; Timberlake
and Kerstein, 1995; Zamir and colleagues,
1998).

SURGICAL ANATOMY

Paired veins form from muscle branches in
the calf and course parallel to the tibial vessels
and coalesce into the popliteal vein, which may
also be paired. The calf is also drained by
numerous subcutaneous veins that flow to
either the greater or the lesser saphenous vein.
The greater saphenous vein joins the common
femoral vein in the groin and the lesser saphenous vein travels proximally along the back
of the calf to join the popliteal vein. Numerous perforating veins connect the greater
saphenous to the deep system. Flow is directed
deep and proximally by valves in both the
superficial and the deep system.
   The popliteal vein transitions the adductor
canal to become the superficial femoral vein.
Numerous muscular branches join this vein.
The profunda femoral vein drains the quadriceps and deep muscles and joins the superficial femoral vein to form a single large
common femoral vein. All of the lower extremity veins collateralize to form an extensive
network of alternative venous drainage routes.
In the absence of disruption of these collaterals, a single-level venous occlusion does not
prevent adequate venous drainage.

EPIDEMIOLOGY AND ETIOLOGY

Venous injury is usually associated with arterial injury and is most commonly due to penetrating trauma. Veins are much more elastic
than arteries and are less frequently injured
in blunt force trauma. Fractures, however, can
lead to lacerations and thrombosis. The low-
pressure venous system allows for tamponade,
and significant external hemorrhage is
uncommon except in large lacerations of the
femoral and popliteal veins.

CLINICAL FEATURES AND DIAGNOSIS

Most clinically significant venous injuries present as persistent hemorrhage of dark red blood from a penetrating wound. In the absence of external hemorrhage or the need for surgical exploration for concomitant arterial trauma, the diagnosis of venous injury is usually delayed. Venous hypertension following major vein injury and thrombosis is usually well tolerated despite causing distal extremity edema. Lower extremity ischemia is rare following venous injury and is the result of extensive soft tissue damage and loss of collateral venous flow. Compartment syndrome is also uncommon and is usually delayed in onset when it occurs.

Duplex scanning is an effective and accurate diagnostic modality to assess venous patency in blunt-force injuries. Most trauma centers periodically perform surveillance duplex scanning of the lower extremities of trauma patients following major injuries. Dynamic computed tomographic scanning and arteriography are rarely used to diagnose venous injuries. Most venous injuries of clinical significance are diagnosed at the time of surgical exploration for arterial trauma due to the high rate of coincidental injuries.

SURGICAL TREATMENT

The veins of the lower extremity are exposed by the same incisions used to expose the associated arteries. Direct pressure and proximal and distal dissection in adjacent tissue allows hemostatic control. Clamp application should be carefully performed or control obtained with Silastic vessel loops to avoid secondary venous trauma.

The choice of technique for venous repair depends on the patient's overall status, the extent of venous and soft tissue injury, and the duration of ischemia from associated arterial injury. Life-threatening associated injuries or hemodynamic instability mandate ligation of venous injuries. Extensive soft tissue injury and loss of collateral venous flow mandate venous reconstruction. Prolonged ischemia from arterial occlusion leads to a dilemma when venous injury is associated. If possible, the vein should be repaired first. Simple lacerations may be repaired by lateral suture, taking care to avoid stenosis. Occasionally, end-to-end repair is possible.

If extensive venous reconstruction is required and associated arterial injury is present, it is best to restore arterial perfusion with a shunt. Venous interposition grafts or venous panel grafts should be used to restore adequate lumen diameter. Panel grafts are constructed by harvesting a sufficient length of contralateral saphenous vein, opening the vein longitudinally, wrapping it in a spiral fashion around an appropriately sized chest tube, and sewing the vein into a conduit for interposition in the injured vein. This tedious and time-consuming procedure requires loupe magnification and precise technique. The use of synthetic grafts for the repair of lower extremity venous injuries is to be avoided because of the certainty of early thrombosis.

The use of small arteriovenous fistula upstream from the venous repair to maintain high flow has been suggested. This technique is time consuming and unproven in its efficacy in the management of venous injuries. A low-molecular-weight dextran infusion to limit platelet adhesion carries a low risk of bleeding complications and may help maintain early patency of the repaired vein. Dextran 40 is infused at 40 mL per hour for 24 hours. Full anticoagulation with intravenous heparin is associated with a significant risk of bleeding and is best reserved for proven deep venous thrombosis.

RESULTS

A traditional skepticism exists among surgeons about the likelihood of venous patency after reconstruction for trauma. Well-performed repairs remain patent at an encouraging rate. Early patency depends on the avoidance of stenosis and prevention of thrombosis. If early thrombosis occurs, recanalization occurs in a significant number of patients. If ligation is required, early postinjury edema can be minimized by placing the lower extremity in a continuous passive mobilization device. Pulmonary emboli are uncommon following venous repair (Nypaver and colleagues, 1992; Timberlake and Kerstein, 1995; Zamir and colleagues, 1998), but chronic venous insufficiency is common.

REFERENCES

Bonanni F, Rhodes M, Lucke JF: The futility of predictive scoring of mangled lower extremities. J Trauma 1993;34:99-105.

Costa MC, Robbs JV: Nonpenetrating subclavian artery trauma. J Vasc Surg 1988;8:71-75.

Endean ED, Veldenz HC, Schwarcz TH, Hyde GL. Recognition of arterial injury in elbow dislocation. J Vasc Surg 1992;16:402-406.

Feliciano DV, Herskowitz K, O'Gorman RB, et al: Management of vascular injuries in the lower extremity. J Trauma 1988;28:319-328.

Feliciano DV, Mattox KL, Graham JM, Bitondo CG: Five-year experience with PTFE grafts in vascular wounds. J Trauma 1985;25:71-82.

Graham JM, Mattox KL, Feliciano DV, DeBakey ME: Vascular injuries of the axilla. Ann Surg 1982;195:232-238.

Granchi T, Schmittling Z, Vasquez J, et al: Prolonged use of intraluminal arterial shunts without systemic anticoagulation. Am J Surg 2000;180:493-497.

Gregory RT, Gould RJ, Peclet M, et al: The mangled extremity syndrome (MES): a severity grading system for multi-system injury of the extremity. J Trauma 1985;25:1147-1150.

Hafez HM, Woolgar J, Robbs JV: Lower extremity arterial injury: results of 550 cases and review of risk factors associated with limb loss. J Vasc Surg 2001;33:1212-1219.

Hardin WD, O'Connell RC, Adinolfi MF, Kerstein MD: Traumatic injuries of the upper extremity: determinants of disability. Am J Surg 1985;150:266-270.

Humphrey PW, Nichols WK, Silver D: Rural vascular trauma: a twenty year review. Ann Vasc Surg 1994;8:179-185.

Johansen K, Daines M, Howey T, et al: Objective criteria accurately predict amputation following lower extremity trauma. J Trauma 1990;30:568-573.

Johnson M, Ford M, Johansen K: Radial or ulnar artery laceration. Repair or ligate? Arch Surg 1993;128:971-975.

Mattox KL, Feliciano DV, Burch J, et al: Five thousand seven hundred sixty cardiovascular injuries in 4459 patients. Epidemiologic evolution 1958 to 1987. Ann Surg 1989;209:698-674.

Meyer J, Walsh J, Schuler J, et al: The early fate of venous repair after civilian vascular trauma. A clinical, hemodynamic, and venographic assessment. Ann Surg 1987;206:458-464.

Nypaver TJ, Schuler JJ, McDonnell P, et al: Long-term results of venous reconstruction after vascular trauma in civilian practice. J Vasc Surg 1992;16:762-768.

Pappas PJ, Haser PB, Teehan EP, et al: Outcome of complex venous reconstructions in patients with trauma. J Vasc Surg 1997;25:398-404.

Rich NM, Baugh JH, Hughes CW: Acute arterial injuries in Vietnam: 1,000 cases. J Trauma 1970; 10:359-369.

Rich NM, Spencer FC: Subclavian artery injuries. In: Vascular Trauma. Philadelphia: WB Saunders, 1978:307-329.

Romanoff H, Goldberger S: Combined severe vascular and skeletal trauma: management and results. J Cardiovasc Surg 1979;20:493-498.

Rosental JJ, Gaspar MR, Gjerdrum TC, Newman J: Vascular injuries associated with fractured femur. Arch Surg 1975;110:494-499.

Rozycki GS, Tremblay LN, Feliciano DV, McClelland WB: Blunt vascular trauma in the extremity: Diagnosis, management, and outcome. J Trauma 2003;55(5):814-824.

Sampson LN, Britton JC, Eldrup-Jorgensen J, et al: The neurovascular outcome of scapulothoracic dissociation. J Vasc Surg 1993;17:1083-1089.

Shackford SR, Rich NM: Peripheral vascular injury. In: Mattox KL, Moore EE, Feliciano DV, eds. Trauma. Philadelphia: WB Saunders, 2001:1011-1046.

Shah DM, Naraynsingh V, Leather RP, et al: Advances in the management of popliteal vascular blunt injuries. J Trauma 1985;25:793-799.

Sparks SR, DeLaRosa J, Bergan JJ, et al: Arterial injury in uncomplicated upper extremity dislocations. Ann Vasc Surg 2000;14:110-113.

Timberlake GA, Kerstein MD: Venous injury: to repair or ligate, the dilemma revisited. Am Surg 1995;61:139-145.

Zamir G, Berlatzky Y, Rivkind A, et al: Results of reconstruction in major pelvic and extremity venous injuries. J Vasc Surg 1998;28:901-908.

SECTION V

SPECIAL PROBLEMS
AND COMPLICATIONS

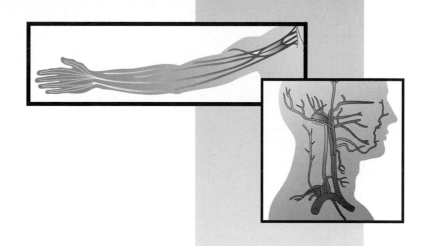

Special Problems

ERIC R. FRYKBERG

There are a number of distinct clinical presentations, problems, and issues in vascular trauma that pose special challenges in diagnosis and management for the surgeon who is confronted with these injuries. Each of these special problems is plagued by relatively poor outcomes, even in the most experienced trauma centers. They tend to be uncommon and complex and require rapid detection and treatment, multidisciplinary prioritization, and innovative management techniques. The purpose of this chapter is to provide a thorough knowledge of the history, epidemiology, current literature, and suggested approaches for some of the most difficult of these problems to optimize outcome.

POPLITEAL ARTERY INJURIES

The special challenge of injury to the popliteal artery lies primarily in the anatomy of this vessel, which begins as the continuation of the superficial femoral artery as it courses through the hiatus of the adductor magnus muscle. Covered proximally by the semimembranosus muscle, it lies only in subcutaneous tissue in the popliteal fossa behind the knee joint, situated between the two heads of the gastrocnemius muscle. It is in this fossa that the popliteal artery is especially vulnerable to stretch and direct injury from extrinsic forces and skeletal distortions, such as fractures and knee dislocations, being tethered proximally and distally to the femur and tibia by tendons of the adductor and soleus muscles. It most often bifurcates twice. As the anterior tibial artery branches laterally through the interosseous septum, the main artery continues for another 2 to 3 cm as the tibioperoneal trunk. This vessel then terminally bifurcates into the peroneal and posterior tibial arteries. Several geniculate, sural, and muscular collateral vessels branch from the popliteal artery behind the knee, which anastomose in a rich network with branches of the profunda femoris artery proximally and tibial arteries distally. However, this collateral supply is frail and subject to obliteration and thrombosis by injury to the main artery and surrounding tissues. These collaterals cannot maintain viability of the leg and foot on their own.

The fact that the popliteal artery is a true end artery with a tenuous collateral support explains why injury to it is so dangerous, and why such injury has long been recognized as the most limb threatening of all peripheral vascular trauma. Nonetheless, several recent advances in diagnosis and treatment of popliteal artery injury have led to dramatic reductions in limb loss and limb morbidity.

History and Epidemiology

General Albert Sidney Johnston died in the American Civil War during the Battle of Shiloh in April 1862 of exsanguination from a gunshot wound to the popliteal artery, an injury that currently would be considered quite treatable and not life threatening. In 1906, the first use of autogenous vein to repair an arterial injury was reported by Goyanes for a traumatic aneurysm of the popliteal artery. Injuries of this artery represented 12% of all arterial injuries in British troops in World War I, 20% of arterial injuries in American troops in World War II, 26% of those in the Korean War, and 217 (21.7%) of 1000 arterial injuries in the Vietnam War. These were virtually all due to penetrating trauma, from bomb and land-mine fragments and high-velocity gunshots. Over the past 25 years, popliteal artery injuries in the civilian sector account for approximately 20% of all extremity arterial injuries reported in the published literature, and as many as 20% to 75% of cases in this setting are caused by blunt mechanisms.

The standard treatment of all extremity arterial trauma before the Korean War was ligation. DeBakey and Simeone (1946) documented this approach to result in limb loss in 72.5% of all popliteal artery injuries in World War II, the highest of any extremity artery. Additionally, many salvaged limbs had severe functional disability. During the Korean and Vietnam Wars, when acute surgical repair replaced ligation for arterial trauma, the incidence of amputation following popliteal artery injury improved substantially to only 29.5%, with fewer problems of morbidity and disability in salvaged limbs. As repair techniques and the use of surgical adjuncts have improved, there has been further substantial improvement in outcome since Vietnam following repair of highly destructive combat injuries of this artery, with limb salvage now approaching 90% (Table 20–1).

As this military experience with arterial repair was adopted in the civilian sector, the same improvements in limb salvage have been realized since the 1950s, despite the higher incidence of more destructive blunt trauma in this setting. Fabian and colleagues (1982) reported 165 civilian popliteal artery injuries treated over 30 years, showing an improvement in amputation rates from 74% to 6% during this period. Daugherty and colleagues (1978) documented a reduction of amputation rates from 54% to 9% among 24 civilian popliteal artery injuries over a 10-year period. Thomas and colleagues (1989) similarly showed a reduction in limb loss from 30% before 1980 to 15% after 1980 in their review of 610 cases of civilian popliteal artery injuries in 25 published series. During the 1980s, four published civilian series reported 78 cases of both penetrating and blunt popliteal artery injury without a single amputation. Although there has been a tendency toward improvement in limb salvage as time has progressed, continued reports of high rates of limb loss even in recent years emphasize how dangerous these injuries remain (Table 20–2).

Diagnostic Issues

GENERAL PRINCIPLES AND MODALITIES

The time interval from popliteal artery injury to repair is the most important factor in limb salvage. Virtually all reports document that the most common reason for limb loss in this setting is a delay in recognition and revascularization. This is because of the time-dependent nature of the major consequences of vascular injury, tissue ischemia, and hemorrhage, to which the popliteal circulation is especially vulnerable. Therefore, a prompt and accurate diagnosis of popliteal artery trauma, within 6 hours of injury, is an extremely important factor influencing outcome.

Diagnosis can be made in most cases by physical examination, as long as the significance of the clinical manifestations of popliteal artery injury is understood. Obvious physical findings of arterial injury, also known as *hard signs,* are present in 70% to 90% of these cases, including active hemorrhage, large, expanding, or pulsatile hematoma, bruit or thrill, absent distal pulses, and distal ischemia (pain, pallor, paralysis, paresthesias, and coolness). These findings must never be ignored. In the setting of uncomplicated penetrating trauma to the lower extremity, any of these signs mandate immediate surgery, because the probability of a major arterial injury requiring repair approaches 100%, and the penetrating wounds clearly show where that

TABLE 20–1
MILITARY EXPERIENCE WITH POPLITEAL ARTERY INJURIES*

Author	Year	Conflict	No. Cases	No. Amputations (%)
Makins	1922	WWI	144	62 (43)
DeBakey, Simeone	1946	WWII	502	364 (72.5)
Hughes	1958	Korea	68	22 (32.4)
Rich	1970	Vietnam	217	64 (29.5)
D'Sa	1980	Ireland	32	4 (12.5)
Sfeir	1992	Lebanon	118	14 (12)
TOTAL			1081	530 (49)

*All injuries were ligated in WWI and WWII and were repaired in all remaining series. WWI, World War I; WWII, World War II.

TABLE 20–2
MANAGEMENT RESULTS OF CIVILIAN POPLITEAL ARTERY INJURIES

Author	Year	No. Cases	No. Penetrating	No. Blunt	No. Amputations (%)
Conkle	1975	27	13	14	12 (44)
Daugherty	1978	24	11	13	8 (33)
O'Reilly	1978	49	49	0	6 (12)
Lim	1980	31	19	12	0
Holleman	1981	32	18	14	4 (12.5)
Fabian	1982	165	125	40	44 (27)
Jaggers	1982	61	49	12	9 (15)
Snyder	1982	110	81	29	14 (13)
McCabe	1983	24	5	19	4 (17)
Orcutt	1983	37	20	17	6 (16)
Yeager	1984	10	5	5	0
Shah	1985	30	0	30	0
Downs	1986	63	10	53	18 (29)
Krige	1987	28	14	14	3 (11)
Weimann	1987	36	11	25	1 (3.6)
Armstrong	1988	76	60	16	9 (12)
Peck	1990	108	32	76	13 (12)
Reed	1990	7	4	3	0
Martin	1994	40	26	14	6 (15)
DeGiannis	1995	35	35	0	5 (14)
Fainzilber	1995	81	63	18	13 (16)
Pretre	1996	31	0	31	6 (19)
Harrell	1997	38	0	38	14 (37)
Melton	1997	102	62	40	25 (25)
Razuk	1998	25	15	10	6 (24)
TOTAL		1270	728 (57%)	543 (43%)	226 (18)

injury is located. Any further diagnostic tests would be superfluous, unnecessarily costly, and potentially dangerous in view of the adverse impact of the inevitable delay on outcome. Exceptions to this include any circumstance in which the physical examination does not clearly reflect the presence or location of arterial injury (e.g., blunt trauma, elderly patient with chronic vascular insufficiency, associated skeletal trauma, shotgun wounds, thoracic outlet wounds, and established complications of delay), in which case arteriographic imaging is warranted.

Arteriography is now known to be unnecessary in injured extremities that do not manifest any hard signs of popliteal artery injury, regardless of mechanism or wound complexity. In the past, all asymptomatic wounds (i.e., those with no hard signs) placing the popliteal artery at risk either were surgically explored or underwent routine arteri-ography. These included penetrating injuries in proximity to the artery and all high-risk blunt trauma, such as lower extremity crush, distal femur or proximal tibia fractures, and posterior knee dislocations. It has long been known that in this setting, occult vascular injury may still be present in 10% to 15% of cases. However, recent studies have shown that such asymptomatic vascular injuries are consistently nonocclusive and have a benign and self-limited natural history with a high rate of spontaneous resolution. They, therefore, require neither surgical repair, nor the considerable expense and resources necessary for routine detection. Virtually all limb-threatening complications of delayed diagnosis of popliteal artery injury are due to overlooked hard signs, rather than an absence of relevant physical findings, on initial presentation.

Noninvasive testing with Doppler pressure measurements and duplex ultrasonography has been applied to the evaluation of injured extremities for popliteal artery trauma, with the potential of being less invasive and less costly than, while equally accurate, as arteriography and surgery. However, these modalities have not realized their theoretical potential for a number of reasons, including equipment expense, lack of round-the-clock availability of the necessary skill and expertise in most hospitals, and a failure to show any advantage over physical examination alone. Several authors have documented these modalities to have no benefit in this setting (Bergstein et al, 1992; Tominaga et al, 1996).

Posterior Knee Dislocation

Posterior knee dislocation has been associated with a substantial incidence of popliteal artery trauma, for which reason mandatory arteriography or popliteal exploration has been advocated to avoid the high risk of limb loss from delayed diagnosis of popliteal artery injury. At least six published studies from the past decade, which report 264 cases of posterior knee dislocation, have related the initial clinical findings to outcome (Table 20–3). The results demonstrate that only 23% (range, 13% to 25%) of all cases present with hard signs of popliteal artery injury, and 70% of this group (range, 18% to 100%) had arterial injury requiring surgical repair (i.e., 30% false-positive rate of physical examination for the detection of surgically significant arterial injury). Among the 77% of all cases of posterior knee dislocation presenting without hard signs, there was not a single popliteal artery injury that required surgical repair, a result confirmed by follow-up studies of up to 1 year. These findings are consistent with those of all other forms of extremity injury in confirming the reliability of physical examination to exclude arterial injury. This has enormous economic implications when considering the expense and morbidity of routine diagnostic workup that can be avoided in such a large majority of patients, especially considering how tight resources are in so many trauma centers and other hospitals. Surgical exploration of the popliteal artery is warranted in the minority of patients presenting with hard signs, especially when obviously due to arterial disruption (e.g., pulsatile hemorrhage and cool ischemic limb without pulses). However, preoperative arteriography in less obvious cases of hard signs (e.g., transient pulse loss

TABLE 20–3
PUBLISHED CASES OF KNEE DISLOCATION RELATING PHYSICAL FINDINGS OF VASCULAR INJURY TO OUTCOME

Author	Year	No. KD	Hard Signs Present			Hard Signs Absent		
			No.	(%)*	No. AIRS (%)[†]	No.	(%)*	No. AIRS
Treiman	1992	115	29	(25)	22 (75)	86	(75)	0[‡]
Kendall	1993	37	6	(16)	6 (100)	31	(84)	0
Kaufman	1992	19	4	(21)	4 (100)	15	(79)	0[§]
Dennis	1993	38	2	(13)	2 (100)	36	(87)	0[‖]
Miranda	2000	32	8	(25)	6 (75)	24	(75)	0
Martinez	2001	23	11	(48)	2 (18)	12	(52)	0[¶]
TOTAL		264	60	(23)	42 (70)	204	(77)	0

*Percentage of total knee dislocations.
[†]Percentage of all patients with hard signs.
[‡]Includes nine minimal arterial injuries with 6 months of average follow-up.
[§]Includes two minimal arterial injuries with 3 and 23 months of follow-up.
[‖]Includes seven minimal arterial injuries with 11.5 months of average follow-up.
[¶]Includes five minimal arterial injuries with 3 months of average follow-up.
AIRS, arterial injuries requiring surgery; KD, knee dislocations.

and hematoma) may allow avoidance of unnecessary vascular exploration in about 20% of cases by demonstrating an intact artery.

Treatment

GENERAL PRINCIPLES AND TECHNIQUES

Prompt transport to the operating room and induction of general anesthesia are necessary once popliteal artery injury has been documented. The patient should be supine and the injured leg should be prepared and draped into the operative field, as should one uninjured extremity in the event that autogenous vein must be harvested. The leg should be abducted and externally rotated with a support under the knee, to facilitate the standard longitudinal medial incision above the knee for optimal popliteal artery exposure. Retraction of the sartorius and semimembranosus muscles posteriorly opens the popliteal space where the artery lies, with the vein and nerve medial and posterior to it. Division of the medial head of the gastrocnemius muscle and tendons of the semimembranosus, semitendinosus, and gracilis muscles allows exposure of the more distal tibioperoneal trunk. Although these structures may be repaired, this is not necessary for an excellent functional result. Arterial repair is performed by the standard techniques of vascular surgery.

Hemorrhage from the injured artery should be controlled by digital pressure until proximal and distal control can be obtained with clamps or vessel loops. Obviously damaged portions of the artery should be débrided back to grossly normal vessel. Balloon catheter thrombectomy should be performed proximally and distally, followed by distal injection of heparinized saline to retard any further thrombus formation. Systemic heparinization may be used if associated injuries permit.

Lateral arteriorrhaphy may be performed with clean lacerations involving less than 30% of the arterial circumference, although only 10% 15% of popliteal artery injuries are amenable to this. Care must be taken to avoid stenosis and thrombosis, and vein patch angioplasty may facilitate this. End-to-end anastomosis is preferred if it can be done without undue tension but is generally not possible if more than 2 cm of artery is lost. Geniculate collaterals should not be divided to achieve mobility because of the detrimental effect this may have on limb perfusion. In this setting, interposition grafting should be performed, preferably using reversed autogenous saphenous vein. Prosthetic grafts across the knee joint tend to have lower patency rates. Arterial anastomosis and repair are performed with a running monofilament nonabsorbable suture, achieving intimal coaptation. Surgical repair should not be considered complete until distal perfusion is clearly documented with palpable pulses in the feet.

SURGICAL ADJUNCTS

A number of measures are available in addition to standard surgical repair of popliteal artery trauma, which should further improve outcome from these dangerous injuries. The liberal use of preoperative and intraoperative systemic and regional anticoagulation with intravenous heparin has been mentioned. Postoperative anticoagulation should almost never be necessary, because it cannot substitute for the meticulous and appropriate technique, which is the most important factor in a successful surgical repair. Any failure of arterial repair should mandate exploration and revision. Completion arteriography is important to ensure patency and distal runoff, especially if there is any doubt about the adequacy of revascularization. This can be done on the operating table by direct needle puncture of the vessel proximal to the injury and injection of water-soluble contrast.

Extra-anatomic bypass should be considered when the native vessel bed is unsuitable for vascular repair, because of contamination, devitalized tissue, or lack of soft tissue coverage. A prosthetic or autogenous vein interposition is tunneled laterally through clean tissue planes from uninvolved proximal and distal portions of the artery, allowing open management of the wound without worry about the vessel.

Fasciotomy to release excessive pressure within the major tissue compartments of the lower leg is a critical adjunct to popliteal artery repair, because injury to this artery poses a high risk of compartmental hypertension and tissue loss (see Chapter 27). Early or prophylactic fasciotomy in this setting has been associated with improved limb salvage and function.

Intraluminal shunting of injured popliteal arteries can be a useful adjunct in those circumstances in which a delay is necessary for skeletal stabilization, soft tissue débridement or vein repair. This immediately restores perfusion, allowing these other problems to be addressed deliberately without ongoing ischemia, before definitive arterial repair is performed.

NONOPERATIVE OBSERVATION

A select group of arterial injuries are nonocclusive and manifest no hard signs, and these have been shown to have a high rate of spontaneous resolution or nonprogression when left untreated. These include intimal flaps, vessel narrowing, and small false aneurysms and arteriovenous fistulas, in which the artery and its runoff remain intact. When found on arteriography, the safety of nonoperative observation of these asymptomatic arterial injuries has been established by long-term follow-up averaging 10 years. This category of arterial injuries exclusively includes the 10% to 15% of arterial injuries known to occur in the setting of asymptomatic lower extremity trauma that places the popliteal artery at risk, such as penetrating proximity wounds and high-risk fractures and posterior knee dislocation. This is what justifies the simple observation of asymptomatic lower extremity trauma without the need for routine surgery or diagnostic imaging for popliteal artery injury (see Table 20–3). The safe avoidance of this routine diagnostic workup on the basis of only a negative physical examination has clear advantages in terms of substantial savings of cost and resource use, as well as reduced limb morbidity.

MANAGEMENT OF VENOUS INJURIES

History and Epidemiology

The evolution of the management principles and techniques for venous injuries has followed the same path as that for arterial injuries, although an appreciation for the distinct differences in venous response to injury and repair did not occur until relatively recently. The first successful surgical repair of a venous injury is credited to the German surgeon Schede in 1882, who reported the lateral suture of a femoral vein. Kummel performed the first successful end-to-end venous anastomosis in 1899, and Goodman reported four cases of lateral venorrhaphy in World War I. Ligation of all injured and uninjured veins adjacent to an arterial injury was advocated by Makins in World War I, to theoretically increase the "dwell time" of blood within the injured extremity after arterial ligation. Venous ligation remained standard practice through World War II and the Korea War, although 20 venous injuries underwent surgical repair in the latter conflict. In the Vietnam War, an aggressive approach toward routine repair of all venous injuries was advocated after reviewing the major complications resulting from venous ligation in the Vietnam Vascular Registry. The overall rate of venous repair rose to 33% in this conflict, and the clear benefits of repair were demonstrated. The fears of previous years that repair would lead to increased levels of thrombophlebitis and embolism were proven groundless and were shown to occur more often when veins were ligated. This military experience rapidly spread into the civilian sector. In 1960, Gaspar and Treiman published the first large series of civilian venous injuries, which confirmed the problems with ligation and the safety and feasibility of routine repair of venous injuries.

The actual incidence of peripheral venous injuries is unknown, because many are known to be asymptomatic, heal spontaneously, and are never discovered. Venous injuries made up 39% of all vascular injuries in the Korean War and 27% of all vascular injuries in the

Vietnam War. They were most often (86%) associated with an adjacent arterial injury in both conflicts. These were largely peripheral in location, because abdominal and cervical venous injuries are highly lethal in military settings, and virtually all were due to destructive and high-velocity penetrating mechanisms. In the civilian sector, venous injuries similarly comprise between 13% and 51% of all vascular injuries, and 35% to 63% of all extremity vascular trauma. In this setting, they also are most commonly due to penetrating, though low-velocity, mechanisms and most commonly occur in association with an adjacent arterial injury. Blunt mechanisms cause 5% to 15% of all civilian venous injuries (Table 20–4). Isolated venous injuries are most likely to result from stab wounds than from other blunt or penetrating agents. Abdominal venous injuries comprise as much as 15% of all civilian vascular trauma. The superficial femoral vein and the popliteal vein are the most commonly injured veins overall in military and civilian series, respectively, consistent with the most common sites of arterial injury. The inferior vena cava is the most common site of abdominal venous injury.

Diagnosis

Peripheral venous injuries are most commonly found incidentally during exploration for an arterial injury. Although they may manifest hard signs, these signs are not specific for venous trauma. Bleeding from the low-pressure venous system is generally easily tamponaded by surrounding structures, which is why venous injuries often are not detected in the absence of arterial injuries. When isolated, venous injuries most commonly present as hemorrhage or large hematoma, which prompts the surgical exploration leading to their detection. Venous trauma is most likely to present with severe bleeding, shock, or hypotension when combined with an arterial injury or when involving one of the major abdominal veins.

Routine venography following extremity trauma has been advocated. Gerlock and colleagues (1976) performed this imaging in 30 consecutive patients with penetrating extremity trauma, detecting five venous injuries (17%). However, four of these five injuries had associated arterial injuries that would have led to their detection without venography. Gagne and colleagues (1995) found venography of injured extremities to be suboptimal and to be difficult to perform, with more than 50% of attempts technically unsuccessful and only 43% of all venous injuries detected. The only benefit of routine venography would be in its detection of previously unsuspected and asymptomatic venous injuries, but there is no evidence to support that such occult venous trauma results in any adverse sequelae when left untreated. In fact, occult venous trauma,

---

TABLE 20–4
EXTREMITY VENOUS INJURIES: MECHANISM AND MANAGEMENT

Author	Year	Total No.	No. Penetrating	No. Isolated	No. Repaired
Rich*	1970	377	377	53	124
Sullivan*	1971	26	26	8	21
Agarwal	1982	57	53	18	34
Phifer	1984	25	25	0	19
Ross	1985	22	0	1	12
Pasch	1986	82	0	4	53
Borman	1987	82	71	20	74
Meyer	1987	36	34	2	36
Yelon	1992	79	78	31	31
Timberlake	1995	322	292	83	98
TOTAL		1108	956 (95%)[†]	220 (20%)	502 (45%)

*Military series.
[†]Based on 1004 injuries that could be evaluated.

even in the inferior vena cava, has been shown to have no long-term complications, suggesting that routine diagnostic imaging for this purpose is unnecessary and not cost effective. On the other hand, Gagne and colleagues (1995) found major thromboembolic complications to occur in 50% of patients with documented asymptomatic venous injuries following penetrating extremity trauma, although whether this was specifically related to the venous trauma is not clear.

Duplex ultrasonography has been applied to the detection of arterial injuries following extremity trauma by several authors. Gagne and colleagues (1995) reported the detection of occult venous injuries in 22% of patients with asymptomatic penetrating extremity trauma, although the benefits of this detection were not clear.

Currently most trauma centers do not perform venous imaging of any sort following torso or extremity trauma. In cases presenting with hard signs, imaging is generally contraindicated, because immediate surgery is warranted. In the absence of hard signs, imaging is unnecessary because there is no clear benefit to intervention for occult venous injury. Only if subsequent symptoms develop, such as venous insufficiency or thromboembolic events, would venous imaging be justified.

Treatment

GENERAL PRINCIPLES

Management of the patient with venous injury is essentially identical to that for any vascular injury. Prompt digital or manual control of any active external bleeding is followed by volume resuscitation through large-bore intravenous catheters placed in uninjured areas. Longitudinal incisions directly over the injured vessels should be made. Digital control of the injury, sponge-stick compression, intraluminal balloon catheters, or occluding clamps are methods that control venous bleeding from the area of injury while the vein is dissected free and formal proximal and distal control can be achieved using clamps or elastic vessel loops.

Unlike arterial trauma, minimal débridement of injured veins is generally necessary. Proximal and distal thrombectomy should be done by gentle milking and the judicious use of balloon catheters, to avoid valvular damage. In combined venoarterial extremity trauma, especially with obvious ischemic changes, intraluminal shunting of the artery restores distal perfusion immediately, allowing deliberate venous repair, as well as any necessary soft tissue or skeletal repairs, without the danger of ongoing ischemia and tissue loss. Another consideration in such combined vascular injuries is to shunt the vein while first repairing the artery, to provide adequate outflow for the artery during its repair and optimizing its success. The shunted vessel in either case then can be definitively repaired.

A variety of techniques that correspond to the same techniques used for arterial injuries have been described for repair of venous injuries. Lateral venorrhaphy, for partial circumferential lacerations, and end-to-end anastomosis, for transections with little loss of vessel length, are the most common methods, as well as the quickest and easiest to perform. Uncommonly used and more difficult and time consuming are interposition grafting with either reversed autogenous vein or prosthetic graft and the construction of spiral grafts or panel grafts from segments of autogenous vein.

VENOUS REPAIR CONSIDERATIONS

The motivation for repair rather than ligation of venous injuries began with the observation of the sequelae of venous hypertension and venous insufficiency following ligation in the Korean War. Rich and colleagues (1976) confirmed these observations during the Vietnam War, noting a substantially greater incidence of extremity edema, stasis dermatitis, ulceration, and chronic venous insufficiency in limbs that underwent major venous ligation compared with those undergoing venous repair. This difference was especially true for the popliteal vein, which provides the major channel for venous drainage from the lower extremity. Several cases of limb amputation were attributed directly to ligation or failed repair of popliteal vein injuries. An aggressive approach toward routine repair of all venous trauma, especially in the popliteal system, led to dramatic improvements in limb salvage and function and dispelled the fears of earlier years that repair would lead to problems with thrombophlebitis and venous thromboembolism. A long-term follow-up of 110 popliteal vein injuries from this conflict (Rich, 1982) demonstrated a reduction of significant limb edema from 51% in cases of vein ligation to only 13% in those undergoing vein repair. The safety and feasibility of venous injury repair had also been shown in the civilian sector by Gaspar and Treiman (1960) and by experimental studies. Repair of the inferior vena cava not only prevents lower limb edema but also restores venous return to the heart to offset hemorrhagic and cardiogenic shock. Pulmonary embolism has been reported in only 2% of these cases.

The natural history of surgically repaired venous injuries is characterized by a substantial rate of thrombosis in the postoperative period that far exceeds that seen following arterial repair. This was documented by Rich (1970) in the Vietnam War in isolated cases. In the civilian sector, Meyer and colleagues (1987) found that 39% of their peripheral venous repairs thrombosed within 1 week by venography, and that this thrombosis rate was higher in complex repairs (59%) than in simple repairs (21%). Hobson and colleagues (1983) reported postoperative thrombosis in 26% of femoral vein repairs, but a significantly higher rate of limb edema (75%) in these occluded repairs than in those remaining patent (23.5%). Agarwal and colleagues (1982) found postoperative thrombosis in 80% of vein repairs followed by venography, and Nypaver and colleagues (1992) found this to occur in 28% of their venous repairs.

Despite these findings, restoration of venous continuity appears to offer major advantages over ligation. Most series have reported few if any adverse sequelae in the limbs of patients with thrombosed venous repairs, indicating that venous repair allows the development of venous collaterals. Also, a number of long-term follow-up studies have shown a high rate of recanalization of thrombosed venous repairs, which cannot occur following ligation.

Nypaver and colleagues (1992) documented that 88% of previously thrombosed vein repairs were subsequently patent by color-flow duplex sonography over a 49-month average follow-up, providing a 90% long-term patency rate. Phifer and colleagues (1985) showed 100% patency of five femoral vein repairs over follow-ups ranging from 6 to 20 years.

These results indicate that veins are extremely sensitive to injury and surgical manipulation, and that meticulous technique is essential to minimize postoperative thrombosis. Gentle handling of venous endothelium, rigorous attention to intimal apposition, and precise suture techniques that restore the vein lumen to its normal diameter without stricture have all been recommended to optimize patency. The use of vein patch or interposition grafting is suggested if simple repair narrows the venous lumen. Completion venography has been recommended to ensure widely patent surgical repairs, but few practice this. Although prosthetic grafts for venous injury repair result in especially high rates of thrombosis, they have the advantage of allowing rapid restoration of continuity and reducing operative bleeding in large open wounds with extensive soft tissue disruption and at fasciotomy sites, by providing immediate venous drainage and avoiding venous hypertension.

A number of adjuncts to venous injury repair have been reported to improve postoperative results. Temporary arteriovenous shunts or arteriovenous fistulas created distal to extremity venous repairs have improved patency rates but have the disadvantages of increased limb edema from the higher venous flow, reduction in arterial flow, and the need for a second operative procedure to take these down. Systemic anticoagulation and antiplatelet therapy has been applied to reduce postoperative thrombosis, but Hobson and colleagues (1973) showed no effect of these measures on improving postoperative patency rates. Intermittent pneumatic compression devices offer theoretical promise but have not been studied for any benefit in this setting.

VENOUS LIGATION CONSIDERATIONS

Clinical experience with the morbid sequelae of the standard practice of ligation of venous injuries during the Vietnam War called this practice into question. Several published experimental studies by Stallworth and colleagues (1967), Barcia and colleagues (1972), Hobson and colleagues (1973), and Wright and colleagues (1973, 1974) documented that acute femoral venous occlusion in uninjured canine limbs resulted in significant reductions in arterial inflow. This reduced flow returned to baseline within 72 hours, suggesting venous collateral development, but the jeopardy this poses to an injured limb, especially in the presence of a fresh arterial repair, is obvious. Clinical investigations from military and civilian settings confirmed these findings in showing increased limb morbidity and limb loss following venous ligation, especially in the popliteal system.

Since the Vietnam War, the enthusiasm for routine repair of venous injuries that these studies fostered has been tempered by several civilian studies showing remarkably uncomplicated outcomes following ligation of major veins in injured extremities. Mullins, Lucas, and Ledgerwood (1980) showed the absence of any clinically significant short- or long-term impairment of limb function in 46 patients undergoing ligation of injured major veins, 70% of which were in the lower extremity. Eight of these patients had moderate edema requiring support stockings, but no limitation of activity. Several other authors have since documented acceptable levels of limb morbidity following lower extremity vein ligation, including inferior vena cava and iliac veins, though with varying levels of postoperative edema in up to 50% of patients. There have been no instances of limb loss attributable to venous ligation in these reports. Studies by Meyer and colleagues (1987), Pasch and colleagues (1986), Yelon and Scalea (1992), and Timberlake and Kerstein (1995) report a total of 440 patients with major peripheral venous injury, including the popliteal and femoral veins, with no limb loss and no significant long-term edema following vein ligation, as well as no difference in outcome between patients undergoing vein ligation and those undergoing vein repair. Ligation of major venous injury is consistently tolerated without problems in the upper extremities and neck, attributable to the greater collateral drainage than that found in the lower extremities.

Recent studies of inferior vena cava and iliac vein injuries show similar results for repair and ligation, although these tend to be more severely compromised patients because of the shock and blood loss accompanying these injuries. Burch and colleagues (1990) reported 161 iliac vein injuries, with a higher rate of venous morbidity (26%) among cases that were ligated (consisting only of limb edema and deep vein thrombosis) than in those repaired (4.9%, two cases edema and two of pulmonary embolism), but without any limb loss.

Successful outcome of limb salvage and function following venous ligation demands an aggressive use of several adjunctive measures to promote venous drainage. These patients should be placed on bed rest, with avoidance of dependent positioning of their limbs. Lower extremities should be wrapped in elastic bandages and elevated for several days before carefully beginning ambulation. Four-compartment lower leg fasciotomy should be applied liberally and prophylactically, to offset the very high probability of development of compartment syndrome. If fasciotomy is not performed, careful serial measurement of compartment pressures is necessary. Routine anticoagulation has no proven benefit.

ROLES OF LIGATION AND REPAIR

Although the published evidence appears contradictory in many ways regarding the relative merits of ligation or repair of venous injuries, each can clearly be successful under certain conditions (see Table 20–4). Which approach is best in any setting requires that the reported differences in outcome be understood and reconciled. Venous ligation results in the worst outcome in military series and experimental models, which can be explained by the greater collateral damage of bone and soft tissue, as well as the total venous outflow occlusion, which occurs in these settings. In actual clinical venous injury in the civilian setting, the better results of ligation can be explained by the simpler, less destructive wounds without major associated trauma and by the fact that ligation of any single vein does not totally occlude limb outflow.

Most authorities agree that all injuries to major veins should undergo surgical repair, unless there are more pressing priorities, such as life-threatening problems, which preclude it. Hemodynamic instability, ongoing hemorrhage, and life-threatening associated injuries to other body systems that require immediate attention are the most common indications to revert to ligation of venous injuries. This is a basic tenet of the damage control approach to severely injured patients, because venous repair always requires more time to accomplish than ligation, and complex repairs take more time than simple repairs. Some authors recommend that ligation be performed if repair requires anything more complex than lateral suture or end-to-end anastomosis, in view of the added time and worse outcome of complex repairs. Deaths have been attributed to ill-considered attempts at complex venous repairs. Ligation of all upper extremity veins and unilateral internal jugular veins can be performed without a problem. Patients generally tolerate ligation of any vein in the body as long as adjunctive measures are properly applied. Also, ligated veins can be reversed by elective definitive repair if necessary in those uncommon instances that severe complications develop in the future.

It is important to recognize those circumstances in which venous repair should be attempted even under suboptimal conditions of patient instability or complex trauma. In patients with injuries involving massive tissue destruction, from blunt or high-velocity penetrating trauma, repair of a major vein may be critical in providing limb outflow, even if that repair must be complex or requires a prosthetic graft. In combined arteriovenous trauma in the same extremity, venous repair should be undertaken to provide outflow for the arterial repair and optimize its success. Any popliteal vein injury merits all possible effort to repair rather than ligate due to the known severe and limb-threatening morbid-

ity that is associated with ligation. Bilateral internal jugular vein injuries in the neck warrant repair of one side to provide critical intracranial venous outflow. In critical circumstances, temporary intraluminal shunts may be used as a damage-control measure to quickly restore venous outflow, allowing definitive repair to be done later when conditions stabilize.

Some authors advocate routine follow-up imaging of repaired venous injuries with venography or duplex scanning, to detect thrombosis early. However, an understanding of the natural history of venous repairs makes clear why this practice is unnecessary and is not used by most centers. The known high incidence of postoperative thrombosis is typically followed by spontaneous recanalization to provide a very high long-term patency. Also, even thrombosed repairs manifest very few clinical problems. Imaging should be applied only to those few patients in whom symptoms of disabling edema and chronic venous insufficiency develop, in which case anticoagulation or surgical revision may be considered.

COMBINED VASCULAR AND SKELETAL EXTREMITY TRAUMA

Extremity trauma that involves both skeletal and vascular injuries poses one of the most difficult management problems. These complex injuries often involve extensive soft tissue and nerve damage as well and are sometimes termed *mangled extremities*. It is important to understand the unique considerations of epidemiology, pathophysiology, prognosis, diagnosis, and multidisciplinary priorities in this setting, to reduce the substantial risks of limb loss that currently prevail.

Epidemiology and Prognostic Factors

Combined vascular and skeletal extremity injuries are relatively uncommon, making up only 0.2% of all military or civilian trauma.

Vascular and trauma surgeons are more likely to see this combined trauma than orthopedic surgeons, because only 1.5% to 6.5% of all extremity skeletal traumas are associated with an arterial injury of the same extremity, whereas 10% to 73% of all extremity arterial injuries may be associated with skeletal fractures and dislocations.

Combined vascular and skeletal extremity injuries pose a substantially increased risk of amputation and limb morbidity than isolated arterial or skeletal injuries. This was documented in several military series dating back to World War II. These reports showed that combined injuries were associated with amputation rates ranging up to ten times those from isolated arterial extremity injuries, even as the outcomes for both simple arterial and com-

bined combat extremity injuries improved over the past 50 years (Table 20–5). McNamara and colleagues (1973) also showed a significantly higher incidence of failed vascular repair among combined extremity injuries (33%) than among isolated arterial injuries of the extremity in the Vietnam War (5%). Similar striking differences have been reported in the civilian sector even in recent years. At a time when isolated arterial or skeletal extremity trauma can be expected to result in limb loss in far less than 5% of civilian cases, the combination of these injuries in the same extremity still are associated with amputation rates up to 68% in the most experienced trauma centers (Table 20–6). Even many salvaged extremities are significantly disabled. These results are largely due to delayed recog-

TABLE 20–5
AMPUTATION RATES (%) FOLLOWING COMBAT EXTREMITY ARTERIAL INJURIES WITH AND WITHOUT ASSOCIATED SKELETAL TRAUMA

Author	Year	Conflict	Isolated Arterial Injury	Combined Injury
DeBakey	1946	World War II	42	60
Spencer	1955	Korea	15	55
McNamara	1973	Vietnam	2.5	23
Romanoff	1979	Israel	11	36
Lovric	1994	Croatia	0	10

TABLE 20–6
MECHANISM AND OUTCOME OF COMBINED CIVILIAN VASCULAR/SKELETAL EXTREMITY TRAUMA

Author	Year	% Penetrating	% Amputation*
Schlickwei	1992	0	45
Van Wijngarden	1993	0	41.5
Alexander	1991	9	28
Johansen	1990	<10	68
Odland	1990	10	35
Lange	1985	13	61
Palazzo	1986	18	7 (0)
Howe	1987	24	43
Bongard	1989	30	18
Drost	1989	36	29
Bishara	1986	57	3 (0)
Attebery	1996	71	7 (0)

*Numbers in parentheses refer to amputations among penetrating injuries only.

nition of vascular injury, major nerve damage, and increased failure of vascular of repair due to disruption of collaterals from soft tissue injury, soft tissue infection from inadequate débridement, failure to provide adequate tissue coverage over sutured vessels, and delayed recognition and treatment of compartmental hypertension.

Mechanism of injury is another important determinant of outcome in this setting. Virtually all combined extremity injuries in military series are due to destructive high-velocity penetrating mechanisms. These approximate the level of tissue damage found in most blunt trauma, which has been the predominant mechanism for this distinct category of extremity trauma in most civilian series. However, an increasing incidence of simple penetrating trauma has been reported as a cause of these injuries in the civilian sector over the past decade, ranging from 18% to 71% of cases. Some correlation is also evident between the extent of penetrating trauma and an improved outcome in these series (see Table 20–6). Among 119 patients with combined vascular and skeletal extremity injuries reported in three of these series (Bishara and colleagues, 1986; Palazzo, 1986; Attebery and colleagues, 1996), 63 cases (53%) were due to penetrating trauma, and the total amputation rate was the lowest ever reported (well below 10%), with no amputations among any of the cases due to penetrating injury.

It is generally accepted that penetrating trauma has a better outcome than blunt trauma, because of less severe and extensive associated tissue damage. Therefore, it should be no surprise that the increasing trend in low-velocity penetration as an etiology for combined vascular and skeletal extremity trauma in the civilian sector appears responsible for the most substantial contribution yet to reducing limb loss from these devastating injuries. Five civilian series of combined extremity trauma have been published since 1986 in which more than 50% of cases were due to penetrating mechanisms (Table 20–7). The overall rate of penetration among all 228 reported cases was 64.5%. The overall amputation rate was 17%, but among penetrating injuries, it was only 6%. Only 23% of all amputations were in patients with penetrating trauma. Among 88 patients with penetrating combined injuries reported in three of these series, remarkably there were no amputations. Although some published series of combined extremity trauma report no difference in outcome between blunt and penetrating mechanisms, and some report a higher amputation rate among penetrating injuries, these series involve small numbers and particularly severe injuries. Nonetheless, they demonstrate that a number of variables other than mechanism affect outcome.

Diagnosis

Prompt and accurate diagnosis of vascular injury is critically important in the setting of

TABLE 20–7

OUTCOME OF PREDOMINANTLY PENETRATING COMBINED CIVILIAN VASCULAR/SKELETAL EXTREMITY TRAUMA

Author	Year	No. Patients	No. Penetrating (%)	No. Amputations (%) Total	Penetrating
Norman	1995	30	30 (100)	0	0
Attebery	1996	41	29 (71)	3 (7)	0
Swetnam	1986	36	24 (67)	16 (44)	8 (33)
Bishara	1986	51	29 (57)	1 (2)	0
Russell	1991	70	35 (50)	19 (27)	1 (3)
TOTAL		228	147 (64.5)	39 (17)	9 (6)

an extremity fracture or dislocation, because prolonged ischemia and delay in restoration of blood flow are cited in most studies as major contributors to limb loss and limb morbidity. The clinical presentation of the patient and the physical examination are the key elements, and in many cases the only elements, necessary for diagnosis or exclusion of vascular injury in this setting. Contrast-enhanced arteriography is the standard imaging modality used to make this diagnosis, although its exact role is debated.

The presence of hard signs (hemorrhage, hematoma, bruit or thrill, absent pulse, distal ischemia) in uncomplicated extremity trauma has been shown to predict major vascular injury with an accuracy approaching 100% and therefore generally mandates immediate operation without any imaging. However, combined skeletal and soft tissue disruption substantially reduces the positive predictive value (i.e., hard signs present) of physical examination for surgically significant vascular injury. Applebaum and colleagues (1990) reported 53 cases of complex blunt extremity trauma, documenting vascular injuries in 39% of all cases manifesting hard signs, but in only 13% of cases did these injuries require surgical repair. This represented an 87% false-positive rate of physical examination for the detection of surgically significant vascular injury, the only ones to require detection and treatment, similar to that reported in other series. This can be explained by the fact that fractures, soft tissue disruption, traction, and distortion of arteries by bony fragments, nerve injuries, and compartment syndrome, all common features of complex limb trauma, can cause hard signs in the absence of injury to a major artery. Arteriography is recommended in complex extremity trauma that manifests hard signs, to exclude an arterial injury to avoid as much as an 87% rate of unnecessary vascular exploration in these already compromised limbs (Figs. 20–1 and 20–2).

On the other hand, arterial imaging does not appear necessary in complex extremity trauma without hard signs. Current evidence indicates that a negative physical examination result (i.e., no hard signs) excludes surgically significant arterial injury as reliably as both

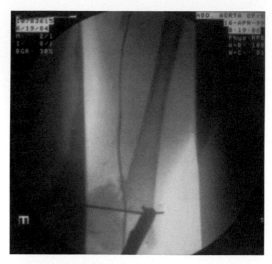

■ **FIGURE 20–1**
Arteriogram performed for displaced supracondylar femur fracture manifesting hematoma and uncertain distal pulses, confirming intact popliteal artery and runoff and sparing unnecessary vascular exploration. ■

arteriography and surgical exploration. Nonocclusive vascular injuries may still occur but are known to have a benign natural history and therefore do not require detection. The economic advantages of avoiding routine arteriography in this group of patients are obvious, as discussed in previous sections of this chapter (see "Popliteal Artery Injuries" and "Posterior Knee Dislocation," earlier in this chapter).

When indicated for complex extremity trauma, arteriography is best performed as a percutaneous hand-injected study right in the trauma center or on the operating table with the extremity already prepared and draped (see Fig. 20–2). This technique is easily performed by any surgeon, using a simple intravenous catheter slipped over a needle directly into the femoral artery at the groin or brachial artery above an occluding blood pressure cuff, with a radiographic plate placed under the injured extremity, and injecting 30 mL of water-soluble contrast while the x-ray film is exposed by a portable unit. Substantial time is saved by this procedure, as formal arteriography in the radiology suite takes at least 1 to 3 hours even in major trauma centers. This

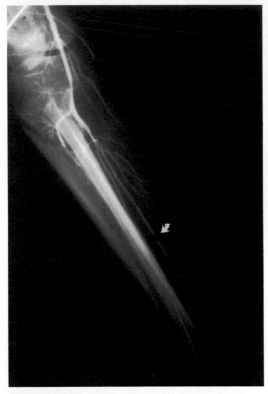

■ **FIGURE 20–2**
Percutaneous one-shot hand-injected
arteriogram on operating table following
comminuted tibial plateau fracture with
hematoma and poorly palpable distal pulses,
showing occluded anterior tibial artery,
narrowed tibioperoneal trunk, and intact
posterior tibial artery with nonocclusive intimal
defect *(arrow)*. No vascular repair was
necessary, skeletal repair was immediately
performed, and distal perfusion remained intact
without subsequent problems. ■

is critical to optimize limb salvage. On-table
arteriography is also highly accurate, provides
excellent resolution, and allows immediate
treatment to begin on either the vascular or
the skeletal injury, depending on the arteriogram results.

Although noninvasive vascular studies with
Doppler pressure monitoring and duplex
ultrasonography have been applied to the evaluation of complex extremity trauma for
vascular injury, there is as yet no clear role for
these modalities. In fact, the expertise
required for interpretation of these tests, their
lack of round-the-clock availability in most

hospitals, and the significant swelling, skeletal disruption, and bulky splints and dressings,
which characterize these extremities, cast
doubt on the utility and accuracy of noninvasive tests in this setting. Any use of these
tests for diagnosis or exclusion of vascular
trauma should be within the context of a controlled study, and their results should be interpreted with caution. Arteriography remains
the standard modality of choice for evaluation of high-risk complex extremity trauma
for vascular injury.

Treatment

Combined vascular and skeletal trauma
requires a multidisciplinary approach to treatment, which can succeed only with the smooth
and coordinated interaction between the
various specialties involved in caring for the
skeletal, soft tissue, and vascular injuries,
as well as for the patient as a whole. All life-
threatening injuries must be treated as a first
priority. Once the extremity is addressed,
orthopedic surgeons and plastic surgeons
should be involved integrally in the treatment
decisions, along with the trauma or vascular
surgeon, as soon as a diagnosis of combined
extremity trauma is established.

Prompt restoration of blood flow within 6
hours of any extremity vascular injury is the
most critical of the many factors that determine limb salvage and function. Clinical and
experimental studies consistently demonstrate a direct linear relationship between the
time interval to extremity reperfusion and the
amputation rate. Associated skeletal and soft
tissue injury makes this time factor even more
important. A small number of retrospective
studies fail to show a correlation between time
delay and outcome, but this again emphasizes
that multiple variables are at play in these devastating extremity injuries. The weight of evidence mandates that rapid diagnosis, based
on the clinical manifestations and selective
application of one-shot on-table arteriography,
be followed as expeditiously as possible by
restoration of blood flow.

Prioritization of management of the vascular and skeletal extremity injuries has been
subject to debate and uncertainty, leading to

wide variations in practice. Early studies recommended that skeletal repair take priority in combined extremity trauma, to avoid the potential disruption of an initial fresh vascular anastomosis by subsequent manipulation of bone fragments or length discrepancies in any initial vascular repair caused by subsequent stabilization of comminuted, unstable skeletal injuries. It was believed that some delay in reperfusion is acceptable in the absence of overt ischemia. However, these conjectures have been refuted by much published evidence. Substantial tissue damage can occur in the absence of signs of ischemia, as has been made clear by our understanding of compartment syndrome. Disruption of an initial vascular repair by subsequent skeletal manipulation occurs only rarely. Snyder and colleagues (1982) reported this to occur in only 7% of cases, and Downs and colleagues (1986) reported this in only 2% of all cases of combined extremity trauma undergoing initial vascular repair, and in each case, the repair was immediately revised with no effect on limb salvage. Howe and colleagues (1987) reported no vascular disruption in 21 such cases. Jahnke and Seeley (1953) generally performed initial vascular repairs in combined extremity injuries in the Korean War without adverse sequelae. Also, the resistance of repaired vessels to disruption has been underestimated. Connolly and colleagues (1969) demonstrated that the strength of fresh anastomoses of transected canine femoral arteries with associated femur fractures approximated that of native vessels, resisting disruption by either 30 pounds of traction or by bone fragment impalement. These data are further supported by clinical studies (Romanoff, 1979; McCabe, 1983), which demonstrate a substantially higher rate of limb salvage among combined extremity injuries in which vascular repair is undertaken first, compared with those in which revascularization is delayed until skeletal stabilization/repair is completed. Most importantly, no disadvantage has ever been documented for initial revascularization, whereas the dangers of delay are well established. Any delay in revascularization must be considered a gamble. Of course, this makes eminent sense, because perfusion, rather than immediate skeletal

continuity, is the *sine qua non* of limb survival. Furthermore, as mentioned earlier, published studies consistently report that the most common reason for limb loss in this setting is delay or failure of revascularization, not of skeletal repair.

It must be emphasized that restoration of extremity perfusion does not always require definitive vascular repair. Temporary plastic or Silastic intraluminal shunts placed in the severed ends of vessels following distal thrombectomy can restore distal perfusion within minutes. In fact, a formal vascular repair should be avoided in the setting of unstable and severely comminuted fractures and dislocations, segmental bone loss, or severe soft tissue disruption and contamination. Shunting in these cases allows deliberate attention to wide débridement and skeletal stabilization and fixation without ongoing ischemia, after which definitive vascular repair can be performed (Fig. 20–3). This avoids major stress on a vascular suture line from bone manipulation or undue tension or slack on the repaired vessel when the limb is fixed at its proper length. Alternatively, initial revascularization can and should be accomplished by immediate definitive arterial repair in the setting of stable skeletal injuries in which minimal subsequent manipulation and length discrepancy is anticipated (Fig. 20–4). The consensus in the literature now strongly favors limb revascularization as the immediate management priority in all combined extremity trauma, as the aforementioned considerations render moot any possible disadvantages. How the revascularization is accomplished is a matter of judgment, which depends primarily on the nature of the skeletal and soft tissue injuries.

Current evidence suggests that asymptomatic nonocclusive arterial injuries found on extremity arteriography are safe to observe nonoperatively in the setting of combined extremity trauma, where they have been shown to have the same benign natural history as in uncomplicated penetrating extremity and neck trauma. Three published series (Applebaum, 1990; Norman, 1995; Attebery and colleagues, 1996) report a total of 98 asymptomatic arterial injuries in extremities with associated skeletal trauma from both

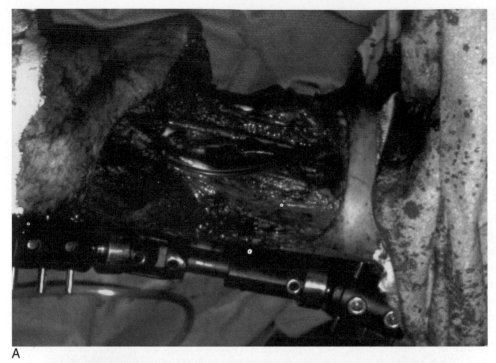

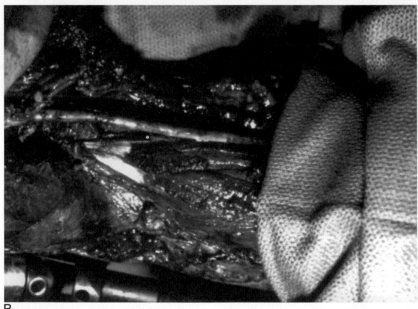

■ **FIGURE 20-3**

A, Unstable elbow dislocation with brachial artery avulsion and loss of overlying skin. Distal perfusion immediately restored by intraluminal brachial artery shunt, allowing cross-joint external fixation and soft tissue débridement. *B,* Artery was then repaired with autogenous vein graft, and a pedicle flap provided immediate coverage. ■

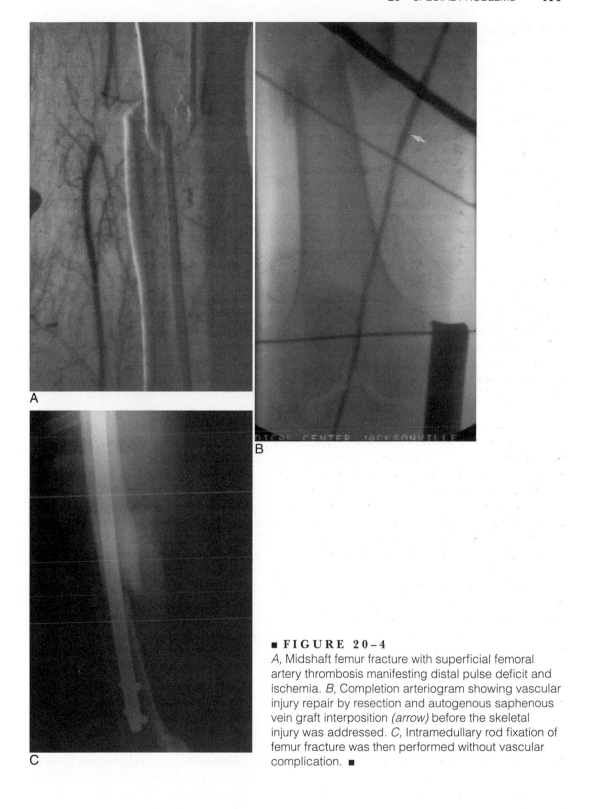

■ **FIGURE 20–4**

A, Midshaft femur fracture with superficial femoral artery thrombosis manifesting distal pulse deficit and ischemia. *B,* Completion arteriogram showing vascular injury repair by resection and autogenous saphenous vein graft interposition *(arrow)* before the skeletal injury was addressed. *C,* Intramedullary rod fixation of femur fracture was then performed without vascular complication. ■

blunt and penetrating mechanisms, of which only one (1%) underwent surgical repair, and that was a nonocclusive intimal flap of the distal radial artery, which was probably unnecessary. There was no limb loss, limb morbidity, or subsequent vascular problems. Attebery and colleagues (1996) followed 15 asymptomatic nonocclusive arterial injuries (35% of all 41 vascular injuries associated with extremity skeletal trauma) for a mean interval of 6.5 months, and none ever required intervention or became symptomatic. This series reported one of the lowest rates of limb loss in this setting (7.3%), and this was attributed in part to the avoidance of unnecessary vascular exploration in so many of these severely injured limbs. These data add support to the avoidance of diagnostic arteriography in complex extremity trauma that does not manifest hard signs of vascular injury.

The optimal method of fracture management in combined vascular and skeletal extremity trauma has evolved over the past few decades. The military experience from the Vietnam War demonstrated substantially higher risks of limb loss following internal skeletal fixation than was found after external fixation (Rich, 1971; McNamara and colleagues, 1973). At least 50% of amputations following internal fixation were due to infection. The civilian experience demonstrates acceptable results with both internal and external fixation, most likely because of the less extensive bone damage in this setting. This evidence suggests that combined extremity injuries with a high risk of infection (e.g., open, contaminated, extensive soft tissue injury), comminuted or unstable skeletal trauma, or those in unstable patients who require rapid treatment undergo external skeletal fixation, either as a definitive or as a temporizing measure. Otherwise internal fixation is appropriate, either immediately or as a later definitive measure.

Liberal use of a variety of surgical adjuncts has shown some correlation with improved limb salvage following combined extremity trauma, just as it has in isolated extremity vascular injuries. Completion intraoperative arteriography should be performed routinely before completing vascular repairs to docu-ment arterial patency and runoff, because any technical errors in this tenuous limb could easily lead to limb loss. Four-compartment fasciotomy should be applied liberally and very early or prophylactically in this setting because of the especially high risk of compartment syndrome following reperfusion. Extra-anatomic bypass or pedicle or free tissue flap coverage may be necessary to protect vascular repairs in the setting of severe contamination and soft tissue injury or loss (see Fig. 20–3).

Indications for Amputation

Extensive and prolonged attempts to salvage extremities with severe and complex injuries may actually harm patients in a variety of ways, especially if these efforts ultimately end in amputation anyway. Financial costs, hospital and intensive care unit days, infectious complications, number of operative procedures, time lost from work, permanent disability, and even death have all been shown to be significantly greater when limb salvage becomes unnecessarily prolonged compared with early amputation. Those combined extremity injuries that ultimately result in limb loss or limb dysfunction can largely be predicted within a few days of injury by a number of prognostic factors that closely relate to outcome. Transected major nerves and Gustilo III-C injuries (open comminuted tibiofibular fractures with arterial injury) are the most common indications for consideration of immediate amputation (Box 20–1). Primary amputation at the time of presentation or early amputation within a few days should be considered strongly whenever these prognostic factors are present. The sophistication of limb prostheses, the early return to work, short hospitalization, and lower costs and complications following early amputation are usually preferable to salvage attempts, which may take months or years and still have uncertain success.

Primary amputation without any attempt at limb salvage is reported in 10% to 22% of cases of complex extremity trauma, and such immediate amputations account for more than 50% of all amputations following these

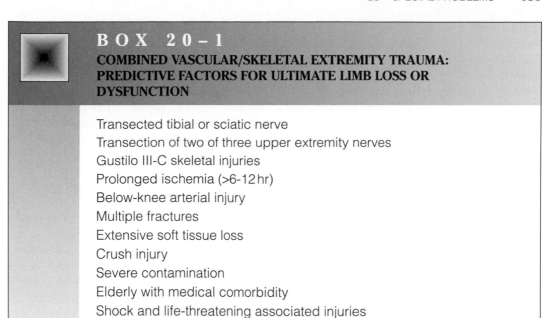

> **BOX 20-1**
>
> **COMBINED VASCULAR/SKELETAL EXTREMITY TRAUMA: PREDICTIVE FACTORS FOR ULTIMATE LIMB LOSS OR DYSFUNCTION**
>
> Transected tibial or sciatic nerve
> Transection of two of three upper extremity nerves
> Gustilo III-C skeletal injuries
> Prolonged ischemia (>6-12 hr)
> Below-knee arterial injury
> Multiple fractures
> Extensive soft tissue loss
> Crush injury
> Severe contamination
> Elderly with medical comorbidity
> Shock and life-threatening associated injuries

injuries. The decision to perform early amputation is one of the most difficult for trauma surgeons. Although a number of predictive scoring indices have been developed, using factors known to correlate with limb salvage (see Box 20–1), none are sufficiently reliable as prospective tools to make the decision for us. In the end, it must be a matter of judgment based on each individual case. This decision should always involve and require the assent of the entire team involved in the care of the patient, including the trauma, vascular, orthopedic, and plastic surgeons, rehabilitation specialist, psychologist, nursing, and especially the patient and family.

A major consideration in the decision for amputation is whether the injury is in the upper or lower extremity. The upper extremity is more tolerant than the lower of deficits in protective sensation, nerve function, and length discrepancy, and prostheses are less satisfactory. Therefore, amputation is generally less necessary in the upper extremity for any given level of tissue damage.

There are extremity injuries of such severity that a decision for primary amputation is not difficult at all (Fig. 20–5). Any obvious impossibility or futility of revascularization,

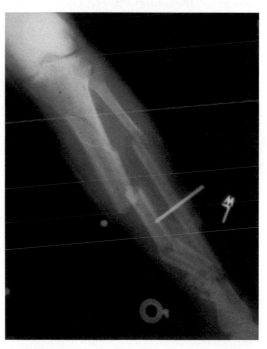

■ FIGURE 20–5
Gustilo III-C complex extremity crush injury in a 64-year-old diabetic man with absent pulses and severe ischemia and no arterial filling on arteriogram. Primary above-knee amputation was performed immediately without attempting limb salvage. ■

transected major nerves, or associated life-threatening injuries that prevent any attention to the limbs are clear indications for immediate amputation. Nerve transection must be confirmed by direct visualization, because vascular insufficiency by itself may cause profound nerve deficits.

However, most complex extremity injuries are not that clear-cut. In these cases, revascularization should be performed immediately to prevent further tissue damage (including aggressive use of surgical adjuncts such as fasciotomy), the skeleton should be quickly stabilized by either traction or external fixation, and the limb then should be observed over the next 48 hours for the level of function that returns. If either revascularization fails, tissue loss is profound or worsens, systemic sepsis or crush syndrome develops, or profound neurologic dysfunction persists, then amputation should be performed. If improvement is noted, each successive stage of limb salvage should be assessed just as critically to minimize unnecessarily prolonged, costly, and futile efforts. The ultimate goal is to return the patient to a comfortable and productive life as quickly as possible.

VASCULAR GRAFTS: ROLE AND COMPLICATIONS

Simple repairs of vascular injuries are always preferred if at all possible, including lateral suture and resection with end-to-end anastomosis. Interposition or patch grafting is used when simple repair is not possible or not preferable, but restoration of the circulation is attainable. Any segmental loss of vessel of more than 2 cm, as is seen in complex injuries with extensive tissue damage, is generally an indication for vascular interposition. In true end arteries, such as the popliteal artery, ligation of tenuous collaterals to achieve adequate mobilization for primary anastomosis is best avoided, and interposition grafting is preferred. Patch grafting of a partially lacerated vessel is occasionally useful to avoid stenosis in smaller vessels such as the brachial or popliteal arteries and allows avoidance of resection.

In the Vietnam War, Rich and colleagues (1970) reported interposition grafting as the most common method of surgical repair of arterial injuries, with autogenous vein being used in 46% of cases and prosthetic grafts in only 0.4%. Several civilian series since then have corroborated these findings. Most authors agree that autogenous reversed saphenous vein is the conduit of choice for arterial interposition grafting because of its high patency rates and low incidence of infection with antibiotic control. Rich and Hughes (1972) reported an 18% amputation rate in Vietnam among arterial repairs undergoing autogenous vein interposition, compared with 12% in Korea. McCready and colleagues (1987) reported an 89.5% long-term patency rate for autogenous vein grafts in 86 cases of extremity arterial injuries, with five graft failures leading to amputation and infection the cause of three graft failures. Keen and colleagues (1991) reported 134 patients with autogenous vein grafts of extremity arterial injuries. In follow-ups ranging up to 24 months, they found a 98% cumulative primary patency rate and 99% cumulative secondary patency rate, with one amputation resulting from graft failure and no perioperative graft infections. Autogenous vein is also the interposition graft of choice for the repair of venous injuries, though having a somewhat higher rate of thrombosis. McCready and colleagues (1987) reported that 17 (77%) of 22 autogenous vein interpositions for extremity vein injuries remained patent.

Prosthetic grafts have been applied increasingly to the repair of vascular injuries over the past 3 decades, following their widespread and successful use in elective vascular surgery. However, the contaminated nature of traumatic wounds led to doubts about the suitability of prosthetic grafting, because of the assumption that these materials are highly prone to infection. Rich and Hughes (1972) reported dismal results using prosthetic grafts in contaminated combat vascular injuries in Vietnam, with a 77% graft failure rate (most commonly from infection and thrombosis) and a 31% amputation rate, significantly worse than autogenous vein in this setting. The lack of an endothelial surface is the most likely explanation for the higher rate of thrombosis of prosthetic grafts. This was supported by some experimental studies in animals in the 1970s.

However, a number of subsequent clinical studies of civilian vascular trauma have demonstrated consistently good results with the use of both polytetrafluoroethylene (PTFE) and Dacron prosthetic grafts placed in contaminated wounds. Shah and colleagues (1984) reported only one arterial and one venous graft thrombosis in 25 vascular reconstructions with PTFE in grossly contaminated wounds with no graft infections. In a report of 236 PTFE grafts placed in contaminated wounds, Feliciano and colleagues (1985) showed a higher graft thrombosis rate than autogenous vein, but no instances of peripheral graft infection in the absence of exposure of the graft or osteomyelitis. The liberal use of antibiotics and adequate full-thickness tissue coverage of these grafts is necessary to achieve these results. Failure to cover any graft and vascular anastomosis inevitably leads to infection, thrombosis, and suture line breakdown.

One advantage of prosthetic grafts over autogenous vein lies in the differential response of these materials to infection. Autogenous vein and arterial homografts both develop transmural necrosis when subject to exposure and/or infection, which leads to sudden blowout of the anastomosis as sutures pull through, with massive life-threatening hemorrhage. Infected prosthetic grafts do not break down in this disastrous way but gradually develop suture pull-through at the anastomosis with native vessel, leading to contained false aneurysm. This allows time for them to be removed electively and new revascularization to be performed. For this reason, prosthetic grafts are considered the material of choice to be used if revascularization must be done in a contaminated field. If they fail, their temporary placement may still allow time to débride devitalized tissue and clean the field of contamination so that vein may be used subsequently.

Other advantages that prosthetic grafts have over autogenous vein for repair of vascular injuries tend to outweigh their higher rate of thrombosis in specific circumstances. They are more suitable for interposition grafting of larger vessels without size discrepancy.

Their ready availability, without the need for harvesting and preparation that autogenous veins require, is preferable when time is an important factor, as in unstable patients. Keen and colleagues (1991) dispute this latter point, reporting an average harvesting time of less than 8 minutes for autogenous veins, which had no adverse impact on limb salvage.

There are circumstances in which prosthetic grafts are best avoided. Injury to small-caliber vessels, such as the brachial or tibial arteries, are more amenable to autogenous vein interposition, because prosthetic grafts smaller than 6 mm in diameter have a prohibitive rate of thrombosis. Grafts that must cross the knee or elbow joint should be autogenous vein, because prosthetic grafts tend to kink and thrombose more readily. Most prosthetic grafts used to repair venous injuries appear to thrombose early, although Feliciano and colleagues (1985) have reported that even their temporary use for this purpose may dramatically diminish hemorrhage from major soft tissue wounds and fasciotomy sites that venous ligation produces, by relieving venous outflow pressure. If used as a venous substitute, prosthetic grafts with external ring support should be applied to enhance their patency.

The proper management of infected prosthetic grafts should begin with measures to prevent infection altogether. Routine coverage of vascular repairs with intravenous broad-spectrum antibiotics, and full-thickness tissue coverage of repairs using primary closure, or pedicled or free flap tissue transfers are essential elements to avoid infection in this setting. If immediate closure of wounds is not possible because of extensive contamination, devitalized tissue, or extensive soft tissue loss, porcine xenografts have been used successfully to temporarily cover vascular repairs until the wound is clean, and primary closure or flap transfers can be done. Extra-anatomic bypass through clean and uninjured tissues is another option for immediate revascularization, which permits adequate coverage despite a hostile wound and allows for appropriately aggressive wound management and an optimal functional and cosmetic result. Autogenous vein is preferred for extra-anatomic bypass, but externally supported prosthetic grafts may also be used.

Graft infection must be assumed whenever obvious purulence is found in its vicinity, especially if it becomes exposed and has failed to incorporate with surrounding tissue. Arterial graft blowout is another manifestation of infection. Immediate excision of the graft is necessary in this setting, and the native vessel should be débrided back to uninvolved tissue and ligated there to prevent secondary hemorrhage. This should be followed by extra-anatomic bypass to restore distal perfusion, leaving the infected bed open for débridement and dressing to ultimately granulate and heal secondarily. Simply placing a new graft in the same infected bed is a futile gesture destined for failure. Although there are isolated reports of successful conservative management of exposed and infected prosthetic grafts, this approach is not recommended.

FAILED RECONSTRUCTION OF ARTERIAL TRAUMA

There are two primary measures of success of peripheral arterial injury management: limb salvage and limb function. Certainly the salvage of a viable extremity is the first goal of arterial injury management, but that does not necessarily mean that a patient is fully restored to their normal lifestyle. The neurologic and skeletal function of the salvaged limb, as well as cosmetic appearance, can have a major impact on the patient's life and may actually be detrimental enough that amputation would be better. Therefore, the ultimate goal of peripheral arterial injury management must be the salvage of a viable, functional, and cosmetically acceptable extremity. The decisions made and the approaches taken in the immediate postinjury period actually have the greatest impact on ultimate outcome.

The first problem that could lead to a failed repair of an arterial injury is delay in its diagnosis and treatment. The direct correlation between delay in revascularization and limb loss is related to irreversible tissue damage that develops with more than 4 to 6 hours of ischemia. Even if the limb remains viable after a treatment delay, permanent disability from nerve and muscle damage is possible even with successful revascularization. Prompt assessment of all injured extremities for hard signs of vascular injury, appropriate and selective use of hand-injected, on-table arteriography, and immediate arterial repair are essential to minimizing delay. Nonvascular tissue damage also adversely affects the salvage of a viable and functional limb in the setting of a concomitant arterial injury. The increased rate of limb loss that occurs in combined vascular and skeletal extremity trauma has been discussed in a previous section of this chapter (Combined Vascular and Skeletal Extremity Trauma). Extensive soft tissue damage disrupts collaterals and increases the sensitivity of an injured extremity to interruption of blood flow. Nerve damage affects the ultimate function of an injured extremity independent of how well it is revascularized. Injury to a major vein in an extremity with arterial injury increases the chance of failure of the arterial repair by jeopardizing venous outflow. In these circumstances, early diagnosis and revascularization and optimal use of surgical adjuncts to improve the success of vascular repair are critically important factors.

Technical errors may lead to failure of arterial repair and to limb loss or limb dysfunction, and therefore must be stringently avoided. Strict attention is necessary to a number of technical factors, including gentle dissection, thorough débridement, appropriate prioritization of multiple injuries, meticulous technique in suturing arteries and veins, proximal and distal thrombectomy, regional and systemic heparinization to prevent further thrombosis, proper choice of repair technique to avoid stenosis, undue tension and collateral damage, full-thickness tissue coverage of the repair, and confirmation of restoration of blood flow by palpation of pulses and clinical signs of normal perfusion. Completion arteriography should be done routinely to detect those unsuspected problems with the vascular repair or distal runoff that even the most experienced centers find in up to 16% of cases, which can be immediately fixed and will avert a subsequent failure of the arterial reconstruction. Certainly, any doubts about the arterial repair must be assessed by an intraoperative arteriogram. Anticoagulation should not be necessary following arterial repairs and cannot substitute for technical perfection.

Postoperative surveillance of the arterial reconstruction with frequent checks of pulses, clinical signs of perfusion, bleeding, and Doppler pressure monitoring is necessary to detect any thrombosis or anastomotic disruption early and permit immediate revisions. Any sign of perfusion deficit or active bleeding must be investigated promptly by arteriography or operative exploration. The cause of a failed reconstruction should be determined, to allow appropriate repair. Any thrombosis must be assumed to be due to technical problems, and the anastomosis or suture lines should be redone following distal thrombectomy. An intraoperative arteriogram must confirm an adequate repair before completion of the surgery. If infection is found as the cause of failed reconstruction, consideration must be given to extra-anatomic bypass following excision of the infected portion of vessel and ligation in a clean field.

Compartment hypertension can be insidious in its presentation and devastating in how much tissue and limb function it can destroy following repair of arterial injuries, even with successful revascularization and in the presence of normal pulses. Any suspicion of this problem mandates immediate and complete fasciotomy of the injured extremity. It is best to perform fasciotomy early, and even prophylactically, in extremities known to be at risk for compartment syndrome, to avert its onset altogether. Those factors posing a high risk for compartment syndrome are well established (see Chapter 27).

Each instance of failure of arterial reconstruction following extremity vascular injury substantially reduces the chance of ultimate limb salvage. Prevention of these failures through optimal diagnosis and initial management is the best way to minimize limb loss. If a failure occurs, limb salvage and good limb function is still possible if recognized and treated promptly.

REFERENCES

Agarwal N, Shah PM, Clauss RH, et al: Experience with 115 civilian venous injuries. J Trauma 1982;22:827.

Alexander JJ, Piotrowski JJ, Graham D, et al: Outcome of complex orrthopedic and vascular injuries of the lower extremity. Am J Surg 1991;162:111.

Applebaum R, Yellin AE, Weaver FA, et al: Role of routine arteriography in blunt lower extremity trauma. Am J Surg 1990;160:221.

Armstrong K, Sfeir R, Rice J, et al: Popliteal vascular and war: Are Beirut and New Orleans similar? J Trauma 1988;28:836.

Attebery LR, Dennis JW, Russo-Alesi F et al: Changing patterns of arterial injuries associated with fractures and dislocations. J Am Coll Surg 1996;183:377.

Barcia PJ, Nelson TG, Whelan TJ: Importance of venous occlusion in arterial repair failure: An experimental study. Ann Surg 1972;175:223.

Barros D'Sa AA, Hassard TH, Livingston RH, et al: Missile-induced vascular trauma. Injury 1980;12:13.

Bergstein JM, Blair JF, Edwards J, et al: Pitfalls in the use of color-flow duplex ultrasound for screening of suspected arterial injuries in penetrated extremities. J Trauma 1992;33:395.

Bongard FS, White GH, Klein SR: Management strategy of complex extremity injuries. Am J Surg 1989;158:151.

Bishara RA, Pasch AR, Lim LT, et al: Improved results in the treatment of civilian vascular injuries associated with fractures and dislocations. J Vasc Surg 1986;3:707.

Bishara RA, Pasch AR, Lim LT, et al: Improved results in the treatment of civilian vascular injuries associated with fractures and dislocations. J Vasc Surg 1976;3:707.

Borman KR, Jones GH, Snyder WH: A decade of lower extremity venous trauma. Am J Surg 1987;154:608.

Burch JM, Richardson RJ, Martin RR, et al: Penetrating iliac vascular injuries: Recent experience with 233 consecutive patients. J Trauma 1990;34:1450.

Conkle DM, Richie RE, Sawyers JL, et al: Surgical treatment of popliteal artery injuries. Arch Surg 1975;110:1351.

Connolly JE, Williams E, Whittaker D: The influence of fracture stabilization on the outcome of arterial repair in combined fracture-arterial injuries. Surg Forum 1969;20:450.

Daugherty ME, Sachatello CR, Ernst CB: Improved treatment of popliteal arterial injuries. Arch Surg 1978;113:1317.

DeBakey ME, Simeone FA: Battle injuries of the arteries in World War II: An analysis of 2,471 cases. Ann Surg 1946;123:534.

DeGiannis E, Levy RD, Sofianos C, et al: Arterial gunshot injuries of the extremities: A South African experience. J Trauma 1995;39:570.

Dennis JW, Frykberg ER, Veldenz HC, et al: Reassessing the role of arteriograms in the management of posterior knee dislocations. J Trauma 1993;35:692.

Downs AR, MacDonald P: Popliteal artery injuries: Civilian experience with sixty-three patients during a 24 year period (1960 through 1984). J Vasc Surg 1986;4:55.

Drost TF, Rosemurgy AS, Proctor D, et al: Outcome of treatment of combined orthopedic and arterial trauma to the lower extremity. J Trauma 1989;29:1331.

Fabian TC, Turkleson ML, Connelly TL, et al: Injury to the popliteal artery. Am J Surg 1982;143:225.

Fainzilber G, Roy-Shapir A, Wall MJ, et al: Predictors of amputation for popliteal artery injuries. Am J Surg 1995;170:568.

Feliciano DV, Accola KD, Burch JM, et al: Extraanatomic bypass for peripheral arterial injuries. Am J Surg 1989;158:506.

Feliciano DV, Cruse PA, Spjut-Patrinely V, et al: Fasciotomy after trauma to the extremities. Am J Surg 1988;156:533.

Feliciano DV, Mattox KL, Graham JM, et al: Five-year experience with PTFE grafts in vascular wounds. J Trauma 1985;25:71.

Frykberg ER: Popliteal vascular injuries. Surg Clin North Am 2002;82(1):67–89.

Frykberg ER, Crump JM, Dennis JW, et al: Non-operative observation of clinically occult arterial injuries: A prospective evaluation. Surgery 1991;109:85.

Gagne PJ, Cone JB, McFarland D, et al: Proximity penetrating extremity trauma: The role of duplex ultrasound in the detection of occult venous injuries. J Trauma 1995;39:1157.

Gaspar MR, Treiman RL: The management of injuries to major veins. Am J Surg 1960;100:171.

Gerlock AJ, Thal ER, Snyder WH: Venography in penetrating injuries of the extremities. AJR 1976;126:1023.

Harrell DJ, Spain DA, Bergamini TM, et al: Blunt popliteal artery trauma: A challenging injury. Am Surg 1997;63:228.

Hobson RW, Croom RD, Rich NM: Influence of heparin and low molecular weight dextran on the patency of autogenous vein grafts in the venous system. Ann Surg 1973;178:773.

Hobson RW, Howard EW, Wright CB, et al: Hemodynamics of canine femoral venous ligation: Significance in combined arterial and venous injuries. Surgery 1973;74:824.

Hobson RW, Yeager RA, Lynch TG, et al: Femoral venous trauma: Techniques for surgical management and early results. Am J Surg 1983;146:220.

Holleman JH, Killebrew LH: Injury to the popliteal artery. Surg Gynecol Obstet 1981;153:392.

Howe HR, Poole GV, Hansen KJ, et al: Salvage of lower extremities following combined orthopedic and vascular trauma: A predictive salvage index. Am Surg 1987;53:205.

Hughes CW: Arterial repair during the Korean War. Ann Surg 1958;147:555.

Jaggers RC, Feliciano DV, Mattox KL, et al: Injury to popliteal vessels. Arch Surg 1982;117:657.

Jahnke EJ, Seeley SF: Acute vascular injuries in the Korean War: An analysis of 77 consecutive cases. Ann Surg 1953;138:158.

Johansen K, Daines M, Howey T, et al: Objective criteria accurately predict amputation following lower extremity trauma. J Trauma 1990;30:568.

Kaufman SL, Martin LG: Arterial injuries associated with complete dislocation of the knee. Radiology 1992;184:153.

Keen RR, Meyer JP, Durham JR, et al: Autogenous vein graft repair of injured extremity arteries: Early and late results with 134 consecutive patients. J Vasc Surg 1991;13:664.

Kendall RW, Taylor DC, Salvian AJ, et al: The role of arteriography in assessing vascular injuries associated with dislocations fo the knee. J Trauma 1993;35:875.

Krige JEJ, Spence RAJ: Popliteal artery trauma: A high risk injury. Br J Surg 1987;74:91.

Lange RH, Bach AW, Hansen ST, et al: Open tibial fractures with associated vascular injuries:

Prognosis for limb salvage. J Trauma 1985;25: 203.

Lim LT, Michuda MS, Flanigan DP, et al: Popliteal artery trauma: 31 consecutive cases without amputation. Arch Surg 1980;115:1307.

Lin C-H, Weif-C, Levin LS, et al: The functional outcome of lower extremity fractures with vascular injury. J Trauma 1997;43:480.

Lovric Z, Wertheimer B, Candrlic K, et al: War injuries of major extremity vessels. J Trauma 1994;36:248.

Makins GH: Injuries to the blood vessels. In: Official History of the Great War Medical Services: Surgery of the War. London: His Majesty's Stationery Office, 1922;170–296.

Martin LC, McKenny MG, Sosa JL, et al: Management of lower extremity arterial trauma. J Trauma 1994;37:591.

Martinez D, Sweatman K, Thompson EC: Popliteal artery injury associated with knee dislocations. Am Surg 2001;67:165.

McCabe CJ, Ferguson CM, Ottinger LW: Improved limb salvage in popliteal artery injuries. J Trauma 1983;23:982.

McCready RA, Logan NM, Dangherty ME, et al: Long-term results with antogenous tissue repair of traumatic extremity vascular injuries. Ann Surg 1987;206:804.

Melton SM, Croce MA, Patton JH, et al: Popliteal artery trauma: Systemic anticoagulation and intraoperative thrombolysis improves limb salvage. Ann Surg 1997;225:518.

McNamara JJ, Brief DK, Stremple JF, et al: Management of fractures with associated arterial injury in combat casualties. J Trauma 1973;13:17.

Meyer J, Walsh J, Schuler J, et al: The early fate of venous repair after civilian vascular trauma: a clinical, hemodynamic, and venographic assessment. Ann Surg 1987;206:458.

Miranda FE, Dennis JW, Veldenz HC, et al: Confirmation of the safety and accuracy of physical examination in the evaluation of knee dislocation for popliteal artery injury: A prospective study. J Trauma 2000;49:375.

Miranda FE, Dennis JW, Veldenz HC, et al: Confirmation of the safety and accuracy of physical examination in the evaluation of knee dislocation for injury of the popliteal artery: A prospective study. J Trauma 2002;52(2):247–251.

Mullins RJ, Lucas CE, Ledgerwood AM: The natural history following venous ligation for civilian injuries. J Trauma 1980;20:737.

Norman J, Gahtan V, Franz M, et al: Occult vascular injuries following gunshot wounds resulting in long bone fractures of the extremities. Am Surg 1995;61:146.

Nypaver TJ, Schuler JJ, McDonnel P, et al: Long-term results of venous reconstruction after vascular trauma. J Vasc Surg 1992;16:762.

Odland MD, Gisbert VL, Gustilo RB, et al: Combined orthopedic and vascular injury in the lower extremities: Indications for amputation. Surgery 1990;108:660.

O'Reilly MJG, Hood JM, Livingston RH, et al: Penetrating injuries of the popliteal artery. Br J Surg 1978;65:789.

Orcutt MB, Levine BA, Root HD, et al: The continuing challenge of popliteal vascular injuries. Am J Surg 1983;146:758.

Palazzo JC, Ristow AB, Cury JM, et al: Traumatic vascular lesions associated with fractures and dislocations. J Cardiovasc Surg 1986;27:688.

Pasch AR, Bishara RA, Schuler JJ, et al: Results of venous reconstruction after civilian vascular trauma. Arch Surg 1986;121:607.

Peck JJ, Eastman AB, Bergan JJ, et al: Popliteal vascular trauma: A community experience. Arch Surg 1990;125:1339.

Phifer TJ, Gerlock AJ, Rich NM, et al: Long term patency of venous repairs demonstrated by venography. J Trauma 1985;25:342.

Pretre R, Bruschweiler I, Rossier J, et al: Lower limb trauma with injury to the popliteal vessels. J Trauma 1996;40:595.

Razuk AF, Nunes H, Coimbra R, et al: Popliteal artery injuries: Risk factors for limb loss. Panam J Trauma 1998;7:93.

Reed MK, Lowry PA, Myers SI: Successful repair of pediatric popliteal artery trauma. Am J Surg 1990;160:287.

Rich NM: Principles and indications for primary venous repair. Surgery 1982;91:492.

Rich NM, Baugh JH, Hughes CW: Acute arterial injuries in Vietnam: 1,000 cases. J Trauma 1970;10:359.

Rich NM, Hobson RW, Collins GJ, et al: The effect of acute popliteal venous interruption. Ann Surg 1976;183:365.

Rich NM, Hughes CW: The fate of prosthetic material used to repair vascular injuries in contaminated wounds. J Trauma 1972;21:459.

Rich NM, Hughes CW, Baugh JH: Management of venous injuries. Ann Surg 1970;171:724.

Rich NM, Metz CW, Hutton JE, et al: Internal versus external fixation of fractures with concomitant vascular injuries in Vietnam. J Trauma 1971; 11:463.

Romanoff H, Goldberger S: Combined severe vascular and skeletal trauma: management and results. J Cardiovasc Surg 1979;20:493.

Ross SE, Ransom KJ, Shatney CH: The management of venous injuries in blunt extremity trauma. J Trauma 1985;25:150.

Schlickewei W, Kuner EH, Mullaji AB, et al: Upper and lower limb fractures with concomitant arterial injury. J Bone Joint Surg 1992;74:181.

Sfeir RE, Khoury GS, Haddad FF, et al: Injury to the popliteal vessels: The Lebanese War experience. World J Surg 1992;16:1156.

Shah DM, Leather RP, Corson JD, et al: Polytetrafluoroethylene grafts in the rapid reconstruction of acute contaminated peripheral vascular injuries. Am J Surg 1984;148:229.

Shah DM, Naraynsingh V, Leather RP, et al: Advances in the management of acute popliteal vascular blunt injuries. J Trauma 1985;25:793.

Spencer FC, Grewe RF: The management of arterial injuries in battle casualties. Ann Surg 1955;141:304.

Snyder WH: Vascular injuries near the knee: An updated series and overview of the problem. Surgery 1982;91:502.

Swetnam JA, Hardin WD, Kerstein MD: Successful management of trifurcation injuries. Am Surg 1986;52:585.

Thomas DD, Wilson RF, Wiencek RG: Vascular injury about the knee: Improved outcome. Am Surg 1989;55:370.

Timberlake GA, Kerstein MD: Venous injury: To repair or ligate–the dilemma revisited. Am Surg 1995;61:139.

Treiman GS, Yellin AE, Weaver FA, et al: Examination of the patient with a knee dislocation: The case for selective arteriography. Arch Surg 1992;127:1056.

Van Wijngaarden M, Omert L, Rodriguez A, et al: Management of blunt vascular trauma to the extremities. Surg Gynecol Obstet 1993;177:41.

Weimann S, San Nicolo M, Sandblicher P, et al: Civilian popliteal artery trauma. J Cardiovasc Surg 1987;28:145.

Wright CB, Hobson RW: Hemodynamic effects of femoral venous occlusion in the subhuman primate. Surgery 1974;75:453.

Yeager RA, Hobson RW, Lynch TG, et al: Popliteal and infrapopliteal arterial injuries: Differential management and amputation rates. Am Surg 1984;50:155.

Yelon JA, Scalea TM: Venous injuries of the lower extremities and pelvis: repair versus ligation. J Trauma 1992;33:532.

Illicit Street Drugs and Vascular Injury

CHARLES E. LUCAS
ANNA M. LEDGERWOOD

INTRODUCTION

The use of illicit street drugs is very common in our society, especially among young people who are most susceptible to trauma. The method of administration and the pharmacologic responses of these drugs produce a unique pattern of vascular injury. This chapter is dedicated to the specific type of vascular problems associated with illicit drug usage.

PERIVASCULAR HEMATOMA AND ABSCESS

A common phenomenon in illicit drug users using intravenous access is a missed venous puncture that results in the needle entering an adjacent artery. This is often recognized by the withdrawal of bright red blood, known as "a pinky" among the users. When recognized, the needle is removed and

421

direct pressure is placed over the puncture site; despite this precaution, a hematoma often results. Treatment consists of observation and oral antibiotics, which are readily available on the street. Formal medical care is avoided unless complications ensue.

Because of the high incidence of contamination associated with the drug preparation including the multiple dilutions, which are performed to maximize profits, the hematoma has a high risk of becoming seeded from the contaminated injectable. This typically leads to infection of the perivascular clot and subsequent abscess formation. Sometimes a fragment of needle will be found within the abscess cavity. Physical examination identifies an area of cellulitis overlying the neurovascular bundle, which commonly is at the wrist or the groin. Transmitted pulsations may lead to the suspicion that this is a false aneurysm. When confusion exists about the nature of the pulsatile inflammatory mass, preoperative arteriography is warranted. During operative evacuation of these abscesses, the surgeon should avoid breaking all the adhesions because one end of the abscess cavity will abut the arterial wall. Overaggressive drainage of abscesses in this setting will lead to bleeding from the adjacent artery, where the puncture site had been sealed by an established platelet and fibrin plug.

Concomitant antibiotic therapy using broad-spectrum coverage is needed. During a 12-month interval at the Detroit Receiving Hospital, 651 patients had abscesses drained by the surgical services; 421 of these patients had abscesses that resulted from illicit street drug use. Most patients who have a single organism cultured will have a *Staphylococcus aureus* infection, which often is resistant to methicillin (methicillin-resistant *S. aureus*). β-streptococcus is also commonly found as an isolated organism. Approximately 25% of patients will have a mixed infection with gram-negative coliform organisms being part of this mixture. Many of the users were using their larger veins (mainlining) so the heroin mix would be injected into the subcutaneous plane (skin-popping). This compromises the surgeon's ability to determine whether the underlying cellulitis is related to the skin-popping or to an arterial injury.

DIRECT ARTERIAL INJECTION

Often patients who hit a "pinky" are already under the influence of alcohol or drugs and do not recognize that the needle has been inserted into an artery. The heroin mix is then injected intra-arterially followed by an immediate burning pain in the distribution area of that artery. This results from the embolization of particulate matter that has been used to dilute the heroin mix, the so-called "mixed jive," which plugs the distal microvascular tree. When small vessel occlusion occurs after a radial artery or ulnar artery injection, the ischemic necrosis typically involves the skin and subcutaneous tissues along the distribution of the thumb or the first and second fingers after a radial artery injection or along the distribution of the third and fourth fingers after an ulnar artery injection. This soft tissue insult is extremely painful. When patients present to an emergency department, the underlying etiology often is not recognized and the patients are treated with oral analgesics and sometimes antimicrobials. When first seen by a surgeon, there is usually evidence of full-thickness skin and sometimes subcutaneous necrosis. The prime therapeutic objectives are prevention of superimposed infection and amelioration of the constant pain. The role of intra-arterial crystalloid irrigation, heparin infusion, or other intra-arterial modalities of treatment have not been successful in this group of patients. Systemic analgesics provide minimal relief. Significant amelioration can be achieved by sympathetic blockade. Transient upper extremity pain relief may be obtained by a stellate block. Patients who experience significant relief on two separate stellate blocks likely will benefit from a dorsal sympathectomy performed through a small transaxillary incision. Patients undergoing sympathectomy in this setting will have increased warmth of the involved hand and a striking but not complete reduction in pain.

Sometimes the ischemic changes are associated with rapidly spreading infection that involves the adjacent muscles and leads to myonecrosis. Such patients will need amputation, which following lower limb or groin injection is a below-knee amputation; seldom is an above-knee amputation needed. When myonecrosis occurs in the hand, individual digits may need amputation. Unfortunately, we have performed several hands and even forearm amputations following wrist injections or brachial artery injections, respectively. Lack of an aggressive approach to myonecrosis after injections with contaminated street narcotics will lead to severe systemic septicemia, rhabdomyolysis, and renal shutdown.

MYCOTIC ANEURYSMS

In 1851 Koch described the first mycotic aneurysm. This occurred in a 22-year-old woman with a history of rheumatic fever with consequent endocarditis. Bacteria embolized from the heart valves into the superior mesenteric artery, which became aneurysmal, ruptured, and caused death. Autopsy demonstrated that the aneurysm was in one of the secondary arcades of the superior mesenteric artery. In 1885 Osler coined the term "mycotic aneurysm" when he described a 30-year-old patient who had a history of rheumatic fever with endocarditis and then developed four thoracic aortic aneurysms. One of these aneurysms ruptured causing death. At postmortem examination, Osler was impressed by the appearance of "fresh fungus vegetations" around the aneurysm. These were not fungus mounds, but inflammatory masses around bacteria-induced infection. The cause for mycotic aneurysm formation was endocarditis, resulting in embolization of bacteria into the vasa vasorum resulting in arterial wall infection and consequent aneurysmal dilation.

Mycotic aneurysms (infected pseudoaneurysms) in drug addicts are due to direct arterial trauma from an errant needle stick resulting in a perivascular hematoma that becomes infected. Huebl and Reid in 1966 described this sequence of events and referred to this entity as "aneurysmal abscess." During a 20-month interval at the Detroit Receiving Hospital, the surgeons excised 52 mycotic aneurysms or aneurysmal abscesses in 50

patients following intra-arterial injection with heroin mix, or "mixed jive." Often, the patient gave a history of a pinky but more often the intra-arterial injection was not recognized. The patient typically presented with pain, swelling, fever, and leukocytosis around the area of injection. About half of the patients had obvious pulsation of the inflammatory mass at the time of the original examination. The duration of symptoms usually was about 1 week. About 25% of patients had a decreased or absent peripheral pulse distal to the inflammatory mass. Few patients (10%) had symptoms of limb ischemia. An associated neural deficit is usually caused by a direct injection into or around the adjacent nerve rather than ischemia. The most common missed diagnosis was cellulitis, especially when not seen promptly by a surgeon. The resultant administration of intravenous antibiotics was followed by a lack of rapid response, which signaled the presence of the mycotic aneurysm.

When mycotic aneurysm is considered, arteriography is recommended. This confirms the diagnosis and serves as a road map defining both the site of leakage and the extent of collateralization. The operative approach should entail careful proximal and distal control of all involved vessels. This often is difficult because of the intense inflammation in the tissues around the abscess. This is due to the multiple prior injections in this area. Extensive fibrosis from repeated soft tissue exposure to mixed jive mistakenly injected around the vein impedes rapid safe dissection. Consequently, one must dissect very slowly after obtaining vascular control, to have as much anatomy displayed as possible before actually getting into the aneurysmal abscess. Very slow and careful dissection helps avoid injury to nearby structures, particularly the adjacent vein, which is often encased in this inflammatory mass.

Once fully exposed, the mycotic aneurysm with the adjacent artery should be excised, followed by proximal and distal ligation of uninvolved arterial wall. Suture ligation of the aneurysm artery without excision likely will lead to rebleeding. Aneurysmectomy will be tolerated without tissue loss in most patients with upper extremity aneurysmal abscesses and in most patients with aneurysmal abscesses involving the superficial femoral artery or the profunda femoral artery. Even the involved popliteal artery has been excised without tissue loss, although this artery is not commonly involved with a mycotic aneurysm. The need to perform aneurysmectomy of the common femoral artery with triple ligation of the common femoral artery, superficial femoral artery, and profunda femoral artery leads to a high incidence of ischemia and necrosis requiring amputation. Attempts to predict, from preoperative arteriographic findings, the level of resultant ischemia after aneurysmectomy are fraught with failure.

VASCULAR RECONSTRUCTION

Ideally, major artery aneurysmectomy is followed by vascular reconstruction. This aim however is hindered after mycotic aneurysmectomy in narcotic addicts by the surrounding inflammation and cellulitis. Efforts at reconstruction therefore must be directed toward extra-anatomic routes. External iliac artery mycotic aneurysms are rare; when such aneurysms are excised, reconstruction is best achieved by a femoral-to-femoral artery bypass if neither groin is involved with drug-related cellulitis. The timing of extra-anatomic reconstruction depends on the patient's presentation. When preoperative ischemic pain exists and there is an available extra-anatomic route, the bypass may be established before aneurysmectomy. When preoperative ischemic pain is absent, aneurysmectomy without bypass is indicated.

When common femoral artery aneurysmectomy with triple ligation leads to ischemia, the patient will wake up complaining of severe, unrelenting pain in the foot. When neither the lower abdominal wall nor the distal thigh has cellulitis, the patient should be taken back to the operating room for placement of an extra-anatomic bypass between the external iliac artery and the distal femoral artery or proximal popliteal artery. The

extra-anatomic bypass is best performed through the obturator foramen. The external iliac artery is most easily exposed through an oblique suprainguinal incision in Langer's lines followed by retroperitoneal dissection, which also allows access to the obturator foramen. The thigh incision must stay distal to the inflammatory changes abutting the groin cellulitis. This procedure is technically challenging and therefore dangerous because of the extensive collateral circulation associated with the groin cellulitis. The surgeon should detach the obturator membrane from its anterior and medial osseous insertion, thereby minimizing the threats of venous hemorrhage and neural contusion. The danger of rerouting through the obturator foramen has resulted in the recommendation that the lateral femoral triangle be used for this bypass. This approach, whereby, the graft goes just medial to the anterior superior spine, is really not extra-anatomic and is prone to failure in patients who have cellulitis involving the femoral triangle. A vein is almost never available in these patients because they have already destroyed their veins with prior injections. Consequently, one must use a synthetic graft. We prefer to use the Dacron graft, although the long-term patency rates between Dacron and PTFE grafts are not different.

The long-term success of extra-anatomic bypass grafts in these patients is directly related to recidivism of the drug usage. Whenever a patient goes back to using heroin mix and resorts to intravascular injection, the likelihood for thrombosis of the obturator foramen bypass graft approaches 100%. When thrombosis does occur, some patients have ischemia that is tolerable and other patients require amputation, which is usually at the below-knee level.

While treating patients with aneurysmal abscesses, antibiotic therapy is necessary. Most patients will have positive culture results for methicillin-resistant *S. aureus,* whereas a significant number of patients will have positive culture results for *Pseudomonas aeruginosa.* About 20% of the patients will have a mixed flora within the aneurysmal abscess, so broad-spectrum antibiotics are necessary. Likewise, the skin over the aneurysmal excision site should be left open to heal by second intent.

MYCOTIC ANEURYSMS OF CAROTID VESSELS

The potential for an infected pseudoaneurysm extends to any artery being injected. Some mainliners have avoided using the groin as a site of injection for fear of losing their legs. Somehow the thought that the blood supply to the brain could be compromised by carotid artery injection is not considered. The differential diagnostic challenge for a mycotic aneurysm involving the common or innominate arteries is the same as in the extremities. The lack of resolution of an inflammatory mass to antibiotic therapy should highlight the fact that this may be an aneurysmal abscess. The principles of treatment are the same. The surgeon must obtain proximal and distal control. Unfortunately, after excision of the infected pseudoaneurysm of the carotid or innominates arteries, there is never a plane that is not involved with cellulitis, so there is no potential for placing a bypass graft. Fortunately, these patients usually have good collateralization and do not develop evidence of cerebral ischemia after mycotic aneurysmectomy of aneurysms of the innominate artery, external carotid artery, common carotid artery, or internal carotid artery. The postoperative care requires the same considerations regarding antibiotics with broad-spectrum coverage and leaving the skin open to heal by second intent.

Occasionally, patients with mycotic aneurysms will have a fistula between the artery and the vein. The principles of care in such patients are the same as those for either a mycotic arterial aneurysm or a venous aneurysm. Proximal and distal control is necessary to get the arterial component isolated. The venous component should then be controlled proximally and distally before entering the artery and doing the aneurysmectomy. The care in dissection is especially important in patients with an arteriovenous fistula.

VENOUS ANEURYSMS

Septic phlebitis is a common coexistent condition in patients with drug injection–related cellulitis caused by mainlining or skin-popping. By the time the patient goes to the emergency department with complications from missed hits, several misses have occurred over the many previous weeks and months. The suspicion that a patient has something more than simple cellulitis is enhanced by the appearance of systemic sepsis that exceeds the severity typical of localized cellulitis. The presence of bilateral lung abscesses typifies the patient who has a venous aneurysm that is embolizing bacteria to the lungs. These changes in the lung are not caused by blood clots but are caused by embolization of bacteria. Anticoagulation should be avoided in this setting because the patient may also have endocarditis and small intracerebral infarcts from bacterial embolization. Anticoagulation may cause one of these intracerebral infarcts to hemorrhage. The surgical approach for mycotic venous aneurysm is excision plus proximal and distal venous ligation. Again, the dissection should be done very carefully to avoid injury to adjacent arteries and nerves. Fogarty catheterization may be helpful in retracting infected clot after venous control is obtained. After excision of a venous pseudoaneurysm, the patient is maintained on antibiotics and the limb is elevated. The skin is allowed to heal by second intent. Long-term care involves support wraps until the wounds have healed, after which time lifelong wearing of a customized venous support hose is necessary. These patients are not candidates for long-term anticoagulation, and they are not candidates for later vein graft inner position for their venous insufficiency.

VASCULAR INJURY FROM COCAINE

Cocaine in various forms has become a very popular substance abuse agent in all walks of life. The vasospastic effects of cocaine produce a multitude of clinical problems that involve the vascular surgeon. The intense vasoconstrictive effects causes multiple-organ dysfunction in young patients. These include myocardial infarction, cardiac arrhythmia, acute renal failure, cerebral vascular ischemia, and rhabdomyolysis. Thrombosis of small vessels is typically associated with ischemia of the distal part and is treated symptomatically with plasma volume expansion and observation. Occasionally, the ischemia will lead to severe myonecrosis, necessitating amputation.

Cocaine may also cause thrombosis of larger vessels including the abdominal aorta. This occlusion is thought to result from spasm of the vasa vasorum, resulting in an intimal injury followed by platelet deposition and clot formation. We treated one patient who had cocaine-induced thrombosis of the abdominal aorta, both renal arteries, the right iliac artery, the profunda femoris artery, and the popliteal artery, in addition to having distal small vessel occlusion with rhabdomyolysis and renal failure. Aggressive surgical therapy was needed to preserve life and threatened tissues. When the cocaine-induced thrombosis threatens the distal part, emergency operation with thrombectomy is indicated. Alternatively, when the occlusion is not associated with distal ischemia, nonoperative therapy with a full course of heparinization will result in complete resolution of the cocaine-induced thrombus. One must be certain that such patients do not have other intracerebral embolic infarcts from prior heroin use before anticoagulation unless the heparinization lead to intracerebral hemorrhage. Fortunately, most patients do not combine cocaine and heroin or use them in temporal proximity.

ACKNOWLEDGMENTS

This work was supported by the Interstitial Fluid Fund (account 4-44966).

REFERENCES

Fromm SH, Lucas CE: Obturator bypass for mycotic aneurysm in the drug addict. Arch Surg 1970;100:82-83.

Huebel H, Read C: Aneurysmal abscess. Minn Med 1966;46:11-16.

Johnson JR, Ledgerwood AM, Lucas CE: Mycotic aneurysm: New concepts in therapy. Arch Surg 1983;118:577-582.

Johnson JE, Lucas CE, Ledgerwood AM, Jacobs LA: Infected venous pseudoaneurysm: A complication of drug addiction. Arch Surg 1984;119:1097-1098.

Koch L: German "Ueber Aneurysma Dir Arteriae Mesenterichae Superioris, Inaug Dural-Abhandlung." Erlangen J Barfus' Schen Universitates-Buchdruckerei 1851:5-23.

Ledgerwood AM, Lucas CE: Mycotic aneurysm of the carotid artery. Arch Surg 1974;109:496-498.

Osler W: The gulstonian lectures on malignant endocarditis. Br Med J 1885;1:467.

Shanti CM, Lucas CE: Cocaine and the injured patient. Crit Care Med 2003;31:

Wallace JR, Lucas CE, Ledgerwood AM: Social, economic and surgical anatomy of a drug-related abscess. Am Surg 1986;52(7):398-401.

Webber J, Kline RA, Lucas CE: Aortic thrombosis associated with cocaine use: Report of two cases. Ann Vasc Surg 1999;13:302-304.

Iatrogenic Vascular Trauma

SAMUEL R. MONEY
MICHAEL R. LEPORE, JR.

INTRODUCTION

Patterns of injury for civilian arterial and venous trauma have long been recognized and discussed in both the vascular and the trauma literature. Most of the discussions are centered around arterial injuries resulting from either blunt or penetrating forces. These mechanisms are usually relatively easy to identify given the circumstances behind a motor vehicle accident or a fall, as is the case in blunt traumatic injury. Identification of the level of injury in the arterial tree, secondary to

427

penetrating trauma, necessitates thorough knowledge of arterial anatomy and recognition of the possible pathway of injury. Iatrogenic patterns of injury are not generally considered in conjunction with vascular trauma. It should, however, be considered as a subheading both trauma and vascular surgery.

These are the injuries that no clinician likes to collect or report in a personal series, but of which the vascular surgeon is well aware. Complications related to arterial access (e.g., pseudoaneurysms, hemorrhage, hematoma, and ischemia) or intra-aortic balloon pump (IABP) placement and venous access (e.g., venous injuries, arterial injuries, and arteriovenous fistula) are not uncommon. In addition, there are patterns of arterial injury that are specific to different surgical procedures and subspecialties such as colorectal, pancreatobiliary, laparoscopic, orthopedic, and neurosurgery. As enthusiasm for new procedures grows, such as endovascular aortic stent grafting for abdominal aortic aneurysms, a new pattern of iatrogenic arterial injuries evolves.

We discuss and illustrate some of the more commonly encountered iatrogenic vascular injuries. Prevention and management of these injuries necessitates an understanding of the mechanism of injury, as it does with all forms of trauma.

PERCUTANEOUS VASCULAR ACCESS

Complications related to percutaneous vascular access are not a new phenomenon. Translumbar aortography was first introduced in the late 1920s and early 1930s by dos Santos. The next generation in the evolution of percutaneous access was fostered by Seldinger who introduced the concept of catheter exchange over a guidewire in 1953. Since that time, technology has continued to advance the field. Percutaneous arterial or venous access has become an almost routine part of clinical patient management.

During the 1990s, there have been major technological advances in the treatment of peripheral vascular and coronary arterial

disease. As a result of these new "endovascular" techniques, various types of sheaths (i.e., crossover sheaths and shuttle sheaths) with increasing diameters have been developed to deliver newer and more complex intraluminal devices for advanced endovascular procedures. Add the increasing use of anticoagulants and the powerful antiplatelet agents (e.g., group IIb/IIIa platelet receptor inhibitors and adenosine diphosphate [ADP] receptor inhibitors) and it is no surprise that the incidence of iatrogenic arterial and venous injuries has mirrored the enthusiasm and growth of percutaneous interventional/endovascular techniques.

The more complex interventions that require larger delivery systems (8- and 9-French sheaths) are mainly performed by femoral arterial approach. Fortunately, for the increasing number of patients undergoing these procedures, vascular occlusion and uncontrolled hemorrhage are the least common complications. Vascular occlusion secondary to thrombosis or dissection does occur but may be treated percutaneously, if recognized, as demonstrated in Figure 22–1. Most surgeons would agree that vascular occlusion or thrombosis that is not amenable to percutaneous therapy requires surgical exploration with treatment dictated by the respective etiology.

Techniques for radial artery access are being used more frequently by interventional cardiologists, mainly for diagnostic coronary studies. As the emphasis toward endovascular intervention continues, peripheral diagnostic angiography and balloon angioplasty via radial arterial access are becoming more prevalent with lower profile percutaneous systems. These procedures are performed through a 6- or 7-French introducer sheath. As a result, such complications as infection, pseudoaneurysm, and thrombosis are not uncommon. Infection may occur and require some local drainage and antibiotics. Pseudoaneurysm of the radial artery can be treated with similar techniques for femoral pseudoaneurysm, discussed later discussion. Thrombosis is typically well tolerated because the ulnar artery is usually the dominant artery of the hand. Thrombosis that leads to symptomatic hand ischemia and/or major vascular

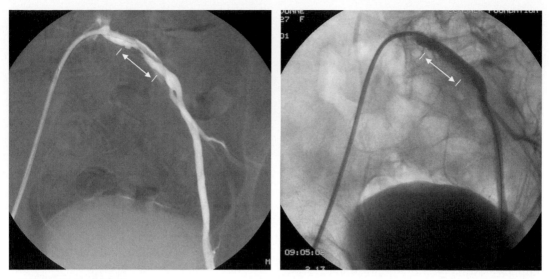

■ **FIGURE 22–1**
Left common iliac dissection secondary to a crossover sheath on right. Left common iliac post—stent placement on right. ■

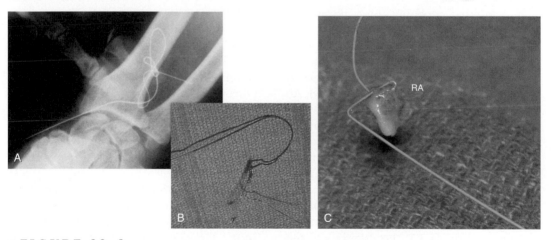

■ **FIGURE 22–2**
A, Wire in radial artery. *B*, Sheath and wire removed. *C*, Wire with piece of radial artery attached. ■

injury (Fig. 22–2) requires immediate surgical intervention using standard techniques of thrombectomy and or arterial reconstruction.

Pseudoaneurysms

Ever since Seldinger's technique for femoral arterial access became more commonplace, pseudoaneurysm has been recognized as one of the most frequently encountered complications. Classic vascular surgical treatment has required open arterial repair, evacuation of the hematoma, and drain placement as needed. In turn, this necessitates further hospitalization for the patient and the accompanying discomfort inherent to recovery from surgery. Open repair still remains the standard of care for more complicated femoral arterial injuries; however, newer and less invasive techniques have been developed.

The technique of ultrasound-guided pseudoaneurysm compression was introduced in the early 1990s. An experienced sonographer is required to apply between 10 and 120 minutes of compression to the "neck" of the pseudoaneurysm. Initial success rates for this procedure have been reported between 60% and 90%, with no further surgical intervention required. Unfortunately, recurrence rates have been reported at 25% to 30%. Many times, the pseudoaneurysm is tender and the patients require significant amounts of sedation before undergoing compression. In addition, ultrasound-guided compression has even lower success rates for patients who are taking anticoagulation or antiplatelet agents. This represents a significant number of patients who undergo percutaneous procedures with concomitant cardiac and peripheral arterial disease.

A combined modality using ultrasound guidance and thrombin injection has been proven more effective in the treatment of pseudoaneurysms. Success rates as high as 96% have been reported even when nearly 25% of the patients were anticoagulated. An experienced sonographer is still required to help identify the respective pseudoaneurysm in the appropriate axis for orientation. The needle is introduced under real-time ultrasonography and the pseudoaneurysm is punctured directly with the needle. Appropriate orientation is crucial because the supplying artery should not be crossed (Fig. 22–3). The thrombin (1000 IU) is then slowly injected into the pseudoaneurysm only, and thrombosis can be seen immediately by ultrasound (Fig. 22–4). Observing the ultrasound during injection ensures instillation of a minimal amount of thrombin. As thrombosis begins to occur, injection can be performed incrementally while the rest of the pseudoaneurysm thromboses. The greatest risk is from direct thrombin injection into the supplying artery, which occurs infrequently given adequate sonographic imaging. Many of the patients simply require some local anesthetic. This is performed as an outpatient procedure and the patients can walk 1 hour after injection.

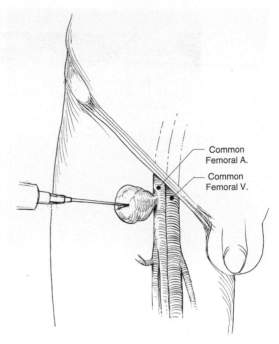

■ FIGURE 22–3
Injection of common femoral artery from lateral approach to avoid intraluminal thrombin injection. ■

Newer echogenic needles can reportedly improve visualization of the needle, avoiding thrombin injection into the supplying artery. We simply use a 22-gauge spinal needle, moving the obturator in and out to improve ultrasonographic visualization before injection.

Enthusiasts of endovascular therapy have reported on the use of covered stents to exclude a pseudoaneurysm or arteriovenous fistula. The early success rates were reasonable, with an 88% immediate result. On initial follow-up, however, there was nearly a 20% failure rate. The use of any stent, covered or uncovered, in the femoropopliteal region has been shown to have relatively poor results when compared to surgery; this is why covered stents should remain investigational in this anatomic region.

Hemorrhage

As discussed earlier, uncontrolled hemorrhage from percutaneous access is not a

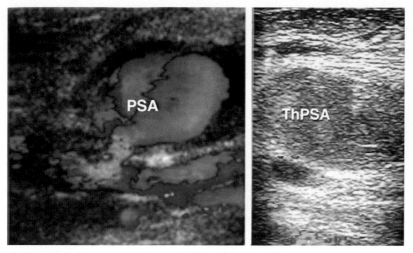

■ **FIGURE 22–4**
Common femoral pseudoaneurysm on left with flow. Thrombosed pseudoaneurysm on right post—thrombin injection. ■

common phenomenon. The patient who has obvious pulsatile bleeding from the puncture site or a growing hematoma should immediately have the hemorrhage controlled with direct pressure on the artery proximal to the puncture, usually over the femoral head. Occasionally the puncture is too cephalad (external iliac) or the femoral artery is damaged too severely for simple compression. This may be the case in the presence of severe arterial laceration or avulsion. Operative repair using the standard vascular principles of adequate exposure and proximal/distal vascular control should be performed immediately.

The more dangerous scenario is that of insidious and unrecognized hemorrhage. Patients who have uncontrolled bleeding without the obvious stigmas (e.g., pulsatile bleeding and expanding hematoma) initially exhibit very subtle clinical signs of hemorrhage. Relative hypotension and mild tachycardia that transiently improves with administration of fluids should alert the astute clinician and necessitate further investigation. Once suspected, a decreasing hemoglobin level verifies the likelihood of a retroperitoneal hematoma. Once again, the location of the puncture may provide some clues (i.e., above the inguinal ligament) to ongoing bleeding. An abdominal computed tomographic (CT) scan will verify the presence, location, and size

of the retroperitoneal hematoma (Fig. 22–5). Surgical exploration should rarely be required, as the retroperitoneum serves to tamponade the bleeding. Adequate resuscitation, reversal of any underlying coagulopathy, and identification and correction of medications that may exacerbate the bleeding (e.g., IIb/IIIa antiplatelet agents) should be first and foremost before any surgical exploration is performed.

Arterial Closure Devices

Given the growing field of endovascular techniques, combined with the accompanying increase in percutaneous access complications, industry has answered with newer products in an attempt to decrease access complications and reduce personnel time holding pressure on groins. The goal is to achieve immediate hemostasis following percutaneous arterial access. Different devices have been designed, each with its own technique toward achieving hemostasis. One approach is to "plug" the hole using collagen-based materials. Another technique involves closing the site with a suture. Still, one other involves using chemicals (procoagulant) to initiate early hemostasis. The development of these devices has created a new set of

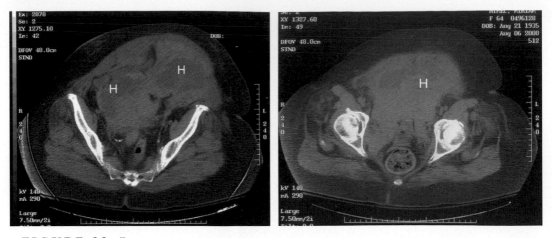

■ **FIGURE 22-5**
Computed tomographic scan of retroperitoneal hematoma (H). ■

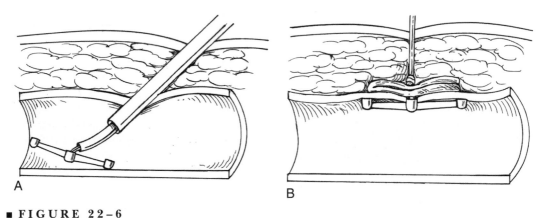

A   B

■ **FIGURE 22-6**
Angio-Seal device in vessel and post-deployment with intraluminal anchor in position. ■

complications. Treating any of the respective complications requires some understanding of how each device functions.

Angio-Seal (Sherwood Davis and Geck, St. Louis, Missouri) makes use of the collagen plug philosophy. The plug is sutured to a small, flat, rectangular anchor that is deployed intraluminally (Fig. 22-6). The plug is "tamped" down and secured extraluminally for near-immediate hemostasis. Initial success rates have been reported in the range of 88% to 92%. Success rates are claimed to improve with experience, as the manufacturers report an inherent learning curve. Given the typical nature of femoral vessels in this patient population, leaving anything intraluminally is disturbing. Rates of infection, stenosis, and

vascular occlusion or acute ischemia have been reported to be 2% to 3%. The risk of infection seems high when compared to simple manual compression. However, it continues to be used by many interventionalists in conjunction with prophylactic antibiotics (not a recommendation of the manufacturer).

The collagen plug technology is shared by VasoSeal (Datascope, New Jersey) but in a different manner. This device requires predilation with measurements of the length of the subcutaneous tract. The plug is then deployed extraluminally (Fig. 22-7) and pressure is applied for 2 to 3 minutes. Immediate success, defined as hemostasis, was achieved in 87% to 95% of the patients. The hematoma rate was alarmingly high, at 21% with

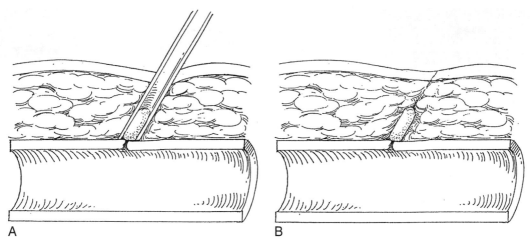

■ **FIGURE 22-7**
VasoSeal device with extraluminal placement of collagen plug. ■

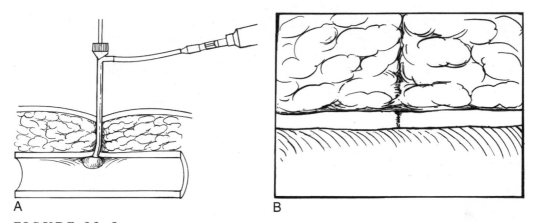

■ **FIGURE 22-8**
Duett device illustrating intraluminal balloon inflated and procoagulant injected after compression on right. ■

1% requiring surgery. If the plug is not adequately placed, then the vessel continues to bleed into the surrounding tissue. This would explain the decreased success rate (58.8%) in obese (>90-kg) patients. The device did not perform as well for patients on anticoagulants or antiplatelet therapy, as success rates were 79%. In addition, embolization of the collagen plug, late bleeding, and infection have required surgical intervention in as many as 5% of patients.

The Duett device (Vascular Solutions, Inc., Minneapolis, Minnesota) makes use of a procoagulant to seal the arterial puncture site. A small balloon is inflated on the luminal side of the puncture site, to avoid introduction of material into the respective vessel, and procoagulant is injected (Fig. 22–8). Once the balloon is deflated, the device is removed and 2 minutes of manual compression is required. A European multicenter registry reported a 96% deployment rate with successful hemostasis in 2 to 5 minutes in 95% of the patients with the Duett device. The overall complication rate was 2.6%, including pseudoaneurysms and complete arterial occlusions. Surgical intervention was required in fewer than 1% of patients. The use of anticoagulants or antiplatelet agents was not an exclusion criterion for the study.

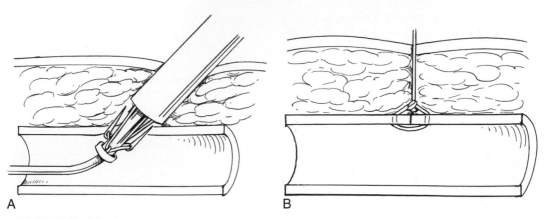

■ **FIGURE 22–9**
A, Perclose device in lumen of the vessel. *B,* Post-deployment with suture in place. ■

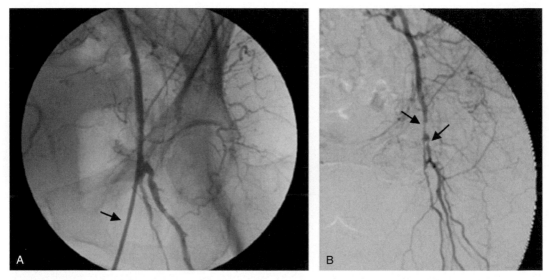

■ **FIGURE 22–10**
A, Angiogram of introducer sheath entering the left common femoral artery just proximal to the profunda femoris artery. *B,* Angiogram exhibiting high-grade stenosis of common femoral and profunda femoris arteries. ■

The last, and probably most frequently used, device uses suture to close the puncture site. Perclose (Perclose Inc., Menlo Park, California) uses two needles and a preloaded suture to puncture the vessel in a cephalad to caudad orientation and close the puncture site (Fig. 22–9). The ends of the suture come out through the device and are tied extracorporeally. A knot pusher then slides the knot down to the vessel. Early success rates are reported at 85% to 90%. Complications are reported at 1.8% and relate to inadequate deployment or pseudoaneurysm formation. Device failures

are usually recognized immediately for lack of hemostasis. Given the size of the needles, the device does not function on thick calcified vessels. We have seen delayed injuries, with development of severe claudication (Fig. 22–10), which ultimately leads to common femoral endarterectomy and profundoplasty.

The aforementioned devices are more frequently being used and this trend will continue. Aside from the acute need for surgical intervention, some delayed complications exist that may mandate surgical intervention. Although none of the studies discuss any of the local tissue changes, we have experiences with all of them at our institution. The surrounding scarring and inflammation encountered when one of these devices has been used is similar to that seen in a "reoperative groin."

Central Venous Access

Venous access by either the internal jugular or the subclavian vein approach has become a frequently performed procedure, with more than 3 million central venous catheters inserted annually. The obvious risk of pneumothorax and/or tension pneumothorax is a well-known complication of this procedure. Prevention of complications requires strict adherence to anatomic landmarks. Most venous injuries will respond to manual digital compression for hemostasis because it is a low-pressure system. The most common complications, however, are from injuries to adjacent structures.

The internal jugular vein can be approached from either side of the neck. It is one of the easiest veins on which to obtain digital compression. The more common significant injury in this location involves the carotid artery, given its proximity (Fig. 22–11). Although it is a higher pressure vessel, again, digital control is relatively easy here. The serious injuries occur with laceration of the vessel or when unrecognized cannulation of the artery occurs with subsequent large-bore dilation for placement of a resuscitation catheter (12 French) or a cordis (8 to 10 French). Additionally, unrecognized cannulation of the internal jugular vein through a portion of the artery may lead to an arteriovenous fistula (Fig. 22–12).

Subclavian venous access has the greater risk of morbidity and mortality. It is more difficult to apply digital pressure to the subclavian vein or the subclavian artery, given their relative anatomic location posterior to the clavicle (Fig. 22–13). Cannulation of the right subclavian vein is felt to be potentially more hazardous secondary to its abrupt angulation into the superior vena cava. Passage of the dilator can lacerate or perforate the vein or the superior vena cava, with an incidence reported as high as 1% of the time, leading

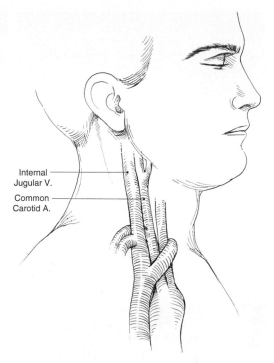

■ **FIGURE 22–11**
Illustration depicting carotid artery and internal jugular vein relationships. ■

to exsanguination and possible death. Passage through the artery into the vein can lead to arteriovenous fistula (Fig. 22–14) formation as well. Aortic perforation and subclavian artery aneurysm, though not common, have been reported as a consequence of central venous access as well.

Intra-Aortic Balloon Pump

The IABP was first instituted, clinically, 30 years ago, and it has become the most widely applied mechanical circulatory assist device, inserted in 2% to 12% of all patients, as an adjunct to heart surgery. However, it has its own set of accompanying vascular complications. Complications have been reported to occur between 12% and 30% of the time.

The most commonly encountered complication is that of ipsilateral lower extremity ischemia. Although most patients will improve with simple removal of the balloon, some patients still require surgical intervention even

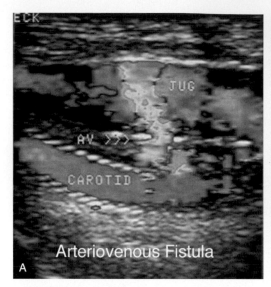
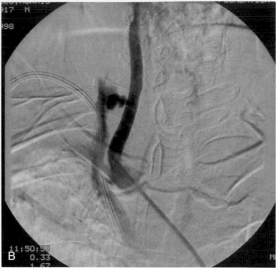

■ **FIGURE 22-12**
A, Duplex ultrasound of carotid/internal jugular vein fistula from access injury. *B,* Corresponding angiogram of fistula filling vein. ■

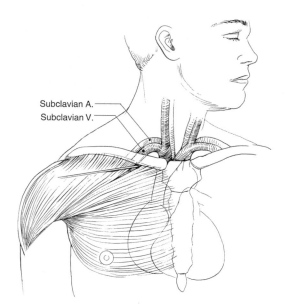

■ **FIGURE 22-13**
Illustration depicts location of subclavian vein and artery behind the clavicle. ■

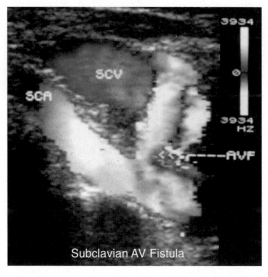

■ **FIGURE 22-14**
Duplex ultrasound of subclavian vein/artery fistula secondary to access. AVF, arteriovenous fistula; SCA, subclavian artery; SCV, subclavian vein. ■

after it is removed. Other patients are just not stable enough to have the balloon removed and may need contralateral placement. Ipsilateral iliac dissection, thrombosis of iliac/femoral arteries, and distal embolization are the most frequently encountered arterial pathology. A dissection may be treated by endovascular techniques and stenting. Thrombosis requires immediate surgical attention and intraoperative decisions dictated by the anatomic location of occlusion. Distal embolization may occur and the severity of distal embolization will dictate treatment. A patient who experiences acute popliteal occlusion leading to a nonviable leg should undergo immediate exploration, thrombectomy, and potentially bypass. In contrast, patients with "blue toes" and intact pulses are best observed for further tissue demarcation and improvement. Luckily, aortic perforation does not occur frequently (<1%) as it carries a near-100% mortality rate in this population.

INTRAOPERATIVE VASCULAR INJURIES

Vascular injuries that occur as a consequence of another operative intervention are more prevalent than is reported. Not many surgeons are willing to report on their series of intraoperative vascular injuries. However, it is well known that certain operations and different procedures have inherent risks of vascular injuries. The injuries that require intraoperative, urgent vascular consultation are usually severe and life threatening, as most surgeons will deal with the less severe injuries themselves.

Colorectal Procedures

Many colorectal operations require dissection into the pelvis. The low anterior resection, total proctocolectomy, abdominoperineal resection, and especially complicated diverticulitis place iliac vascular structures at risk. The arterial injuries are usually fairly simple to recognize and repair following standard vascular surgical principles. However, venous injuries to the iliac veins or inferior vena cava may be more challenging and can lead to significant blood loss. Simple ligation or oversewing of the bleeding may slow the bleeding enough that compression or packing of the pelvis may stop the hemorrhage. By the time a vascular surgeon is called, the patient has usually bled significantly. Initial packing of the pelvis, while resuscitation and correction of an underlying coagulopathy can begin, is the most prudent first step in this situation. Once corrected, the packing can be removed in a systematic fashion to identify the source of

bleeding for subsequent repair. All venous repairs should use pledgeted sutures of fine Prolene.

Pancreatobiliary Procedures

Pancreatobiliary operations can be difficult without a thorough understanding of the anatomy of the region. The pancreatobiliary structures lie in a peritoneal and retroperitoneal location (Fig. 22–15) that places them in proximity to the superior mesenteric, splenic, renal, and portal veins, as well as the superior mesenteric, celiac, splenic, and hepatic arteries, in addition to the vena cava and aorta. Even though these vascular injuries are not often reported, it has been estimated that they may approach 4%.

Injuries of aforementioned vessels occur most frequently to the portal vein, followed by superior mesenteric vein, right hepatic artery, splenic vein, superior mesenteric artery (SMA), and common hepatic artery. Injury patterns will be dictated by the types and frequency of the pancreatobiliary operation (e.g., Whipple versus laparoscopic cholecystectomy) performed. Sometimes these vascular injuries are recognized only after the retractors have been pulled back and the bowel is ischemic (SMA injury).

In the trauma setting of a severely injured patient, many injuries may be ligated or oversewn. However, elective pancreatobiliary surgery often destroys the collateral connections that are required to maintain viability after simple ligation. For this reason, it is advisable to repair these injuries when recognized and feasible. Venous injuries may require simple venorrhaphy or mobilization and primary anastomosis. In the case of arterial injuries, primary repair is the goal, but not always possible given the type of resection and length of remaining artery. Autogenous reconstruction with saphenous vein is our preferred method of repair in this setting.

Laparoscopic Procedures

Laparoscopic surgery has become routine in surgical practice. Some of the early

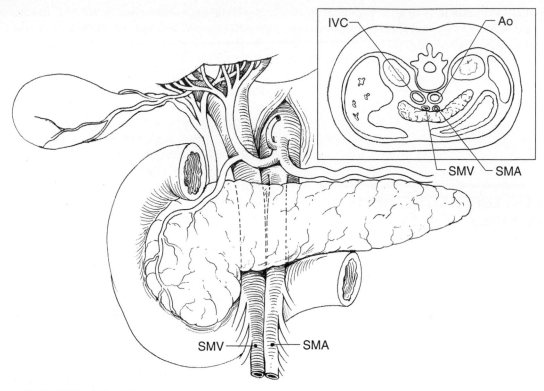

■ **FIGURE 22-15**
Pancreatobiliary anatomic relationships and in cross section. Ao, aorta; IVC, inferior vena cava; SMA, superior mesenteric artery; SMV, superior mesenteric vein. ■

complications from this "minimally invasive" technique have completely disappeared. However, some of the vascular complications have persisted over the years. The mechanism of injury has not changed, even today.

The overall vascular complication rate is quite low (0.08% to 0.1%) when compared with that of many other operations. Most commonly, vascular injuries reported in the largest series continue to be to the distal abdominal aorta, iliac arteries, inferior vena cava, and iliac veins. These structures are susceptible to injury from introduction of the Veress needle, for blind abdominal insufflation, or trocars into the lower abdomen. The distance, after compression of the periumbilical region with a Veress needle or trocar, between the abdominal wall and the vessels during insertion is generally not appreciated by the inexperienced laparoscopist (Fig. 22–16). The result is major vascular injury. It is usually

immediately recognized though, requiring conversion to open laparotomy with repair of the respective vascular injury.

Vascular/Endovascular Surgery

Iatrogenic vascular injuries during vascular procedures are again an area that is likely unreported for two reasons. The first is that the vascular surgeon is going to repair the injury at the time it occurs and the second involves the lack of willingness to report vascular complications. Nonetheless, some well-established injuries are known to be associated with different operations and have been discussed for many years. For example, iliac vein injury during aortobiliary bypass for aneurysmal disease. Endovascular surgery has borne out a whole new set of complications relative to aortic-stent grafts that are still in the

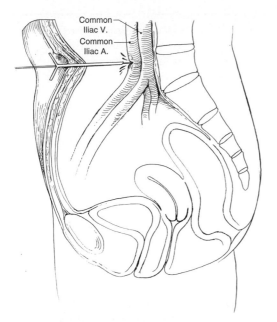

■ **FIGURE 22–16**
Iliac artery injury from Veress needle
placement. ■

discovery phase. The complications associated
with percutaneous access have been discussed
at length.

Thoracoabdominal aortic operations are
generally recognized, by most, as one of the
highest risk operations a vascular surgeon

performs. The large experience of E. Stanley
Crawford and colleagues at Baylor/Methodist
set the standard for this procedure. Respiratory failure, renal failure, cardiac complications, and stroke have all been well established
and are beyond the scope of this chapter. Thorough familiarity with retroperitoneal anatomy
is imperative if one is to perform these operations safely. Some of the most dangerous
bleeding involves the network of veins that
should be avoided while approaching the
aorta. Examples include the lumbar and
gonadal veins behind the left kidney (Fig.
22–17) and the azygous system. As in transabdominal aortic operations, the vena cava
and iliac veins can lead to massive exsanguination and even intraoperative death if
injured. These vessels are difficult to control
and should be packed/compressed initially.
If the injury is too large, then adequate exposure with ligation and/or oversewing still
remains the standard treatment for these
dreaded injuries.

Endovascular aortic aneurysm repair is
still in its infancy in the United States. The
Europeans, however, have been using multiple devices since the early 1990s. Certain complications such as iliac limb occlusion, distal
migration, and device malfunction are

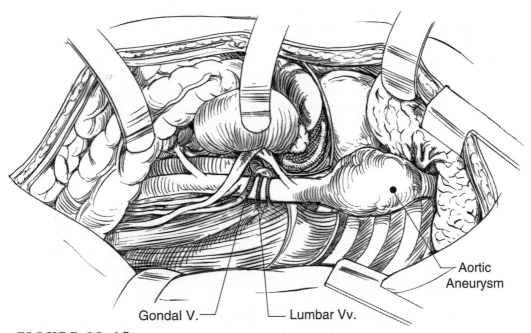

■ **FIGURE 22–17**
Gonadal and lumbar veins to be avoided during thoracoabdominal exposure of the aorta. ■

specific to different devices, the subject of another chapter. Identification of common vascular complications to the procedure itself is more important. The Eurostar Collaborators, 56 European centers, identified a 3% vascular complication rate in more than 1500 patients. These complications were identified as (1) arterial rupture, perforation, or dissection; (2) thrombus, obstruction, or stenosis; (3) embolization; (4) occlusion of renal artery; and (5) other injuries. This does not include the need for open conversion, which was required in 2.5% of the patients, or late ruptures as a result of endoleaks.

The Fogarty balloon catheter was first introduced in 1963. Although it is an instrumental part of the vascular surgical armamentarium, some potential complications are associated with its use. The most common injuries that have been documented include (1) perforation of the artery by the catheter tip, (2) rupture of the artery resulting from overinflation of the balloon, (3) disruption or injury to the arterial intima, (4) embolization of fragments of the ruptured balloon or catheter tip, (5) arteriovenous fistula, and (6) pseudoaneurysm formation.

Many of these injuries are the result of overzealous inflation and thrombectomy by the operator, which can be avoided as follows: (1) Before using the balloon in the vessel, place a 3-way stopcock on the end of the catheter to inflate the balloon to the proper volume (size) under direct visualization, then turn the stopcock to expel the excess saline; (2) tactile feel of catheter resistance to withdrawal in conjunction with careful control of the syringe to avoid overinflation; (3) if significant resistance is encountered and the anatomy unclear, then dilute the syringe with some contrast and monitor balloon passage fluoroscopically. Another method would be to simply proceed with an intraoperative angiogram and use an "over-the-wire" balloon thrombectomy catheter.

Orthopedic Surgery

Common vascular injuries that occur secondary to orthopedic injuries such as fractures and dislocations have been well recognized and reported. Given the nature of a subspecialty that requires placement of rods and screws for fixation of fractures, it is amazing that iatrogenic vascular injuries are not more common. Aside from complete misplacement of a rod, the most common injuries are reported with arthroplasty.

Total knee arthroplasty has been performed for more than 30 years now. The incidence of vascular injury is reported to be as low as 0.03%. This operation is typically performed under tourniquet control, so the injury may not be recognized initially. The mechanism of injury, when direct trauma is not involved, has been theorized to be secondary to arterial stretching or disruption of arterial plaques from the tourniquet placement. A thorough preoperative vascular assessment for reference is not always available when one is consulted on these patients acutely. In this case, the best approach is to determine the viability of the affected leg and compare it to the uninvolved extremity as a baseline. The most common complication is that of acute occlusion of the popliteal artery, requiring immediate exploration with thrombectomy or potential bypass.

One of the other well-established vascular injuries occurs secondary to screw placement for total hip arthroplasty. The vascular injuries that have been reported are related to intrapelvic extrusion of cement or damage to the common iliac vein during reaming for prosthesis placement. Orthopedic surgeons are well acquainted with the structures that are anterior, superior, and posterior to the acetabulum but are relatively unaware of those that lie medial to it. During the developmental period of total hip arthroplasty, after some catastrophic complications, it became widely recognized that the screws for the acetabular component placed medial structures at risk. Medial to the acetabulum lie the external iliac vein, obturator artery, and obturator vein. The anterior part of the acetabulum became recognized as the danger zone with the highest risk for vascular injury during screw placement. Through education, this complication has been reduced dramatically.

Neurosurgery

Neurosurgical vascular emergencies are not common. Intracranial vascular complications will be primarily handled by the neurosurgeon and obviously not the vascular surgeon. Back operations, such as disk surgery or corrective scoliosis surgery, have the highest potential for iatrogenic vascular complications in neurosurgery. Typically, large multilevel spine operations require adequate exposure. It is not uncommon for a general surgeon or a vascular surgeon to provide anatomic exposure for the neurosurgeon.

In the case of scoliosis surgery, prevention of major vessel injury during anterior exposures to the spine is of major concern. Given their anatomic proximity to the spine, the aorta and vena cava are at greatest risk. Typically, laceration or avulsion type of injuries occur secondary to rigorous retraction. Penetrating injuries may occur during removal of the rim of the disk annulus by the neurosurgeon. The recommended preventive technique is for placement of an elevator between the vessels and the spinal column during disk removal. Appropriate-length screws will avoid further vascular injury as well. However, late hemorrhage resulting from erosion, leakage, or false aneurysm of adjacent vessels has been reported. Retroperitoneal exposure to the spine is fraught with the same hazards as those discussed earlier with relation to thoracoabdominal exposure. The lumbar veins and arteries are the most commonly injured vessels because of avulsion or laceration. Digital pressure should be attempted initially, followed by suture ligation if unsuccessful. These can be troublesome injuries that result in a significant amount of blood loss.

Vascular injuries in lumbar disk surgery are rare (0.05%) but serious complications. They may be delayed in presentation or difficult to recognize given the anatomic approach. The most commonly seen vascular injuries are lacerations of the iliac veins, lumbar veins, abdominal aorta, median sacral artery, and arteriovenous fistulas. Because of the relative rarity of these injuries, no large series has been published that discusses the surgical approach to any of these injuries. It is important to keep the possibility in the back of one's mind, when recent back surgery has been performed, that the potential for vascular injury exists.

Early recognition of these injuries will help avoid unrecognized and ongoing hemorrhage.

SUMMARY

Any busy vascular surgeon is fully aware that a number of iatrogenic vascular injuries occur with varying frequencies based on anatomic location. However, reliable data about to the true incidence of these complications are not easily obtained. As previously discussed, this is not a series that any surgeon in any subspecialty would like to collect and report. The incidence and prevalence of iatrogenic vascular injuries are likely even higher than has been reported.

Our population continues to age and the greater percentage of the population will be older than 55 years within 10 years. That translates into more general, vascular, and cardiovascular disease. In turn, a greater number of operations are likely to be performed in all of the surgical subspecialties. As technologic advances continue to develop more devices for performance of endovascular techniques, there will continue to be a concomitant increase in the iatrogenic vascular injuries that accompany these techniques. The vascular surgeon will need to be well trained to handle different types of injuries that will continue to evolve with advancing technology. This will require a current knowledge base regarding to this ever-changing and rapidly developing technology.

REFERENCES

Arafa OE, Pedersen TH, Svennevig JL, et al: Vascular complications of the Intraaortic balloon pump in patients undergoing open heart operations: 15-year experience. Ann Thorac Surg 1999;67:645-651.

Bridwell KH, DeWald RL: The Textbook of Spinal Surgery, 2nd ed. Philadelphia, Lippincott—Raven Publishers, 1997.

Buth J, Laheij RJF, et al: Early complications and endoleaks after endovascular abdominal aortic aneurysm repair: Report of a multicenter study. J Vasc Surg 2000;31:134-146.

Cikrit DF, Dalsing MC, Sawchuk AP, et al: Vascular injuries during pancreatobiliary surgery. Am Surg 1993;59:692-697.

Fruhwith J, Koch G, Mischinger HJ, et al: Vascular complications in minimally invasive surgery. Surg Laparosc Endosc 1997;7(3):251-254.

Gonze MD, Sternbergh WC II, Salartash K, et al: Complications associated with percutaneous closure devices. Am J Surg 1999;178:209-211.

Goyen M, Manz S, Kroger K, et al: Interventional therapy of vascular complication caused by the hemostatic puncture closure device Angio-Seal. Cathet Cardiovasc Intervent 2000;49:142-147.

Kang SS, Labropoulos N, Mansour MA, et al: Expanded indications of ultrasound-guided thrombin injection of pseudoaneurysms. J Vasc Surg 2000;31:289-298.

Keating ME, Ritter MA, Faris PM: Structures at risk from medially placed acetabular screws. J Bone Joint Surg 1990;72-A(4):509-511.

Lazarides MK, Tsoupanos SS, Georgopoulos SE, et al: Incidence and patterns of iatrogenic arterial injuries. A decade's experience. J Cardiovasc Surg 1998;39:281-285.

Menlhorn U, Kroner A, de Vivie ER: 30 years clinical intra-aortic balloon pumping: Facts and figures. Thorac Cardiovasc Surg 1999;47 (Suppl):298-303.

Robinson JF, Robinson WA, Cohn A, et al: Perforation of the great vessels during central venous line placement. Arch Intern Med 1995;155:1225-1228.

Silber S, Tofte AJ, Kjellevand TO, et al: Final report of the European multi-center registry using the Duett vascular sealing device. Herz 1999;24(8):620-623.

Sorell KA, Feinberg RL, Wheeler JR, et al: Color-flow duplex-directed manual occlusion of femoral false aneurysms. J Vasc Surg 1993;17:571-577.

Svensson LG, Crawford ES, Hess KR, et al: Experience with 1509 patients undergoing thoracoabdominal operations. J Vasc Surg 1993;17:357-370.

Compartment Syndromes

THOMAS S. GRANCHI
PRISCILLA GARCIA
KENNETH L. MATTOX
MICHAEL E. DEBAKEY

Compartment syndrome occurs when pressure in a rigid compartment exceeds perfusion pressure. It can occur in any limb, the anterior chamber of the eye, the spinal canal, the pericardium, or in the abdomen and is seen in many clinical settings, threatening life, limb, sight, and/or neurologic function. Despite technology advances in noninvasive measurements and a better understanding of the anatomy, biology, and chemistry of reperfusion injury, diagnosis of this complication may still be missed or delayed. Operative decompression of the compartment is the mainstay of treatment. Fasciotomy treats compartment syndrome in limbs, laparotomy is the treatment for abdominal compartment syndrome, pericardiotomy treats cardiac tamponade, and spinal canal decompression has been used to treat reperfusion-related spinal compartment syndrome. For these reasons, compartment syndrome poses many potential pitfalls for trauma, vascular, and orthopedic surgeons. Medical treatments to reduce swelling and protect against cellular injury may have adjunct roles but do not replace the timely operative decompression.

Common clinical presentations include reperfusion injury after blunt trauma, vascular injury and repair, closed fractures, and electrical injuries. Additionally, compartment syndromes have been reported following use of compressive devices, such as the military antishock trousers. In these clinical settings, the astute clinician suspects compartment syndrome on initial physical examination and must then develop diagnostic and therapeutic actions, to include serial examinations of the involved region or extremity, serial pressure measurements, and/or use of new machines that evaluate tissue perfusion.

Excessive pain and loss of motor and sensory function in a limb are late clinical findings. In patients with a high risk for compartment syndrome, but in who repeated examination is not feasible, immediate compartment pressure measurement or immediate prophylactic fasciotomies should be considered. Pressure measurements can be graded, but a direct pressure of 25 cm H_2O or a pressure differential between mean arterial pressure and compartment pressure of more than 50 mm Hg indicates the need for immediate decompression.

Pericardial compartment syndrome is associated with increasing pressures in the pericardial sac and can be secondary to venous, arterial, or cardiac injury. Beck's triad of elevated central venous pressure, hypotension, and muffled heart sounds is a late manifestation of the pericardial compartment syndrome. Early detection of post-traumatic hemopericardium should lead to immediate thoracic decompression before the late manifestations develop. Narrowed pulse pressure and cardiac arrest from pericardial tamponade are very late manifestations and usually occur in patients with multisystem injury where the attention of the examining physician has been diverted, causing delayed or missed diagnosis of the compartment syndrome.

Spinal compartment syndrome has been evaluated most often in patients undergoing operation for extensive thoracoabdominal aortic surgery, where drainage of cerebrospinal fluid and reducing the spinal canal pressure are performed to reduce the incidence of paraplegia. Post-traumatic paraplegia, even associated with treatments of blunt injury of the descending thoracic aorta, has not been treated with spinal canal decompression. However, because paraplegia is associated with increased pressures in a closed compartment, decreasing pressure differentials, spinal cord swelling, and ischemia/reperfusion conditions undoubtedly conforms to the definition of a compartment syndrome. Further research in patients with thoracic aortic injury, post-traumatic paraplegia, and direct spinal column injury is required to define the post-traumatic spinal cord compartment syndrome. One might raise the argument that any potential value of use of corticosteroids in paraplegia following blunt injury to the spinal cord is actually an attempt to treat a spinal compartment syndrome.

Abdominal compartment syndrome can occur in patients with intra-abdominal injuries and hemorrhagic shock but is not directly related to these conditions. Abdominal compartment syndrome also occurs in some patients with no abdominal injury but who have treatment for remote conditions, such as cardiopulmonary bypass and excessive fluid resuscitation. In the abdomen, elevated compartment pressure is manifested by the following triad:

- Oliguria
- Reduced cardiac output that does not improve with intravascular fluid replacement
- Increased airway pressures

Organ impairment and increased airway pressure can be detected at intra-abdominal pressures as low as 15 mm Hg. At 25 to 30 mm Hg, organ failure is evident and immediate laparotomy should be performed (Burch and colleagues, 1996). Measuring intra-abdominal pressures will confirm an already suspected clinical diagnosis.

PRESENTATION

Surgeons caring for trauma patients most commonly diagnose and treat compartment syndromes, because this condition is often seen in association with injury. Pediatric, orthopedic, plastic, replantation, microvascular, vascular, and thoracic surgeons also often encounter compartment syndromes. Arterial or venous occlusion followed by reperfusion injury is a common presentation, whether occlusion is secondary to injury or vascular control during attempted reconstruction. Long bone fractures often precipitate compartment syndrome because of hematoma and tissue swelling at the site. Traditionally, calf compartment syndromes have been the most commonly diagnosed, treated, and reported. Gulli and Templeton (1994) report that compartment syndrome occurs in 3% to 17% of closed tibia fractures. Compartment syndrome associated with femur injuries is rare if the fracture occurs at the shaft and absent associated vascular injuries (Schwartz and colleagues, 1989; Russel and colleagues, 2002). Compartment syndrome occurring in the thigh is often overlooked because of other life-threatening injuries that distract the surgeon.

Pericardial compartment syndromes are often detected during the surgeon performed ultrasound examination in the emergency center. Rarely, a patient with unexplained continuing hypotension in the operating room following laparotomy will be found to have an occult pericardial compartment syndrome.

Although most cases of compartment syndrome from vascular etiologies occur with arterial injuries, it can also occur with venous pathology. There are many reports of compartment syndrome occurring with phlegmasia cerulea dolens (Dennis, 1945; Cywes and Louw, 1962; Wood and colleagues, 2000). Venous bleeding in the calf, thigh, abdomen, arm, and neck has also produced compartment syndromes. The individual fascial and muscle compartments in each of these areas deserve careful attention.

In the upper arm and forearm, compartment syndrome may occur with supracondylar humerus fractures, intravenous drug abuse, electrical injuries, intravenous line insertion site complications, prolonged tourniquet use, and even weight lifting (Moore and Friedman, 1989). Historically, when home washing machines had mechanical wringers attached to the machine, children getting arms caught in the wringer was an extremely common cause of both humeral fracture and compartment syndrome, known then as *Volkmann's ischemic contracture*. Many of these patients will present in ambulatory settings, where the index of suspicion may be low. Deep pain and tense swelling of the limb should prompt further investigation.

Abdominal compartment syndrome often develops in trauma patients who have undergone recent laparotomy and been excessively resuscitated for hemorrhagic shock using large volumes of crystalloid solution. The abdominal cavity will stretch anteriorly and superiorly (along the diaphragm) to accommodate visceral edema or accumulating blood until it reaches the limits of its compliance. At this point, the abdomen becomes a rigid compartment and pressure rises sharply, impairing organ function. Increased vascular resistance and reduced venous return impair cardiac output. Reduced renal perfusion pressure causes oliguria. Much of the post-traumatic renal failure reported in the literature during the 1960s and 1970s appears now to have been secondary to an abdominal compartment syndrome, which at that time had not yet been described. Transference of the abdominal pressure to chest and tension on the diaphragm increase ventilator and airway pressures. Loss of functional residual capacity and ventilation-perfusion mismatch causes hypoxia (Ivatory, Sugerman, and Peiztman, 2001).

Several systemic diseases are associated with compartment syndromes. Rutgers, van der Harst, and Koumans (1991) reported four cases on nontraumatic rhabdomyolysis and compartment syndrome in young male alcoholics receiving treatment with benzodiazepines. Ergotamine use and cocaine intoxication have also been implicated in the development of compartment syndrome (Gilman, Goodman, and Murad, 1989). Patients with type I diabetes mellitus can suffer spontaneous compartment syndrome (Lafforgue and colleagues, 1999; Smith and Laing, 1999; Silberstein and colleagues, 2001). Systemic diseases or drugs that cause vasoconstriction can induce muscle ischemia and subsequent compartment syndrome. Local factors including hematoma, fluid injection, infection, and metastatic melanoma that increase mass within the inelastic fascial compartments can also raise intracompartment pressure sufficiently to cause the feared syndrome (Simmons, 2000).

ANATOMY

Calf

The four muscle compartments of the calf are the anterior, lateral, superficial posterior, and deep posterior. The anterior compartment is bounded by the tibia medially, the interosseous membrane posteriorly anterior crural intermuscular septum laterally, and the crural fascia anteriorly. It contains the tibialis anterior, the extensor digitorum longus, and the extensor hallucis longus muscles. It also contains the

anterior tibial artery and vein, as well as the deep peroneal nerve. The lateral compartment contains the peroneus longus and brevis muscles and the superficial peroneal nerve. The superficial posterior compartment contains the bulky soleus muscle. The deep posterior compartment encloses the tibialis posterior, flexor digitorum longus, and flexor hallucis longus muscles. The posterior tibial vessels and the tibial nerve run within this compartment. Note that the saphenous vein courses in the subcutaneous tissue along the medial border of the superficial compartment. It can be damaged during fasciotomy if care is not taken to protect it. Also, the sural nerve runs along the posterior lateral border of the superficial posterior compartment (Clemente, 1981). Lateral and medial incisions are made throughout the extent of the calf, with retraction of the more superficial muscles to expose the deep compartment so that all compartments are decompressed. Historically, small skin incisions with incisions in the superficial fascia only and use of a lateral fibulectomy fasciotomy did not adequately decompress all calf fascial compartments. These procedures have little utility in today's trauma armamentarium.

Thigh

The thigh has three muscle compartments: anterior, medial, and posterior. The anterior compartment contains the quadriceps, sartorius, iliacus, and psoas muscles, as well as the femoral vessels and nerve and the lateral cutaneous nerve. The medial compartment encloses the adductor muscles, and the posterior compartment encircles the biceps femoris muscle and the sciatic nerve. Compartment syndrome of the thigh usually involves the anterior and lateral compartments (McGee and Dalsey, 1992). The gluteal muscle group also constitutes a compartment that is enclosed by the fascia lata. Gluteal compartment syndrome occurs but is often diagnosed late (Hill and Bianchi, 1997). A liberal lateral fasciotomy will usually decompress a thigh compartment syndrome.

Arm/Hand

The muscles of the arm, forearm, and hand are also grouped into compartments but are not as defined by tight investing fascia as those of the calf (Doyle, 1998). The arm has anterior and posterior compartments. The anterior compartment contains the biceps muscle, the brachial vessels, and the median, ulnar, and musculocutaneous nerves. The posterior compartment contains the triceps muscle and the radial nerve. The forearm has three compartments the volar, dorsal, and the "mobile wad." The volar compartment contains the flexor and pronator muscles, the radial and ulnar arteries, and the median and ulnar nerves. The dorsal compartment contains the extensor muscles. The "mobile wad" is closely associated with the dorsal compartment and contains the radial nerve. The hand has four compartments: the central, thenar, hypothenar, and interossei. The thick retinaculum cutis and the carpal tunnel serve as a venous obstruction at the wrist for compartment syndromes of the forearm and hand. Fasciotomies of the forearm, usually carried out with "zig-zag" and "straight" incisions, are carried across the carpal tunnel onto the hand to achieve a complete decompression (Fig. 23–1).

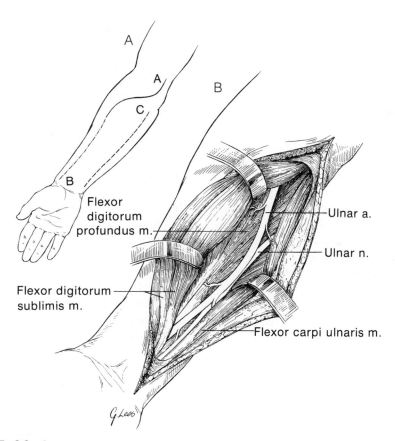

■ **FIGURE 23–1**

Elective incisions that can be used for approach to the radial and ulnar arteries. *A,* An *S*-type incision starting along the course of the distal brachial artery, carried throughout the antecubital fossa and continued down on the forearm will give excellent exposure of the proximal ulnar and radial arteries as well as the origin of the common interosseous artery (A). An extension of this incision (B) along the course of the radial artery can be used for exposure to the wrist level. A separate incision can be used over the course of the ulnar artery (C). *B,* This drawing demonstrates exposure of the ulnar neurovascular bundle within the deep muscle layers, which have been split proximally. ■

Abdomen

The abdominal viscera are encircled with peritoneum and the intra-abdominal contents are contained within the endoabdominal fascia, named in various locations as the transversalis fascia or Gerota's fascia. This investing fascia is contiguous with the esophageal hiatus and abdominal outlets at the groins. Numerous layers of muscles exist outside the endoabdominal fascia. Both the retroperitoneal and intraperitoneal organs are within this fascia. Swelling, gaseous distention, tissue edema, and hemorrhage are contained within this fascia. Although having great capacity to contain large quantities of fluid, tissue edema combined with large volumes of fluid increases abdominal pressure.

Spinal Cord

The spinal cord is surrounded by thick dura and is contained within a bony encasement. It is supplied by radicular arteries from the thoracic and abdominal aorta. A single radicular artery from the segmental arteries divides into anterior and posterior radicular arteries. The anterior radicular artery feeds a single anterior spinal artery, and the posterior radicular artery feeds paired posterior spinal arteries. The anterior spinal artery is more rudimentary and may even be interrupted, thus explaining the more common anterior spinal artery syndrome. Nine paired segment arteries arise in the chest, although the number may ranges from three to twelve. On occasion, one of the segmental arteries off of the aorta is much larger than the others and has been called the artery of Adamkiewicz. This variation is not consistent. Any condition from swelling of the spinal cord to pericord hematomas can contribute to a spinal column compartment syndrome.

Pericardium

Contained within the pericardial sac are the heart, ascending aorta, intrathoracic inferior vena cava, superior vena cava, pulmonary artery, right and left main pulmonary arteries, azygous vein, lymphatic channels, and pericardial vessels. Any condition that results in increasing fluid within the pericardial sac may contribute to hemopericardium and the development of pericardial compartment syndrome. Concomitant injury to the anterior pericardium and internal mammary arteries can also produce hemopericardium. Iatrogenic causes of hemopericardium, such as puncture of the heart or vessels during pericardiocentesis or trocar chest tube insertion, have been described.

DIAGNOSIS

The symptoms of deep muscle pain, pain on passive motion, muscle weakness or paralysis, hyperesthesia, and tense muscle compartments have been well described and repeated to generations of surgery residents (Matsen, Windquist, and Krugmire, 1980; Perry, 1988; Velmahos and Toutouzas, 2002). Recognition of the symptom constellation should prompt immediate measurement of compartment pressure, using any of the several accurate devices available. If accurate measurements cannot be performed, or if the results are conflicting, a clinical diagnosis of compartment syndrome should lead to strong consideration for compartment decompression. Once diagnosis is made, immediate release of pressure is indicated.

Abdominal compartment syndrome should be suspected in the patient with a tense, distended abdomen within a few hours of laparotomy for trauma or massive bleeding. Visceral swelling or continued bleeding push abdominal compliance beyond its limits. Oliguria that does not respond to fluid boluses or frequent ventilator alarms should prompt immediate measurement of the intra-abdominal pressure. This can be accomplished easily at the bedside by measuring the bladder pressure through a Foley catheter (Burch and colleagues, 1996; Ivatury, Sugerman, and Peiztman, 2001).

Extremity Compartment Measurements

There are several techniques for measuring extremity compartment pressures (Matsen and colleagues, 1976; Perron, Brady, and Keats, 2001; Hargens and colleagues, 1977). There are two variations of the catheter technique, the wick and the slit catheters. The catheters are inserted into the muscle through large-bore needles and then connected to a pressure transducer or manometer via saline-filled tubing. Because insertion and connection of the catheters are cumbersome, measuring several compartment pressures is difficult. The new electronic transducer-tipped catheter is promising but shares many of the shortcomings with the other catheter techniques, such as need for tubes, catheter kinking, and poor placement beneath the fascia (Willy, Gerngross, and Sterk, 1999). Commercial devices for measuring compartment pressures are readily available at the bedside and are easier to use.

Manufactured pressure monitors such as the Stryker (Stryker Instruments, Kalamazoo, Michigan) and Ace (Ace Medical Company, Los Angeles, California) instruments employ modifications of the needle technique and measure pressure directly through a needle inserted into the muscle compartment. These self-contained units require no assembly, making multiple measurements at different sites and times easier.

Regardless of the device used, multiple measurements should be taken at various sites in the muscle and in different compartments. Pressure is not uniformly distributed throughout each compartment, and measurements can be highly variable. In the calf, the anterior and deep posterior compartments, at least, should be measured. The highest measurement in each compartment should be used for clinical decisions.

Noninvasive Assessment of Compartment Compromise

The persistent trend in medicine toward noninvasive diagnosis and treatment extends to compartment syndrome. Several techniques that have clinical utility in other settings have been tried here, including near-infrared spectroscopy (NIRS), have been studied (Garr and colleagues, 1999; Giannotti and colleagues, 2000; Gentilello and colleagues, 2001). NIRS measures muscle perfusion, not pressure, and can reliably diagnose ischemic tissue. Oxyhemoglobin saturation of less than 60% correlates with muscle compromise of compartment syndrome. Champions for its use argue that it directly identifies ischemic tissue rather than compartment pressure, which is a proxy for tissue compromise. If clinicians monitor for tissue ischemia rather than a rise in pressure, unnecessary fasciotomies might be prevented. Conversely, skeptics argue that waiting until ischemia is manifest may delay surgery. Also, the probe's range is limited to 2 cm or less below the skin surface. Therefore, it may miss deep muscle ischemia. Of the noninvasive tests discussed, NIRS holds the most promise. It reliably identifies ischemic tissue and can provide continuous measurements. The latter makes it particularly attractive for use in the operating room and intensive care unit, where serial physical examinations are difficult on unconscious and or multi-injured patients. Continuous monitoring may identify development of compartment syndrome while surgeons are occupied with other injuries. Reliable measurements and safe thresholds for operation may reduce the unnecessary prophylactic fasciotomies. Studies of these questions continue.

Continuous compartment pressure or NIRS monitoring may influence the decision to refrain from fasciotomy. If the surgeon has continuous reliable monitoring, an operation should not be performed unless pressure or tissue perfusion reaches the threshold. However, the risk of compartment syndrome must be recognized and frequent or continuous measurements must be undertaken, always keeping in focus the clear indications for fasciotomy and the consequences of failing to act expeditiously.

Although it has been suggested, digital pulse oximetry is not sensitive in diagnosing compartment syndrome and muscle ischemia. It relies on pulsatile arterial flow to the distal digit to accurately measure the hemoglobin oxygen saturation. Because the arterial blood measured in the toe or finger bypasses the muscle compartments, measuring the former gives little useful information of the latter (Mars and Hadley, 1994).

Scintigraphy using technetium-99 methoxy-isobutyl isonitrile (^{99m}Tc-MIBI) has been used to diagnose chronic exertional compartment syndrome (Edwards and colleagues, 1999; Owens and colleagues, 1999). The study requires a stable, ambulating patient, a trip to the nuclear medicine department, and a subsequent study the next day with the patient at rest. With these limitations, this study cannot diagnose acute compartment syndrome in time to save the limb. We found no reports that it has been studied in acute compartment syndromes.

Laboratory Evaluation

There are no laboratory tests that will predict or diagnose early compartment syndrome. Serum creatinine phosphokinase, a marker for muscle cell injury, is a finding in late or missed compartment syndrome (Robbs and Baker, 1979; Moore and Friedman, 1989). Postoperative levels may be useful in monitoring response to treatment.

Similarly, myoglobinuria is a marker for muscle injury. It often occurs with crush or electrical injuries, which often lead to compartment syndrome. The presence of myoglobinuria in such patients does not per se diagnose compartment syndrome. The muscle injury may follow from direct trauma rather than ischemia secondary to elevated compartment pressures. Therefore, myoglobinuria has little value in diagnosing acute early compartment syndrome.

Pathophysiology

Restoration of oxygenated blood flow to an ischemic limb often worsens the initial cellular damage. The reperfused tissue suffers from the initial ischemia and from free radical toxicity. If microvascular flow slows or stops, then ischemia recurs and free radicals accumulate,

compounding the injury. This sequence of events produces reperfusion injury, which is a common etiology of compartment syndrome.

The cellular damage and capillary leak result from oxygen free radical and neutrophil activity. Hypoxanthine accumulates as a product of dephosphorylated adenosine and is converted to urate in the presence of xanthine oxidase and oxygen. The enzyme xanthine oxidase also catalyzes the reduction of molecular oxygen to superoxide and hydrogen peroxide. These radicals contribute to increased microvascular permeability. Superoxide can also generate the hydroxyl radical in the presence of Fe^{3+}, which is reduced to Fe^{2+}. The hydroxyl radical is highly cytotoxic through lipid peroxidation of the cell membrane. Neutrophils adhere to damaged microvascular endothelium and release superoxide radicals and proteases, contributing further to reperfusion injury (Granger, 1988).

TREATMENT OF EXTREMITY COMPARTMENT SYNDROME

Surgery has and continues to be the mainstay of treatment of compartment syndromes. Releasing the pressure through generous fascial incisions restores microvascular flow and rescues the threatened tissue. Nonoperative therapies received minimal theoretical initial enthusiasm and support; however, to date, none have demonstrated adequate efficacy. Choices in operative treatment are choices of incision and wound closure. The necessity of fasciotomy for diagnosed compartment syndrome remains unassailable. Indications for prophylactic fasciotomies, however, have been questioned (Field and colleagues, 1994; Velmahos and colleagues, 1997; Velmahos and Toutouzas, 2002).

Prophylactic fasciotomies in the calves have been advocated for combined popliteal artery and vein injuries and for ischemic times of more than 6 hours. Advocates argue that while waiting for compartment pressures to reach threshold for precise diagnosis may lead to severe dysfunction or need for an amputation; therefore, Hofmeister and Shin (1998) recommend liberal fasciotomies, especially in the anesthetized or comatose patient.

Hofmeister and Shin (1998) recommend prophylactic fasciotomy of all muscle compartments of the arm after replantation, because replantation requires 5 to 10 hours to accomplish, and the already compromised muscle relies on tenuous arterial and venous anastomosis. Fasciotomy, therefore, should be performed before compartment syndrome develops (Hofmeister and Shin, 1998). Under these circumstances, fasciotomy is prudent.

Technique of Decompression

The four compartments of the lower leg can be decompressed through a single lateral incision (Fig. 23–2) or through lateral and medial incisions (Fig. 23–3). The two-incision technique is more common because it is technically easier to reach the posterior compartments through the medial incision. Fibulectomy has been described but abandoned because easier and less morbid operations accomplish adequate decompression (Mubarak and Owen, 1977; Gulli and Templeton, 1994). Care must be taken at the upper end of a lateral calf fasciotomy incision to avoid injury to the peroneal nerve. Likewise, care must be taken to not incise or damage the long saphenous vein while making a medial calf fasciotomy incision.

Less invasive methods have been attempted. Surgical textbooks of the 1960s showed drawings of small skin incisions, and using long scissors, a continuous medial and lateral fascial incisions would be made. As the fascial compartments then had increased swelling,

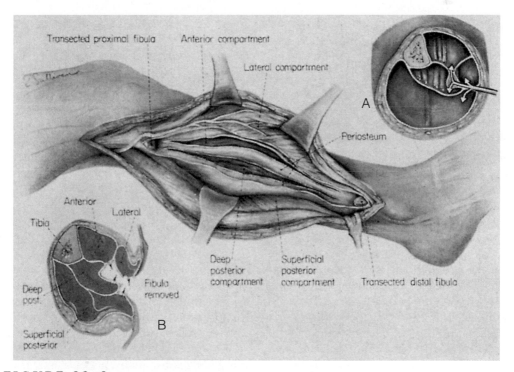

■ **FIGURE 23–2**
In selected patients, a fasciotomy by means of the subperiosteal fibulectomy technique may have merit in obtaining adequate decompression of all four major compartments of the leg. The completed fibulectomy/fasciotomy is shown. *A,* A cross section at the midcalf level, showing *(arrows)* the direction to be followed for four-compartment decompression. *B,* The area decompressed. (From Ernst CB, Kauder HJ: Fibulectomy-fasciotomy. An important adjunct in the management of lower extremity arterial trauma. J Trauma 1971;11[3]:365-380.) ■

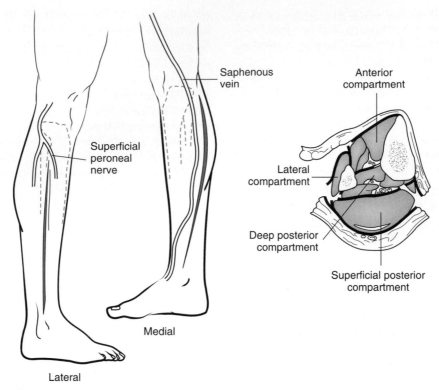

■ FIGURE 23–3

Drawing depicting medial and lateral calf incisions to decompress four of the fascial compartments of the lower leg. Specifically, note the proximity of the superficial peroneal nerve and saphenous vein, which must be protected. (Redrawn from Baylor College of Medicine, 1987.) ■

the skin became an investing constriction. Ota and colleagues (1999) described endoscopic release of the anterior leg compartment using an arthroscope and a transparent outer tube for chronic compartment syndrome in an athlete. The patient enjoyed relief of symptoms postoperatively, and the compartment pressures diminished (Ota and colleagues, 1999). Other authors have been less enthusiastic about endoscopic fasciotomies. Havig, Leversedge, and Seiler (1999) compared endoscopic and open forearm fasciotomies in cadavers. They found the endoscopic procedure reduced compartment pressures, but not as dramatically as the open procedure, and cautioned against using the endoscopic forearm fasciotomy in the clinical setting.

After diagnosing compartment syndrome and performing fasciotomy, the surgeon faces a large problematic wound. Primary closure is usually impossible because of exuberant muscle swelling. Delayed primary closure or later skin grafting is the most common method of wound closure.

Advocates of liberal fasciotomies tend to discount the morbidity of the scars. Conversely, other experts hold that complications from fasciotomies, including prophylactic ones, can be significant (Field and colleagues, 1994; Velmahos and colleagues, 1997; Fitzgerald and colleagues, 2000). Wound complications include ulcers, skin tethering to the muscle, paresthesias, pruritus, muscle herniation, and disfigurement. Fitzgerald and colleagues (2000) report that unsightly scars resulted in life changes for many patients and recommend primary closure of the wounds whenever possible.

Delayed primary closure of extremity wounds offers the benefit of a smaller scar but is usually labor intensive. This method involves some daily manipulation of sutures, wires, or elastic bands. Steri-Strips (3M Surgical Products, St. Paul, Minnesota) have been used for gradual approximation of skin edges, closing the wound in 5 to 8 days (Harrah and colleagues, 2000). Chiverton and Redden (2000) used subcuticular polypropylene sutures to achieve skin closure. Harris (1993) described using rubber vessel loops stretched between skin staples in shoelace fashion. One historic technique involved using interrupted wires stretched between skin staples, but this technique has been abandoned because of the difficulty endured by physician, patient, and nurses. The technique required adding tension daily by twisting of 20 to 30 interrupted wires spanning the incisions. The theory was attractive, but the practice was arduous.

Wound closure with split-thickness skin grafts is accomplished in 5 to 7 days after the fasciotomy. This method requires little bedside wound manipulation and achieves closure of large wound. It requires an additional general anesthetic for the patient and produces a significant scar. Skin grafting, however, is a mainstay in this setting because of its simplicity and coverage of large wound areas.

Because of the morbidity of fasciotomy, medical treatments have been researched in animals. The results are equivocal. Most are used to ameliorate the damage from oxygen free radicals (Hofmeister and Shin, 1998). They include deferoxamine to chelate iron, xanthine oxidase inhibitors, such as allopurinol, to block production of hypoxanthine, and superoxide dismutase, an enzyme to catalyze the superoxide radical to hydrogen peroxide. These antioxidants have been studied in many animal models, but not in humans. Currently, such nonprocedural therapies are not recommended.

In the abdomen, primary closure of the fascia is usually impossible, and sometimes, a skin-only closure can be accomplished. The most common forms of closure after laparotomy for abdominal compartment syndrome involve some form of temporary prosthesis such as a "Bogota bag" or vacuum pack (Burch and colleagues, 1996; Ivatury, Sugerman, and Peiztman, 2001). These prostheses maintain protection of the visceral while allowing loss of domain and effectively increasing the volume of the abdominal cavity. Removal of the prosthesis may be accomplished when swelling recedes. If delayed primary closure cannot be performed, skin grafting or component separation can cover the viscera. For the most severe forms of abdominal compartment syndrome in patients with multisystem trauma and prolonged intensive care unit stays, secondary reconstruction of the abdominal wall, using prosthetic material sewn to the fascia, may be accomplished several months later, often longer than 12 months.

SUMMARY

Compartment syndrome, if not detected early, can result in loss of limb, organ function, and even life. Effective treatment relies on early diagnosis through clinical examination and bedside measurements of compartment pressures. Measurements are accomplished using one of several commercially available devices. NIRS may have benefit as a noninvasive harbinger of muscle compromise. Although research has mapped the complex reactions in reperfusion injury, it has not produced a means for prevention or effective medical treatment.

Once diagnosis is made, the surgeon must perform expeditious decompression. A variety of incisions have been described. In the lower leg, median and lateral longitudinal incisions are most commonly used. In the forearm, volar and radial incisions are preferred. For the abdomen, a midline laparotomy accomplishes decompression. Pericardiotomy relieves compartment syndrome of the pericardium.

Prophylactic fasciotomy for high-risk patients is common. With newer, more reliable methods of tissue perfusion and compartment pressure measurements, prophylactic fasciotomy may be performed less commonly. Obviously, unnecessary fasciotomy should be avoided if possible. However, if muscle, organ, or limb loss is the alternative, decompression of the compartment is always indicated.

REFERENCES

Burch JM, Moore EE, Moore FA, Franciose R: The abdominal compartment syndrome in complex and challenging problems in trauma surgery. Surg Clin North Am 1996;76(4):883-843.

Chiverton N, Redden JF: A new technique for delayed primary closure of fasciotomy wounds. Injury 2000;31(1):21-24.

Clemente C: Anatomy, a Regional Atlas of the Human Body, 2nd ed. Baltimore: Urban & Schwarzenberg, 1981.

Cywes S, Louw JH: Phlegmasia cerulea dolens: successful treatment by relieving fasciotomy. Surgery 1962;51:169-172.

Dennis C: Disaster following femoral vein ligation for thrombophlebitis; relief by fasciotomy; clinical case of renal impairment following crush injury. Surgery 1945;17:264-269.

Doyle J: Anatomy of the upper extremity muscle compartments. Hand Clin 1998;14:343-364.

Edwards PD, Miles KA, Owens SJ, et al: A new noninvasive test for detection of compartment syndromes. Nuclear Med Commun 1999;20(3):215-218.

Field CK, Senkowsky J, Hollier LH, et al: Fasciotomy in vascular trauma: is it too much, too often? Am Surg 1994;60(6):409-411.

Fitzgerald AM, Gaston P, Quaba A, McQueen MM: Long term sequelae of fasciotomy wounds. Br J Plast Surg 2000;53:690-693.

Garr JL, Gentilello LM, Cole PA, et al: Monitoring for compartmental syndrome using near-infrared spectroscopy: a noninvasive, continuous, transcutaneous monitoring technique. J Trauma Injury Infect Crit Care 1999;46(4):613-618.

Gentilello LM, Sanzone A, Wang L, et al: Near-infrared spectroscopy versus compartment pressure for the diagnosis of lower extremity compartment syndrome using electromyography-determined measurements of neuromuscular function. J Trauma Injury Infect Crit Care 2001;51(1):1-9.

Giannotti G, Cohn SM, Brown M, et al: Utility of near-infrared spectroscopy in the diagnosis of lower extremity compartment syndrome. J Trauma Injury Infect Crit Care 2000;48(3):396-401.

Gilman AG, Goodman LS, Murad F: Goodman and Gilman's The Pharmacological Basis of Therapeutics, 8th ed. New York: Macmillan, 1989.

Granger DN: Role of xanthine oxidase and granulocytes in ischemia-reperfusion injury. Am J Physiol 1988;246:H1269-H1275.

Gulli B, Templeton D: Compartment syndrome of the lower extremity. Orthoped Clin North Am 1994;25(4):677-684.

Hargens AR, Mubarak SJ, Owen CA, et al: Interstitial fluid pressure in muscle and compartment syndromes in man. Microvasc Res 1977;14:1-10.

Harrah J, Gates R, Carl J, Harrah JD: A simpler, less expensive technique for delayed primary closure of fasciotomies. Am J Surg 2000;180(1):55-57.

Harris I: Gradual closure of fasciotomy wounds using a vessel loop shoelace. Injury 1993;24(8):565-567.

Havig MT, Leversedge FJ, Seiler JG 3rd: Forearm compartment pressure: an in vitro analysis of open and endoscopic assisted fasciotomy. J Hand Surg Am 1999;24(6):1289-1297.

Hill SL, Bianchi J: The gluteal compartment syndrome. Am Surg 1997;9:823-826.

Hofmeister EP, Shin AY: The role of prophylactic fasciotomy and medical treatment in limb ischemia and revascularization, in compartment syndrome and Volkmann's ischemic contracture. Hand Clin 1998;14(3):457-465.

Ivatury RR, Sugerman HJ, Peiztman AB: Abdominal compartment syndrome: recognition and management. In: Advances in surgery, vol. 35. St. Louis, MO: Mosby, 2001:251-269.

Lafforgue P, Janand-Delenne B, Lassman-Vague V, et al: Painful swelling of the thigh in a diabetic patient: Diabetic muscle infarction. Diabetes Metab 1999;25(3):255-260.

Mars M, Hadley GP: Failure of pulse oximetry in the assessment of raised limb intracompartmental pressure. Injury 1994;25(6):379-381.

Matsen FA, Mayo KA, Sheridan GW, Krugmire RB: Monitoring of intramuscular pressure. Surgery 1976;79(6):702-709.

Matsen FA, Windquist RA, Krugmire RB: Diagnosis and management of compartmental syndromes. J Bone Joint Surg Am 1980;62:286.

McGee DL, Dalsey WC: The mangled extremity; compartment syndrome and amputations, in soft tissue emergencies. Emerg Med Clin North Am 1992;10(4):783-800.

Moore RE III, Friedman RJ: Current concepts in pathophysiology and diagnosis of compartment syndromes. J Emerg Med 1989;7:657-662.

Mubarak SJ, Owen CA: Double-incision fasciotomy of the leg for decompression in compartment syndromes. J Bone Joint Surg 1977;59A:184-187.

Ota Y, Senda M, Hashizume H, Inoue H: Chronic compartment syndrome of the lower leg: a new diagnostic method using near-infrared spectroscopy and a new endoscopic fasciotomy. Arthroscopy 1999;15(4):439-443.

Owens S, Edwards P, Miles K, et al: Chronic compartment syndrome affecting the lower limb: MIBI perfusion imaging as an alternative to pressure monitoring: two case reports. Br J Sport Med 1999;33(1):49-51.

Perron AD, Brady WJ, Keats TE: Orthopedic pitfalls in the ED: acute compartment syndrome. Am J Emerg Med 2001;19(5):413-416.

Perry MO: Compartment syndromes and reperfusion injury. Vasc Trauma Surg Clin North Am 1988;68(4):853-864.

Robbs JV, Baker LW: Late revascularization of the lower limb following acute arterial occlusion. Br J Surg 1979;78:490-493.

Russel GV, Kregor PJ, Jarret CA, Zlowodowski M: Complicated femoral shaft fractures, in treatment of complex fractures. Orthop Clin North Am 2002;33(1):1-17.

Rutgers PH, van der Harst E, Koumans RKJ: Surgical implications of drug induced rhabdomyolysis. Br J Surg 1991;78:490-492.

Schwartz JT Jr, Brumback RJ, Lakatos R, et al: Acute compartment syndrome of the thigh, a spectrum of injury. J Bone Joint Surg Am 1989;71:392-400.

Silberstein L, Britton KE, Marsh FP, et al: An unexpected cause of muscle pain in diabetes. Ann Rheum Dis 2001;60(4):310-312.

Simmons DJ: Compartment syndrome complicating metastatic malignant melanoma. Br J Plast Surg 2000;53(3):255-257.

Singhal P, Horowitz B, Quinones QC, et al: Acute renal failure following cocaine abuse. Nephron 1989;52:76-78.

Smith AL, Laing PW: Spontaneous tibial compartment syndrome in type I diabetes mellitus. Diabetes Med 1999;16(2):168-169.

Velmahos GC, Theodorou D, Demetriades D, et al: Complications and nonclosure rates of fasciotomy for trauma and related risk factors. World J Surg 1997;21:247-253.

Velmahos GC, Toutouzas KG: Vascular trauma and compartment syndromes, in vascular trauma: complex and challenging injuries, part II. Surg Clin North Am 2002;82(1):125-141.

Willy C, Gerngross H, Sterk J: Measurement of intracompartmental pressure with use of a new electronic transducer-tipped catheter system. J Bone Joint Surg Am 1999;81(2):158-168.

Wood KE, Reedy JS, Pozniak MA, Coursin DB: Phlegmasia cerulean dolens with compartment syndrome: a complication of femoral vein cauterization. Crit Care Med 2000;28(5):1626-1630.

Historic Review of Arteriovenous Fistulas and Traumatic False Aneurysms

NORMAN M. RICH

ARTERIOVENOUS FISTULA

> If it should be found by experience, that a
> large artery, when wounded, may be healed
> up by this kind of suture, without becoming
> impervious, it would be an important
> discovery in surgery. It would make the
> operation for the Aneurysm still more
> successful in the arm, when the main trunk
> is wounded; and by this method, perhaps,
> we might be able to cure the wounds of
> some arteries that would otherwise require
> amputation, or be altogether incurable.
> Lambert, 1762; quoted in Hallowell, 1762

It is generally accepted that the first successful arterial repair was performed by Hallowell in 1759. His comments emphasize his realization that repair of false aneurysms and arteriovenous fistulas (AVFs) could be valuable. The diagnosis, pathophysiology, and surgical management of AVFs and false aneurysms have stimulated the intellectual curiosity and challenged the technical abilities of surgeons for more than 200 years. These lesions are often found in association, and they are often discussed together, despite the variable aspects that exist. Appropriate emphasis is given where indicated.

Because of the outstanding contributions of Matas, Halsted, Reid, Holman, Elkin, Shumacker, Hughes, and others and a plethora of reports from three major armed conflicts in this century, considerable documentation exists regarding principles of diagnosis and management of AVFs and false aneurysms. During the Korean Conflict, Hughes, Jahnke, and Spencer documented that arterial repair could be successful, even in a combat zone. Consequently, more vascular repairs were done at the time of initial wounding, with a resultant decrease in the number of AVFs and false aneurysms that required later repair. With the rapid progress that was made in vascular surgery in the 10 years preceding the increased American military involvement in Southeast Asia in 1965, hundreds of well-trained young surgeons from both military and civilian training programs were available

and eager to perform vascular repairs during the fighting in the Republic of South Vietnam.

With the establishment of the Vietnam Vascular Registry at Walter Reed Army Medical Center in 1966, an effort was made to document as accurately as possible all vascular injuries that occurred among American casualties in Southeast Asia and to provide long-term follow-up of these casualties. The initial analysis was important in providing guidelines for determining the ultimate success or failure following various types of repairs. It was believed that there would be relatively few AVFs and false aneurysms, compared with other recent wars. Nevertheless, it was recognized that a number of factors, such as multiple wounds and other more serious problems, might lead to delayed recognition of both AVFs and false aneurysms. In later follow-up from the registry, it was shown that there were more AVFs and false aneurysms than initially anticipated. The registry report provided an analysis of information gathered over 9 years for nearly 7500 records of American casualties, showing that there were 558 AVFs and false aneurysms among 509 combat casualties (Rich, Hobson, and Collins, 1975) (Fig. 24–1).

History

Hunter (1757, 1762) provided documentation more than 200 years ago that the heart enlarged in a patient with an AVF and that the arterial dilation occurred proximal to an arteriovenous communication (Table 24–1). Norris (1843) noted the recurrence of physical findings associated with an arteriovenous aneurysm 10 days after ligation of the artery above and below the fistula. Nicoladoni (1875) and Branham (1890) described slowing of the heart with pressure occlusion of an arteriovenous communication, and their names are often associated with this physical finding (the Nicoladoni-Branham sign). Annandale (1875) described the successful management of a popliteal AVF by the ligature of the popliteal artery and vein. Eisenbrey (1913) described pathologic changes associated with arteriovenous aneurysms of the superficial femoral

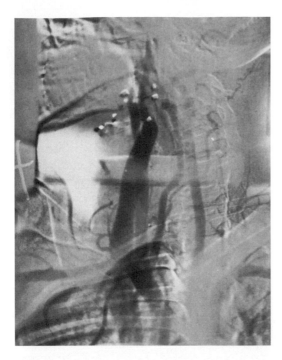

■ **FIGURE 24–1**

Multiple fragments from various exploding devices were responsible for the majority (87.3%) of arteriovenous fistulas and false aneurysms in this study. The subtraction study of an arch angiogram helped confirm the clinical impression of an arteriovenous communication in the patient's right neck at the level of the common carotid bifurcation. Excision of the fistula with ligation of the external jugular vein was performed at Walter Reed Army Medical Center in 1971. (From Rich NM, Hobson RW II, Collins GJ Jr: Traumatic arteriovenous fistulas and false aneurysms: A review of 558 lesions. Surgery 1975;78:817-828.) ■

TABLE 24–1

ACHIEVEMENTS AND UNDERSTANDING IN TREATING ARTERIOVENOUS FISTULAS: REPRESENTATIVE HISTORICAL NOTES

Author (Yr)	Contribution
Hunter (1757)	Recognized an abnormal communication between an artery and vein. Described the associated thrill and bruit. Eliminated the thrill and bruit by pressure over the proximal artery or site of communication. Noted tortuosity and dilation of the artery proximal to the fistula.
Norris (1843)	Cured an arteriovenous fistula by double arterial ligation.
Breshet (1833)	Described two patients in whom ligation of the artery proximal to the arteriovenous communication was followed by gangrene.
Nicoladoni (1875)	The first to demonstrate the remarkable slowing of the pulse rate by compression of the artery proximal to the arteriovenous fistula.
Branham (1890)	Emphasized the slowing of the pulse rate by obliterating a large acquired arteriovenous fistula (Branham-Nicoladoni sign).
Stewart (1913)	Noted that the heart diminished in size within 10 days after elimination of the arteriovenous fistula.
Gunderman (1915)	The first to mention an increase in blood pressure on obliteration of an acquired arteriovenous fistula.
Reid (1920)	Presented experimental evidence of cardiac enlargement in the presence of an arteriovenous fistula.
Nanu and colleagues (1922)	Accurately described the effect on the blood pressure of closure of the arteriovenous fistula.
Franz	Observed an increase in skin temperature and an increase in extremity growth in the presence of a femoral fistula of 18 months' duration in a 12-year-old boy.
Holman (1937)	Clarified many of the anatomic and hemodynamic variations seen with arteriovenous fistulas.

vessels (Fig. 24–2). Holman (1937), in his classic monograph, described the pathophysiology associated with abnormal communications between arterial and venous circulations. Holman (1940, 1962) has also provided reviews of the pathophysiology of AVFs. Osler (1893, 1905) made a number of early observations on AVFs. His respect for these lesions is exemplified by a quotation from an article written in 1905, "The great danger of operating is in the gangrene which is apt to follow."

Halsted made numerous contributions in the field of vascular surgery, including the management of AVFs. He referred to case presentation by Bernheim in 1916, when the latter used an interposition autogenous saphenous vein graft as a replacement for a popliteal repair (Halsted, 1916). He noted the important contributions of Carrel and specifically stated that the operation of Lexer, which Bernheim also was advocating, was the "the ideal operation." Reid, in two important contributions (1920, 1925), described abnormal arteriovenous communications. Using the vast World War II experience, Elkin (1945), Elkin and DeBakey (1955), and Shumacker (1946, 1950) documented a number of important

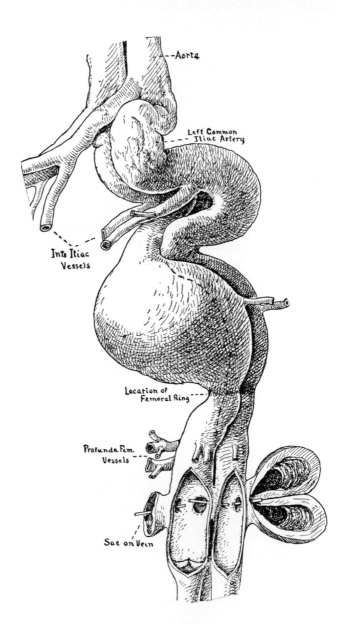

■ **FIGURE 24–2**
An arteriovenous communication with extensive vascular alterations. (From Eisenbrey AB. JAMA 1913;61:2155-2157.) ■

findings. Shumacker (1946) outlined the surgical approach to various AVFs and false aneurysms. He recognized the important work by Matas (1901, 1908), who made significant contributions to the present management of both AVFs and false aneurysms. The management of 215 AVFs and false aneurysms during the Korean Conflict was reported by Hughes and Jahnke (1958).

Incidence

It is difficult to determine the true incidence of AVFs. Some series combine congenital with traumatic lesions. False aneurysms may or may not be included. Some reports of arterial lesions include AVFs and others do not. Often the diagnosis is not made until years later. As an example, AVFs are still diagnosed at this time among World War II veterans, more than 30 years after their original injury.

Encouraged by Halsted, Callander (1920) made a literature review of 447 AVFs to 1914, including some from World War I. In the earliest reports of management of combat-incurred AVFs, Soubbotitch (1913) reported a insignificant percentage of vascular injuries: 77 injuries to large blood vessels among 20,000 wounded. The numerous separate reports by Elkin, Shumacker, Freeman, and others from their vast experience during World War II are included in a final bound report (Elkin and DeBakey, 1955). A total of 593 AVFs were treated; however, no incidence was given for these lesions among World War II combat casualties. In the Korean Conflict, 202 patients were treated for 215 AVFs and false aneurysms, with notation made for incidence among all combat casualties (Hughes and Jahnke, 1958).

The only statistic from the Vietnam experience of any value was an incidence of approximately 7% of AVFs and false aneurysms among nearly 7500 American casualties in Southeast Asia who suffered some type of vascular trauma. When Heaton and colleagues (1966) evaluated the initial military surgical practices of the U.S. Army in Vietnam, they recorded the following:

The lessons learned in Korea, the advances made in the techniques of vascular surgery, the increased numbers of surgeons trained in vascular techniques, plus rapid evacuation, new instruments and antibiotics have resulted in practically all arterial injuries occurring in Vietnam being repaired primarily with a high degree of success, so that only rarely do patients develop an arteriovenous fistula or false aneurysm.

The factors mentioned certainly played a significant role in limiting the number of AVFs and false aneurysms. With time, however, an increasing number of AVFs and false aneurysms were recorded. In many cases, these occurred in patients sustaining multiple small fragment wounds over a large portion of the body, which made it impractical to explore every artery in which a vascular injury might be present.

Hewitt and Collins (1969) reported a 10% incidence of AVFs among 60 patients with arterial injuries treated between December 1966 and October 1967, at the Eighteenth Surgical Hospital and during November 1967 at the Seventy-first Evacuation Hospital in Vietnam. Five of the six lesions were acute AVFs, which were noted on admission of the patients to the hospital within 1 to 6 hours after injury.

Civilian reports of vascular trauma have increased in the past 40 years, and some include reviews of experience in managing AVFs. Patman, Poulos, and Shires (1964) included six patients with AVFs among their 256 patients with civilian arterial injuries, an incidence of 2.3%. Drapanas and colleagues (1970) stated that because the immediate repair of all acute arterial injuries is advocated, the development of serious delayed complications, including AVFs and false aneurysms, should largely be prevented. They found that chronic AVFs and false aneurysms declined noticeably during the last period of their study, between 1958 and 1969 at Charity Hospital in New Orleans (Fig. 24–3). Hewitt, Smith, and Drapanas (1973) reported a 6.8% incidence, with 14 cases of acute AVFs among 206 patients with acute arterial injuries treated

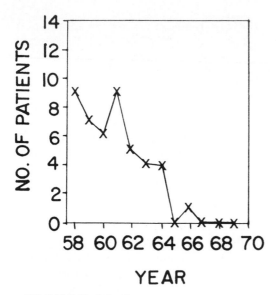

■ **FIGURE 24–3**
The number of patients with chronic arteriovenous fistulas and false aneurysms admitted to Charity Hospital in New Orleans on the Tulane Service between 1958 and 1969. There has been a notable decline in the incidence of these vascular injuries with delayed recognition. (From Drapanas T, Hewitt RL, Weichert RF, Smith AD: Civilian vascular injuries: A critical appraisal of three decades of management. Ann Surg 1970;172:351-360.) ■

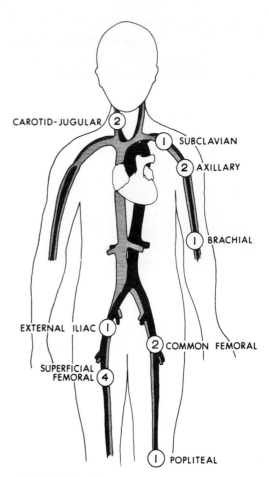

■ **FIGURE 24–4**
Distribution of acute arteriovenous fistulas in 14 of 206 patients with acute civilian arterial injuries in New Orleans: an incidence of 6.8%. (From Hewitt RL, Smith AD, Drapanas T: Acute traumatic arteriovenous fistulas. J Trauma 1973;13:901-906.) ■

on the Tulane University Surgical Service (Fig. 24–4).

The incidence of AVFs compared to that of false aneurysms has varied from one series to another. Shumacker and Carter (1946) studied 364 AVFs and false aneurysms in 351 individuals. There were 245 AVFs and 119 aneurysms, with 206 and 82, respectively, operated upon at one of the three Vascular Centers, Mayo General Hospital, established by the Army Surgeon General during World War II (Fig. 24–5; Table 24–2). In the 1964 series of Patman, Poulos, and Shires from Dallas, there were 17 patients who developed late complications, but only five AVFs were reported, compared with 12 false aneurysms. Thus, in their series, the false aneurysms outnumbered the AVFs by 2:1, a ratio opposite to that reported by Hughes and Jahnke (1958) from the Korean experience.

Seeley and colleagues (1952) reported that AVFs occurred in at least twice as often as false aneurysms in 106 cases seen at Walter Reed General Hospital. Most of the patients sustained their injury in the earlier part of the Korean Conflict. The incidence was nearly equal in the Vietnam experience (Rich, 1975), although there were fewer AVFs than false aneurysms (Table 24–3). AVFs and false aneurysms are often found together in various anatomic configurations (Figs. 24–6 and 24–7). Shumacker and Wayson (1950) outlined the development of AVFs, showing that pulsating hematomas may present initially, with well-formed saccular aneurysms developing subsequently. Notes made at the time

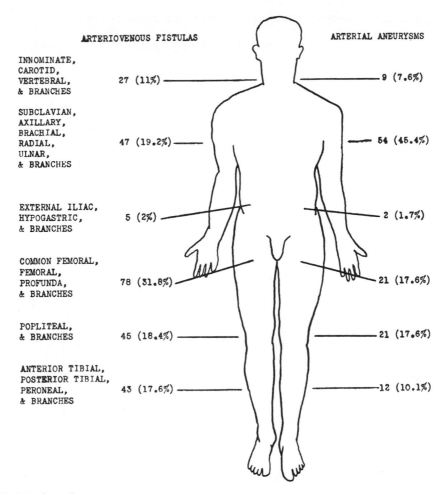

ARTERIOVENOUS FISTULAS   ARTERIAL ANEURYSMS

INNOMINATE,
CAROTID,
VERTEBRAL,   27 (11%) ———————————————————— 9 (7.6%)
& BRANCHES

SUBCLAVIAN,
AXILLARY,
BRACHIAL,
RADIAL,   47 (19.2%) ——————   54 (45.4%)
ULNAR,
& BRANCHES

EXTERNAL ILIAC,
HYPOGASTRIC,   5 (2%) ——————————   2 (1.7%)
& BRANCHES

COMMON FEMORAL,
FEMORAL,
PROFUNDA,   78 (31.8%) ——————   21 (17.6%)
& BRANCHES

POPLITEAL,
& BRANCHES   45 (18.4%) ——————————   21 (17.6%)

ANTERIOR TIBIAL,
POSTERIOR TIBIAL,
PERONEAL,   43 (17.6%) ——————————   12 (10.1%)
& BRANCHES

■ **FIGURE 24-5**
General distribution of arteriovenous fistulas and false aneurysms in a study from the Mayo General Hospital during World War II. (From Shumacker HB Jr, Carter KL: Arteriovenous fistulas and false aneurysms in military personnel. Surgery 1946;20:9-25.) ■

TABLE 24–2
COMPARISON OF INCIDENCE OF ARTERIAL ANEURYSMS AND ARTERIOVENOUS FISTULAS IN THE MAIN PERIPHERAL ARTERIES: MAYO GENERAL HOSPITAL, WORLD WAR II

Involved Artery	Arteriovenous Fistulas		Arterial Aneurysm	
	No.	%	No.	%
Subclavian	10	4.1	5	4.2
Axillary	12	4.9	15	12.6
Brachial	13	5.3	28	23.5
Common femoral and femoral	66	26.9	17	14.3
Popliteal	42	17.1	21	17.6

From Shumacker HB Jr, Carter KL: Arteriovenous fistulas and false aneurysms in military personnel. Surgery 1946;20:9-25.

TABLE 24–3
ARTERIOVENOUS FISTULAS AND
FALSE ANEURYSMS: VIETNAM
VASCULAR REGISTRY

Lesions	No.	%
False aneurysms	296	53.1
Arteriovenous fistulas	262	46.9
TOTAL	558	100.0

From Rich NM, Hobson RW II, Collins GJ Jr: Traumatic
arteriovenous fistulas and false aneurysms: A review of
558 lesions. Surgery 1975;78:817-828.

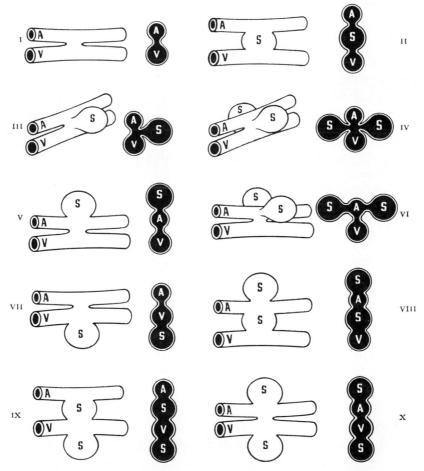

■ **FIGURE 24–6**
This diagrammatic representation of various types of arteriovenous fistulas and associated
aneurysms evolved from a study of 195 cases of arteriovenous fistulas. There was an associated
aneurysm in 60% of the arteriovenous fistulas. A, artery; S, sac; V, vein. (From Shumacker HB Jr,
Wayson EE: Spontaneous cure of aneurysms and arteriovenous fistulas, with some notes on
intravascular thrombosis. Am J Surg 1950;79:532-544.) ■

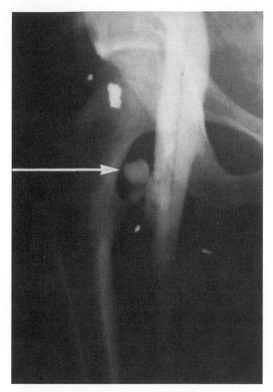

■ **FIGURE 24–7**
Femoral angiogram demonstrating an arteriovenous fistula at the level of the right common femoral arterial bifurcation. There is an associated false aneurysm *(arrow).*
Arteriorrhaphy of the origin of the profunda femoris artery and venorrhaphy of the common femoral vein were successfully accomplished at Walter Reed Army Medical Center in 1970. (From Rich NM, Hobson RW II, Collins GJ Jr: Traumatic arteriovenous fistulas and false aneurysms: A review of 558 lesions. Surgery 1975;78:817-828.) ■

TABLE 24–4
ARTERIOVENOUS FISTULAS AND FALSE ANEURYSMS; MULTIPLE LESIONS AT VARIOUS ANATOMIC SITES: VIETNAM VASCULAR REGISTRY

Patients	Lesions	Total
468	1	468
35	2	70
4	3	12
2	4	8
509		558

From Rich NM, Hobson RW II, Collins GJ Jr: Traumatic arteriovenous fistulas and false aneurysms: a review of 558 lesions. Surgery 1975;78:817-828.

TABLE 24–5
LOCATION OF ARTERIOVENOUS ANEURYSMS: BAYLOR UNIVERSITY COLLEGE OF MEDICINE AFFILIATED HOSPITALS

Location	No.
Popliteal	9
Femoral	9
Brachial	6
Common carotid	5
Radial	2
Subclavian	2
External carotid	2
Internal carotid	2
Posterior tibial	2
Temporal	2
Aortic arch	1
Internal iliac	1
External iliac	1
Occipital	1
Internal maxillary	1
Thyrocervical	1
Uterine	1
Peroneal	1
Medial circumflex femoral	1
TOTAL	50

From Beall AC Jr, Harrington BO, Crawford ES, DeBakey ME: Surgical management of traumatic arteriovenous aneurysms. Am J Surg 1963;106:610-618.

of operation and on examination of the excised specimen permitted an analysis of the presence or absence of an aneurysms in 195 cases of AVFs. There was no associated aneurysms in 78 cases, or 40%. The 60% majority had one or more aneurysm. Multiple lesions may also exist in various anatomic sites (Table 24–4).

A wide variation exists in the regional distribution of AVFs. This may include specific arteries, as well as regional areas. During a 15-year period from 1947 through 1962, 50 patients with AVFs were admitted to the Baylor University College of Medicine–affiliated hospitals in Houston. The greatest

number of these lesions were found in the extremities, with the lower extremities being more commonly involved than the upper (Table 24–5). Vollmar and Krumhaar (1968) found that nearly 50% of the AVFs in their series were localized in the lower extremities (Fig. 24–8). Next in frequency were fistulas of the upper extremities and shoulders (27%), head and neck (22.5%), and trunk (2%). Table 24–6 outlines representative World War II statistics concerning predominantly lower extremity injuries, specifically those involving the femoral and popliteal vessels. Involvement of major (Table 24–7) and minor (Table 24–8) vessels was outlined from the Korean experience by Hughes and Jahnke (1958). The Vietnam data centered around lower extremity involvement (Table 24–9), with the superficial femoral and popliteal arteries being most commonly injured (Table 24–10).

There are hundreds of reports of specific or unusual AVFs. Complete analysis is beyond the scope of this review. Creech, Gantt, and Wren (1965) presented a series of traumatic AVFs at unusual sites, including the superior gluteal, hepatic-portal, coronary, and vertebral vessels. Conn and colleagues (1971) reported challenging arterial injuries, including an aortocaval fistula, an iliac AVF, and a mesenteric AVF in eight patients.

Other representative reports include the following (additional information can be found in specific chapters): Hunt and colleagues (1971) reported their experience in managing five AVFs of major vessels in the abdomen.

LOCALIZATION OF 200 TRAUMATIC ARTERIOVENOUS FISTULAE

(Surg. Clin of the Univ. of Heidelberg, 1939 - 1967).

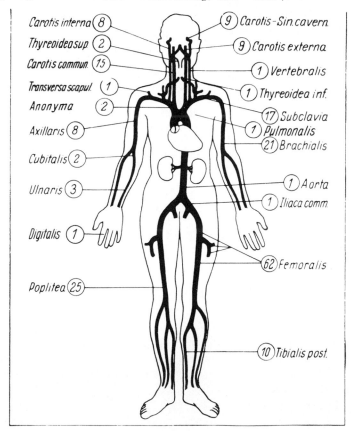

■ **FIGURE 24–8**

In the cases seen at Heidelberg University, nearly 50% of the arteriovenous fistulas were found in the lower extremities. (From Vollmar J, Krumhaar D: In: Hiertonn T, Rybeck B, eds. Traumatic arterial lesions. Stockholm, Sweden: Research Institute of National Defense, 1968.) ■

TABLE 24–6

DISTRIBUTION OF FALSE ANEURYSMS AND ARTERIOVENOUS FISTULAS: MAYO GENERAL HOSPITAL

Involved Artery	Arteriovenous Fistulas: No. of Cases			Arterial Aneurysms: No. of Cases		
	Operation at Mayo General Hospital	Operation Elsewhere	"Spontaneous Cure"	Operation at Mayo General Hospital	Operation Elsewhere	"Spontaneous Cure"
Aorta	1					
Innominate				1		
Internal carotid	3			2		
External carotid	3					
Common carotid	6		1	1	1	2
Vertebral	4					
Lingual	1					
Occipital	1					
Cirsoid, nose, ear	2					
Superior temporal	2			1		
Transverse cervical	1	1				
Deep cervical				1		
Internal mammary	1					
Subclavian	6	3	1	5		
Axillary	12			13	2	
Branch axillary	4			2		
Brachial	11	1	1	22	5	1
Radial	1	1		2		
Ulnar	4	2		2		
External iliac		1		1		
Hypogastric	1					
Superior gluteal	2			1		
Obturator	1					
Common femoral	3	2				1
Femoral	47	13	1	6	9	1
Profunda femoris	6			2		
Branch profunda	2	2	1	2		
Popliteal	41	1		14	6	1
Geniculate	4					
Posterior tibial	21	5		1	4	2
Anterior tibial	5	1		2	1	
Peroneal	5	1			1	
Branches in calf	5			1		
TOTAL	206	34	5	82	29	8

From Shumacker HB Jr, Carter KL: Arteriovenous fistulas and arterial aneurysms in military personnel. Surgery 1946;20:9-25.

TABLE 24–7
LOCATION OF TOTAL MAJOR VESSEL LESIONS: ARTERIOVENOUS FISTULAS; KOREAN EXPERIENCE

Vessel	Arteriovenous Fistulas	False Aneurysms	Total
Common carotid	7	2	9
Internal carotid	3	—	3
Subclavian	6	2	8
Axillary	9	11	20
Brachial	10	9	19
Iliac	3	1	4
Common femoral	7	1	8
Superior femoral	24	7	31
Popliteal	22	10	32
TOTAL	91	43	134

From Hughes CW, Jahnke EJ Jr: The surgery of traumatic arteriovenous fistulas and aneurysms: A five-year followup study of 215 lesions. Ann Surg 1958;148:790-797.

TABLE 24–8
LOCATION OF ARTERIOVENOUS FISTULAS: TOTAL MINOR VESSEL LESIONS TREATED; KOREAN EXPERIENCE

Vessel	Lesions			Treatment		
	Arteriovenous Fistulas	False Aneurysms	Ligation	Spontaneous Closure	Anastomosis	Total
Occipital	1	1	2	—	—	2
Supraorbital	—	1	1	—	—	1
Superior temporal	2	1	3	—	—	3
Vertebral	3	—	3	—	—	3
Superior thyroid	—	1	—	1	—	1
Inferior thyroid	2	—	2	—	—	2
Thoracoacromial	2	—	2	—	—	2
Thoracodorsal	2	1	3	—	—	3
Posterior humeral circumflex	1	1	2	—	—	2
Subscapular	1	—	—	—	1	1
Profunda brachii	—	1	1	—	—	1
Radial	2	4	5	—	1	6
Ulnar	2	2	4	—	—	4
Posterior interosseous	1	—	1	—	—	1
Anterior interosseous	2	—	2	—	—	2
Digital	—	1	1	—	—	1
Profunda femoris	10	—	10	—	—	10
Muscular branch femoral	—	1	1	—	—	1
Circumflex femoral, lateral	1	1	2	—	—	2
Inferior genu	2	1	3	—	—	3
Posterior tibial	11	2	12	1	—	13
Peroneal	8	1	9	—	—	9
Anterior tibial	3	3	6	—	—	6
Dorsalis pedis	—	1	1	—	—	1
Deep mantar	1	—	1	—	—	1
TOTAL	57	24	77	2	2	81

From Hughes CW, Jahnke EJ Jr: The surgery of traumatic arteriovenous fistulas and aneurysms: A five-year followup study of 215 lesions. Ann Surg 1958;148:790-797.

TABLE 24–9
ARTERIOVENOUS FISTULAS AND FALSE ANEURYSMS: ANATOMIC LOCATION; VIETNAM VASCULAR REGISTRY

Location	No.	%
Head/neck	42	7.5
Upper extremity	134	24.0
Thorax	17	3.1
Abdomen	22	3.9
Lower extremity	343	61.5
TOTAL	558	100.0

From Rich NM, Hobson RW II, Collins GJ Jr: Traumatic arteriovenous fistulas and false aneurysms: A review of 558 lesions. Surgery 1975;78:817-828.

TABLE 24–10
ARTERIOVENOUS FISTULAS AND FALSE ANEURYSMS: ARTERIAL INJURIES; VIETNAM VASCULAR REGISTRY

Artery	Arteriovenous Fistulas	False Aneurysms	Total	%
Common carotid	6	5	11	2.0
Internal carotid	2	4	6	1.1
External carotid	2	3	5	0.7
Vertebral	6	2	8	1.4
Subclavian	1	7	8	1.4
Axillary	10	8	18	3.2
Brachial	22	33	55	9.9
Radial	2	25	27	4.8
Ulnar	8	15	23	4.1
Innominate	1	1	2	0.4
Thoracic aorta	0	2	2	0.4
Abdominal aorta	0	1	1	0.2
Common iliac	1	1	2	0.4
External iliac	0	6	6	1.1
Internal iliac	0	1	1	0.2
Common femoral	4	7	11	2.0
Superficial femoral	57	31	88	15.8
Deep femoral	17	20	37	6.6
Popliteal	41	28	69	12.4
Posterior tibial	30	33	63	11.3
Anterior tibial	20	18	38	6.8
Peroneal	12	12	24	4.3
Miscellaneous	20	33	53	9.5
TOTAL	262	296	558	100.0

From Rich NM, Hobson RW II, Collins GJ Jr: Traumatic arteriovenous fistulas and false aneurysms: A review of 558 lesions. Surgery 1975;78:817-828.

One of the cases was unique in that the authors could find no previous report of successful repair of a fistula between the aorta, the renal vein and the portal vein (Fig. 24–9). They also described immediate repair of a mesenteric AVF and other fistulas involving the portal and renal veins. Dillard, Nelson, and Norman (1968) reported one case in which a 29-year-old woman was stabbed in the right flank and 3 years later was found to have severe hypertension. After correction of the renal AVF, the patient's blood pressure returned to normal.

Etiology

Although AVFs may be either acquired or congenital, we are essentially concerned with those that are acquired by trauma. On the other hand, one cannot be knowledgeable about acquired AVFs without also understanding the anatomic and pathophysiologic aspects of congenital AVFs (Table 24–11). Long-standing acquired AVFs must be differentiated from congenital AVFs, because there is a considerable difference in their surgical management, as well as the final results. An

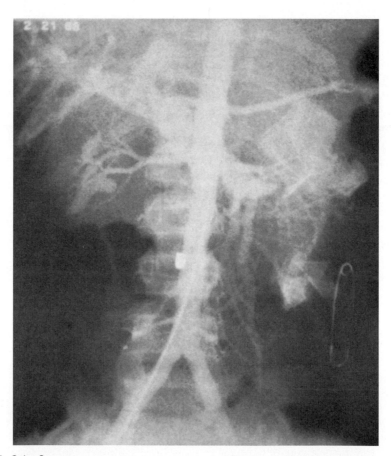

■ **FIGURE 24-9**
Abdominal aorta injured by a small-caliber bullet. This angiogram reveals the tip of the catheter in the area of injury; the portal vein fills selectively. The additional injury to the renal vein could not be shown simultaneously in this unique lesion involving the aorta, the renal vein, and the portal vein. (From Hunt TK, Leeds FH, Wanebo HJ, Blaisdell FW: Arteriovenous fistulas of major vessels in the abdomen. J Trauma 1971;11:483-493.) ■

TABLE 24–11
ARTERIOVENOUS FISTULAS: 10-YEAR EXPERIENCE AT THE MAYO CLINIC

	Congenital	Acquired
AV fistulas of the extremities	80	17
Aorta–inferior vena cava fistulas	0	7
Pulmonary AV fistulas	47	0
Renal AV fistulas	0	6
AV fistulas of the portal system	0	1
AV fistulas of the neck and face	11	4
Pelvic AV fistulas	1	5
AV fistulas of the chest wall	0	2
TOTAL	139	42

AV, arteriovenous.
Modified from Gomes MMR, Gernatz PE: Arteriovenous fistulas: A review and 10-year experience at the Mayo Clinic. Mayo Clin Proc 1970;45:81-102.

acquired AVF can have one, or possibly two, communications, whereas the communication between the arteries and the veins in the congenital type of AVF may be myriad.

Usually an AVF results from a simultaneous injury of an artery and adjacent vein, which permits blood to flow directly from the injured artery into the vein. Penetrating injuries are usually responsible for these lesions. In military injuries, penetrating missiles are the major cause, and in civilian injuries, stab wounds, as well as missile wounds, are associated with these lesions. The largest series of AVFs have been associated with recent combat wounds that have occurred during wars in the past century (Table 24–12). Both gunshot and fragment wounds have created AVFs that have been recognized either in the immediate or in the acute state or after a delayed period of several weeks or months. One of the ironies of the combat situation in Vietnam, where modern weapons have been employed, is that the primitive punji stick has also caused AVFs. I saw such an injury of the anterior tibial artery and vein at the Second Surgical Hospital in 1966.

Vollmar and Krumhaar (1968), based on their experience with 200 traumatic AVFs

TABLE 24–12
ARTERIOVENOUS FISTULAS AND FALSE ANEURYSMS: ETIOLOGY OF INJURY; VIETNAM VASCULAR REGISTRY

Wounding Agent	No.	%
Fragment	487	87.3
Bullet	59	10.6
Blunt	7	1.2
Punji stick	5	0.9
TOTAL	558	100.0

From Rich NM, Hobson RW II, Collins GJ Jr: Traumatic arteriovenous fistulas and false aneurysms: a review of 558 lesions. Surgery 1975;78:817-828.

treated at the Surgical Clinic at the University of Heidelberg between 1939 and 1967 (Table 24–13), reported that two world wars greatly increased the incidence of traumatic AVFs.

In civilian experience, many AVFs result from stab wounds, although they can also be caused by bullets. However, these are usually low-velocity gunshot wounds. Beall (1963) reported that 36 of 50 of AVFs in their 15-year study of vascular injuries resulted from gunshot wounds (Table 24–14).

Sako and Varco (1970) reported their experience in managing 57 patients with congenital and acquired AVFs of the extremities, abdomen, and chest wall during a 20-year

TABLE 24–13
ETIOLOGY OF 200 TRAUMATIC ARTERIOVENOUS FISTULAS; SURGICAL CLINIC OF THE UNIVERSITY OF HEIDELBERG: 1939-1967

Wounding Agent	No.	%
War projectiles	177	88.5
Fractures	10	5.0
Stab wounds	7	3.5
Iatrogenic trauma	4	2.0
Gunshot wounds (civil)	2	1.0
TOTAL	200	100.0

From Vollmar J, Krumhaar D: In: Traumatic Arterial Lesions. Hiertonn T, Rybeck B, eds. Stockholm, Sweden: Research Institute of National Defense, 1968.

TABLE 24–14

TYPES OF INJURIES RESULTING IN ARTERIOVENOUS ANEURYSMS: BAYLOR UNIVERSITY COLLEGE OF MEDICINE AFFILIATED HOSPITALS

Type of Injury	No.
Gunshot wounds	36
Stab wounds and lacerations	10
Shrapnel injuries	3
Blunt trauma	1
TOTAL	50

From Beall AC Jr, Harrington OB, Crawford ES, DeBakey ME: Surgical management of traumatic arteriovenous aneurysms. Am J Surg 1963;106:610-618.

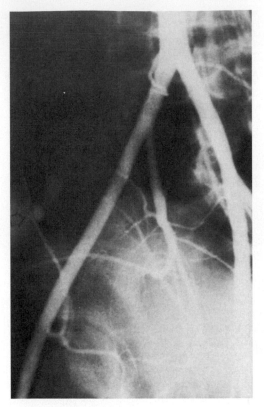

■ **FIGURE 24–10**
Arteriogram of the aortoiliac vessels demonstrating an inferior epigastric artery false aneurysm, which occurred as a complication of abdominal retention sutures. (From Ello FV, Nunn DB: False aneurysm of the inferior epigastric artery as a complication of abdominal retention sutures. Surgery 1973;74:460-461.) ■

period (1949 to 1969). Fewer than 50%, or 25 patients, had acquired AVFs. The etiology of these injuries included small-arms fire in nine, penetration with a knife or glass in six, a shell fragment or land mine explosion in three, multiple puncture for cardiac catheterization in two, blunt injury of the hand in one, pelvic fracture in one, renal needle biopsy in one, rupture of an aneurysm in one, and following gastrectomy in one.

Though uncommon, traumatic AVFs have been reported after both major and minor surgical procedures (Fig. 24–10). The vessels that have been involved include the superior thyroid (Ranshoff, 1935), renal (Muller and Goodwin, 1956), intercostal (Reid and McGuire, 1938), uterine (Elkin and Banner, 1946), and aortocaval (DeBakey, 1958). Pridgen and Jacobs (1962) reviewed three postoperative AVFs treated in a 3-year period at Vanderbilt University. They emphasized the necessity for exercising extreme care to avoid accidental injury to vessels during any surgical procedure. In one of their cases, they also emphasized that *en masse* ligation must be carefully avoided. They felt that the suture ligature had passed through the right superior epigastric artery and vein in one of their patients to result in an arteriovenous communication. AVFs have occurred following mass ligature of the renal vessels during nephrectomy and of the blood supply to the thyroid gland during lobectomy. One case report from Walter Reed General Hospital documented the development of an AVF following subtotal gastric resection (Blackmore and Whelan, 1965) (Fig. 24–11).

Beattie, Oldhan, and Ross (1961) presented the case of a 25-year-old man with an AVF of the superior thyroid vessels. Approximately 18 months earlier, he had a partial thyroidectomy for primary thyrotoxicosis. The superior thyroid pedicles were each ligatured with one ligature of no. 40 linen thread. Approximately 5 months after his partial thyroidectomy, the patient noted swelling in his neck and was aware of a "humming" in the region of the swelling. After angiographic demonstration of the superior thyroid AVF between the superior thyroid artery and vein,

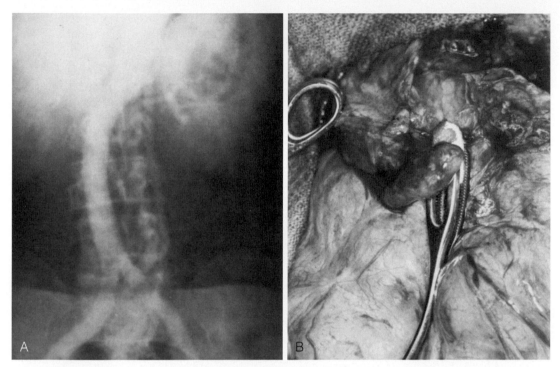

■ **FIGURE 24-11**
A, Antegrade aortogram showing larger anomalous artery to the left of the aorta communicating with veins in the lower part of the abdomen. *B,* The specimen in situ showing the artery ending in a cul-de-sac communicating with dilated veins. The Kütner dissector has been placed beneath the arteriovenous fistula. The transverse colon and mesocolon lie inferior to the fistula. (From Blackwell TL, Whelan TJ: Arteriovenous fistulas as a complication of gastrectomy. Am J Surg 1965;109:197-200.) ■

excision of the remnant of the left lobe of the thyroid gland was accomplished.

There have been unusual forms of AVFs reported following essentially every type of surgical operation and every type diagnostic or therapeutic procedure: For example, an AVF was reported following removal of an intervertebral disk with injury to the iliac artery and vein. Another such fistula occurred following a percutaneous transaxillary angiogram performed at Walter Reed General Hospital. Lester (1966) described AVFs as a complication of selective vertebral angiography. One of these lesions has also been treated at Walter Reed General Hospital.

White, Talbert, and Haller (1968) stated that there was an increasing awareness of peripheral arterial injuries in infants and children. One of their patients, a 3-month-old female, had a right femoral vein right heart catheterization to investigate a small ventricular septal defect and mild pulmonic stenosis. Over the following 3 years, she developed borderline heart failure, with a pulse rate of 120 and an increase in her heart size. At the age of 4.5 years, a thrill was noted over the left groin, and the left leg was 2 cm longer than the right. The proximal fibula was present on the left and not on the right. A large AVF (Fig. 24-12) was demonstrated between the profunda femoris artery and profunda femoris vein. Arterial blood gases had been measured and samples obtained from arterial punctures of the right femoral artery. The needle must have been inserted in a lateral and downward direction, penetrating the femoral vein before puncturing the femoral artery for the blood samples. A direct AVF was created by the needle. After ligation of this fistula and without sacrifice of either the artery or the

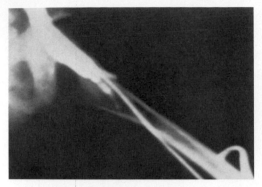

■ **FIGURE 24–12**
Angiogram demonstrating an arteriovenous communication between the right profunda femoris artery and the deep femoral vein following arterial puncture for blood gas analysis. Over the subsequent 3 years, the patient was in borderline heart failure, with an increased heart rate and increased growth in her lower extremity. (From White JJ, Talbert JL, Haller JA Jr. Peripheral arterial injuries in infants and children. Ann Surg 1968;167:757-766.) ■

vein, over the next several months, her pulse rate gradually returned to normal and her cardiac failure decreased.

Lord, Ehrenfeld, and Wylie (1968) presented the case of a profunda femoris AVF caused by passage of a Fogarty arterial catheter. At the time of their report, they stated that there were two other similar incidences in the literature. Subsequent reports include those of Rob and Battle (1971) and Gaspard and Gaspar (1972).

AVFs occasionally occur with fractures (additional details are given in Chapter 5). Harris (1963) reported an AVF following closed fracture of the tibia and fibula in a 35-year-old man (Fig. 24–13). Vascular injuries have occurred with orthopedic procedures rather than those involved in the management of fractures. Ferguson (1914) presented an infant who developed an AVF following an osteotomy of the femur genu valgum.

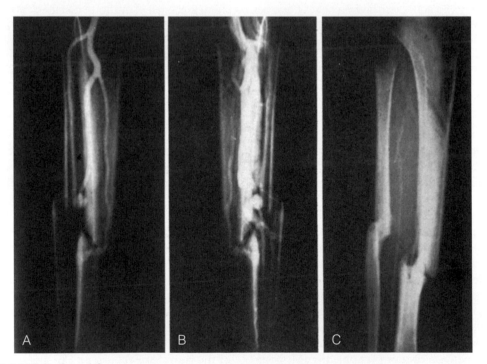

■ **FIGURE 24–13**
A, Closed fracture of the tibia and fibula; the arteriogram shows an arteriovenous fistula of the peroneal artery and the arterial phase of filling. *B,* The arteriogram shows the venous phase of filling of the peroneal arteriovenous fistula. *C,* A postoperative arteriogram following excision of the fistula. Note the rapid advance and union of the fracture of the tibia and fibula following excision of the fistula. (From Harris JD: A case of arteriovenous fistula following closed fracture of tibia and fibula. Br J Surg 1963;50:774-776.) ■

Anthopoulos, Johnson, and Spellman (1965) reported on the unusual case of 23-year-old woman who at age 9 years had sustained a human bite at the base of the finger. The authors believed that the AVF of the fifth finger developed as a complication of the human bite. There was spontaneous, periodic subungual spurting of the arterial blood, as well as increased growth, venous distention, increased local temperature, and more rapid growth of the nail. Surgical excision of the aneurysmal sacs and ligation of visible communications on two separate occasions resulted in relief of symptoms and enabled the patient to resume her occupation as a typist.

Pathophysiology

As a student at the Johns Hopkins Medical School in 1917, my curiosity about arteriovenous fistulas was aroused and repeatedly whetted by Doctor Halsted's recurrent expressions of great puzzlement at the occasional massive enlargement of the heart to the point of cardiac failure and at the marked dilatation of the proximal artery that could accompany an arteriovenous fistula, usually one long duration. Equally puzzling was the fact that this heart enlargement and arterial dilatation occurred with some but not all fistulas.
Holman, 1971

There is a sense of anatomic and pathologic changes that evolve when an AVF is produced (Fig. 24–14). An AVF is an abnormal communication between the arterial and venous systems that creates a shorter circuit in relation to the heart by allowing blood to pass from the higher peripheral resistance of the arterial system to the lower peripheral resistance of the venous system (Fig. 24–15). The secondary circuit, which has a constant tendency to divert the arterial blood into the lower resistance venous system through the fistula, causes a number of hemodynamic disturbances. The effective systemic blood flow is reduced, and there is a decreased mean sys-

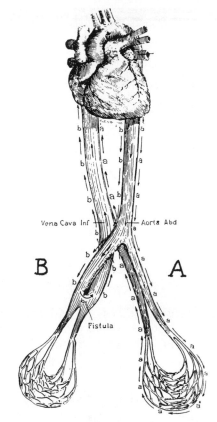

■ FIGURE 24-14
This schema shows the circulation in the presence of a right femoral arteriovenous fistula establishing a second circuit of blood. A progressively increasing volume of blood is sequestered in circuit B as long as resistance in the fistula circuit is less than resistance in the capillary bed in circuit A. (From Holman E: Arteriovenous aneurysms: Abnormal communication between the arterial and venous circulations. New York: Macmillan, 1937.) ■

temic arterial pressure. However, there is an increase in the blood volume, total cardiac output, stroke volume, heart rate, left arterial pressure and pulmonary arterial pressure, as has been described by Holman (1937, 1968). Holman also emphasized that the size of the AVF, the location of the communication in the vascular tree and the distensibility of the vascular rim are the factors that determine the volume of the blood that is diverted through the AVF's border permits progressive increase of the blood shunted through the secondary circuit of the fistula, with additional

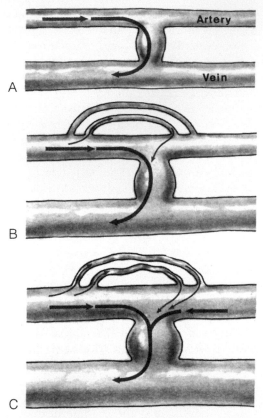

■ FIGURE 24–15
A, Immediately following the development of an
arteriovenous fistula, there is shunting of blood
from the artery through the fistula into the vein,
from which it returns to the heart. This results in
a decrease in peripheral vascular resistance, a
decrease in diastolic blood pressure, and an
increase in heart rate. The venous pressure
rises in the involved vein. Peripheral blood flow
is decreased in the involved artery. *B,* After
several weeks, collateral circulation enlarges
around the fistula because of the decreased
vascular resistance at the site of the fistula. As
the collateral circulation develops, the involved
artery and vein also dilate, increasing the
amount of blood flowing through the fistula.
C, After several years, extensive dilation may
develop about a fistula with marked
enlargement of collateral circulation. In
addition, there is enlargement of the artery
immediately distal to the fistula, through which
blood flows in a retrograde fashion through the
fistula toward the heart. The vein may enlarge
to marked proportions, creating varicosities in
the extremity. Ultimately such progressive
dilation after some years may result in
congestive heart failure from the increased
cardiac output. (From Spencer FC, Schwartz
SI: Principles of surgery. New York: McGraw-
Hill, 1974.) ■

increase in the blood volume and dilatation
of the heart. Lewis (1940) demonstrated that
the entire circuit gradually dilates to accommodate the increased volume of blood flow;
this includes dilatation of the cardiac chambers, the arterial tree proximal to the fistula,
the proximal vein and vena cava and even the
AVF itself. Nakano and DeSchryver (1964)
studied the effects of AVFs on systematic and
pulmonary circulation and stated that the
increase in cardiac output was essentially a
result of the increase in stroke volume, noting
that the heart rate may change very little.

Holman (1965) reviewed abnormal arteriovenous communications with particular reference to the delayed development of cardiac
failure. He emphasized that low resistance in
the venous system to the shunt of blood at the
site of the fistula and the decrease in peripheral perfusion distal to the AVF were strong
stimuli for the development of collateral
circulation. Holman (1940) documented
significant structural changes in both the
arteries and the veins associated with the
hemodynamic disturbances of an AVF. With
a small communication, the vein gradually
assumes the appearance of an artery, and it
may not be easily distinguished from the artery
at the end of 6 to 9 months. In contrast, with
larger fistulas, the vein may become so distended that it appears to be a false aneurysmal sac. As has been known since the first
description by Hunter in 1757, the artery proximal to the AVF can be dilated; however,
Holman (1940) stated that the dilatation of
the artery can also occur distal to the fistula.
It is not the initial injury that creates the AVF;
the arterial walls at the fistula or proximal to
it may become rigid as a result of deposition
of fibrous tissue, or the lumen may even
become stenotic by contraction of surrounding fibrous tissues.

AVFs may be associated with decreased
resistance in the peripheral arterial tree. The
consequent enlargement of superficial venous collaterals can be mistaken for changes
associated with chronic venous insufficiency.
One Vietnam casualty seen subsequently at
Walter Reed General Hospital had been
treated for varicose veins of his left lower
extremity for 5 years, when in actuality the
increase in his left thigh and associated

superficial varicosities were associated with an acquired femoral AVF.

According to Petrovsky and Milinov (1967), the structural changes that occur in the walls of both the arteries and the veins associated with an AVF are called "venization" of arteries and "arterialization" of veins. The alterations in the venous walls are easier to understand because they can be caused by an abrupt increase in the venous pressure and can be a consequence of adaptions. There is more difficulty in understanding the changes in Petrovsky and Milinov (1967)—performed experiments, which showed thickening of the media of the venous wall due to an increase in the amount of muscular and connective tissue elements, marked elastosis of all layers of the vessel wall, intimal thickening, and an increase in the vasa vasorum, which made it resemble the wall of an artery. They saw an increase in muscular fibers and fibrosis in the arterial wall, with a corresponding increase of mucopolysaccharides and extracellular fibers, elastosis and later dystrophy of the elastic fibers, focal necrosis of connective tissue elements in the adventitia, and diminution of the vasa vasorum. It was felt that a decrease in the oxidative process accounted for the accumulation of mucopolysaccharides, the extracellular fibrosis, and the elastolysis (decrease in oxidative process and tissue hypoxia, which results from a decreased blood supply in the arterial wall).

Holman (1940) stated that hemodynamic changes caused by AVFs were reversible. However, some structural changes may not be reversible, such as dilatation of the proximal artery associated with a long-standing AVF, which may not regress if aneurysmal deterioration of the wall has occurred. Also, cardiac enlargement associated with long-standing AVFs and dilatation may not revert to normal.

Eisenbrey (1913) emphasized the extensive alterations in both the artery and the vein up to the bifurcation of the aorta and vena cava in a patient with a superficial femoral AVF (see Fig. 24–2). The patient complained of shortness of breath and presented symptoms of cardiac insufficiency. Eighteen years earlier, the patient had been shot in the thigh with a small-caliber (probably .22-caliber) rifle bullet. Terminal illness allowed necropsy

examination of the aneurysmal dilatation and tortuosity of the artery and vein.

Subsequent studies have augmented the original and monumental contributions of Holman. Schenk and colleagues (1957) evaluated the regional hemodynamics of experimental acute AVFs. Their objective was to use the newer electronic methods for pressure and flow measurements to investigate the pressure-flow changes that occurred immediately upon opening an experimental fistula. Figure 24–16 summarizes the pressure-flow data in a representative model.

Johnson, Peters, and Dart (1967) studied the cardiac vein negative pressure in AVFs with a plastic model. They demonstrated creation of negative pressure in the cardiac vein, the result of transformation of energy, and explained this by the use of the principles of flow through a conduit (Fig. 24–17).

Johnson and Blythe (1970) evaluated eight patients with AVFs created for hemodialysis over a period of 3 years. Their study demonstrated that peripheral AVFs created for hemodialysis in patients with chronic renal failure result in a slight increase in cardiac output and pulse rate and a decrease in the total peripheral resistance. Although these alterations in hemodynamics did not lead to perceptible cardiac strain, a warning was

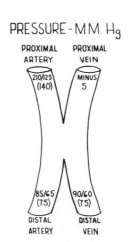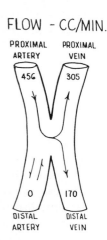

■ **FIGURE 24–16**
Schematic summary of pressure-flow data in a representative animal after a large femoral arteriovenous fistula was opened. (From Schenk WG Jr, Bahn RA, Cordell A, Stephens JG: Surg Gynecol Obstet 1957;105:733.) ■

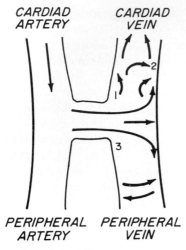

■ **FIGURE 24–17**
Flow pattern through fistula. In model, pressure at 1 was –10 mmHg, at 2 it was –5 mmHg, and at 3 it was –4 mmHg, emphasizing the negative pressure in the cardiac vein and arteriovenous fistula. (From Johnson G Jr, Peters RM, Dart CH Jr: A study of cardiac vein negative pressure in arteriovenous fistula. Surg Gynecol Obstet 1967;124:82-86.) ■

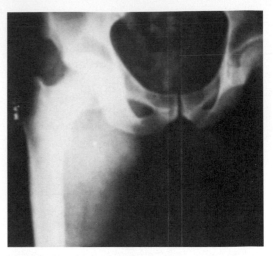

■ **FIGURE 24–18**
This small fragment wound of the upper right thigh created an arteriovenous fistula that was not diagnosed initially. The surrounding increased density on the roentgenogram was caused by an associated pulsating hematoma. (From Rich NM: Vascular trauma in Vietnam. J Cardiovasc Surg 1970;11:368-377.) ■

made that physicians managing these patients should be cognizant of this possibility, especially in patients on long-term hemodialysis.

Clinical Pathology

The capillary circulation is bypassed in an AVF when there is a direct communication between an artery and a vein. Although this type of communication can be a normal function of the microcirculation, the AVF becomes pathologic when its size or location causes significant hemodynamic alterations. An AVF may be established immediately after a penetrating injury in which blood flows directly from the injured artery into the vein. On the other hand, thrombus may surround the AVF, and the communication may not be obvious until days or weeks later when the surrounding clot becomes liquefied (Fig. 24–18).

Once a traumatic AVF has been established, there is usually little difficulty in its recognition. The previous history of trauma, the finding of a prominent pulsation and palpable thrill, and the presence of an audible machinery-like murmur, or any combination of these findings should alert one to the presence of an AVF. A bruit often appears over the sight of arteriovenous communications within a matter of hours after the establishment of the lesion. Other signs and symptoms that can develop distal to an AVF include intermittent claudication, edema (Fig. 24–19), and prominent veins (Fig. 24–20), which are often accompanied by bluish discoloration of the skin and venous stasis. The last two findings result from shunting of the arterial blood into the venous system.

More than 200 years ago, in 1757 William Hunter recognized an abnormal communication between an artery and a vein and accurately described the thrill and bruit associated with the communication. He noted that he can eliminate both the thrill and the bruit by pressure over either the proximal artery or the site of the communication. He also documented his observation of tortuosity and dilation of the artery proximal to the fistula.

Nicoladoni in 1875 is generally given credit for being the first to demonstrate the remarkable fact that the pulse rate could be lowered

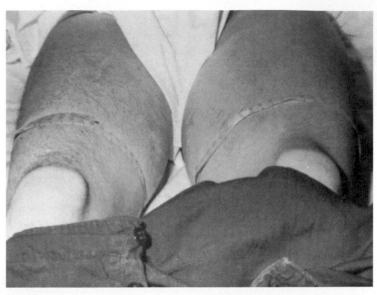

■ **FIGURE 24–19**
Edema can be associated with arteriovenous fistulas. The massive swelling of the left lower extremity in this Vietnam casualty is obvious. He had a femoral arteriovenous fistula of 5 years' duration; however, he had been treated as a patient with varicose veins. (NMR Vietnam Vascular Registry #630 1972.) ■

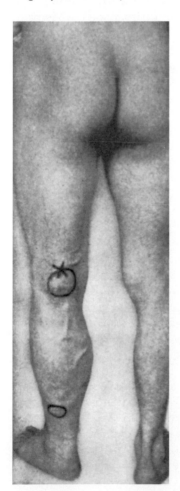

■ **FIGURE 24–20**
The position of an arteriovenous fistula and pulsating venous lakes *(circled);* note the difference in size of the two lakes. The site of the fistula is indicated by a cross. (From Holman EF: Arch Surg 1923;7:64-82.) ■

by compression of the artery proximal to the AVF. Fifteen years later, in 1890 Branham again called attention to the reduction of the pulse rate by obliteration of a large acquired AVF. This phenomenon is frequently referred to as the "Branham-Nicoladoni sign."

> The most mysterious phenomenon connected with the case, one which I have not been able to explain myself, or to obtain a satisfactory reason for from others, was slowing of the heart's beat, when compression of the common femoral was employed. This began to be noticeable after the wound had entirely healed. The patient was apparently well, with exception of the injured vessel, which necessitated his confinement to bed. This symptom became more marked until pressure of the artery above the wound caused the heart's beat to fall from 80 to 35 to 40 per minute, and so remain until the pressure was relieved.
> Harris H. Branham, 1890

While working as a student of Halsted, Reid (1920) established that there was enlargement of the heart in the presence of an AVF. In 1913, Stewart noted that the heart diminished in size within 10 days after elimination of the fistula.

Clinical Features

If the patient has had a penetrating injury, the possibility of an AVF must be recognized; however, this may not be immediately obvious. As previously noted, if the arteriovenous communication has surrounding thrombus, the classic findings of the thrill and bruit may not exist until several days or weeks later. There may be little evidence of vascular trauma in the way of blood loss or loss of peripheral pulses (Fig. 24–21). The patient may or may not be aware of a buzzing sensation when his fingers are placed over the area of the arteriovenous communication. One patient in the registry had originally been wounded in Korea; however, it was nearly 15 years later, when he was piloting a helicopter in Vietnam, that he noticed a buzzing sensation in his popliteal fossa. It may be more unusual for the patient to present with one of the complications of AVF, such as infection within the

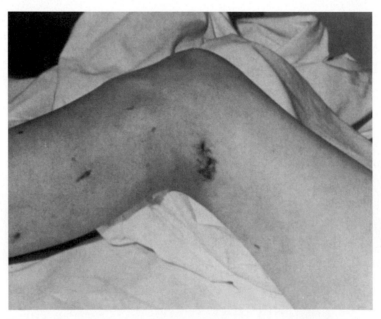

■ **FIGURE 24–21**
A small wound may deceive the casual observer as to the extent of underlying vascular pathology. (NMR Vietnam Vascular Registry #2513 1971.) ■

vascular system, peripheral embolization, or congestive heart failure.

Errors in diagnosis can exist. Patients with AVFs have been treated for years for varicose veins (see Fig. 24–19). Venous hypertension with resultant varices, peripheral pigmentation, and ulceration from venous insufficiency can confuse the diagnosis; however, the classic findings of a thrill and bruit should be carefully sought.

There may or may not be a soft diffuse mass on physical examination. Depending on the period of time that the AVF has existed, dilated veins may surround the area. A thrill, with its maximal component during systole, is usually felt very easily on palpation. A "machinery murmur" is usually heard easily on auscultation, the loudest part of the continuous murmur occurring during systole. Detection of this classic finding differentiates an AVF from an arterial false aneurysm. The Nicoladoni-Branham sign, which has been previously described, is another significant finding if a slowing pulse can be demonstrated when the fistula is obliterated by digital compression. Ironically, this test was not positive in many of the Vietnam casualties with AVFs. The peripheral resistance increases when the fistula is digitally occluded, causing the blood pressure to rise, with reflex slowing of the heart rate and consequent slowing of the pulse. The temporary bradycardia results from a neurogenic reflex mediated through pressure-sensitive receptors in the carotid sinuses and great vessels.

With large AVFs and large shunting of blood, cardiac enlargement and, more rarely, cardiac failure may occur (Fig. 24–22). Smith (1963) found the most serious complication of AVF, left ventricular myocardial failure, in two of their patients. One of these was a 16-year-old male who had been shot in the right thigh with a .22-caliber rifle bullet. Nine days after the accident, the patient developed a gallop rhythm and severe dyspnea. A chest roentgenogram revealed a marked enlargement of the cardiac shadow. An emergency operation was performed to correct a common femoral arteriovenous communication. The signs of congestive cardiac failure regressed in 3 weeks. The authors pointed out that there was a regrettable error of omission

in the immediate exploration of the wound. They felt that the rapid development of cardiac decompensation, which made surgical intervention most urgent, was an unusual aspect of the case.

Diagnostic Considerations

The history of a penetrating injury and the classic physical findings usually establish the diagnosis of an AVF. Establishment of the diagnosis may be more difficult if the lesion is within the thoracic or abdominal cavity. Angiography readily demonstrates the rapid filling of an adjacent vein and increased collateral circulation (Fig. 24–23). Angiographic demonstration of most arteriovenous lesions is usually not necessary from the diagnostic standpoint, but it may be helpful in planning the surgical correction. This is particularly true if multiple arteriovenous communications exist, or if one or more false aneurysms are associated with the arteriovenous communication (Fig. 24–24). Bell and Cockshott (1965) demonstrated the angiographic features found in patients with both acute and chronic AVFs.

Cardiac enlargement may be noted on roentgenogram of the chest. Shumacker and Stahl (1949) evaluated the cardiac frontal area in patients with AVFs to determine the heart size before and after operative obliteration of the fistula in a large group of patients. They studied 185 soldiers with traumatic peripheral AVFs of relatively short duration. Cardiac enlargement was noted in a large number before operative excision of the fistula, and the reduction in the heart size occurred in a comparable number after operation. These authors believe that the location of the fistula, the size of the artery involved, the size and age of the fistula, and the magnitude of the pulse and blood pressure response to temporary occlusion of the fistula could be correlated with the tendency toward early development of cardiac enlargement. These studies showed conclusively that demonstrable evidence of cardiac enlargement was present in approximately 50% of young subjects with peripheral AVFs of relatively short duration; however, few had symptoms of

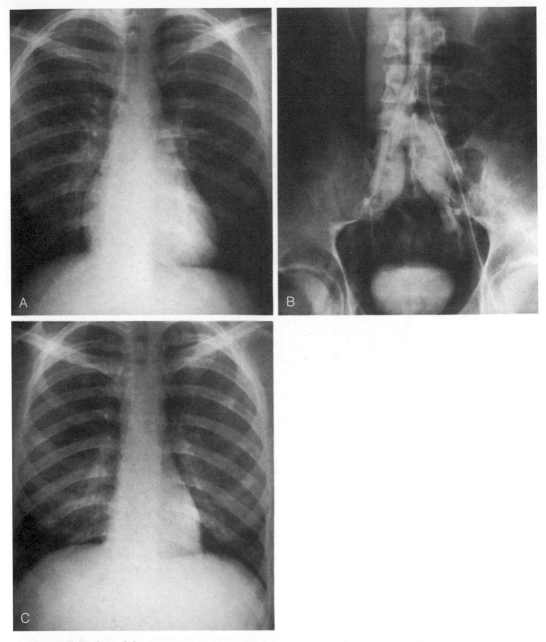

■ **FIGURE 24–22**

A, Cardiac enlargement may occur with large arteriovenous fistulas and occasionally progress to cardiac fistulas and occasionally progress to cardiac failure. *B,* This patient had an arteriovenous fistula 1.0 × 1.5 cm between the right common iliac artery and the left common iliac vein following disk surgery. *C,* The heart returned to normal size limits after closure of the fistula by lateral suture of the vein and resection of a small segment of artery followed by end-to-end anastomosis. (From Jarstfer BS, Rich NM: The challenge of arteriovenous fistula formation following disk surgery: A collective review. J Trauma 1976;16:726-733.) ■

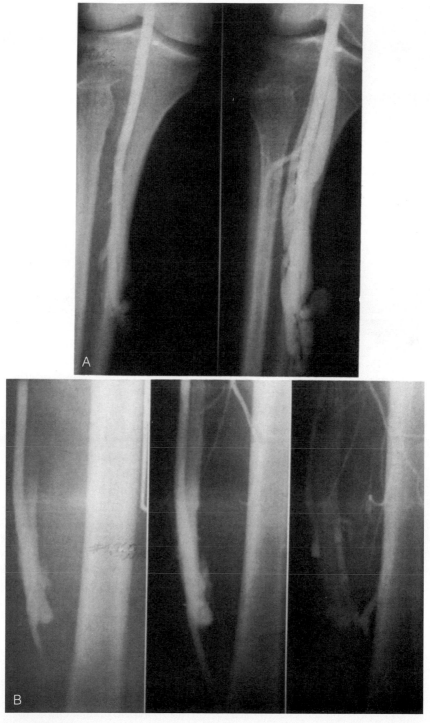

■ **FIGURE 24-23**

A, Angiography is helpful in identifying the site of communication in an arteriovenous fistula. *Left,* Contrast media descends in the artery to the fistula. *Right,* The dilated veins are then rapidly visualized by passage of contrast media through the fistula. *B,* From left to right, the distal superficial femoral artery is visualized angiographically with rapid filling of the adjacent vein. (*A,* From NMR, Vietnam Vascular Registry #7182; *B,* from Vietnam Vascular Registry #2760, Walter Reed General Hospital.) ■

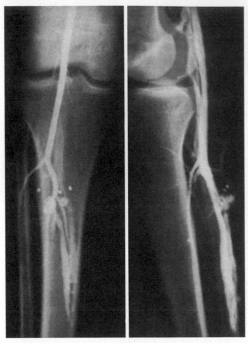

■ **FIGURE 24–24**
Multiple false aneurysms and arteriovenous
fistulas were demonstrated angiographically in
this Vietnam casualty. The extent of pathologic
involvement of the posterior tibial and peroneal
vessels could not be determined clinically.
(From Vietnam Vascular Registry #2761, Walter
Reed General Hospital.) ■

cardiac strain, and there was essentially no
evidence of cardiac failure. This fact was
confirmed by a measurable reduction in cardiac size after operation in a comparable percentage. Cardiac failure has been reported in
a series of 14 patients (Pate and colleagues,
1965).

Surgical Treatment

A literature review and a successful personal
repair of an AVFs prompted Stewart (1913)
to write, "With angiorrhaphy the aneurysm
can be dealt with radically and the vessels
conservatively, thus effecting cure without
interrupting the bloodstream and without producing gangrene."

Despite his interest in repair of AVFs, he
noted that suture of vessels was not always pos-

sible. He cited that in a number of instances,
the surgeon had planned to repair the vessel
but was forced to abandon the idea because
of hemorrhage (Delanglade), friability of
the artery, (Thompson), the large size of
the opening (Mignon), dense adhesions
(Cranwell), or obliteration of the sutured
vessel (Cestan).

Shumacker (1948) stated, "It has long been
recognized that the ideal method of treating
aneurysms and arteriovenous fistula involving
important arteries is the extirpation of the
lesion combined with some procedure which
permits maintenance or re-establishment of
the continuity of the affected artery."

The best time for surgical cure of a traumatic AVF is immediately after the establishment of the communication.

There has been a period of profound
changes in the surgical management of AVFs.
Surgeons' energies were formally directed
toward the selection of a time when maximal
collateral circulation would have developed.
If the intervention was properly timed and
if the collateral circulation was adequate,
ligation of the four component vascular
trunks without excision of the fistula cured
the lesion, the extremity remaining viable
despite the fact that there might be some arterial and venous insufficiency. The important
change, which was strongly influenced by the
experience at Walter Reed General Hospital
in managing Korean battle casualties, con-
centrated on dissection of the proximal and
distal communicating artery and vein with
repair of defects in both vessels (Seeley and
colleagues, 1952).

The initial treatment of AVFs included a
delay of 2 to 6 months to allow collateral circulation to develop. It was anticipated that this
would improve extremity survival after ligation of the involved artery. However, it should
be emphasized that some of the earliest
vascular repairs, including venorrhaphy and
arteriorrhaphy, of this century involved AVFs.
At present, division of the fistula with venous,
as well as arterial, repair is preferred. Excision with multiple ligations is accepted for
smaller vessels not essential to normal circulation, such as one of the tibial arteries or veins.
There is currently an interest in treating AVFs
when they are initially diagnosed. If the lesion

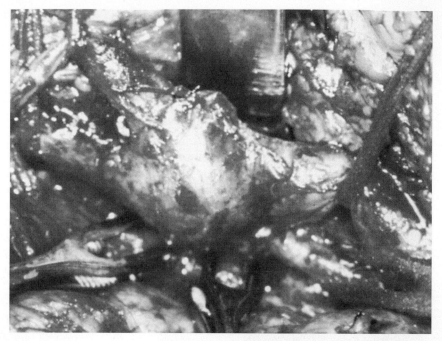

■ **FIGURE 24–25**
Proximal and distal control of both the artery and the vein is important in the successful
management of arteriovenous fistulas. It was possible to repair the popliteal vein by lateral suture
and the popliteal artery by an end-to-end anastomosis to correct the arteriovenous fistula. (From
Rich NM: In: Beebe HG, ed. Complications in vascular surgery. Philadelphia: JB Lippincott,
1973.) ■

is discovered on the third or fourth day after
an injury, it is usually better to wait until 3
weeks have passed to allow soft tissue healing
to occur and edema to subside.

Elective incisions should be used, as was
emphasized for arterial repair and for venous
repair. Adequate exposure of the artery and
vein proximal and distal to the fistula should
be accomplished before the fistula is directly
approached (Fig. 24–25). When these vessels
are isolated and temporarily occluded, the
arteriovenous communication can be incised
and directly isolated (Fig. 24–26). There
usually is a small lesion between the artery
and the vein, and the size of the surrounding
false sac may vary greatly. Nevertheless, a small
segment of the artery is usually involved, the
remainder of the artery being freed from the
false sac during mobilization to perform the
arterial repair. Lateral venorrhaphy is usually
possible. Only in large arteries is arteriorrhaphy by lateral suture possible. Frequently,
minimal excision of the damaged artery and

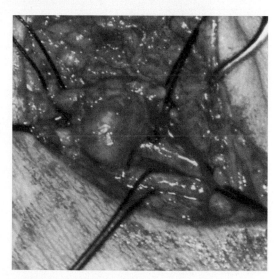

■ **FIGURE 24–26**
Proximal and distal control of both artery and
vein has been obtained with silk suture loops in
place. Multiple ligatures with excision of the
arteriovenous fistula and false aneurysm were
elected for this distal posterior tibial lesion.
(From NMR, Vietnam Vascular Registry #1806,
1969.) ■

end-to-end anastomosis are possible. Otherwise, segmental replacement with autogenous greater saphenous vein is preferred.

Intra-arterial balloon catheter control of hemorrhage and many other useful techniques used in arterial repair are covered in more detail in Chapter 19 and in the discussions of specific arteries. LeVeen and Cerruti (1963) described a method for intra-arterial balloon tamponade of blood vessels in the surgical management of AVFs (Fig. 24–27). Noon (1969) emphasized the use of balloon catheters to provide temporary arterial occlusions for control of hemorrhage. The use of

multiple balloon catheters to control intra-arterial hemorrhage and venous bleeding has been successful in the management of Vietnam casualties with AVFs at Walter Reed Army Medical Center (Fig. 24–28).

Spontaneous Cure

Shumacker and Wayson (1950) evaluated spontaneous cure of aneurysms and AVFs. They studied 122 aneurysms and 245 AVFs. Thrombosis appeared to be responsible for the obliteration of the lesions. Fibrosis can also

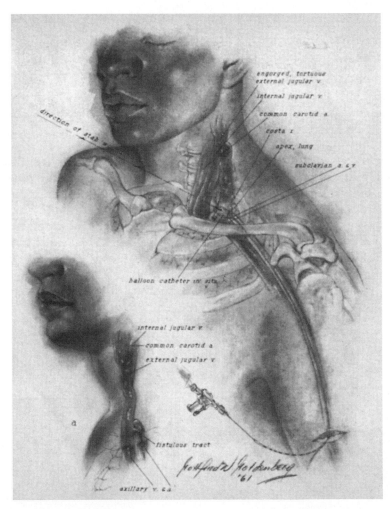

■ **FIGURE 24–27**
A Woodruff catheter was inserted through the open brachial artery and the balloon inflated at the region of the arteriovenous fistula. *A,* Dilated vessels anterior to the fistula. This was a method for intra-arterial balloon tamponade of blood vessels in the surgical management of arteriovenous fistulas. (From LeVeen HH, Cerruti MM: Surgery of large inaccessible arteriovenous fistulas. Ann Surg 1963;158:285-289.) ■

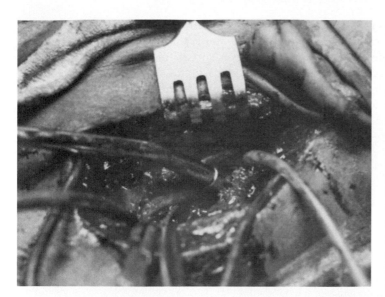

■ **FIGURE 24-28**
Intraoperative photograph showing a Fogarty balloon catheter in the distal internal carotid artery for intraluminal arterial control of hemorrhage *(small arrow)* and a Foley balloon catheter inserted into the adjacent internal jugular vein for temporary control of venous hemorrhage during repair of a distal carotid–internal jugular arteriovenous fistula. (From NMR, Walter Reed General Hospital, 1972.) ■

occur as a more gradual process. Because there are only five spontaneous cures, only 2% of the 245 AVFs (four of five arteriovenous lesions that healed spontaneously did so suddenly and within three months of the original injury), the authors stated, "Satisfactory spontaneous cures occurred in our series so infrequently as to make consideration of this possibility of little or no importance in reaching a decision as to the necessity for or the proper time for surgical treatment of the lesion."

Spontaneous closure of the AVFs has been a relatively unusual event. Billings, Nasca, and Griffin (1973) reported one such instance in a 19-year-old Marine who had sustained multiple fragment wounds from a land mine explosion in August 1970 while on duty in the Republic of Vietnam. In September, a 3-cm pulsating mass was noted in the right axilla, and there was continuous bruit and thrill over the mass. An axillary AVF was demonstrated by angiography (Fig. 24–29). Treatment of other multiple wounds was carried out, and during the first week in November, the axillary mass was no longer palpable. A second arteriogram demonstrated that there had been spontaneous closure of the AVF (Fig. 24–30). Two similar patients—Vietnam

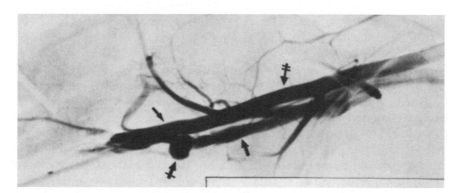

■ **FIGURE 24-29**
Subtraction print demonstrating the early arterial phase of an arteriogram performed via subclavian injection. The right axillary artery (↦) communicates with the axillary vein (→) through a large arteriovenous fistula (↔). (From Billings KJ, Nasca RJ, Griffin HA: Traumatic arteriovenous fistula with spontaneous closure. J Trauma 1973;13:741-743.) ■

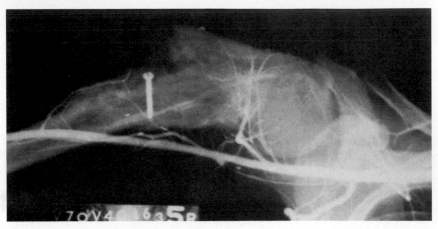

■ **FIGURE 24–30**
A second arteriogram performed 6 weeks later, demonstrating that the arteriovenous communication in the axillary vessels (see Fig. 24–29) is no longer present. Elective operative closure had not been performed because of a wound infection. The site of "thrombosis" is visible as a small, contrast-filled saccule on the inferior surface of the axillary artery. (From Billings KJ, Nasca RJ, Griffin HA: Traumatic arteriovenous fistula with spontaneous closure. J Trauma 1973;13:741-743.) ■

casualties—were seen at Walter Reed General Hospital.

Results

Annandale (1875) reported the successful ligature of a popliteal artery and vein in the treatment of a traumatic popliteal AVF. Pick (1883) reported the case of a 28-year-old man who sustained a gunshot wound of the thigh with a resultant AVF of the femoral vessels. He stated that the only operative procedure that appeared to hold any hope for success was ligature of the artery above and below the point of communication. According to Murphy (1897), Von Zoege-Manteuffel successfully repaired a femoral arteriovenous aneurysm by lateral suture of the wall in 1895. When the first end-to-end arterial anastomosis in a human was reported by Murphy (1897), he described his successful treatment in 1896 of a common femoral AVF. In addition to the end-to-end arterial anastomosis following resection of the damaged portion of the artery, he closed the wound in the vein by lateral venorrhaphy. Bickham (1904) suggested that Matas endoaneurysmorrhaphy could be employed for the intravascular repair of AVFs. He also recommended transverse closure of the defects in the vascular walls as a practical method of preserving the continuity of both the injured artery and the injured vein. Matas emphasized the reason for failure when partial ligation was used in the treatment of AVFs was the remaining patency in other vessels not ligated (Fig. 24–31).

Soubbotitch (1913) reported on the military experience in the Serbo-Turkish and Serbo-Bulgarian Wars. There were 16 different surgeons who performed ligation of large vessels on 41 arteries and 4 veins and partial suture on 17 vessels—8 arteries and 9 veins. Circular suture was employed on 15 vessels—11 arteries and 4 veins—to bring the total number of vessels sutured to 32 (19 arteriorrhaphies and 13 venorrhaphies). The 60 arteries and 17 veins made of a total 77 injuries to the larger blood vessels among 20,000 wounded. Osler (1915) stated that there was agreement with a conclusion arrived at by Soubbotitch, senior surgeon at the Belgrade State Hospital, from his experience in the Balkan War, "that arteriovenous aneurysms should be operated upon, as they offer small prospect of spontaneous cure, although they often remain stationary for a long time and cause relatively little trouble."

World War I contributed little significant data compared to World War II. Because competent vascular surgeons had chosen to head three centers for vascular surgery during

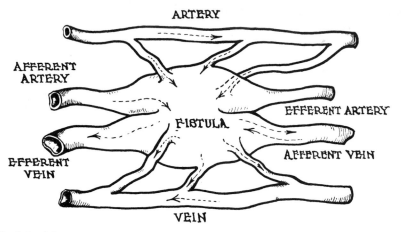

■ **FIGURE 24–31**

Schematic drawing showing the communications of an arteriovenous fistula and the necessity of not only quadruple ligation but also complete excision including all branches. (From Matas R: Military surgery of the vascular system. In: Keene's surgery, vol. 7. Philadelphia: WB Saunders, 1921.) ■

World War II, a large number of AVFs and arterial aneurysms were managed. Elkin and Shumacker (1955) outlined the techniques of operative treatment of 585 AVFs (Table 24–15). Arterial repair was used in only 34 lesions.

The representative material that follows covers a small portion of the World War II experience. Freeman and Shumacker (1955) outlined various approaches in the management of AVFs. Figure 24–32 shows one of the approaches, which involved the following:

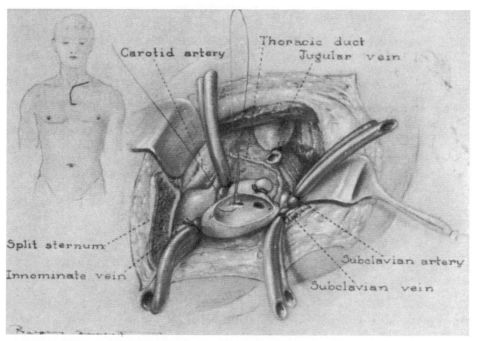

■ **FIGURE 24–32**

Transvenous repair of an arteriovenous fistula involving the left subclavian artery and innominate vein. Insert shows the surgical approach to the lesion that was used to manage a World War II combat casualty at DeWitt General Hospital in 1945. (From Freeman NE, Shumacker HB Jr, DeBakey ME: Vascular surgery. Washington, DC: US Government Printing Office, 1955.) ■

TABLE 24–15

TECHNIQUES OF OPERATIVE TREATMENT IN 585 ARTERIOVENOUS FISTULAS: WORLD WAR II EXPERIENCE

Location	Arterial Repair	Quadruple Ligation and Excision	Ligation Alone (Mass Proximal, Distal, or Proximal and Distal)	Total Cases
Upper extremity				
Axillary	—	32	—	32
Brachial	—	29	—	29*
Cervical, transverse	—	1	—	1†
Humeral, posterior circumflex	—	1	—	1
Interosseous, common	—	1	—	1
Radial	—	2	—	2
Scapular, transverse	—	2	—	2
Subclavian	1	16	1	18‡
Ulnar	—	9	—	9
Lower extremity	—	—	—	—
Calf, to muscles of	—	4	—	4
Circumflex, lateral	—	1	—	1
Femoral	16	124	1	141§
Geniculate	—	5	—	5
Gluteal, inferior	—	1	—	1
Gluteal, superior	—	3	—	3
Peroneal	—	24	1	25
Plantar	—	6	—	6
Popliteal	11	91	—	102
Profunda femoris	—	19	—	19
Profunda branch	—	2	—	2
Tibial	—	87	—	87
Head and neck				
Carotid	5	29	14	48‡
Cirsoid	—	9	—	9
Lingual	—	1	—	1
Occipital	—	1	—	1
Temporal, superficial	—	3	2	5
Vertebral	—	8	5	13
Trunk				
Aorta–vena cava	1	—	—	1
Hypogastric	—	1	—	1
Iliac	—	9	—	9
Innominate	—	—	1	1
Mammary, internal	—	1	—	1
Obturator–iliac vein	—	1	—	1
Subscapular	—	2	—	2
Thoracoacromial	—	1	—	1
TOTAL	34	526	25	585

*This total does not include two fistulas: one in which the method of management was not stated and one in which spontaneous cure occurred.

†This total does not include one fistula in which the method of management was not stated.

‡This total does not include one fistula in which spontaneous cure occurred.

§This total does not include three fistulas: one in which methods of management were not stated and two in which spontaneous cure occurred.

From Elkin DC, Shumacker HB Jr: In: Vascular Surgery in World War II. Elkin DC, DeBakey ME, eds. Washington, DC: Government Printing Office, 1955.

1. Mass ligation of the fistula
2. Quadruple ligation and division of the main vessels with excision of the fistula
3. Transvenous closure of the arterial opening
4. Repair of the opening in both the artery and vein

Shumacker (1948) stressed the importance of maintaining arterial continuity in the repair of aneurysms and AVFs. In his early experience, he performed only four reparative procedures, with 2.9% of 138 cases involving the innominate, common carotid, extracranial internal carotid, subclavian, axil-lary, brachial, iliac, common femoral, femoral, and popliteal arteries. In later experience, he repaired 52.6% of the arteries: 30 of 57 cases. This included lateral arteriorrhaphy, end-to-end anastomosis, and vein graft repair (Table 24–16). The types of autogenous interposition venous grafts used range from the saphenous to a branch of the femoral. Figures 24–33 and 24–34 reveal patency of the venous grafts and no dilatation of the grafts in the early follow-up period of 7 to 10 weeks.

Shumacker (1948) also used oscillometry to evaluate the patency of arterial repair (Table 24–17). The results of oscillometry were good in those cases in which arterial repairs

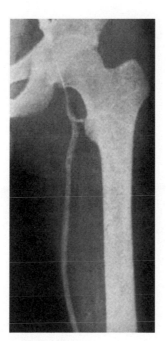

■ **FIGURE 24–33**
This arteriogram taken 10 weeks after repair of a fistula between the femoral and profunda femoral arteries and the femoral vein, with resection and end-to-end anastomosis of the profunda femoral artery proximally to the superficial femoral artery distally, shows no narrowing at the suture line after 70% Diodrast was injected into the common femoral artery. (From Shumacker HB Jr: Problems of maintaining continuity of artery in surgery of aneurysms and arteriovenous fistulae; notes on development and clinical application of methods of arterial suture. Ann Surg 1948;127:207-230.) ■

TABLE 24–16
CASES IN WHICH CONTINUITY OF ARTERY WAS RESTORED BY VEIN TRANSPLANTATION

Case No.	Age of Patient	Duration of Lesion (Months)	Type of Lesion	Location of Lesion	Preoperative Sympathectomy	Length of Vein Graft (cm)	Source of Vein Graft	Period of Follow-Up (Months)	Result
1	26	4.2	AV and saccular aneurysms	Femoral, distal third	0	2	Saphenous	3	Excellent
2	19	5	AV	Femoral, middle third	0	2	Branch of femoral	3	Excellent
3	26	4	AV	Femoral, distal third	+	5	Saphenous	3	Excellent
4	35	?	Saccular aneurysm	Popliteal, middle third	+	2	Small saphenous	4	Excellent
5	36	6 yr	Saccular aneurysm	Femoral, proximal third	0	2.5	Femoral	1.5	Excellent
6	24	5.3	Saccular aneurysm	Brachial, middle third	0	2.5	Saphenous	1.2	Thrombosis; good circulation maintained

AV, arteriovenous.
From Shumacker HB Jr: Problems of maintaining continuity of artery in surgery of aneurysms and arteriovenous fistulas; notes on development and clinical application of methods of arterial suture. Ann Surg 1948;127:207-230.

TABLE 24–17
OSCILLOMETRIC STUDIES AFTER ARTERIAL REPAIR

Type of Repair	Artery Repaired	No. of Cases	Oscillometry at Ankle or Wrist		Oscillometry at Calf or Forearm		Oscillometry at Thigh or Arm	
			Reading Average	Percentage of Reading in Contralateral Limb	Reading Average	Percentage of Reading in Contralateral Limb	Reading Average	Percentage of Reading in Contralateral Limb
Ligation of fistula	Femoral	5	2.3	96	5.1	96	3.5	95
	Popliteal	4	5.1	75	7.6	95	—	—
Lateral arteriorrhaphy	Subclavian	2	2.5	83	3.8	70	4.5	88
	Axillary	2	1.0	37	1.5	41	2.2	44
	Brachial	4	2.5	83	2.8	51	—	—
End-to-end suture	Femoral	1	3.0	60	4.5	50	7	100
	Femoral	4	3.1	67	4	50	4	67
Vein transplantation	Popliteal	1	2.0	67	3	43	—	—
Successful repairs	Total	24	2.9	79	4.3	68	4.0	68
Unsuccessful repairs	Total	5	1.0	17	0.9	16	0.5	18

From Shumacker HB Jr: Problems of maintaining continuity of artery in surgery of aneurysms and arteriovenous fistulae; notes on development and clinical application of methods of arterial suture. Ann Surg 1948;127:207-230.

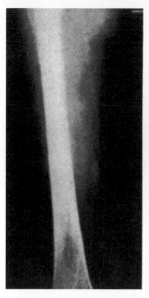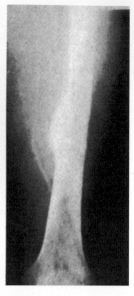

■ **FIGURE 24-34**

Left, Arteriogram, taken 7 weeks after repair of an arteriovenous fistula between the superficial femoral artery and vein, with interposition of a segment of a large branch of the femoral vein 2 cm in length, reveals that the venous insert and the artery have relative diameters about equal to those observed at completion of the operation (case 2). *Right,* Arteriogram showing no dilatation of the venous segment of a 2-cm piece of saphenous vein used to reconstruct the superficial femoral vessels (case 1). There was no dilatation at the completion of the anastomosis, and no dilatation was seen on this arteriogram performed 10 weeks later. (From Shumacker HB Jr: Problems of maintaining continuity of artery in surgery of aneurysms and arteriovenous fistulae; notes on development and clinical application of methods of arterial suture. Ann Surg 1948;127:207-230.) ■

remained patent and poor in those in which arterial repair failed due to thrombosis.

Hughes and Jahnke (1958) performed end-to-end anastomosis in the majority of AVFs (61/134) from the Korean Conflict (Table 24–18). As a result of the Korean Conflict, more than 200 patients with false aneurysms and AVFs, 133 of the injuries involving major vessels, were seen at Walter Reed General Hospital. The lesions were excised, with reparative or reconstructive surgery of the major vessel, without loss of a single limb. Treatment

of minor vessel lesions has previously been outlined in Table 24–8. Repair of major veins was performed whenever possible to prevent venous insufficiency. This venous repair was possible in about 30% of major veins involved in fistula formation. Cardiac dilatation was common with large fistulas; however, only two patients showed cardiac failure.

Rich, Hobson, and Collins (1975) reported the experience from Vietnam. Of 558 lesions identified in 509 patients, there was almost an equal number of AVFs (262 AVFs) and false aneurysms (296 false aneurysms). As might be anticipated by the number of American troops committed to Southeast Asia in that year, the largest number of lesions resulted from wounds in 1968 (Table 24–19). There was also a relatively large number of similar wounds in 1967 and 1969. The time from injury to recognition of the lesion was arbitrarily divided into four categories: immediate, early, delayed, and remote. The largest number of lesions was recognized in the early period of 1 to 30 days: 273, or 48.9% (Table 24–20). Nearly an equal number was diagnosed in the delayed period between 1 and 6 months. In the remote group, all but 7 of the 35 patients had recognition and treatment of their lesions in less than 2 years. Only two had recognition and treatment of their lesions after more than 5 years following the initial injury, and both were treated in less than 6 years. Nearly an equal number of lesions were treated in the intermediate hospitals in Japan and similar Far West locations as were treated in the continental United States (Table 24–21). Several hundred surgeons were involved in these repairs. Approximately one fifth of these operations were performed at Walter Reed Army Medical Center.

Table 24–22 outlines the method of treatment used for the various arterial and venous injuries. Arterial ligation was used in 290 lesions, or 52.0%. Compelling problems often caused this method to be used over the favored and desired arterial repair. Infection, associated injuries, poor general condition of the patient, and involvement of smaller caliber arteries were considered. The overall mortality rate for the 509 patients was 1.8%, or 7 deaths (Table 24–23). Even considering this low mortality rate, only two deaths could be directly

TABLE 24–18

TOTAL OPERATIONS FOR MAJOR VESSEL LESIONS: MILITARY SERIES FROM KOREAN CONFLICT

Vessel	Ligation and Excision	Anastomosis	Vein Graft	Artery Graft	Lateral Repair	Division of Fistula	Spontaneous Closure	Total
Common carotid	—	6	—	—	—	1	2	9
Internal carotid	2	—	—	—	—	—	—	3
Subclavian	3	2	—	1	1	1	—	8
Axillary	4	8	2	1	2	—	3	20
Brachial	6	9	1	1	1	1	—	19
Iliac	—	3	—	1	—	—	—	4
Common femoral	—	3	2	1	—	2	—	8
Superficial femoral	6	14	9	—	—	2	—	31
Popliteal	9	16	3	1	—	2	1	32
TOTAL	30	61	17	6	4	10	6	134

From Hughes CW, Jahnke EJ Jr: The surgery of traumatic arteriovenous fistulas and aneurysms: A five-year followup study of 215 lesions. Ann Surg 1958;148:790-797.

TABLE 24–19

ARTERIOVENOUS FISTULAS AND FALSE ANEURYSMS BY YEAR: VIETNAM VASCULAR REGISTRY

Year	No.	%
1963	1	0.2
1964	0	0.0
1965	11	2.0
1966	44	7.9
1967	116	20.8
1968	249	44.6
1969	124	22.2
1970	5	0.9
1971	7	1.2
1972	1	0.2
TOTAL	558	100.0

From Rich NM, Hobson RW II, Collins GJ Jr: Traumatic arteriovenous fistulas and false aneurysms: A review of 558 lesions. Surgery 1975;78:817-828.

TABLE 24–20

ARTERIOVENOUS FISTULAS AND FALSE ANEURYSMS, BY TIME OF DIAGNOSIS: VIETNAM VASCULAR REGISTRY

Time	No.	%
Immediate (24 hr)	22	3.9
Early (1-30 days)	273	48.9
Delayed (1-6 mo)	228	40.9
Remote (>6 mo)	35	6.3
TOTAL	558	100.0

From Rich NM, Hobson RW II, Collins GJ Jr: Traumatic arteriovenous fistulas and false aneurysms: A review of 558 lesions. Surgery 1975;78:817-828.

attributed to the vascular problem. The morbidity rate of 6.8% included 35 complications: hemorrhage in 14, thrombosis in 12, stenosis in 2, and persistent, immediately adjacent, or recurrent AVFs requiring additional operations in 7.

Experience in the civilian hospitals is increasing. Hershey (1961) encountered a technical complication. The artery proximal to the AVF had dilated and become fragile; it was crushed by clamp, and a hematoma developed (Fig. 24–35).

Beall (1968) repaired 8 of 50 AVFs within 24 hours of injury; an additional 17 were repaired within 24 hours to 3 months following injury. However, there was a delayed repair

TABLE 24–21
ARTERIOVENOUS FISTULAS AND FALSE ANEURYSMS, BY HOSPITAL LOCATION FOR REPAIR: VIETNAM VASCULAR REGISTRY

Location	No. of Repairs	%
Vietnam	57	10.2
Japan, etc.	238	42.7
CONUS	251	45.0
No repair	12	2.1
TOTAL	558	100.0

From Rich NM, Hobson RW II, Collins GJ Jr: Traumatic arteriovenous fistulas and false aneurysms: a review of 558 lesions. Surgery 1975;78:817-828.

TABLE 24–23
ARTERIOVENOUS FISTULAS AND ANEURYSMS, MORTALITY AND MORBIDITY RATES: VIETNAM VASCULAR REGISTRY

	No.	%
Deaths	7	1.8
Morbidity		
Amputations	8	1.7
Complications	35	6.3

From Rich NM, Hobson RW II, Collins GJ Jr: Traumatic arteriovenous fistulas and false aneurysms: a review of 558 lesions. Surgery 1975;78:817-828.

TABLE 24–22
ARTERIOVENOUS FISTULAS AND FALSE ANEURYSMS, BY METHOD OF MANAGEMENT: VIETNAM VASCULAR REGISTRY

Type	No.	%
Arterial		
Ligation	290	52.0
End-to-end anastomosis	143	25.6
Vein graft	57	10.2
Lateral suture	40	7.2
Prosthesis	2	0.3
Miscellaneous	26	4.7
TOTAL	558	100.0
Venous		
Ligation	138	52.7
Suture	79	30.1
Miscellaneous	45	17.2
TOTAL	262	100.0

From Rich NM, Hobson RW II, Collins GJ Jr: Traumatic arteriovenous fistulas and false aneurysms: a review of 558 lesions. Surgery 1975;78:817-828.

of more than 3 months following injury for 23, or nearly 50%, of these lesions. No repair was performed for two of the AVFs. Excision and repair was used for 27 lesions and ligation and excision for 17 lesions. No deaths were reported. There were no amputations required. Not counting two patients lost in follow-up who had no treatment, 42 were asymptomatic. Six patients were symptomatic after their original definitive surgical procedure, and three required subsequent operations.

In the civilian series of 61 arterial injuries reported by Smith, Foran, and Gaspar (1963), approximately two thirds of the 33 chronic or late lesions were AVFs. They mentioned that the time interval from original injury to treatment varied considerably from a few days to 29 years, with most patients, 57%, being treated after 1 year. Of the six patients with AVFs reported by Patman, Poulos, and Shires (1964), five did not have initial explorations of the area. The remaining patient did have initial exploration; however, the AVFs were not diagnosed until 4 hours after injury. The authors stressed that this development demonstrated the rapidity with which an AVF can develop. The common and superficial femoral arteries were involved in AVFs. The remaining four fistulas were equally divided among the smaller radial and posterior tibial arteries. There were no deaths, amputations, or other significant complications in any of the patients.

Dillard, Nelson, and Norman (1968) reported a number of AVFs including (1) a 29-year-old female who was stabbed in the right flank and 3 years later was found to have severe hypertension; after correction of the renal AVF, the patient's blood pressure returned to normal; (2) a patient with severe leg ulcers that healed only after correction of an AVF in

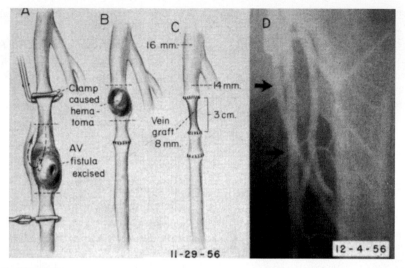

■ **FIGURE 24–35**

A, Artist's sketch of a superficial femoral arteriovenous fistula. *B,* End-to-end anastomosis after excision of the fistula. An intraluminal hematoma developed at the site of a Blalock clamp. *C,* Sketch of the vein graft after excision of the hematoma, showing size discrepancies. *D,* Postoperative arteriogram showing *(arrows)* the site of anastomosis. (From Hershey FB: Secondary repair of arterial injuries. Am Surg 1961;27:33-41.) ■

the same extremity between the common femoral artery and vein; and (3) a patient with an AVF between the popliteal artery and vein, which resulted in amputation. Two of the nine AVFs reported by Dillard, Nelson, and Norman (1968) involved high-output failure. One of these fistulas occurred between the subcapsular artery and the axillary vein, and the other between the right iliac artery and the left common iliac vein.

Sako and Varco (1970) reported corrective procedures in 25 patients with acquired AVFs. Excisions of the fistula with arterial and venous repair were performed in more than 50%, or 16 lesions. Quadruple ligation was used in six and multiple ligation in two, and included in the arterial repairs were 13 primary anastomoses, 3 autologous venous grafts, and 1 homograft. All of the acquired fistulas were cured by the surgical procedures described without a death.

Gaspard and Gaspar (1972) reported two patients who developed AVF after Fogarty catheter thrombectomy in the lower extremity. They emphasized that neither of their patients required immediate operation for limb salvage or had an operation performed subsequently. They cited the report by Rob

and Battle (1971) in which correction of the AVF 26 days after the use of the Fogarty catheter was mandatory because the distal extremity was in jeopardy.

Hewitt, Smith, and Drapanas (1973) advocated immediate repair of acute AVFs. This was possible in 13 of the 14 patients in their series, and they reported satisfactory results in all repairs, including resection with end-to-end anastomosis in 6, saphenous vein graft in 2, saphenous vein patch graft in 2, and lateral suture repair in 3, with ligation being required only for one distal internal carotid artery.

In addition to the anticipated complications of cardiac enlargement, cardiac failure, endocarditis, and proximal arterial aneurysm formation, unusual complications have been reported. Rhodes, Cox, and Silver (1973) reported a case of a 53-year-old male with a 10-day history of bruising easily, hematoma, and bleeding from his tongue. The patient was involved in a shooting accident 17 years previously and had acquired an AVF between the left subclavian artery and vein as a result. The authors attributed the local sustained intravascular coagulation that caused a man's symptoms to turbulence from the fistula and

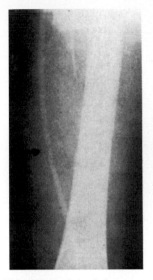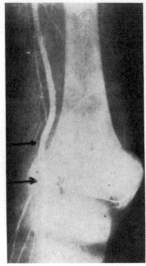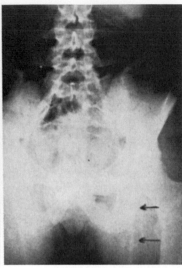

■ **FIGURE 24–36**

A, Arteriography after excision and anastomosis of the superficial femoral artery shows an excellent lumen. A vein graft inserted into the popliteal artery is demonstrated by angiography approximately 6 months after operation. *B,* Examination of this patient 5.5 years after operation showed the vein graft to be functioning perfectly without clinical evidence of dilatation. *C,* Arteriography was used to demonstrated an arterial homograft that replaced the common femoral artery. These angiograms were part of the follow-up of Korean casualties who had repair of arteriovenous fistulas. (From Hughes CW, Jahnke EJ Jr: The surgery of traumatic arteriovenous fistulas and aneurysms: A five-year follow up study of 215 lesions. Ann Surg 1958;148:790-797.) ■

stasis from the aneurysm. The coagulopathy and bleeding responded to surgical elimination of the fistula and aneurysm. The authors felt that this was the first report of a consumption coagulopathy resulting from an AVF and false aneurysm.

Follow-up

Hughes and Jahnke (1958) included a 5-year follow-up of 148 lesions treated during the Korean Conflict, with satisfactory results being obtained in most of the patients (Fig. 24–36).

The Vietnam Vascular Registry continues to follow patients included in the report by Rich (1975). More than one fourth—149 patients or 29.3%—have been evaluated in the vascular clinic at Walter Reed Medical Center. Many of these patients can be expected to live 50 years or more (Fig. 24–37).

Sako and Varco (1970) reported long-term follow-up of 14 of 25 patients with acquired AVFs who were cured of their lesions for 5 to 16 years. Seven additional patients were followed for more than 2 years and were all cured. One patient in this group had a portion of the anterior tibial artery repaired after excision of the fistula, but the artery was occluded within the first year. Two were lost to follow-up after the first year, and one had quadruple ligation of the subclavian AVF. When last seen, he had symptoms indicating some ischemia of the arm. The other patient lost to follow-up had quadruple ligation of the gluteal AVF. The remaining two patients who had an aneurysmal dilatation in the proximal artery excised and replaced with prosthetic graft were well 8 and 11 years after the operation (Fig. 24–38). The other two patients with aneurysmal dilatation of the artery proximal to the fistula had not yet had these corrected.

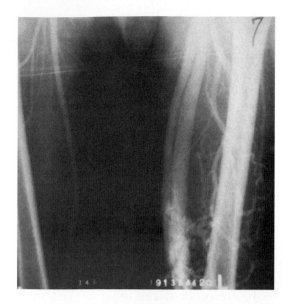

■ **FIGURE 24–37**
This angiogram corroborated the clinical impression of a left femoral arteriovenous fistula. Additional assistance, however, was provided to establish that the communication involved a muscular branch of the superficial femoral artery and the superficial femoral vein. Note the development collaterals. Also note the proximal arterial dilatation of the superficial femoral artery in this former soldier who had been wounded 5 years before this study. (From Rich NM: In: Beebe HG, ed. Complications in vascular surgery. Philadelphia: JB Lippincott, 1973.) ■

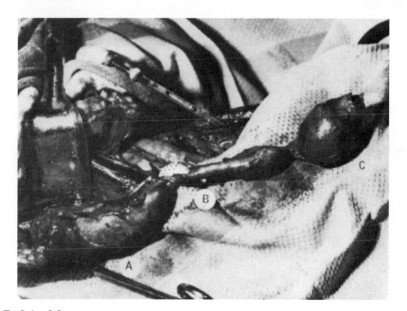

■ **FIGURE 24–38**
In this operative photograph, aneurysmal dilatation of the superficial femoral artery *(A)*, the narrowed segment *(B)* where the artery traversed Hunter's canal, and a popliteal aneurysm *(C)* are demonstrated. This patient had closure of an arteriovenous fistula of 21 years' duration, which involved the anterior tibial vessels. Fourteen years after the fistula closure, multiple aneurysms of femoropopliteal arteries developed. (From Sako Y, Varco RL: Arteriovenous fistula: Results of management of congenital and acquired forms, blood flow measurements, and observations on proximal arterial degeneration. Surgery 1970;67:40-61.) ■

TRAUMATIC FALSE ANEURYSMS

> *He was bled at his own desire by a bleeder who had performed the same operation for him, and generally in the same arm, some 30 or 40 times. Bleeding from an orifice was done by firm compression, and on the day following finding the bandage tight, he removed it, and found the orifice to be completely closed. A short time after this, a small pulsating swelling was observed by him at this point which slowly increased till a day or two previous to my seeing him when after some exertion with his arm he observed a very considerable augmentation of its size.*
> Norris, 1843

History

Since antiquity, the management of false aneurysms has been closely allied to vascular surgery. It has been repeatedly recorded that Antyllus in the second century treated an arterial aneurysm by ligature above and below the lesion, with incision of the aneurysm and extraction of the clot. Schwartz (1958) reported that Antyllus treated small peripheral traumatic aneurysms by ligating both ends and puncturing the center; however, he advised against this practice in large aneurysms. Figure 24–39 shows some of the early methods of treatment of aneurysms. Hunter electively ligated the femoral artery proximal to a popliteal aneurysm in 1786 to reduce blood loss during subsequent attempts at excision of the aneurysm. Pick (1873) provided an interesting and detailed account of his management of a large femoral false aneurysm by digital compression, which had

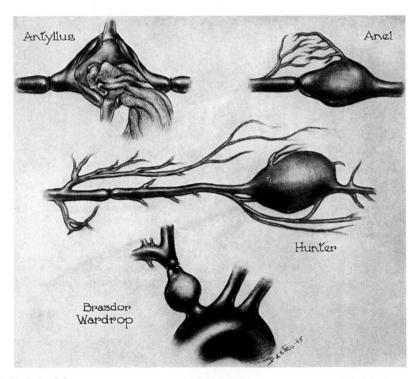

■ **FIGURE 24–39**
Various types of operations employed for the treatment of aneurysms before the introduction of Matas' endoaneurysmorrhaphy in 1888. (From Elkin DC: Traumatic aneurysms; Matas operation—57 years after. Surg Gynecol Obstet 1946;82:1-12.) ■

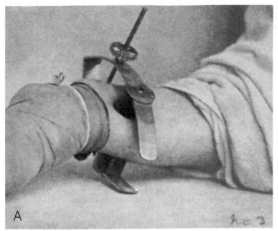

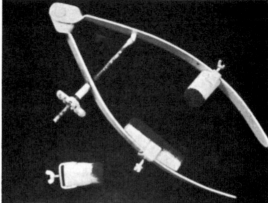

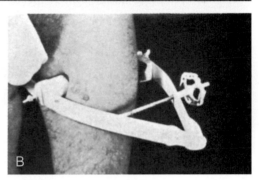

■ **FIGURE 24-40**
A, Matas used a contemporary compressor applied to the femoral artery at Hunter's canal to test the collateral circulation in lesion such as this popliteal aneurysm. *B,* In World War II, Elkin found the Matas compressor to be an inexpensive and easily constructed instrument that could compress various arteries to determine the development of collateral circulation. (*A,* From Matas R: Keene's surgery, vol. 7. Philadelphia: WB Saunders, 1921; *B,* from Elkin DC: Vascular injuries of warfare. Ann Surg 1944;120:284-310.) ■

disastrous final results. This digital compression directly over the pulsating mass was applied fairly continuously initially and then for a considerable period of the waking hours until 4 days later when the area became so tender that the compression had to be discontinued. Not only did this initiate thrombus formation in the false aneurysm, but it also became evident in less than 1 week that the distal pulses could not be felt over either the anterior or the posterior tibial artery. Gangrene developed approximately 3 weeks after the initiation of the digital compression, an amputation was performed at the hip level. The patient had a stormy postoperative course for approximately 3 hours before he died.

Matas (1888) described an endoaneurysmorrhaphy operation, a method of intrasaccular suture, for the treatment of a brachial arterial aneurysm. Within a few years, Matas (1903) also recommended restoration of circulation through the damaged artery as the ideal treatment for arterial aneurysms. He developed a compressor (Fig. 24–40) to test

the development of collateral circulation before performing his endoaneurysmorrhaphy. His approach to widely open the aneurysm and to suture the communications into the artery (Fig. 24–41) was the standard treatment, with minimal modification, for more than 50 years, a period that included World War II.

Despite the acceptance of the Matas endoaneurysmorrhaphy during World War I and World War II, interest in preserving arterial continuity was maintained. Lexer (1907) was the first to use a segment of saphenous vein as an interposition graft in an arterial defect caused by excision of a traumatic axillary aneurysm. Some of the problems associated with arterial repair have been detailed in Chapter 1. Individual series of successful arterial repairs have been reported. Soubbotitch (1913) used suture repair, as has previously been described in Chapter 1. Elkin (1946) emphasized that all of the previous approaches outlined by Antyllus, Anel, Hunter, and Brasdor and Wardrop were frequently followed by infection, hemorrhage, gangrene, or failure to cure the false aneurysm. Only the Matas procedure avoided these complications during the World War II experience. The following methods of managing arterial aneurysms were outlined by Freeman and Shumacker (1955):

1. Endoaneurysmorrhaphy of Matas
2. Measures designed to produce clot in the aneurysmal sac or to induce formation of fibrous tissue about it to prevent further expansion and possible rupture
3. Obliteration of the sac by closure of the offending vessel
4. Extirpation of the aneurysm-bearing is portion of the artery
5. Extirpation of the lesion, combined with some procedure to permit maintenance or to reestablish continuity of the affected artery.

The extensive World War II experience is documented in detail by Elkin, by Shumacker, and by DeBakey and Elkin (1955).

Since the Korean Conflict in which arterial repair was emphasized, vascular recon-struction has become the procedure of choice in restoring arterial continuity in the repair of false aneurysms, in both the military and the civilian situation. Hughes and Jahnke (1958) reviewed the Korean experience and provided a 5-year follow-up. A similar extensive review has been completed recently for the Vietnam experience (Rich, 1975).

As might be anticipated, a smaller number of false aneurysms have been documented in civilian experience than in recent military experience. Patman, Poulos, and Shires (1964) reported 12 patients who developed false aneurysms in their series of 256 patients with civilian arterial injuries in Dallas, an incidence of 4.7%. None of these patients had an initial exploration. Among the major vessels that developed false aneurysms were the aorta (1), subclavian (1), axillary (2), superficial femoral (1), and popliteal (1). There were also three radial artery false aneurysms and single false aneurysms of the profunda femoris, anterior tibial, and posterior tibial arteries. The ratio of false aneurysms to AVFs was 2:1 in their series, which was the opposite of the ratio reported by Hughes and Jahnke (1958) from the Korean experience.

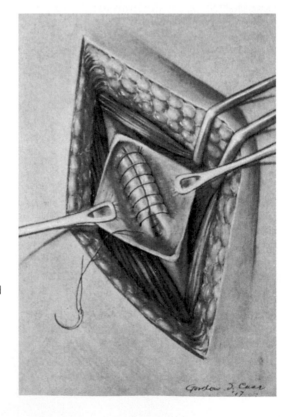

■ **FIGURE 24–41**
This diagram illustrates the obliterative endoaneurysmorrhaphy of Matas. Although Matas also believed in the reconstructive endoaneurysmorrhaphy, he elected to use the obliterative technique in this case in 1917 involving a gunshot wound of the superficial femoral artery because collateral circulation had been established and the obliterative suture could be applied with safety to the limb. A continuous intrasaccular silk suture obliterated the orifices of the communication with the main artery, both proximally and distally. (From Matas R: Keene's surgery, vol. 7. Philadelphia: WB Saunders, 1921.) ■

Incidence

With the increased interest in primary arterial repair of injured arteries during the past 25 years, many anticipated that there would be a resultant decrease in false aneurysms. This was particularly true in Vietnam (Rich 1975). However, considering the various etiologic factors, remaining diagnostic problems, and priorities of managing a patient with multiple life-threatening injuries, it should be obvious that the treatment of false aneurysms remains an important aspect of vascular surgery.

Similar to the varying incidence of arterial injuries in the injured patient in general and of AVFs, there is considerable disparity in the reported incidence of false aneurysms, in both civilian and military experience. One explanation for this is at times false aneurysms are included in series of arterial trauma and at other times they are not. Also, some series do not distinguish AVFs from false aneurysms in combined reports.

Shumacker and Carter (1946) compared the incidence of arterial aneurysms and AVFs in large caliber peripheral arteries in their World War II experience (see Table 24–2). Brachial false aneurysms were more prevalent than brachial AVFs, and the converse was true with femoral AVFs and false aneurysms. Hughes and Jahnke (1958) found that there were approximately twice as many AVFs as false aneurysms in the Korean experience. When major vessel lesions were considered (see Table 24–7), they also noted fewer femoral false aneurysms than AVFs. Rich (1975) reported a somewhat different experience in Vietnam, where there were slightly more false aneurysms than AVFs (see Table 24–3).

In the relatively small series of arterial injuries reported by Dillard, Nelson, and Norman (1968), false aneurysms (nine injuries) were more common than AVFs (seven injuries) in their civilian experience in St. Louis.

Etiology

Penetrating injuries are usually responsible for a false aneurysm, or traumatic aneurysm, which is produced by a tangential laceration through all three layers of the wall of an artery. In the military experience, fragments from various exploding devices and bullets account for the penetrating missile wounds (Fig. 24–42). In Civilian experience, stab wounds, in addition to low-velocity bullet wounds, are often associated with false aneurysms.

The increased use of fragmenting missiles in combat parallels the relatively high incidence of the development of these aneurysms in a number of wars, particularly before the advent of vascular repair. Hughes (1954) noted that 85% of the vascular wounds in Korea resulted from fragmenting missiles, with only 15% being from bullets. Rich (1975) found that a similar percentage, about 87%, of fragment wounds were responsible for 558 false aneurysms and AVFs (see Table 24–12).

Diagnostic and therapeutic procedures can result in false aneurysms if the placement of

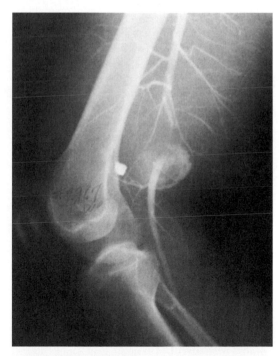

■ **FIGURE 24–42**
Representative of military wounds associated with false aneurysms is this large fragment wound of the popliteal fossa with a large false aneurysm of the popliteal artery demonstrated angiographically. (From Vietnam Vascular Registry #2967, NMR, Walter Reed General Hospital.) ■

needles and catheters injures the arteries. The first lesions that were successfully treated by Lambert (1759) and Norris (1843) resulted from bloodletting. At Walter Reed General Hospital, four false aneurysms developed following catheterization for angiographic procedures (Rich, 1975). Postoperative false aneurysms, other than anastomotic false aneurysms, have been associated with many operations. Smith (1963) cited development of a false aneurysm of the common femoral artery following an inguinal herniorrhaphy. There was sudden profuse arterial bleeding in the course of the herniorrhaphy, and hemostasis was eventually secured by multiple silk sutures. Approximately 2 weeks after the operation, a pulsatile, firm, and tender mass measuring 8 by 6 by 4 cm was palpated in the area of the left inguinal ligament. Despite tile fact, there was a purulent exudate surrounding the area of the 1-cm tear in the common femoral artery where a number of sutures had been placed in the defect. It was elected to excise the traumatized area and perform an end-to-end anastomosis. Five days after this second procedure, severe hemorrhage occurred and it was necessary to ligate the common femoral artery. Nevertheless, viability of the extremity persisted.

The fact that a false aneurysm can develop following the operative removal of a herniated nucleus pulposus was documented by Seeley (1954). Seeley mentioned treating a 20-year-old patient with a right common iliac artery aneurysm who had been operated on the L4-5 intervertebral space 1 month before his admission at Walter Reed General Hospital. Six weeks following the initial disk operation, a second operation was performed and an enormous false sac was found surrounding a right common iliac artery defect (Fig. 24-43). It was necessary to restore arterial continuity by inserting a 2-cm homologous arterial graft. Subsequent complications associated with disruption of the graft necessitated ligation of the right common iliac artery and vein. Fortunately, viability of the extremity was maintained.

Fractures can be associated with false aneurysm formation. Cameron, Laird, and Carroll (1972) presented an interesting review of 10 cases of false aneurysms complicating

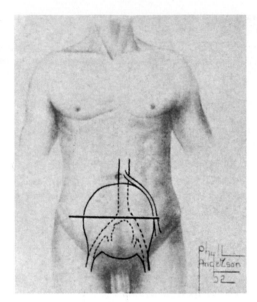

■ **FIGURE 24–43**
An enormous false aneurysm from a defect in the right common iliac artery was operated on at Walter Reed General Hospital 6 weeks after the initial disk operation. The right ureter was displaced laterally by the mass. The segment of the artery with the posterior defect was excised, and the hypogastric artery ligated. A 2-cm homologous arterial graft was used to bridge the defect. (From Seeley SF, Hughes CW, Jahnke EJ Jr: Major vessel damage in lumbar disc operation. Surgery 1954;35:421-429.) ■

closed fractures in a variety of anatomic locations (Table 24–24). Singh and Gorman (1972) emphasized that the formation of a false aneurysm as a result of a closed trauma to the lower extremity was unusual. They presented a case of a 51-year-old man who sustained a closed fracture at the junction of the middle and distal thirds of the tibia and fibula when his leg was caught by an encircling boat cable in a ship-building yard in 1966. Initially, a closed reduction of the fracture was performed, with immobilization of the limb in a long leg cast. This was replaced by a walking cast, which was kept on for 6 months before it was determined that the fracture was healed. At that time, the patient noted superficial varicosities. The examining physician stated that his extremity had the typical postphlebitic syndrome appearance, except that

TABLE 24–24
REPORTED CASES OF FALSE ANEURYSMS COMPLICATING CLOSED FRACTURES

Author	Year	Artery Involved	Fracture
Robson	1957	Fourth lumbar artery	Fractured spinous processes and traumatic spondylolisthesis
Crellin	1963	Anterior tibial artery	Fracture upper third tibia
Meyer and Slager	1964	Profunda femoral artery	Subtrochanteric osteotomy
Dameron	1964	Profunda femoral artery	Screwn blade plate
Staheli	1967	Popliteal artery	Fracture distal femoral shaft
Smith	1963	One false aneurysm with closed fracture in 61 arterial injuries; site not stated	—
Stein	1958	Anterior tibial artery	Fracture of tibial plateau
Bassett and Houck	1964	Profunda femoral artery	Blade plate for subtrochanteric osteotomy
Bassett and Silver	1966	Thoracic aorta	Eleventh dorsal vertebra
Harrow	1970	Right internal iliac artery	Pelvis

Modified from Cameron HS, Laird JJ, Carroll SE: False aneurysms complicating closed fractures. J Trauma 1972;12:67-74.

there was a pulsatile mass with a bruit located over the posteromedial aspect of the distal tibia. A femoral arteriogram revealed a large false aneurysm and an AVF of the distal part of the posterior tibial artery and accompanying veins (Fig. 24–44). It was possible to perform a lateral repair of the posterior tibial artery with interruption of the venous component. Six months later, the patient was asymptomatic with no extremity edema.

Blunt trauma without an associated fracture can also result in a false aneurysm. Lai, Hoffman, and Adamkiewicz (1966) presented an unusual case of dissecting aneurysm of the cervical carotid artery in a 21-year-old male following a hyperextension neck injury sustained in an automobile accident. The patient presented at the Johns Hopkins Hospital with a chief complaint of pain of the left side of his head and neck 6 months after the car he was driving collided with a truck. A firm, tender, 4-by-4 cm mass high in the left cervical area was obvious, and a bruit was heard over the mass. A left carotid angiogram revealed considerable lateral displacement of the internal carotid artery, and the mass promptly filled with contrast media. A 4-by-6 cm dissecting aneurysm of the internal carotid artery was found at the time of exploration, with the hypoglossal nerve, the vagus nerve, and the spinal accessory nerve all being displaced by the aneurysmal sac. Because

the superior portion of the aneurysmal sac approached the base of the skull, it was necessary to ligate the internal and external carotid arteries. The patient had an uneventful postoperative recovery with no abnormal neurologic findings other than the cranial nerve deficits present before surgery.

Clinical Pathology

A false aneurysm, or traumatic aneurysm, is caused by trauma that lacerates or ruptures all three layers of the wall of an artery. Arterial flow through the artery is usually maintained, and the extravasated blood through the laceration is contained by surrounding tissues to become a pulsating hematoma and subsequently an encapsulated false aneurysm. The hematoma that is formed compresses and seals the point of injury. Within days to weeks later, the thrombus gradually liquefies. False aneurysms are distinguished from true aneurysms. Whether the true aneurysm is congenital in origin, arteriosclerotic, mycotic, syphilitic, or caused by unusual systemic diseases such as polyarteritis nodosa, the true aneurysm has a sac composed of one or more layers of the artery rather than a rupture through all of the walls of the artery, as occurs in the traumatic false aneurysm. Indirect or blunt trauma can actually cause a true

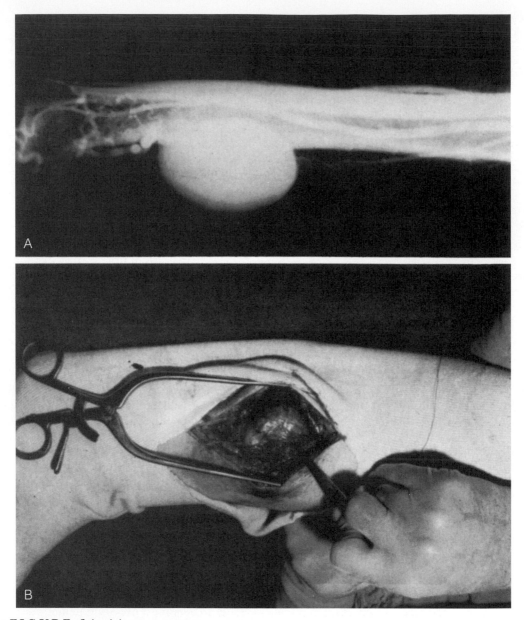

■ **FIGURE 24–44**
A, A large false aneurysm of the posterior tibial artery and a posterior tibial arteriovenous fistula were demonstrated angiographically in a 51-year-old man who sustained a closed fracture at the junction of the middle and distal thirds of the tibia and fibula. *B,* The large posterior tibial false aneurysm was demonstrated at the time of surgical exploration. (From Singh I, Gorman JF: Vascular injuries in closed fractures near junction of middle and lower thirds of the tibia. J Trauma 1972;12:592-598.) ■

aneurysm. True traumatic aneurysms caused by blunt, nonpenetrating trauma form a small group compared to traumatic false aneurysms. Blunt trauma causes a confusion of the arterial wall, with the damaged arterial segment progressively dilating and forming a true

aneurysm. Early recognition and treatment are rarely possible because the injury will usually not be apparent until a true aneurysm develops to a significant size. Only pathologic evaluation may differentiate a traumatic true aneurysm from a traumatic false aneurysm.

An unrepaired laceration of an artery with an inevitable periarterial hematoma usually has partial liquefaction of the latter, and a communication is established between the artery and the hematoma. A pseudocapsule of connective tissue forms gradually, and the pulsating hematoma becomes a false aneurysmal sac. The lesion will usually continue to expand, often causing pressure symptoms. One of the most easily recognizable results of pressure is a neuropathy, such as the easily recognizable neurologic deficits that develop in the hand from pressure on the median nerve by a false aneurysm (Fig. 24–45). False aneurysms may eventually rupture. The potential for exsanguinating hemorrhage endangers not only the limb but also the patient's life. If there is an associated infection, the threat of rupture is even greater (Fig. 24–46).

The size, configuration, and location of false aneurysms can vary greatly. The false aneurysm can be one single sac (Fig. 24–47) or it can be bilobed (Fig. 24–48). The distribution of 82 false aneurysms treated in World War II shows that the brachial artery was involved most often, followed by the popliteal

artery (see Table 24–6). The anatomic region most often involved with 558 false aneurysms and AVFs in Vietnam casualties was the lower extremity (see Table 24–9). The most common involved arteries were the posterior tibial and brachial, followed closely by the superficial femoral and popliteal arteries (see Table 24–10). Multiple lesions can exist. Table 24–4 shows that 41 out of the 509 Vietnam casualties had two or more lesions, for a total of 90 separate lesions (Fig. 24–49).

Expanding false aneurysms can cause neurologic changes due to direct pressure on major nerves (Fig. 24–50). Shumacker and Carter (1946) emphasized the high frequency of false aneurysms of upper extremity major arteries with associated nerve lesions that required operations (Table 24–25).

Usual pathologic changes can occur with false aneurysms. Distal embolization of a thrombus (Fig. 24–51) from a false aneurysm (Fig. 24–52) is unusual, but the potential threat with possible disastrous sequelae always exists. Sachtello, Ernst, and Griffen (1974) described the case of one patient with a false subclavian aneurysm who had distal embolism

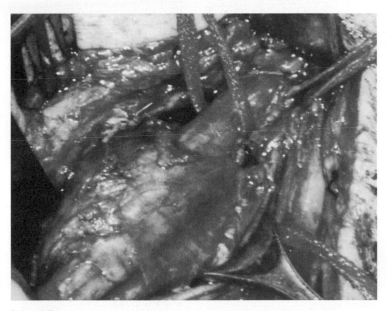

■ **FIGURE 24–45**
Pressure from a false aneurysm can compress an adjacent nerve. Fairly rapid expansion of the false aneurysm of the brachial artery caused external compression of both the median and the ulnar nerves with resultant neurologic deficit. (From Rich NM: In: Beebe HG, ed. Complications in vascular surgery. Philadelphia: JB Lippincott, 1973.) ■

508 V • SPECIAL PROBLEMS AND COMPLICATIONS

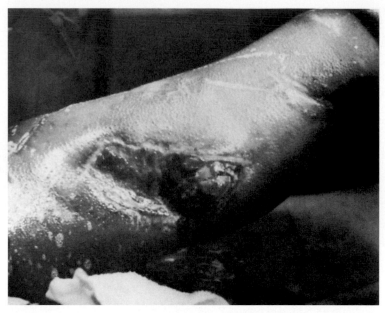

■ **FIGURE 24–46**
A false aneurysm associated with surrounding infection has an increased potential for rupture and exsanguinating hemorrhage. An infected false aneurysm of the superficial femoral artery resulted in intermittent hemorrhage through the open wound of the thigh in a Vietnam casualty. (From NMR, Vietnam Vascular Registry #837.) ■

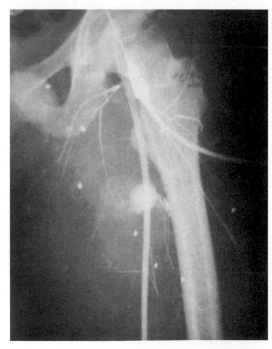

■ **FIGURE 24–47**
A false aneurysm can exist in a large variety of sizes and configurations. It may be a single sac, as shown in this arteriogram. (From NMR, Vietnam Vascular Registry #2590.) ■

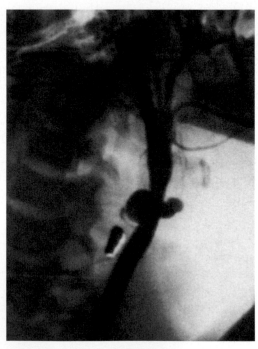

■ **FIGURE 24–48**
Among the variety of configurations of false aneurysms is a double or bilobed sac, as shown in this arteriogram of the common carotid artery. The offending fragment is seen adjacent to the carotid artery. (From NMR, Vietnam Vascular Registry #826.) ■

TABLE 24–25

PERIPHERAL NERVE LESIONS ASSOCIATED WITH ARTERIAL ANEURYSMS

Artery Involved	Nerve Lesion Requiring Operation		Nerve Lesion Not Requiring Operation		No Nerve Lesion	
	No.	%	No.	%	No.	%
Brachial	24	85.7	1	3.6	3	10.7
Axillary	11	73.3	1	6.7	3	20.0
Subclavian	3	60.0	1	20.0	1	20.0
Popliteal	2	9.5	6	28.6	13	61.9
Femoral	1	6.2	3	18.8	12	75.0
Others	7	13.0	13	24.0	34	63.0
TOTAL	48	40.3	25	21.0	66	38.7

Modified from Shumacker HB Jr, Carter KL: Arteriovenous fistulas and arterial aneurysms in military personnel. Surgery 1946;20:9-25.

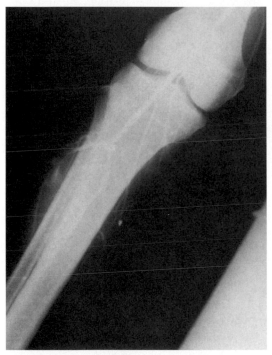

■ **FIGURE 24–49**
Multiple lesions can occur, as evidenced by this Vietnam casualty who had a false aneurysm of the anterior tibial artery, which was obvious, and a false aneurysm of the distal popliteal artery, which was diagnosed only by angiography. (From NMR, Vietnam Vascular Registry #5189.) ■

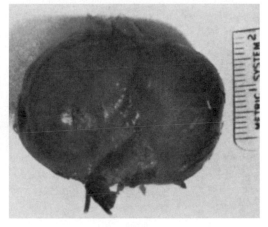

■ **FIGURE 24–50**
There is a groove made by the median nerve in the excised axillary false aneurysm. Direct pressure on the median nerve had resulted in a neuropathy. (From Elkin DC: Vascular injuries of warfare. Ann Surg 1944;120:284-310.) ■

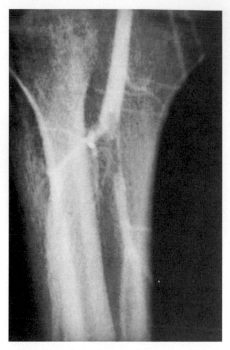

■ **FIGURE 24–51**
Mural thrombus may embolize from either a false aneurysm or an arteriovenous fistula. This angiogram demonstrates an embolus from a proximal popliteal artery false aneurysm to the distal popliteal and proximal posterior tibial arteries. (From Rich NM: In: Beebe HG, ed. Complications in vascular surgery. Philadelphia: JB Lippincott, 1973.) ■

from a thrombus within a false aneurysm. They managed the problem by resection of the clavicle, resection of the subclavian false aneurysm with vein graft replacement and brachial arterial embolectomy. Pulses were restored. Rhodes, Cox, and Silver (1973) reported the unusual complication of consumption coagulopathy, which developed in a patient with a false aneurysm and an AVF.

Clinical Features

The most obvious clinical finding with a false aneurysm is a mass that is usually pulsatile. There is often evidence of a penetrating wound (Fig. 24–53). The mass may or may not be painful. On examination, the borders of the mass can be ill defined because the false aneurysm is beneath the deep fascia. Depending on the amount of thrombus within the false aneurysm, the mass may or may not be pulsatile. There is often an associated systolic bruit over the mass, and there can be considerable radiation of the bruit into the surrounding anatomy.

Gradual enlargement of the false aneurysm may occur (Fig. 24–54), with the development

■ **FIGURE 24–52**
Except for 14% of the lesions that were associated with external hemorrhage into open wounds, there were rare preoperative complications associated with arteriovenous fistulas and false aneurysms in this series. One of these was embolization of thrombus from popliteal arterial false aneurysm, identified in the arteriogram with its adjacent wounding fragment. In 1968 at Walter Reed Army Medical Center, the false aneurysm was resected, the thrombus was removed with a Fogarty catheter, and arterial continuity was reestablished by end-to-end anastomosis. (From Rich NM, Hobson RW II, Collins GJ Jr: Traumatic arteriovenous fistulas and false aneurysms: A review of 558 lesions. Surgery 1975;78:817-828.) ■

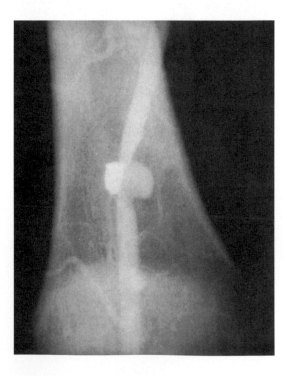

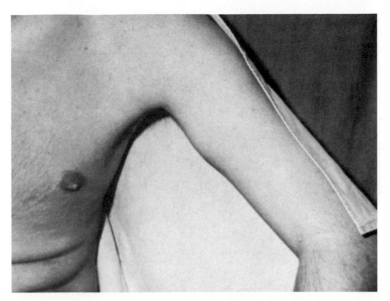

■ **FIGURE 24–53**
The diagnosis of a false aneurysm may be obvious with the physical finding of a pulsating mass.
There is usually evidence of a penetrating wound. (From NMR, Vietnam Vascular Registry #3273.) ■

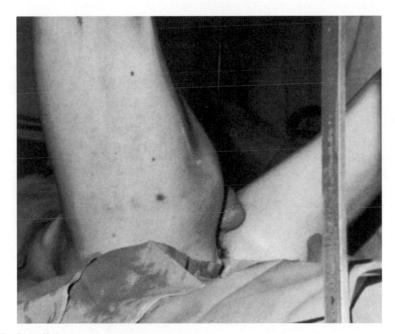

■ **FIGURE 24–54**
Enlargement of a false aneurysm may be gradual, or there may be rapid expansion of a mass. The
size of the mass may also be quite variable, as in this large false aneurysm of the profunda femoris
artery. The mass may be painful, and there may be warmth and tenderness on examination. (From
NMR, Vietnam Vascular Registry #3159.) ■

of a firm, warm, tender area. Confusion with an abscess has occurred in the differential diagnosis. A stable false aneurysm of longer duration can also be confused with a cyst or neoplasm.

If the false aneurysm is associated with an AVF, a continuous bruit and thrill over the sight of injury may also be present. As previously noted, pressure on adjacent nerves may result in neurologic deficits, and the first symptom or physical finding may result from neuropathy. Distal pulses are usually intact and considered to be normal on examination.

Diagnostic Considerations

Diagnosis is usually made by physical examination of a pulsatile mass. Roentgenograms in the anteroposterior and lateral views might identify an offending metallic foreign body in the anatomical location of an artery.

Nevertheless, angiography may be necessary to establish the diagnosis (Fig. 24–55). The size of the false aneurysm may be misleadingly small because of the amount of laminated clot filling the sac (Fig. 24–56). Angiography may delineate a clinically unsuspected adjacent AVF (Fig. 24–57) or multiple vascular lesions, as demonstrated in Fig. 24–49.

Angiography may be necessary to make the diagnosis of the false aneurysms in arteries that are not easily acceptable to physical examination, such as those within the chest and abdomen (Fig. 24–58).

Newer investigative techniques, such as sonography, can also be valuable in determining the size and location of false aneurysms. This was emphasized by Bole, Purdy, and Munda (1976) (Fig. 24–59). The diagnostic value of sonography for both true aneurysms and false aneurysms has been demonstrated with increasing utilization of this modality at Walter Reed General Hospital.

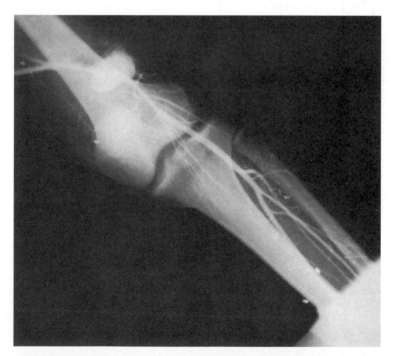

■ FIGURE 24–55
Preoperative angiography is helpful in confirming clinical impressions, outlining the site of the vascular defect, and ruling out additional adjacent vascular injuries. When not preoperatively available or practical, angiograms can be obtained easily. This one demonstrates a popliteal arterial false aneurysm seen at Walter Reed Army Medical Center in 1969 before resection and end-to-end anastomosis. Similar angiograms in the operating room immediately after repair have helped establish the status of vascular repair. (From Rich NM, Hobson RW II, Collins GJ Jr: Traumatic arteriovenous fistulas and false aneurysms: A review of 558 lesions. Surgery 1975;78:817-828.) ■

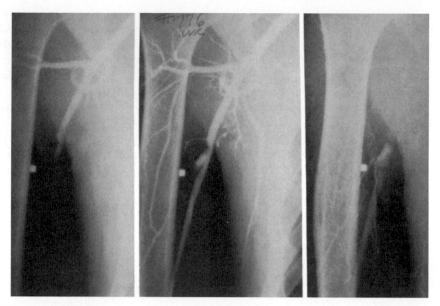

■ **FIGURE 24–56**

This series of film in an angiogram of the right brachial artery demonstrates early filling of the false aneurysm adjacent to the offending fragment *(left);* the obvious false aneurysm, which was angiographically much smaller than the large palpable mass because of the laminated clot that filled the false aneurysm sac *(middle);* and residual contrast in the false aneurysm sac *(right).* (From NMR, Vietnam Vascular Registry #3159.) ■

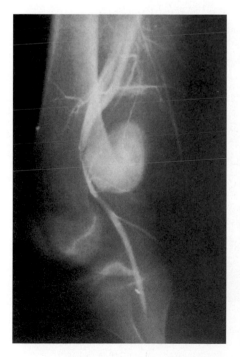

■ **FIGURE 24–57**

A large false aneurysm, such as this one demonstrated angiographically, can cause local arterial compression. In this Vietnam casualty, the large false aneurysm of the popliteal artery compressed the artery sufficiently to nearly obliterated the associated arteriovenous fistula. There was no associated classic "machinery-type" bruit, and the arteriovenous fistula was diagnosed angiographically. Also, the patient had weak pedal pulses because of the compression of the popliteal artery by the large false aneurysm, in contrast to what has previously been described in most patients who have intact distal pulses. (From NMR, Vietnam Vascular Registry #2513159.) ■

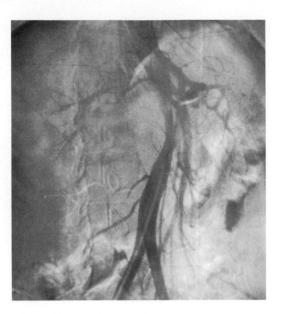

■ **FIGURE 24–58**
Compression and lateral displacement of the abdominal aorta toward the patient's left side are demonstrated in this subtraction study of an angiogram of the aorta. The offending fragment from an M26 grenade caused a large false aneurysm of the aorta, which was repaired by lateral suture technique with interrupted sutures at Walter Reed Army Medical Center in 1967. (From Rich NM, Hobson RW II, Collins GJ Jr: Traumatic arteriovenous fistulas and false aneurysms: a review of 558 lesions. Surgery 1975;78:817-828.) ■

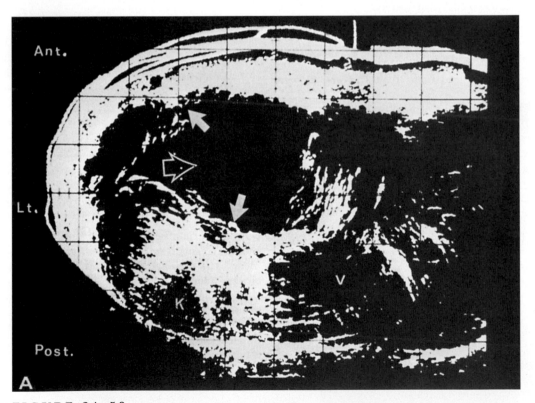

■ **FIGURE 24–59**
Ultrasonic tomography of the upper abdomen in a transverse plane showing the pseudoaneurysm *(open arrow)* in a patient with nonpulsatile diffuse mass. Thrombus echoes and irregular contour of the aneurysm are noted *(solid arrows)*. Vertebral body *(V)* and the left kidney *(K)* are also visualized. (From Bole PV, Purdy RT, Munda R, et al: Traumatic pseudoaneurysms: A review of 32 cases. J Trauma 1976;16:63-70.) ■

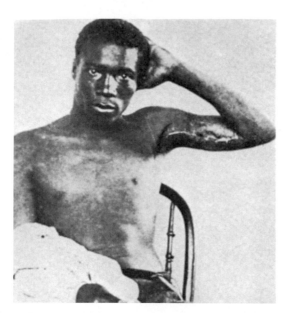 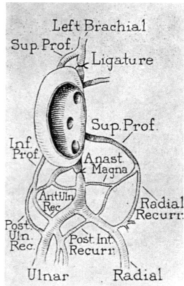

■ **FIGURE 24–60**

The original photograph and drawing shown in the report of Dr. Matas, *Philadelphia Medical News*, October 27, 1988, when he proposed his endoaneurysmorrhaphy approach to the management of false aneurysms. (From Elkin DC: Traumatic aneurysm; Matas operation—57 years after. Surg Gynecol Obstet 1946;82:1-12.) ■

Surgical Treatment

The report of the first operation performed by Matas in 1888 was presented again by Elkin (1946) to emphasize that the Matas operation has stood the test of time for 57 years and had had a profound impact on the surgery of blood vessels (Fig. 24–60).

On April 6, 1988, I operated on a young male Negro for a very large traumatic (multiple gunshot) aneurysm of the brachial artery, extending from the armpit to the elbow, which opened my eyes to the possibilities of an entirely new method of conservative treatment, which was to revolutionize my previous notions of aneurysmal surgery. In this case, successive ligation of the main artery on the proximal and distal poles of the aneurysm had been followed by relapse, and it seemed to me that I had no other alternative but to extirpate the sac. When I exposed the sac and emptied its contents, the failure of the ligations to control the circulation was easily explained by the appearance in the bottom of the sac of the large orifices corresponding to the collateral branches, which opened into the sac in the segment of the artery included

in between the ligatures (Fig. 24–61). It was evident that it was these collateral orifices that fed the sac despite the ligatures that had been placed at each one of its poles. I, at first, intended to secure these collaterals by excising the sac, but the branches of the brachial plexus of nerves were so densely incorporated in its walls that I could have not dissected them and detached them, without serious damage, thereby paralyzing the arm. It occurred to me then that the easiest way out of this awkward dilemma was to steal the orifices of all the bleeding collaterals by suturing them as we would an intestinal wound, leaving the sac attached and undisturbed in the wound. This procedure was at once put into effect and the hemostasis was so perfect and satisfactory that it seemed to me strange that no one should have thought of so simple an expedient before.

Matas used the intrasaccular suture (see Figs. 24–41 and 24–61); however, he was also interested in reconstructive endoaneurysmorrhaphy (Fig. 24–62).

In the management of a false aneurysm, repair of the arterial defect is usually the goal that should be sought. An elective incision

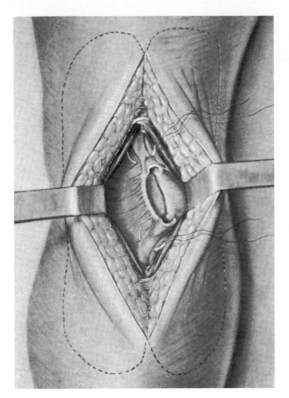

■ **FIGURE 24–61**
The Matas obliterative aneurysmorrhaphy is
demonstrated in this intrasaccular suture
ligature of a ruptured popliteal aneurysm. The
dotted line shows the area of extravasation
filled with clot. Arterial reconstruction was
considered impractical in this specific case,
and the distal and proximal popliteal arteries
were obliterated with encircling sutures.
Collateral circulation was adequate to maintain
extremity viability. (From Matas R: Surgery, vol.
7. Philadelphia: WB Saunders, 1921.) ■

should be made that will allow adequate exposure for proximal and distal control. Examples were afforded by the extensive World War
II experience. Shumacker (1946) described
in detail the incisions that could be successfully employed in the surgical approach to
aneurysms, especially those in antecubital
(Fig. 24–63) and popliteal (Fig. 24–64) fossae.
His report was based on his extensive
experience in managing false aneurysms in
hundreds of American combat casualties.
Specifically, these incisions were devised to
replace longitudinal incisions across the
popliteal and antecubital creases, which were
often associated with heavy scars or keloids,

contracture, or ulceration. Although resection
of the false aneurysm is often recommended,
an alternative plan that is presently employed
has several advantages. The laminated clot
within the false aneurysm should be evacuated
after temporary proximal and distal control
is obtained with vascular clamps, but the majority of the sac can usually be left in place. This
will shorten the length of the operative procedure and decrease the possibility of damage
to associated structures, such as tearing of the
popliteal vein, which has become closely
adherent and attenuated to an adjacent
popliteal arterial false aneurysm. If the false
aneurysm is inadvertently entered before
obtaining proximal and distal control, digital
control will usually suffice as an expedient
measure. Unnecessary resection of normal
artery can also be avoided if careful dissection of both the proximal and the distal artery
toward the side of the defect is carried out.
In this manner, a more limited resection of
artery will be necessary.

Occasionally, lateral suture of a punctuate
wound of an artery is possible, without constriction of the arterial lumen. However,
limited arterial resection and end-to-end anastomosis is usually the procedure of choice. If
it is necessary to use an arterial replacement,
an autogenous vein graft is usually preferred.
This graft should be placed in tissue as normal
as possible, which is often difficult because of
considerable inflammation and cicatrix. If
there is extensive scarring, it might be possible to place a graft in an extra-anatomic area
of adjacent tissues in a position away from the
usual course of the major vessel. In the case
of noncritical arteries, such as the radial artery
or distal posterior tibial artery, ligation is
usually satisfactory. This is particularly important if there is an infected false aneurysm.
However, arterial repair is preferred even in
small caliber arteries.

Surgical correction of a false aneurysm
should be performed as soon as possible after
the diagnosis is made to prevent the complications of rupture or rapid expansion with
resultant pressure on adjacent nerves. Immediate surgery should be advocated if neurologic symptoms develop.

Additional information related to specific
arterial false aneurysms, such as those of the

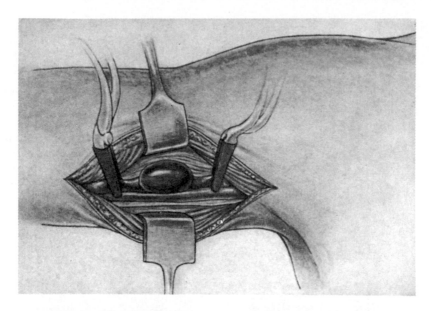

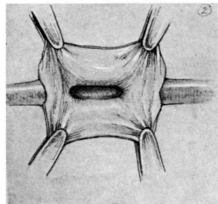 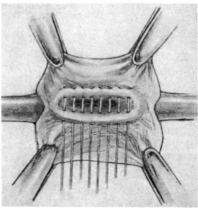

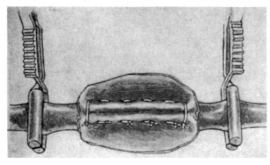 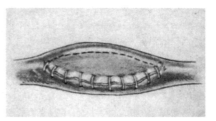

■ **FIGURE 24–62**

In addition to the obliterative aneurysmorrhaphy for the treatment of the false aneurysms, Matas encouraged selective reconstructive endoaneurysmorrhaphy, as was used in this repair of a false aneurysm of the brachial artery. (From Matas R: Surgery, vol. 7. Philadelphia: WB Saunders, 1921.) ■

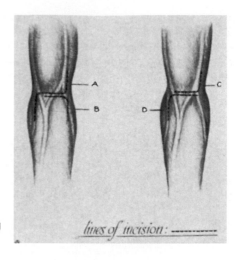

■ **FIGURE 24–63**
Incisions used in exposure of vessels in the antecubital fossa. *A,* The usual incision for exposure of brachial vessels in antecubital space. *B,* Incision used when the lesion is suspected in proximal portion of ulnar vessels. *C,* Incision used when brachial vessels are involved just proximal to antecubital creased. *D,* Incision used for exploration of distal end of brachial or proximal end of radial vessels. (From Shumacker HB Jr: Incisions in surgery of aneurysms, with special reference to exploration in antecubital and popliteal fossae. Ann Surg 1946;124:586-598.) ■

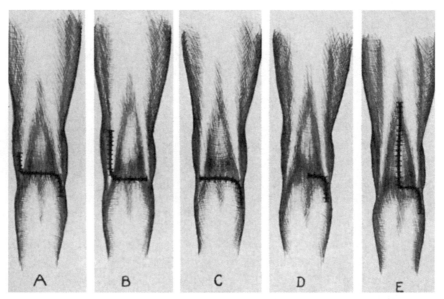

■ **FIGURE 24–64**
Skin incisions used in exploring the popliteal vessels in the surgical approach to false aneurysms in World War II. *A,* Incision used when the lesion exists in the midpopliteal space. *B,* Incision used when the lesion is higher in the popliteal fossa. *C* and *D,* Incisions used for exploring the distal popliteal vessels. *E,* A modified incision useful when associated nerve lesion require exploration. (From Shumacker HB Jr: Incisions in surgery of aneurysms, with special reference to exploration in antecubital and popliteal fossae. Ann Surg 1946;124:586-598.) ■

subclavian artery, can be found in specific chapters. Details of arterial repair and specific techniques, such as intraluminal control of hemorrhage with a balloon catheter, are to be found in Chapter 19.

Elkin (1946) reported the results of operating on 106 false aneurysms at the Ashford General Hospital Vascular Center in White Sulfur Springs, West Virginia, in a 30-month period. The Matas procedure was employed in 61 of the operations, and some other type of operation, usually complete excision of a small sac, was employed in the remaining 45 cases. There were no deaths in his series, no recurrence of the false aneurysm, and no incidence of gangrene. Table 24–26 shows

TABLE 24–26
LOCATION OF INJURY AND NUMBER OF PATIENTS TREATED BY MATAS ENDOANEURYSMORRHAPHY: ASHFORD GENERAL HOSPITAL VASCULAR CENTER, WHITE SULFUR SPRINGS, WORLD WAR II EXPERIENCE

Artery Involved	Cases
Axillary	5
Brachial	14
Femoral	11
Iliac	2
Peroneal	1
Popliteal	7
Profunda femoris	3
Radial	4
Superior gluteal	1
Tibial, anterior	3
Tibial, posterior	8
Ulnar	2
TOTAL	61

From Elkins DC: Traumatic aneurysm; Matas operation—57 years after. Surg Gynecol Obstet 1946;82:1-12.

the location and number of injuries treated by endoaneurysmorrhaphy. Elkin and Shumacker (1955) outlined the operative treatment of 209 arterial aneurysms (Table 24–27). Nearly an equal number were treated by endoaneurysmorrhaphy as by excision. Shumacker (1948) reported successful results with vein graft repair of arteries that had false aneurysms (see Table 24–16).

De Takats and Pirani (1954) stated that Herlyn, a pupil of Stich in Göttingen, reported he performed 164 ligatures and 230 reconstructive operations in World War II. This emphasized that the trend in German was surgery, and Herlyn felt that the artery should never be ligated for traumatic aneurysm unless it was small or the patient's life was in danger.

Hughes and Jahnke (1958) reported on 215 false aneurysms and AVFs treated at Walter Reed Army Medical Center in the early 1950s, mainly in casualties from the Korean Conflict. The various operations used in managing 43 false aneurysms and 91 AVFs in large vessels are reviewed in Table 24–18. Similar data con-

cerning smaller caliber arteries are given in Table 24–8.

Rich, Hobson, and Collins (1975) reported the experience from the Vietnam War. There were 296 false aneurysms among 558 AVFs and false aneurysms identified in 509 patients. As might be anticipated by the number of American troops committed in Southeast Asia, the largest number of lesions resulted from wounds during 1968, with a relatively large number of lesions in 1967 and 1969. The time from injury to recognition of the AVFs and false aneurysms was arbitrarily considered to be immediate if recognized within the first 24 hours, early if recognized between the second and thirtieth day, delayed if recognized between the second through the sixth month, and remote if recognized after 6 months. In this study, the largest number of lesions (273 or 48.9%) was recognized in the early period (see Table 24–20). A nearly equal number of lesions, 228, was recognized in the delayed period. In the immediate group, there were 22 acute lesions operated on in Vietnam. In the remote group, all but 7 of the 35 patients had recognition and treatment of their lesions in less than 2 years. Only two had recognition and treatment of their lesions more than 5 years following the initial injury, and both were less than 6 years. Nearly an equal number of operations were performed in the intermediate hospitals, mainly in Japan, and in hospitals in the continental United States (see Table 24–21). Several hundred surgeons were involved in performing the repairs. Table 24–22 outlines the methods of treatment used for the various repairs. Arterial ligation was used in 290 lesions, 52%. The overall morbidity rate for the 509 patients was 1.8% (seven deaths) (see Table 24–23). Only two of these deaths could be directly attributed to the vascular problem. One patient died from a ruptured external iliac arterial false aneurysm. The overall morbidity included five complications, for a morbidity rate of 6.3%. Hemorrhage occurred in 14, thrombosis in 12, and stenosis in 2.

The numerous reports of the management of false aneurysms from civilian experience range from individual case reports to reports of 20 to 30 lesions. However, the civilian experience has not been as extensive as the warfare

TABLE 24–27

TECHNIQUES OF OPERATIVE TREATMENT IN 209 ARTERIAL ANEURYSMS: WORLD WAR II EXPERIENCE

Location	Endoaneurysmorrhaphy	Excision	Proximal Ligation	End-to-End Anastomosis	Total No. Cases
Upper extremity					
Axillary	10	24	1	—	35
Brachial	16	30	—	1	47*
Radial	7	5	—	—	12
Subclavian	2	10	1	—	13†
Ulnar	3	4	—	—	7
Lower extremity:					
Femoral	14	4	—	—	18‡
Gastrocnemius, muscle branch	—	1	—	—	1
Peroneal	2	—	—	—	2
Popliteal	19	2	—	—	21§
Profunda femoris	6	—	—	—	6
Profunda branch	2	—	—	—	2
Tibial, anterior	5	—	—	—	5
Tibial, posterior	7	8	—	—	15¶
Head and neck:					
Carotid	—	5	8	—	13¶
Cervical, deep	1	—	—	—	1
Temporal, superficial	—	2	—	—	2
Trunk:					
Gluteal, superior	2	—	—	—	2
Iliac	2	1	1	—	4
Innominate	1	—	—	—	1
Thoracic, lateral	—	1	—	—	1
Thoracoacromial	—	1	—	—	1
TOTAL	99	98	11	1	209

*This total does not include one aneurysm in which cure occurred spontaneously.
†This total does not include two aneurysms in which methods of management were not stated.
‡This total does not include two aneurysms in which cure occurred spontaneously.
§This total does not include three aneurysms: two in which methods of management were not stated and one in which spontaneous cure occurred.
¶This total does not include two aneurysms in which cure occurred spontaneously.
From Elkin DC, Shumacker HB Jr: In: Vascular Surgery in World War II. Elkin DC, DeBakey ME, eds. Washington, DC: US Government Printing Office, 1955.

experience in this century. Examples of the civilian experience are the reports of Lloyd (1957), Baird and Doran (1964), Engelman, Clements, and Herrmann (1969), and Bole, Purdy, and Munda (1976). Particularly noteworthy is the report of the management of 23 traumatic false aneurysm in 23 patients treated in New York City over a 5-year period starting in 1968. Table 24–28 outlines the method of management of these false aneurysms, with lateral suture repair, resection and end-to-end anastomosis, and ligation being used almost equally. These authors reported no mortality, no recurrence, and no distal edema or arterial insufficiency. They did have two patients who continued to have pain, and three wound infections occurred.

TABLE 24–28
TYPE OF REPAIR: CIVILIAN EXPERIENCE IN NEW YORK CITY

Resection and end-to-end anastomosis	8
Resection and graft replacement	1
Lateral repair	7
Ligation	5
Spontaneous closure	1
Refused treatment	1
TOTAL	23

From Bole PV, Munda R, Purdy RT, et al: Traumatic pseudoaneurysms: a review of 32 cases. J Trauma 1976;16:63-70.

Spontaneous Cure

Shumacker and Wayson (1950) evaluated spontaneous cure of false aneurysms and AVFs. They studied 122 aneurysms and 245 AVFs. They felt that thrombosis was responsible for the obliteration of these lesions. Because there were only eight satisfactory spontaneous cures of false aneurysm—6.6% of 22 lesions—these authors though that there was little merit in awaiting the possibility of this occurrence. This was only slightly better than the 2% spontaneous cure for AVFs. Although some case reports have been documented, recent experience has not witnessed a change in the low incidence of spontaneous cure of false aneurysms. This is undoubtedly also affected by early surgical intervention for the mass majority of false aneurysms.

Follow-up

Hughes and Jahnke (1958) provided a 5-year follow-up study of 250 AVFs and false aneurysms treated at Walter Reed Army Medical Center. Most of the patients had been injured during the Korean Conflict. This long-term follow-up was one of the first and one of the few extensive follow-up studies to be conducted. This study emphasized the difficulty in evaluating vascular trauma in combat casualties because of the many associated injuries. Neither of the two deaths in this follow-up

study were related to vascular problems following repair of false aneurysms. Residual pain, coldness, and claudication in the involved extremity were noted; however, no distinction was made between those patients treated for AVFs and those treated for false aneurysms. In the follow-up of the Vietnam casualties through the Vietnam Vascular Registry, more than one fourth—29.3%—or 149 of the 509 patients with AVFs and false aneurysms have been evaluated at Walter Reed Army Medical Center. In the long-term follow-up, which extends to 10 years for many patients, additional problems and symptomatic residuals have been limited. Unfortunately, some of these patients have been lost to the long-term follow-up effort because of untimely deaths. One patient was killed in subsequent action during a second tour in Vietnam, and another patient died in an automobile accident. In the civilian reports, there are very limited data regarding long-term follow-up of patients who have false aneurysms. While few wanted to be reminded of the unfortunate Vietnam experience for more than 25 years in the United States, as we enter the twenty-first century, there is a realization that data in the Vietnam Vascular Registry are of value. A concerted effort is being developed to expand the long-term follow-up, which will be helpful to collective experiences in the civilian community and in responding to military interventions.

REFERENCES

Albuquerque FC, Javedan SP, McDougall CG: Endovascular management of penetrating vertebral artery injuries. J Trauma 2002;53(3):574-580.

Annandale T: Traumatic popliteal arterio-venous aneurysm treated successfully by ligature of the popliteal artery and vein. Lancet 1875;1:568.

Anthopoulos LP, Johnson JB, Spellman M: Arteriovenous fistula in multiple saccular arterial aneurysms of a finger, following childhood human bite. Angiology 1965;16:89.

Baird RJ, Doran ML: The false aneurysm. Can Med Assoc J 1964;91:281-284.

Bassett FH, Houck WS: False aneurysm of profunda femoris artery after subtrochanteric osteotomy and nail-plate fixation. J Bone Joint Surg 1964; 46A:583-585.

Bassett FH, Silver D: Arterial injury associated with fractures. Arch Surg 1966;92:13-19.

Beattie EJ Jr, Oldham JB, Ross JA: Superior thyroid arteriovenous aneurysm. Br J Surg 1961;48:456-457.

Bell D, Cockshott WP: Angiography of traumatic arterio-venous fistulae. Clin Radiol 1965;16:241-247.

Bickham WS: Arteriovenous aneurysm. Ann Surg 1904;39:767-775.

Billings KJ, Nasca RJ, Griffin HA: Traumatic arteriovenous fistula with spontaneous closure. J Trauma 1973;13:741-743.

Blackmore TL, Whelan TJ: Arteriovenous fistula as a complication of gastrectomy. Am J Surg 1965; 109:197.

Bole PV, Munda R, Purdy RT: Traumatic pseudoaneurysms: A review of 32 cases. J Trauma 1976;16:63-70.

Bole PV, Purdy RT, Munda RT, et al: Civilian arterial injuries. Ann Surg 1976;183:13-23.

Branham HH: Aneurysmal varix of the femoral artery and vein following a gunshot wound. Int J Surg 1890;3:250.

Callander CL: Study of arteriovenous fistula with an analysis of 447 cases. Ann Surg 1920;19:428-459.

Cameron HS, Laird JJ, Carroll SE: False aneurysms complicating closed fractures. J Trauma 1972; 12:67-74.

Conn JH, Hardy JD, Chavez CM, Fain WR: Challenging arterial injuries. J Trauma 1971;11:167-177.

Creech O Jr, Gantt J, Wren H: Traumatic arteriovenous fistula at unusual sites. Ann Surg 1965;161:908-920.

Dameron TB Jr: False aneurysm of femoral profundus artery resulting from internal-fixation device (screw). J Bone Joint Surg 1964;46A:577-580.

De Takats G, Pirani C: Aneurysms: General considerations. Angiology 1954;5:173-208.

Dillard BM, Nelson DL, Norman HG: Review of 85 major traumatic arterial injuries. Surgery 1968; 63:391-395.

Drapanas T, Hewitt RL, Weichert RF III, Smith AD: Civilian vascular injuries: A critical appraisal of three decades of management. Ann Surg 1970; 172:351-360.

Eisenbrey AB: Arteriovenous aneurysm of the superficial femoral vessels. JAMA 1913;61:2155-2157.

Elkin DC: Arteriovenous aneurysm. Surg Gynecol Obstet 1945;80:217-224.

Elkin DC: Traumatic aneurysm: the Matas Operation 57 years after. Surg Gynecol Obstet 1946;82:1-12.

Elkin DC, Banner EA: Arteriovenous aneurysms following surgical operations. JAMA 1946;131:1117-1119.

Elkin DC, DeBakey ME: Vascular surgery in World War II. Washington, DC, US Government Printing Office, 1955.

Engleman RM, Clements JM, Herrmann JB: Stab wounds and traumatic false aneurysms in the extremities. J Trauma 1969;9:77-87.

Ferguson WM: Arteriovenous aneurysm following osteotomy for genu valgum. Lancet 1914;1:532.

Freeman NE, Shumacker HB Jr: Vascular surgery. In Elkin DC, DeBakey ME (eds): Washington, DC, US Government Printing Office, 1955.

Gaspard DJ, Gaspar MR: Arteriovenous fistula after Fogarty catheter thrombectomy. Arch Surg 1972;105:90-92.

Hallowell. Extract of a letter from Mr. Lambert, surgeon at Newcastle upon Tyne, to Dr. Hunter, giving an account of new method of treating an aneurysm. Med Obser Inq 1762;30:360.

Halsted W: Discussion in Bernheim, BM. Bull Johns Hopkins Hosp 1916;27:93.

Harris JD: A case of arteriovenous fistula following closed fracture of tibia and fibula. Br J Surg 1963;50:774-776.

Heaton LD, Hughes CW, Rosegay H, et al: Military surgical practices of the United States Army in Vietnam. In Current Problems in Surgery. Chicago, Year Book Medical Publishers, 1966.

Hershey FB. Secondary repair of arterial injuries. Am Surg 1961;27:33-41.

Hewitt RL, Collins DJ: Acute arteriovenous fistulas in war injuries. Ann Surg 1969;169:447-449.

Hewitt RL, Smith AD, Drapanas T: Acute traumatic arteriovenous fistulas. J Trauma 1973;13:901-906.

Holman E: Arteriovenous Aneurysms: Abnormal Communication between the Arterial and Venous Circulations. New York, Macmillan, 1937.

Holman E: Clinical and experimental observations on arteriovenous fistulae. Ann Surg 1940;112:840-875.

Holman E: Contributions to cardiovascular physiology gleaned from clinical and experimental observations of abnormal arteriovenous communications. J Cardiovasc Surg 1962;3:48-63.

Holman E: Abnormal arteriovenous communications. Great variability of effects with particular reference to delayed development of cardiac failure. Circulation 1965;32:1001-1009.

Holman E: Abnormal Arteriovenous Communications: Peripheral and Intracardiac, Acquired and Congenital, 2nd ed. Springfield, Ill, Charles C Thomas, 1968.

Holman EF: Physiology of an arteriovenous fistula. Arch Surg 1971;7:64-82.

Hughes CW: Acute vascular trauma in Korean War casualties: An analysis of 180 cases. Surg Gynec Obstet 1954;99:91-100.

Hughes CW, Jahnke EJ Jr: The surgery of traumatic arteriovenous fistulas and aneurysms: A five-year follow up study of 215 lesions. Surg Clin North Am 1958;148:790-797.

Hunt TK, Leeds FH, Wanebo HJ, Blaisdell FW: Arteriovenous fistulas of major vessels of the abdomen. J Trauma 1971;11:483-493.

Hunter W: The history of an aneurysm of the aorta, with some remarks on aneurysms in general. Med Obs Soc Phys Lond 1757;1:323.

Hunter W: Further observations upon a particular species of aneurysm. Med Obs Soc Phys Lond 1762;2:390.

Johnson G Jr, Blythe WB: Hemodynamic effects of arteriovenous shunts used for hemodialysis. Ann Surg 1970;171:715-723.

Johnson G Jr, Peters RM, Dart CH Jr: A study of cardiac vein negative pressure in arteriovenous fistula. Surg Gynecol Obstet 1967;124:82-86.

Lai MD, Hoffman HB, Adamkiewicz JJ: Dissecting aneurysm of internal carotid artery after nonpenetrating neck injury. Acta Radiol Diag 1966;5:290-295.

Lester J: Arteriovenous fistula after percutaneous vertebral angiography. Acta Radiol Diag 1966;5:337-340.

LeVeen H, Cerruti M: Surgery of large inaccessible arteriovenous fistulas. Ann Surg 1963;158:285-289.

Lewis T: The adjustment of blood flow to the affected limb in arteriovenous fistula. Clin Sci 1940;4:277-285.

Lexer E: Die ideale operation des arteriellen und des arteriell-venosen aneurysma. Arch Klin Chir 1907;83:459-477.

Lord R, Ehrenfeld W, Wylie EJ: Arterial injury from the Fogarty catheter. Med J Aust 1968;2:70-71.

Matas R: Traumatic aneurysm of the left brachial artery—Incision and partial excision of sac: Recovery. Phil Med News 1888;53:462-466.

Matas R: Traumatic arteriovenous aneurysms of the subclavian vessels, with an analytical study of fifteen reported cases, including one operated. Trans Am Surg Assoc 1901;19:237.

Matas R: An operation for radical cure of aneurysm based on arteriography. Ann Surg 1903;37:161-196.

Matas R: Recent advances in the technique of thoracotomy and pericardiotomy for wounds of the heart. South Med J 1908;1:75-81.

Meyer TJ, Slager R: False aneurysm following subtrochanteric osteotomy. J Bone Joint Surg 1964;46:581-582.

Muller WJ, Goodwin W: Renal arteriovenous fistula following nephrectomy. Ann Surg 1956;144:240-244.

Murphy J: Resection of arteries and veins injured in continuity end-to-end suture. Exp Clin Res Med Rec 1897;51:73-104.

Nakano J, DeSchryver C: Effects of arteriovenous fistula on systemic and pulmonary circulations. Am J Physiol 1964;207:1319.

Nicoladoni C: Phlebarteriectasie der rechten oberen extremitat. Arch Klin Chir 1875;18:252.

Norris G: Varicose aneurysm at the bend of the arm: Ligature of the artery above and below the sac; secondary hemorrhages with a return of the aneurysm thrill on the tenth day; cure. Am J Med Sci 1843;5:17.

Osler W: Case of arterio-venous aneurysm of the axillary artery and vein of 14 years duration. Ann Surg 1893;17:37-40.

Osler W: Report of a case of arteriovenous aneurysm of the thigh. Johns Hopkins Hosp Bull 1905;16:119.

Osler W: Remarks on arteriovenous aneurysm. Lancet 1915;1:949.

Pate J, Sherman R, Jackson T, Wilson H: Cardiac failure following traumatic arteriovenous fistula: A report of 14 cases. J Trauma 1965;5:398-403.

Patman R, Poulos E, Shires G: The management of civilian arterial injuries. Surg Gynecol Obstet 1964;118:725-738.

Petrovsky B, Milinov O: "Arterialization" and "venization" of vessels involved in traumatic arteriovenous fistulae: Aetiology and pathogenesis (an experimental study). J Cardiovasc Surg 1967;8:396-407.

Pick T: On partial rupture of arteries from external violence. St George's Hosp Rep (Lond) 1873;6:161.

Pick T: A clinical lecture of a case of arterio-venous aneurysm. Lond Med Times Gaz 1883;2:677.

Pridgen W, Jacobs J: Postoperative arteriovenous fistula. Surgery 1962;51:205.

Ranshoff J: Arteriovenous aneurysm of the superior thyroid artery and vein. Surg Gynecol Obstet 1935;61:816.

Reid M: The effect of arteriovenous fistula upon the heart and blood vessels: An experiment and clinical study. Bull Johns Hopkins Hosp 1920;31:43-50.

Reid M: Abnormal arteriovenous communications. Acquired and congenital, II. The orgin and nature of arteriovenous aneurysms, cirsoid aneurysms and simple angiomas. Arch Surg (Chicago) 1925;10:996-1009.

Reid M, McGuire J: Arteriovenous aneurysm. Ann Surg 1938;108:643-693.

Rhodes G, Cox C, Silver D: Arteriovenous fistula and false aneurysm as the cause of consumption coagulopathy. Surgery 1973;73:535-540.

Rich NM, Hobson RW II, Collins GJ Jr: Traumatic arteriovenous fistulas and false aneurysms: A review of 558 lesions. Surgery 1975;78:817-828.

Rob CG, Battle S: Arteriovenous fistula following the use of the Fogarty balloon catheter. Arch Surg 1971;102:144-145.

Sachtello C, Ernst CB, Griffen WJ: The acute ischemic upper extremity: Selected management. Surgery 1974;76:1002.

Sako Y, Varco R: Arteriovenous fistula: Results of management of congenital and acquired forms, blood flow measurements and observations on proximal arterial degeneration. Surgery 1970;67:40-61.

Schenk WJ, Bahn RA, Cordell A, Stephens J: The regional hemodynamics of acute experimental arteriovenous fistulas. Surg Gynecol Obstet 1957;105:733.

Schwartz A: The historical development of methods of hemostasis. Surgery 1958;44:604.

Seeley S: Vascular surgery at Walter Reed Army Hospital. US Armed Forces Med J 1954;8.

Seeley S, Hughes CW, Cooke F, Elkin DC: Traumatic arteriovenous fistulas and aneurysms in war wounded. Am J Surg 1952;83:471-479.

Shumacker HB Jr: Incisions in surgery of aneurysm: With special reference to explorations in the antecubital and popliteal fossae. Ann Surg 1946;124:586-598.

Shumacker HB Jr: Problem of maintaining the continuity of artery in surgery of aneurysms and arteriovenous fistulae; notes on the development and clinical application of methods of arterial suture. Ann Surg 1948;127:207-230.

Shumacker HB Jr, Carter KL: Arteriovenous fistulas and false aneurysms in military personnel. Surgery 1946;20:9-25.

Shumacker HB Jr, Stahl N: A study of the cardiac frontal area in patients with arteriovenous fistulas. Surgery 1949;26:928-944.

Shumacker HB Jr, Wayson EE: Spontaneous cure of aneurysms and arteriovenous fistulas, with some notes on intravascular thrombosis. Am J Surg 1950;79:532-544.

Singh I, Gorman JF: Vascular injuries in closed fractures near junction of middle and lower thirds of the tibia. J Trauma 1972;12:592-598.

Smith L, Foran R, Gaspar MR: Acute arterial injuries of the upper extremity. Am J Surg 1963;106:144-151.

Soubbotitch V: Military experiences of traumatic aneurysms. Lancet 1913;2:720-721.

Stewart F: Arteriovenous aneurysm treated by angiography (angiorrhaphy). Abb Surg 1913;57:247-254.

Vollmar J, Krumhaar D: Surgical experience with 200 traumatic arteriovenous fistulae. In Hiertonn T, Rybeck B (eds): Traumatic Arterial Lesions. Stockholm, Försvarets Forskningsanstalt, 1968.

White J, Talbert J, Haller JA Jr: Peripheral arterial injury in infants and children. Ann Surg 1968;167:757-766.

Thromboembolic Complications in Trauma Patients

M. MARGARET KNUDSON

HISTORICAL PERSPECTIVES

In the 1934 volume of the *American Journal of Pathology*, McCartney initially suggested that there was an association between trauma and death from pulmonary embolism (PE), and that this association was particularly strong in patients with lower extremity fractures. This observation was followed by a number of autopsy studies that not only confirmed the relationship between injury and throm-

525

boembolic complications but also further suggested that these thromboembolic events were rarely diagnosed premortem. These preliminary studies stimulated the sentinel work by Freeark, Boswick, and Fardin (1967), who performed venograms on 124 trauma patients, demonstrating venous thrombosis in 35% of fracture patients. Thrombus formation was observed within 24 hours of injury and involved both the injured and the uninjured extremity. More than two thirds of the patients with roentgenographic evidence of deep venous thrombosis (DVT) had no symptoms or physical findings to suggest its occurrence. These authors were among the first to advocate studies to examine the effectiveness of prophylactic measures in reducing postinjury thromboembolism.

PATHOPHYSIOLOGY

The basic factors leading to the development of venous thrombosis have long been defined by the Virchow triad, which includes stasis, endothelial damage, and a prothrombotic state. In the microcirculation, a series of steps linking thrombosis and inflammation has been suggested. This inflammatory process involves platelets, neutrophils, monocytes, and substances released from the activated platelets and neutrophils, such as adenosine diphosphate, neutrophil-activating peptide-2, and cathepsin G. More recently, direct injury to the venous endothelium, induced by the venodilation that occurs under anesthesia, has been implicated as the initiating step in this inflammatory process. The exposed subendothelial surface acts as a nidus for platelets and leukocytes, thus setting the stage for clot formation.

Trauma patients are at risk for thromboembolic complications for a number of reasons. Trauma patients are normally in a hypercoagulable state by the third day after trauma and often have depressed levels of antithrombin. Most trauma patients are immobilized for at least some period, and many are paralyzed to facilitate respiratory care or secondary to neurologic injuries. Additionally, many trauma patients have direct venous injuries either associated with fractures or following penetrating trauma. We have detected lower extremity thrombi by duplex sonography within 12 hours of injury, and other investigators have documented that 6% of post-traumatic pulmonary emboli occur on day 1 following injury. Many of these injured patients are young and have no known pre-existing risk factors for thromboembolism. It is thus imperative that research in this field be directed toward understanding both the pathogenesis and the prevention of post-traumatic thromboembolism.

CLINICAL EPIDEMIOLOGY AND RISK FACTOR ANALYSIS

The overall incidence of post-traumatic DVT is estimated to be between 10% and 20% in patients who are not receiving any method of prophylaxis. The actual incidence will vary with such factors as the age of the patient, the nature of the injuries, the geographic location, and the method used to detect occult DVT. In addition to its association with potentially fatal PE, undetected (and thus untreated) DVT can also result in permanent postphlebitic changes. PE occurs in at least 1% to 2% of injured patients, with an associated mortality as high as 50%. The true incidence of PE is probably much higher, as most PEs in trauma patients are clinically silent. Additionally, a practical method of screening high-risk trauma patients for PE has not been developed. Importantly, many of the deaths attributable to PE occur in trauma patients who would otherwise recover fully from their injuries. This recognition has inspired many clinical investigators to attempt to describe the risk factors associated with the development of post-traumatic thromboembolic complications as the first step in preventing them.

As mentioned, early autopsy studies documented the association between injured patients with fractures and deaths from PE. Burned patients were also found to be at high risk for thromboembolism. More recently, various investigators have identified increased age, the presence of head injury, spinal cord injury with paralysis, and prolonged immobilization as important risk factors for post-traumatic thromboembolism. Direct venous injury, either resulting from the trauma itself or induced by large-caliber venous access devices, has also been implicated. Burch and colleagues (1990) were among the first to warn of the risk of DVT and/or fatal PE following ligation or repair of penetrating iliac vascular injuries. A report from Sue, Davis, and Parks (1995) supports the concept that direct iliac venous injuries are associated with a significant risk for thromboembolic complications.

In a recent study that used venography to identify distal (calf) and proximal (thigh/pelvic) lower extremity DVT, the incidence of DVT was found to be 54% in patients with head injuries and 62% in those with spinal injuries. Sixty-nine percent of injured patients with lower extremity or pelvic fractures who underwent venography had evidence of DVT within 14 to 21 days after the injury. The overall incidence of *proximal* DVT was 18%. Prophylaxis against thromboembolism was not used in any of the patients in this study.

A group of investigators dedicated to the field of thromboembolic research in injured patients recently collaborated in compiling a risk factor assessment scale. The risk factors included underlying conditions, iatrogenic factors, injury-related factors, and age (Table 25–1). Each factor was given a weight, based on the perceived association with the development of DVT/PE (i.e., a weight of 2 was relatively low risk and a score of 4 represented the highest risk factors). When adding up the weighted scores for each patient, a trauma patient with a score of 5 or greater was considered at high risk for thromboembolic complications and a candidate for prophylaxis. Further research by this group, using a prospective study, confirmed that five of these factors were significantly associated with the development of post-traumatic DVT. Patients with one or more of these five factors had an overall rate of DVT at 10% despite aggressive prophylaxis. It should be noted that although the authors of this particular study did not find spinal cord injury to be a significant risk factor, this likely represents a type II statistical error due to a low number of patients

TABLE 25–1
RISK ASSESSMENT PROFILE

Risk Factors	Points Assigned
Underlying condition	
Obesity*	2
Malignancy	2
Abnormal coagulation	2
History of thromboembolism	3
Iatrogenic factors	
Femoral venous lines	2
Transfusion > 4 units*	2
Operation > 2 hours*	2
Major venous repair	3
Injury-related factors	
Chest AIS > 2	2
Abdomen AIS > 2	2
Head AIS > 2*	2
Spinal fractures	3
Glasgow Coma Scale score < 8	3
Severe lower extremity fracture*	4
Pelvic fracture	4
Spinal cord injury	4
Age (yr)	
40-59	2
60-74	3
≥75	4

*Factors found to be *significantly* associated with deep venous thrombosis/pulmonary embolism on subsequent prospective analysis.
AIS, Abbreviated Injury Severity Score.
From Greenfield LJ, Proctor MC, Rodriguez JL, et al: Post-traumatic thromboembolic prophylaxis. J Trauma 1997;42:100-103.

(seven total) enrolled with this injury. All other studies have included patients with spinal cord injuries as among the highest risk patients, with rates of DVT approaching 80% and PE rates at 5%. In fact, PE is one of the most common causes of death following spinal cord injury.

PROPHYLACTIC MEASURES

Definitive randomized controlled clinical studies on prophylactic measures in trauma patients with multiple injuries do not exist. Unlike other surgical patients with isolated disease (e.g., hip-replacement patients and colectomy patients), the injured patients are a heterogeneous group and difficult to "categorize." They can have isolated injuries or any combination of injuries, making stratification extremely difficult. Additionally, many patients are excluded from one type of prophylactic measure or another by the very nature of their injuries. For example, bilateral leg compression devices cannot be used with external fixators, and some head-injured patients cannot receive anticoagulants. Considering all of these factors, a large multicenter trial with thousands of patients and defined endpoints would be needed to definitively answer the questions of which trauma patients need prophylaxis and which prophylactic measures are effective for a given combination of traumatic injuries. To date, no funding source for this important study has been identified. However, several smaller prospective studies on injured patients have been attempted, and recommendations can be made based on the best available data.

Prophylactic measures can generally be divided into two categories: mechanical and pharmacologic. Mechanical measures are aimed at reducing stasis, whereas drug therapy attempts to alter some part of the extrinsic clotting system. An extreme example of a mechanical measure is a "prophylactic" vena cava filter (VCF), placed before the development of PE/DVT in a high-risk patient. Each of these methods is described in the following sections.

Mechanical Prophylactic Devices

The mechanical devices, which vary from a simple elastic stocking to a full-length sequential compression sleeve, are attractive because of their safety. Few if any complications can be attributed to the use of these devices if they are properly fit according to the directions supplied by the manufacturer for each patient and used appropriately. The only real "complication" is the lack of compliance in patients who are awake enough to remove the devices. Despite their widespread use, however, there are no level I trials demonstrating protection

from DVT/PE in trauma patients using any type of mechanical device. Knudson and colleagues (1991) demonstrated that the sequential pneumatic compression device (SCD) was more effective than no prophylaxis in head-injured patients, but not in trauma patients with other injuries. In another study, which included trauma patients without orthopedic injuries, 62 were randomized to wear calf-thigh sequential pneumatic compression and 62 wore plantar compression devices ("foot pumps") only. DVT developed in 21% of the patients wearing the plantar device and in 6.5% of those wearing the calf-thigh device ($P = .009$). Studies by Ginzburg and colleagues (2001) and Knudson and colleagues (1996) have demonstrated clearly that compression devices are less effective than low-molecular-weight heparin (LMWH) in preventing thromboembolic complications after trauma. No data exist on the use of mechanical devices combined with anticoagulant therapy in patients with multiple injuries, and there is no documented benefit in compressing only one leg or an arm, in hopes of stimulating fibrinolytic activity. Based on the current available data, trauma patients who are considered at risk for DVT/PE and who cannot safely be given an anticoagulant drug should receive bilateral whole leg pneumatic compression. Anything short of that should be considered inadequate protection.

Unfractionated Heparin

Of all the methods of prophylaxis, low-dose unfractionated heparin (LDUH, 5000 units given subcutaneously 2 hours before surgery and then every 12 hours for 7 days postoperatively) has been the most widely studied and the most effective method of preventing thromboembolic complications in surgical patients. In 20 trials in which more than 8000 general surgery patients were enrolled, LDUH reduced the incidence of leg DVT from 25% to 8% and consistently reduced the incidence of *fatal* PE by 50%. Unfortunately, in patients undergoing elective hip and knee surgery, in which the risk of proximal DVT is more than 30% and fatal PE up to 6%, LDUH does not offer sufficient protection. Similarly, in trauma patients, LDUH does not appear to be any more effective than no prophylaxis, and its use in trauma patients as the sole method of protection should be discouraged.

Low-Molecular-Weight Heparin

LMWHs are fragments of unfractionated heparin, induced by a controlled enzymatic or chemical depolymerization process that yields chains of glycosaminoglycans with a mean molecular weight of around 5000. These shorted chains retain their anticoagulant activity by their ability to interact with antithrombin but have relatively less activity against thrombin and platelets. LMWH has a more predictable anticoagulant response than LDUH because of increased bioavailability, longer half-life, and dose-independent clearance. Thus, LMWH results in improved anticoagulant activity while causing less bleeding. In hip and knee replacement surgery, LMWH has been demonstrated to be highly effective in preventing DVT/PE even when given postoperatively.

To date, only the LMWH enoxaparin (Lovenox) has been studied in trauma patients. However, two large prospective studies have documented the effectiveness of the LMWH enoxaparin in preventing posttraumatic thromboembolism. Geerts and colleagues (1994) compared LDUH with LMWH (30 mg given subcutaneously every 12 hours), both started within 36 hours after injury, in 344 major trauma patients without frank intracranial bleeding. Bilateral contrast venography was performed between postinjury days 10 and 14. The proximal DVT rate was 15% with LDUH and 6% with LMWH (risk reduction with LMWH of 58%, $P = .01$). The overall rate of major bleeding was less than 2% with no significant differences between the groups, thus demonstrating both the efficacy and the safety of LMWH in trauma patients. The study by Knudson and colleagues (1996) included 372 patients with multiple trauma and compared LMWH to mechanical compression. Patients were followed with serial duplex ultrasound examinations. Of the 120 patients who were randomized to receive LMWH, only 1 developed DVT by ultrasound (0.8%). In the mechanical compression group (199 patients), the incidence of DVT was 2.5%. Only one patient had a major bleeding complication with LMWH. Although LMWH was withheld in patients with injuries to the spleen and/or liver who were being managed without operation, recent data suggest that LMWH can be given safely in these situations, without inducing bleeding. In patients with major head injury and evidence of bleeding on a head computed tomographic (CT) scan, LMWH is generally withheld until the injury has been demonstrated to be stable. For now then, LMWH is considered the most effective form of prophylaxis against DVT/PE in trauma patients and it should be initiated once bleeding is under control and early postinjury coagulopathy has been corrected.

Prophylactic Vena Cava Filters

The effectiveness of a VCF in the prevention of PE in patients with proximal DVT has been well established. Traditionally, these filters have been placed in patients with acute proximal DVT or a recent PE who have a contraindication to anticoagulation. Filters can be placed percutaneously with relative ease and have long-term patency rates of more than 95%. Some trauma surgeons have advocated the *prophylactic* placement of a VCF in high-risk trauma patients, especially in those patients who have relative contraindications to anticoagulation. A recently described technique of placing Inferior Vena Cava (IVC) filters at the bedside using ultrasound guidance makes it even easier to advocate for an aggressive approach in critically injured patients.

The problems associated with the use of IVC filters in trauma patients include the following:

1. *Recurrent PE:* Despite the presence of a filter, recurrent PE occurs in 3% of trauma patients. This complication may result from filter tilt or strut malposition and has been fatal in a few reported injured patients.

2. *DVT:* An IVC filter does nothing to prevent DVT and, in fact, may promote thrombosis. In studies reported by Rodriquez and colleagues (1996), 10% of injured patients who had a prophylactic filter demonstrated caval thrombosis and 50% of these patients had long-term lower extremity edema.

3. *Permanence:* Because all currently marketed VCFs are designed to be permanently implanted, patients are at risk for complications for their lifetime. In addition to filter-associated thromboembolic events and filter migration, complications with vascular access procedures including trapping of the guidewire in the filter have been described.

4. *Timing:* We and others have documented PE as early as 12 to 24 hours postinjury. In the study by Owings and colleagues (1997), 4 (6%) of 63 patients had embolism within 1 day of their trauma. It would be highly unlikely that a prophylactic filter would be placed within such a narrow time frame in patients with multiple trauma who are in need of various other procedures to address their injuries.

No data support the routine use of prophylactic VCFs in high-risk trauma patients. Their use should be restricted to the occasional injured patients who are at prolonged exceedingly high risk for PE, as described in Table 25–1, and in whom no other prophylactic measures can be used.

DIAGNOSIS AND TREATMENT OF POST-TRAUMATIC THROMBOEMBOLIC COMPLICATIONS

Most venous thrombi are clinically silent, presumably because they do not totally obstruct the vein and because of the existence of collateral circulation. Even when symptoms do develop, they are nonspecific and may include pain, swelling, or fever. In trauma patients, these symptoms may be totally overlooked or attributed to bone or soft tissue injury. In most trauma patients, DVT is clinically occult. The symptoms associated with PE depend on the quantity of the embolus involved and the cardiopulmonary status of the patient. Signs and symptoms may include chest pain, dyspnea, tachypnea, anxiety, cyanosis, and fever. Arterial blood gas analyses may reveal hypoxia and an acute decrease in carbon dioxide. Unfortunately, the first sign of PE in many injured patients is sudden death.

For many years, the standard diagnostic test for DVT was ascending phlebography (venography). Venography can reliably detect both proximal (pelvic, thigh, popliteal) and distal (calf) thrombosis. Side effects include allergic reactions to the contrast, renal toxicity, and a 2% to 3% incidence of contrast-induced DVT. Additionally, venography cannot easily be repeated and is thus impractical for surveillance in high-risk patients. Thrombi have also been visualized incidentally during computerized scanning of the abdomen or pelvis performed for other indications. Recently, duplex ultrasound (color flow Doppler [CFD] imaging) has become the method of choice for detecting DVT in many centers. CFD imaging allows information on flow to be overlaid onto the real time two-dimensional image of the vein. Venous sonography is 90% sensitive (100% specific) in detecting proximal DVT in symptomatic patients, but the sensitivity drops significantly in asymptomatic patients, most likely related to the small size of the clot in this latter group of patients. The most reliable sign of DVT is lack of compressibility of the vein on ultrasound imaging (Fig. 25–1). Other signs of acute DVT include the loss of flow augmentation with the Valsalva maneuver or with muscle contraction and the presence of a homogenous thrombus with low echogenicity. The involved vein is distended and noncompressible, with decreased or absent flow and no collateral channels. The limitations of color duplex sonography include the difficulty in imaging pelvic veins and the fact that the quality of the examination is highly dependent on the experience and expertise of the sonographer.

We have performed venous ultrasound examinations on hundreds of trauma patients during our research studies investigating thromboembolism prophylaxis. DVT detected

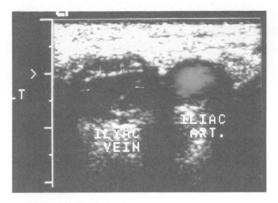

■ **FIGURE 25-1**
Appearance of a clot in the iliac vein by color flow duplex sonography. ■

via ultrasound was the main outcome measure in three prospective studies on trauma patients at our center, and we have been impressed with our ability to detect clinically silent DVT with surveillance scanning. Our results have been confirmed by other investigators, in which color flow imaging surveillance in high-risk trauma patients revealed an overall DVT incidence of between 10% and 18%. Interestingly, up to 30% of the cases of DVT involved the upper extremity, an area not routinely studied with venography. Some authors have argued that there is no need to detect clinically occult DVT, and that the number of cases detected does not justify the expense of surveillance. Most would agree, however, that given the incomplete protection offered by available methods of prophylaxis, some type of surveillance is warranted in extremely high-risk trauma patients (see Fig. 24–3). Treatment of occult DVT is most likely the key factor contributing to the low incidence in of PE in our center and in other centers that perform venous imaging liberally in trauma patients.

Pulmonary angiography remains the gold standard for the diagnosis of pulmonary emboli. Ventilatory-perfusion scans have not been useful in trauma patients, primarily because few trauma patients at risk for PE have a normal chest x-ray film. Additionally, the risks associated with full-dose anticoagulation in injured patients are significant, and the diagnosis must be secured by the most sensitive and specific study. Pulmonary angiography

requires transportation to the radiology suite, and there is the potential for allergic reactions, contrast-induced nephropathy, or vascular injuries during the procedure. Combining noninvasive diagnostic tests has been advocated for critically ill patients who cannot be moved out of the intensive care unit. For example, the combination of a positive ultrasound of the lower extremities and a transthoracic echocardiogram showing right ventricular hypokinesis is pathognomonic for PE. Whole-blood D-dimer levels are always elevated in patients with thrombosis, but this test is not very specific. Still, the combination of a normal D-dimer level and a negative venous ultrasound examination virtually rules out PE. Recently, calculation of the late pulmonary dead space fraction, calculated from the CO_2 expirogram, was found to be valuable as a bedside screening technique for detection of PE.

Spiral CT of the chest with contrast is another excellent screening tool for PE. This study is most sensitive (90%) in detecting emboli that are located in the proximal pulmonary vascular tree. In the presence of a positive CT scan, anticoagulant therapy should be initiated immediately (Fig. 25–2). If more distal emboli are suspected and the initial CT scan is negative, pulmonary angiography should be performed. In a recent analysis of 15 combinations of diagnostic tests (spiral CT, lower limb ultrasonography, ventilation-perfusion scintigraphy, pulmonary arteriography, and D-dimer plasma levels), the combination of spiral CT and lower limb ultrasonography was found to be the least morbid and the most cost-effective combination of studies per life saved.

Heparin remains the first line of treatment for both DVT and PE. In patients with DVT, a bolus of heparin (5000 units) is given immediately, followed by a continuous drip of 18 U/kg per hour. The heparin dose is adjusted to keep the partial thromboplastin time twice normal or between 60 and 80 seconds. For PE, especially when accompanied by hypoxia, a bolus of 10,000 units of heparin is initiated, followed by a continuous drip. Alternatively, a fully anticoagulating dose of enoxaparin (1 mg/kg given subcutaneously twice daily) has been found to be effective

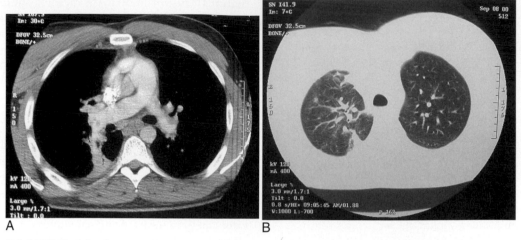

■ **FIGURE 25-2**
A, Spiral computed tomographic scan of the chest demonstrating pulmonary emboli in the right pulmonary artery. *B,* Lung window on the same patient. Note the area of infarction in the right lower lobe. ■

treatment for both DVT and PE. The advantage of enoxaparin is the ability to treat DVT as an outpatient with twice-daily injections performed by the patient. We have used this approach in patients with venous injuries who are anticoagulated for a short period (1 to 2 months). For documented cases of DVT/PE however, we advocate anticoagulation for 6 months, and this is best accomplished by converting the patient from heparin (either unfractionated or LMWH) to Coumadin before discharge from the hospital. In patients with documented DVT and/or PE who cannot receive full-dose anticoagulation because of the nature of their injuries, a VCF should be placed. On rare occasions, trauma patients with life-threatening PE and persistent hypoxia may be candidates for transvenous catheter embolectomy.

OUTCOMES RESEARCH IN PREVENTION OF THROMBOEMBOLISM IN TRAUMA PATIENTS

As mentioned, no large-scale, prospective, randomized trials that definitively establish the safety and effectiveness of any prophylactic measures have been performed in trauma patients. Several investigators have attempted to review all of the data available to assist in the development of outcome-driven guidelines for DVT/PE prophylaxis in injured patients. Brasel, Borgstrom, and Weigelt (1997) used decision-tree analysis to compare three approaches for PE prevention in trauma patients: no intervention, surveillance ultrasound, and VCF. The probabilities in each subtree were taken from available published data. Their findings support the use of surveillance duplex ultrasound examinations, with a cost/PE prevented of $46,300 compared to $93,700 per PE prevented with the use of a prophylactic VCF. However, these costs were based on the assumption that the filter was placed in the radiology suite and that the patient was hospitalized for at least 2 weeks. A VCF may be more cost-effective in patients requiring prolonged hospitalization.

Three other groups have attempted to develop cost-effective guidelines for DVT prevention in trauma patients by employing Cochrane-type principles in literature reviews. These groups include the Eastern Association for the Surgery of Trauma (EAST), the American College of Chest Physicians (ACCP), and the Southern California Evidence-Based Practice Center (SCEPC). The recommendations developed by each of these groups are

TABLE 25–2

SUMMARY OF RECOMMENDATIONS FOR THROMBOEMBOLIC PROPHYLAXIS FOR THREE INDEPENDENT REVIEWS

Group	LDUH	SCD	LMWH	Foot Pump	IVC Filter	Ultrasound
EAST	N/R	Level II	Level II	Level III	Level II	Level II
ACCP	N/R	Level II	Level I	N/A	Level III	Level III
SCEPC	Equal to LMWH	R	Equal to LDUH	N/A	No data	N/A

ACCP, American College of Chest Physicians; EAST, Eastern Association for the Surgery of Trauma; IVC, Inferior Vena Cava; LDUH, low-dose unfractionated heparin; LMWH, low-molecular-weight heparin; N/R, not recommended; R, recommend use; SCD, sequential pneumatic compression device; SCEPC, Southern California Evidence-Based Practice Center.

summarized in Table 25–2. The EAST guidelines recommend LMWH for patients with one of the following injury patterns: (1) pelvic fractures requiring operative fixation or prolonged bed rest (>5 days); (2) complex lower extremity fractures (defined as open fractures or multiple fractures in one extremity) requiring operative fixation or prolonged bed rest (>5 days); and (3) spinal cord injury with complete or incomplete motor paralysis. SCDs were recommended for high-risk patients with head injuries, spinal cord injuries, or pelvis or hip fractures. Foot pumps were given only a level III recommendation, due to insufficient data. Prophylactic VCFs in trauma patients *without* established PE or DVT were recommended only in patients who (1) could not receive anticoagulation because of increased bleeding risk *and* (2) who had one of the following injuries:

- Severe closed head injury (Glasgow Coma Scale score <8)

- Incomplete spinal cord injury with paraplegia or quadriplegia

- Complex pelvic fracture with associated long bone fractures

- Multiple long bone fractures

These recommendations are based on class II/III data. The ACCP recommendations are similar to EAST. However, the SCEPC investigators concluded that there was no evidence that any existing method of prophylaxis was clearly superior to other methods or even to no prophylaxis. They concluded that LMWH was not superior to LDUH and they could

make no conclusions on the role of IVC filters, based on their review of the literature. Although I do not agree with the conclusions drawn by the SCEPC investigators, I do agree that a large, multicenter, prospective trial on prophylactic methods in trauma patients is long overdue.

CURRENT RECOMMENDATIONS AND FUTURE DIRECTIONS

At the San Francisco General Hospital, we have had a long-standing interest in the prevention of thromboembolic complications in trauma patients. Before implementing a standardized protocol for DVT/PE prevention, our incidence of DVT was 10% (established by surveillance ultrasound scanning). Since 1992, we have prospectively followed more than 12,000 patients for the *clinical* development of DVT or PE and used a standardized management algorithm for DVT prophylaxis (Fig. 25–3). Our overall incidence of DVT is 0.003% and the PE rate is 0.002%. The death rate for PE, however, was 17%. In a detailed audit of our patients, we found that 20% of the time, trauma clinical case managers had to intervene to ensure that the house staff ordered the proper prophylactic measure. All cases of DVT/PE are thoroughly reviewed to assess whether the protocol was implemented and followed correctly. In our experience, in most patients in whom thromboembolic complications occurred, prophylactic measures were inappropriately withheld early in the patients' postinjury course. Only one patient with PE

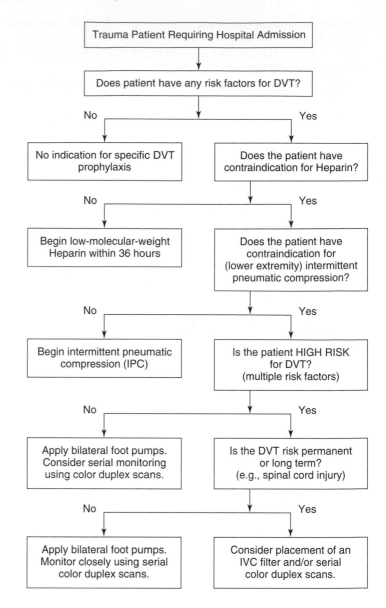

■ **FIGURE 25-3**
Algorithm for deep venous thrombosis prophylaxis in the trauma patient from the San Francisco General Hospital. ■

fell outside of our established risk factors and thus did not receive prophylaxis. We encourage other institutions to prospectively study the guidelines in place at their institution, so that high-quality, evidence-based outcome data will be available for analysis.

Future investigations will include new and potentially more effective drugs that target not only the various steps in the coagulation cascade, but perhaps even the venous wall itself. One such agent, Aristra/Xantidar, a synthetic pentasaccharide that acts as an indirect inhibitor of factor Xa, has recently been shown to be more effective than LMWH in the

prevention of DVT following orthopedic surgery. In the area of mechanical prophylaxis, a prototype removable IVC filter has been developed. This Tulip filter can be used as either a permanent or a temporary device and has been removed from a small number of patients as early as 5 days after insertion without injuring the vena cava. A temporary filter would obviously be more attractive in young trauma patients in whom the risk of developing thromboembolic complications is also temporary. Armed with an appreciation for and a better understanding of thromboembolism in trauma patients, and coupled with effective and safe prophylactic measures, we should be able to offer our future trauma patients protection from both the morbidity of DVT and the risk of a premature death from PE.

REFERENCES

Anderson JT, Owings JT, Goodnight JE: Bedside noninvasive detection of acute pulmonary embolism in critically ill surgical patients. Arch Surg 1999;134:869-875.

Brasel KJ, Borgstrom DC, Weigelt JA: Cost-effective prevention of pulmonary embolus in high-risk trauma patients. J Trauma 1997;42:456-462.

Burch JN, Richardson RJ, Martin RR, Mattox KL: Penetrating iliac vascular injuries: recent experience with 233 consecutive patients. J Trauma 1990;30:1450-1990.

Claget GP, Anderson FA, Geerts W, Heit JA, Knudson MM et al: Prevention of venous thromboembolism. Chest 1998;114:531S-560S.

Coon WW: Risk factors in pulmonary embolism. Surg Gynecol Obstet 1976;143:385-390.

Elliott CG, Dudney TMN, Egger M, et al: Calf-thigh sequential pneumatic compression compared with plantar venous pneumatic compression to prevent deep-vein thrombosis after non-lower extremity trauma. J Trauma 1999;47:25-32.

Freeark RJ, Boswick J, Fardin R: Posttraumatic venous thrombosis. Arch Surg 1967;95:567-573.

Gearhart MM, Luchette FA, Proctor MA, et al: The risk assessment profile score identified trauma patients at risk for deep vein thrombosis. Surgery 2000;128:631-640.

Geerts WH, Code KI, Jay RM, et al: A prospective study of venous thromboembolism after major trauma. N Engl J Med 1994;331:1601-1606.

Merli G, Geerts W, Ginzburg E, et al: for the Spinal Cord Injury Thromboprophylaxis Investigators: Prevention of venous thromboembolism in the acute treatment phase after spinal cord injury: A randomized multicenter trial comparing low-dose heparin plus intermittent pneumatic compression with Enoxaparin. J Trauma 2003; 54:1116-1126.

Knudson MM, Lewis FR, Clinton A et al: Prevention of venous thromboembolism in trauma patients. J Trauma 1994;37:480-487.

Knudson MM, Morabito D, Paiement GD, Shackleford S: Use of low-molecular-weight heparin in preventing thromboembolism in trauma patients. J Trauma 1996;41:446-459.

McCartney JS: Pulmonary embolism following trauma. Am J Pathol 1934;10:709-710.

Meredith JW, Young JS, O'Neil EA, et al: Femoral catheters and deep venous thrombosis: a prospective evaluation with venous duplex sonography. J Trauma 1993;35:187.

Millward SF, Bhargava A, Aquino J, et al: Gunther Tulip filter: preliminary clinical experience with retrieval. JVIR 2000;11:75-82.

Owings JT, Kraut E, Battistella F et al: Timing of occurrence of pulmonary embolism in trauma patients. Arch Surg 1997;132;862-867.

Roergs FB, Cipolli MD, Velmahos GC, et al: Practice guidelines for the prevention of venous thromboembolism in trauma patients: The EAST Practice Management Guidelines Work Group. J Trauma 2002;53:142-164.

Rodriquez JL, Lopez JM, Proctor MC, et al: Early placement of prophylactic vena caval filters in injured patients at high risk for pulmonary embolism. J Trauma 1996;40:797-804.

Rogers FB, Cipolle MD, Velmahos G, et al: Practice management guidelines for the prevention of venous thromboembolism in trauma patients: The EAST practice management guidelines work group. J Trauma 2002;53(1): 142-164.

Rogers FB, Shackford ST, Ricci MA, et al: Routine prophylactic vena cava filter insertion in severely injured trauma patients decreases the incidence of pulmonary embolism. J Am Coll Surg 1995;180:641-647.

Sevitt S, Gallagher N: Venous thrombosis and pulmonary embolism: a clinico-pathological study in injured and burned patients. Br J Surg 1960;48:475-488.

Sue LP, Davis JW, Parks SN: Iliofemoral venous injuries: an indication for prophylactic caval filter placement. J Trauma 1995;39:693-695.

Turpie AGG, Gallus AS, Hoek JA: A synthetic pentasaccharide for the prevention of deep vein thrombosis after total hip replacement. N Engl J Med 2001;344:619-625.

Van Erkel AR, van Rossum AB, Bloem JL, et al: Spiral CT angiography for suspected pulmonary embolism: a cost-effectiveness analysis. Radiology 1996;201:29-36.

Velmahos GC, Kern JK, Chan LS et al: Prevention of venous thromboembolism after injury: an evidence-based report. J Trauma 2000:49:132-144.

THE RICH
REFERENCE COLLECTION

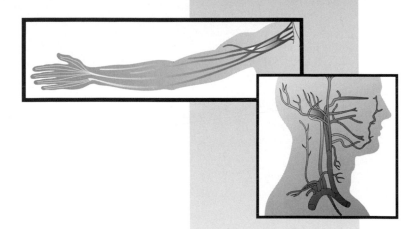

26

Rich's Historic Collection of Vascular References

Aaland M, Bryan FC, Sherman R: Two dimensional echocardiogram in hemo-dynamically stable victims of penetrating precordial trauma. Am Surg 1994;60:412-415.

Aarabi B, McQueen JD: Traumatic internal carotid occlusion at the base of the skull. Surg Neurol 1978;10:233-236.

Abbe R: The surgery of the hand. N Y Med J 1894.

Abbott JA, Cousineau M, Cheitlin M, et al: Late sequelae of penetrating cardiac wounds. J Thorac Cardiovasc Surg 1978;75:510-518.

Abbott WM, Darling RC: Axillary artery aneurysms secondary to crutch trauma. Am J Surg 1973;125:515-520.

Abdo F, Massad M, Slim M, et al: Wandering intravascular missiles: Report of five cases from the Lebanon war. Surgery 1988;103:376-380.

Abdul-Razek MS, Mnaymneh W, Yacoubian HD: Acute injuries of peripheral arteries with associated bone and soft tissue injury. J Trauma 1973;13:907-910.

Abouljoud M: Arterial injuries of the thoracic outlet: A ten-year review. Am Surgeon 1993;59:590-595.

Accola KD, Feliciano DV, Mattox KL, et al: Management of injuries to the superior mesenteric artery. J Trauma 1986;26:313-317.

Accola KD, Feliciano DV, Mattox KL, et al: Management of injuries to the suprarenal aorta. Am J Surg 1987;154:613-618.

Adar R, Bass A, Walden R: Five years' experience in general and vascular surgery in a university hospital. Ann Surg 1982;196:725-729.

Adar R, Nerubay J, Katznelson A: Management of acute vascular injuries. J Cardiovasc Surg 1970;11:435-439.

Adar R, Schramek A, Khodadadi J, et al: Arterial combat injuries of the upper extremity. J Trauma 1980;20:297-302.

Adebonojo SA: Management of chest trauma: A review. West Afr J Med 1993; 12:122-132.

Adinolfi MF, Hardin WD, O'Connell RC, Kerstein MD: Amputations after vascular trauma in civilians. South Med J 1983;76:1241-1248.

Adkins RB Jr, Bitseff EL Jr, Meacham PW: Abdominal vascular injuries. South Med J 1985;78:1152-1160.

Adkins RB, Whiteneck JM, Woltering EA: Penetrating chest wall and thoracic injuries. Am Surg 1985;51:140-148.

Agee CK, Metzler MH, Churchill RJ, Mitchell FL: Computed tomographic evaluation to exclude traumatic aortic disruption. J Trauma 1992;33:876-881.

Agnew D II: The Principles and Practice of Surgery. Philadelphia, JB Lippincott Co, 1978.

Agrwal N, Shah PM, Clauss RH, et al: Experience with 115 civilian venous injuries. J Trauma 1982;22:827-832.

Aitken RJ, Matley PJ, Immelman EJ: Lower limb vein trauma: A long-term clinical and physiological assessment. Br J Surg 1989;76:585-588.

Akins CW, Buckley MJ, Daggett W, et al: Acute traumatic disruption of the thoracic aorta: A ten-year experience. Ann Thorac Surg 1981;31:305-309.

Akins EW, Carmichael MJ, Hill JA, Mancuso AA: Preoperative evaluation of he thoracic aorta using MRI and angiography. Ann Thorac Surg 1987;44:499-507.

Al Zharani HA: False aneurysm of the abdominal aorta after blunt trauma. Eur J Vasc Surg 1991;5:685-687.

Alberty RE, Goodfried G, Boyden AM: Popliteal artery injury with fracture dislocation of the knee. Am J Surg 1981;142:36-40.

Albo D Jr, Christensen C, Rasmussen BL: Massive liver trauma involving the suprarenal vena cava. Am J Surg 1969;118:960-963.

Albrik MH, Rodriguez E, England GJ, et al: Importance of designated thoracic trauma surgeons in the management of traumatic aortic transection. South Med J 1994;87:497-501.

Alexander EL, Szentpetery S, Greenfield L: Posttraumatic thoracic aortic aneurysm associated with a diaphragmatic hernia. Ann Thorac Surg 1985;40:195-198.

Alexander JJ, Imbembo AL: Aorta-vena cava fistula. Surgery 1989;105:1-12.

Ali IS, Fitzgerald PG, Gillis DA, Lau HYC: Bunt traumatic disruption of the thoracic aorta: A rare injury in children 10-year-old. J Pediatr Surg 1992;27:1281-1284.

Ali J, Vanderby B, Purcell C: The effect of the pneumatic antishock garment (PASG) on hemodynamics, hemorrhage, and survival in penetrating thoracic aortic injury. J Trauma 1991;31:846-851.

Allen MJ, Stirling AJ, Crawshaw CW, Barnes MR: Intracompartmental pressure monitor of leg injuries: An aid to management. J Bone Joint Surg 1985;67-B:53-57.

Allen MJ, White GH, Harris JP, et al: Iatrogenic vascular trauma associated with intra-aortic balloon pumping: Identification of risk factors. Am Surg 1993;59:813-817.

Allen RE, Blaisdell FW: Injuries to the inferior vena cava. Surg Clin North Am 1972;52:699-710.

Allen TR, Franklin JD, Withers EH, Davis JL: Extremity salvage utilizing microvascular free tissue transfer. Surgery 1981;90:1047-1054.

Allen TW, Reul GJ, Morton JR, Beall AC Jr: Surgical management of aortic trauma. J Trauma 1972;12:862-868.

Alpert J, Bhaktan EK, Gielchinsky I: Vascular complications of intra-aortic balloon counterpulsation. Arch Surg 1976;111:1190-1195.

Alpert J, O'Donnell JA, Parsonnet V, et al: Clinically recognized limb ischemia in the neonate after umbilical artery catheterization. Am J Surg 1980;140:413-418.

Alpert J, Parsonnet V, Goldenkranz RJ, et al: Limb ischemia during intra-aortic balloon pumping: Indication for femoro-femoral crossover graft. J Thorac Cardiovasc Surg 1980;79:729-734.

Alsofrom DJ, Marcus NH, Seigel RS, et al: Shotgun pellet embolization from the chest to the middle cerebral arteries. J Trauma 1982;22:155-157.

Althaus SJ, Keskey TS, Harker CP: Percutaneous placement of self expanding stent for acute traumatic arterial injury. J Trauma 1996;41:145-148.

Amato JJ, Billy LJ, Gruber RP, et al: Vascular injuries: An experimental study of high and low velocity missile wounds. Arch Surg 1970;101:167-174.

Amato JJ, Billy LJ, Gruber RP, Rich NML: Temporary cavitation in high velocity pulmonary missile injury. Ann Thor Surg 1974;18:565-570.

Amato JJ, Billy LJ, Lawson NS, Rich NM: High velocity missile injury. Am J Surg 1974;127:454-459.

Amato JJ, Rich NM: Temporary cavity effects in blood vessel injury by high velocity missiles. J Cardiovasc Surg 1972;13:147-155.

Amato JJ, Rich NM, Billy LJ, et al: High velocity arterial injury: A study of the mechanism of injury. J Trauma 1971;11:412-416.

Amato JJ, Syracuse D, Seaver PR Jr, Rich NM: Bone as a secondary missile: An experimental study in the fragmenting of bone by high missiles. J Trauma 1989;29:609-612.

Amato JJ, Vanecko RM, Yao JST, Weinberg M Jr: Emergency approach to the subclavian and innominate vessels. Ann Thorac Surg 1969;8:537-541.

Amin A, Alexander JB, O'Malley KF, Doolin E. Blunt abdominal aortic trauma in children: Case report. J Trauma 1993;34:293-297.

Amine ARC, Sugar O: Repair of severed brachial plexus: A plea to emergency room physicians. JAMA 1976;235:1039.

Ammons MA, Moore EE, Moore FA, Hopeman AR: Intra-aortic balloon pump for combined myocardial contusion and thoracic aortic rupture. J Trauma 1990;30:1606-1608.

Anamah NV, Konstam PG: Traumatic dissecting aneurysm of the abdominal aorta. Br J Surg 1965;52:981-982.

Anastasia LF: Traumatic disruption of the thoracic aorta treated with external shunt. Am J Surg 1970;120:810-812.

Anderson RJ, Hobson RW II, Lee BC, et al: Reduced dependency on arteriography for penetrating extremity trauma: Influence of wound location and non-invasive vascular studies. J Trauma 1990;30:1059-1065.

Anderson RJ, Hobson RW II, Padberg FT Jr: Reduced dependency on arteriography for penetrating extremity trauma (PET): Influence of wound location and noninvasive studies. J Trauma 1989;29:1024.

Anderson RJ, Hobson RW II, Padberg FT Jr, et al: Penetrating extremity trauma: Identification of patients at high-risk requiring arteriography. J Vasc Surg 1990;11:544-548.

Andrade-Alegre R, Mon L: Subxiphoid pericardial window in the diagnosis of penetrating cardiac trauma. Ann Thorac Surg 1994;58:1139-1141.

Anfossi A, Bertoglio C, Iurilli L, et al: Delayed development and rupture of an aortic aneurysm after closed abdominal trauma. J Cardiovasc Surg 1987; 28:35-37.

Annandale T: Traumatic popliteal arteriovenous aneurysm treated successfully by ligature of the popliteal artery and vein. Lancet 1875;1:568.

Anthopoulos LP, Johnson JB, Spellman M: Arteriovenous fistula in multiple saccular arterial aneurysms of a finger, following childhood human bite. Angiology 1965;16:89.

Anton GE, Hertzer NR, Beven EG, et al: Surgical management of popliteal aneurysms: Trends in presentation, treatment, and results from 1952 to 1984. J Vasc Surg 1986;3:125-134.

Antonovic R, Rosch J, Dotter CT: Complications of percutaneous transaxillary catheterization for arteriography and selective chemotherapy. Am J Roentgenol 1976;126:386-393.

Antunes MJ: Acute traumatic rupture of the aorta: Repair by simple aortic cross-clamping. Ann Thorac Surg 1987;44:257-259.

Antunes MJ, Fernandes LE, Oliveira JM: Ventricular septal defects and arteriovenous fistulas, with and without valvular lesions, resulting from penetrating injury of the heart and aorta. J Thorac Cardiovasc Surg 1988; 95:902-907.

Antyllus. Oribasius 4:52 (Daemberg Edition). Cited by: Olser. Lancet 1915;1:949.

Appelbaum A, Karp RB, Kirklin JW: Surgical treatment for closed thoracic aortic injuries. J Thorac Cardiovasc Surg 1976;71:458-460.

Applebaum R, Yellin AE, Weaver FA, et al: Role of routine arteriography in blunt lower-extremity trauma. Am J Surg 1990;160:221.

Aprahamina C, Thompson BM, Towne JB, Darin JC: The effect of a paramedic system on mortality open intra-abdominal vascular trauma. J Trauma 1983;23:687-690.

Arajarvi E, Santavirta S: Chest injuries sustained in severe traffic accidents by seatbelt wearers. J Trauma 1989;29:37-41.

Arajarvi E, Santavirta S, Tolonen J: Aortic ruptures in seat belt wearers. J Thorac Cardiovasc Surg 1989;98:355-361.

Archambault R, Archambault HA, Mizeres NJ: Rupture of the thoracoacromial artery and anterior dislocation of the shoulder. Am J Surg 1959;97:782-783.

Armstrong K, Sfeir R, Rice J, Kerstein M: Popliteal vascular injuries and war: Are Beirut and New Orleans similar? J Trauma 1988;28:836-839.

Arnon RG, Allen RG: Traumatic aortic aneurysm in a child. J Pediatr Surg 1981;16:72-74.

Arom KV, Richardson JD, Webb G, et al: Subxyphoid pericardial window in patients with suspected traumatic pericardial tamponade. Ann Thorac Surg 1977;23:545-549.

Aronstam EM, Gomez AC, O'Connell TJ, Geiger JP: Recent surgical and pharmacologic experience with acute dissecting and traumatic aneurysms. J Thorac Cardiovasc Surg 1970;59:231-238.

Aronstam EM, Strader LD, Geiger JP, Gomez AC: Traumatic left ventricular aneurysms. J Thorac Cardiovasc Surg 1970;59:239-242.

Artz T, Huffer JM: A major complication of the modified Bristow procedure for recurrent dislocation of the shoulder. J Bone Joint Surg 1972;54-A:1293-1296.

Asensio J, Hanpeter D, Demetriades D: The Futility of Liberal Utilization of Emergency Department Thoracotomy: Proceedings of the American Association for the Surgery of Trauma, 58th Annual Meeting. 1998, p 210.

Asensio J, Ierardi R: Exsanguination: Evolving issues in emergency trauma. Emerg Care Q 1991;9:59-75.

Asensio J, Murray J, Demetriades D: Penetrating cardiac injuries: A prospective study of variables predicting outcomes. JACS 1998;186:24-34.

Asensio JA: Exsanguination from penetrating injuries. Trauma Q 1989;16:1-25.

Asensio JA, Berne JD, Chahwan S, et al: Traumatic injury to the superior mesenteric artery. Am J Surg 1999;178:235-239.

Asensio JA, Berne JD, Demetriades D: One hundred five penetrating cardiac injuries. J Trauma 1998;44:1073-1082.

Asensio JA, Britt LD, Borzotta A: Multi-institutional experience with the management of superior mesenteric artery injuries. J Am Coll Surg 2001;193:354-366.

Asensio JA, Chahwan S, Hanpeter D. Operative management and outcome of 302 abdominal vascular injuries: AAST-OIS Correlates well with mortality. Am J Surg 2000;180:528-534.

Asensio JA, Forno W, Gambaro E, et al: Abdominal vascular injuries: The trauma surgeon's challenge. Anales Chirurgiae Gynaecol 2000;89:71-78.

Asensio JA, Lejarraga M: Abdominal vascular injury. In Demetiades D, Asensio JA (eds). Trauma Handbook. Austin, Tex, Landes Bioscience, 2000, pp 356-362.

Asensio JA, Stewart BM, Murray J: Penetrating cardiac injuries. Surg Clin North Am 1996;76:685-724.

Asensio JA, Voystock J, Khatri VJ, Kerstein MD: Toracotomia en el Centro de Urgencias. Procedimientos en el Paciente Critico 1993;III:337-341.

Asensio JA, Wall M, Minel J: Practice management guidelines for emergency department thoracotomy. J Am Coll Surg 2001;193:303-309.

Asfaw I, Arbulu A: Penetrating wounds of the pericardium and heart. Surg Clin North Am 1977;57:37-48.

Asfaw I, Ramadan H, Talbert JG, Arbulu A: Double traumatic rupture of the thoracic aorta. J Trauma 1985;25:1102-1104.

Ashbell TS, Kleinert HE, Kutz JE: Vascular injuries about the elbow. Clin Orthop 1967;50:107-127.

Ashton F, Slaney G: Arterial injuries in civilian surgical practice. Injury 1970;1:303-314.

Ashworth EM, Daising MC, Glover JL, Reilly MK: Lower extremity vascular trauma. J Trauma 1988;28:329-336.

Assalia A, Schein M: Resuscitation of haemorrhagic shock. Br J Surg 1993;80:213.

Attar S, Ayella RJ, McLaughlin JS: The widened mediastinum in trauma. Ann Thorac Surg 1972;13:435-449.

Aufranc OE, Jones WN, Stewart WG Jr: Common fracture with unusual associated vascular injury. JAMA 1965;191:1073-1075.

Aust JC, Bredenberg CE, Murray DG: Mechanisms of arterial injuries associated with total hip replacement. Arch Surg 1981;116:345-349.

Austin JH, Carsen GM: Acute traumatic hematoma of aorta. J Thorac Cardiovasc Surg 1976;71:321.

Ayella RJ, Hankins JR, Turney SZ, Cowley RA: Ruptured thoracic aorta due to blunt trauma. J Trauma 1977;17:199-205.

Ayres ML, Winspur I: Major injuries and bullet wounds. Injury 1976;7:221-224.

Ayuyao AM, Kaledzi YL, Parsa MH, Freeman HP: Penetrating neck wounds: Mandatory versus selective exploration. Ann Surg 1985;202:563-567.

Baadsgaard SE, Bille S, Egeblad K: Major vascular injury during gynecologic laparoscopy: Report of case and review of published cases. Acta Obstet Gynecol Scand 1986;68:283-285.

Babu SC, Piccorelli GO, Shah PM, et al: Incidence and results of arterial complications among 16,350 patients undergoing cardiac catheterization. J Vasc Surg 1989;10:113-116.

Bacharach JM, Garratt KN, Rooke TW: Chronic traumatic thoracic aneurysm: Report of two cases with the question of timing for surgical intervention. J Vasc Surg 1993;17:780-783.

Baek SM, Brown RS, Shoemaker WC: Cardiac tamponade following wound tract injection. J Trauma 1973;13:85-87.

Baik S, Uku JM, Joo KG: Seat belt injuries to the left common carotid artery and left internal carotid artery. Am J Forens Med Pathol 1988;9:38-39.

Bailey H: Wounds of the neck. In Bailey H (ed): Surgery of Modern Warfare. Edinburgh, E & S Livingston, 1944.

Baillot R, Dontigny L, Verdant A, et al: Penetrating chest trauma: A 20-year experience. J Trauma 1987;27:994-997.

Baillot R, Dontigny L, Verdant A, et al: Intrapericardial trauma: Surgical experience. J Trauma 1989;29:736-740.

Baird RJ, Doran ML: The false aneurysm. Can Med Assoc J 1964;91:281-284.

Baker CC, Thomas AN, Trunkey DD: The role of emergency room thoracotomy on trauma. J Trauma 1980;20:848-855.

Baker MS: Recognition of vascular injury in the trauma patient. Milit Med 1990;155:225.

Baker SP, O'Neill B, Haddon W Jr, Long WB: A method for describing patients with multiple injuries and evaluating emergency care. J Trauma 1974;14:187-196.

Bakker FC, Patka P, Haarman HJ: Combined repair of a traumatic rapture of the aorta an anterior stabilization of a thoracic spine fracture: Case report. J Trauma 1996;40:128-129.

Bakker KW, Gast LF: Retroperitoneal haemorrhage from the superior gluteal artery: A late complication of total hip arthroplasty. Clin Rheumatol 1990;9:249.

Ballance C: The surgery of the heart (Bradshaw Lecture). Lancet 1920;1:1.

Baltsch J, Klose KJ, Gonninger J: Angiography in acute arterial trauma of peripheral vessels and the aorta. Vasa 1987;16:246-250.

Bandt RL, Foley WJ, Fink GH, Regan WJ: Mechanism of perforation of the heart with production of hydropericardium by a venous catheter and its prevention. Am J Surg 2001;33:311-316.

Banks E, Chun J, Weaver FA: Chronic innominate artery dissection after blunt thoracic trauma: Case report. J Trauma 1995;38:975-978.

Barcia PJ, Nelson TG, Whelan TJ: Importance of venous occlusion in arterial repair failure: An experimental study. Ann Surg 1972;175:223-227.

Barcia TC, Livoni JP: Indications for angiography in blunt thoracic trauma. Radiology 1983;147:15-19.

Baret AC, DeLong RP, Tukanowicz SA, Blakemore WS: Transfixation of the aorta accompanied by a Browne-Syndrome: A case report. J Trauma 1958;35:359-362.

Barker NW, Hines EA Jr: Arterial occlusion in the hands and fingers associated with repeated occupational trauma. Proc Staff Meet Mayo Clin 1944;19:345-349.

Barker JE, Knight KR, Romeo R, et al: Targeted disruption of the nitric oxide synthase 2 gene protects against ischaemia/reperfusion injury to skeletal muscle. J Pathol 2001;194:109-115.

Barkun JS, Terazza O, Daignault P, et al: The fate of venous repair after shock and trauma. J Trauma 1988;28:1322-1329.

Barner HB: Sutureless intraluminal aortic prosthesis in traumatic aortic rupture: Is it appropriate? J Trauma 1988;28:1607-1608.

Barnes RW, Petersen JL, Krugmire RB, Strandness DE Jr: Complications of percutaneous femoral arterial catheterization: Prospective evaluation with the Doppler ultrasonic velocity detector. Am J Cardiol 1974;33:259-263.

Barone GW, Kahn MB, Cook JM, et al: Traumatic left renal artery stenosis managed with splenorenal bypass: Case report. J Trauma 1990;30:1594-1596.

Barros D'Sa AAB: A decade of missile-induced vascular trauma. Ann Surg 1981;64:37-44.

Barros D'Sa AAB: Management of vascular injuries of civil strife. Injury 1982;14:51-57.

Barros D'Sa AAB: The Rationale for Arterial and Venous Shunting in the Management. Belfast, Northern Ireland, Grune &Stratton, 1989.

Barros D'Sa AAB, Hassard TH, Livingston RH, Irwin JW: Missile-induced vascular trauma. Injury 1980;12:13-30.

Bass A, Papa M, Morag B, Adar R: Aortic false aneurysm following blunt trauma of the abdomen. J Trauma 1983;23:1072-1073.

Bass A, Allison EJ, Reines HD: Thigh compartment syndrome without lower extremity trauma following application of pneumatic antishock trousers. Ann Emerg Med 1983;12:382-384.

Bassett FH, Houck WS: False aneurysm of profunda femoris artery after subtrochanteric osteotomy and nail-plate fixation. J Bone Joint Surg 1964;46A:583-585.

Bassett FH, Silver D: Arterial injury associated with fractures. Arch Surg 1966;92:13-19.

Batt M, Hassen-Khoudja R, Bayada JM, et al: Traumatic fistula between the aorta and the left renal vein: Case report and review of the literature. J Vasc Surg 1989;9:812-816.

Batzdorf U, Bentson JR, Machleder HI: Blunt trauma to the high cervical carotid artery. Neurosurgery 1979;5:192-201.

Baumgartner F, White GH, White RA, et al: Delayed, exsanguinating pelvic hemorrhage after blunt trauma without bony fracture: Case report. J Trauma 1990;30:1603-1605.

Baxter BT, Moore EE, Synhorst DP, et al: Graded experimental cardiac contusion: Impact on cardiac rhythm, coronary artery flow, ventricular function, and myocardial oxygen consumption. J Trauma 1988;28:1411-1417.

Beall AC Jr: Penetrating wounds of the aorta. Am J Surg 1960;99:770-774.

Beall AC Jr, Arbergast NR, Hallman GL: Complete transection of the thoracic aorta due to rapid deceleration. Am J Surg 1967;114:769-773.

Beall AC Jr, Arbergast NR, Ripepi AC, et al: Aortic laceration due to rapid deceleration. Arch Surg 1969;98:595-601.

Beall AC Jr, Crosthwait RW, Crawford ES, DeBakey ME: Gunshot wounds of the chest: A plea for individualization. J Trauma 1964;4:382.

Beall AC Jr, Diethrich EB, Cooley DA, DeBakey ME: Surgical management of penetrating cardiovascular trauma. South Med J 1967;60:698-704.

Beall AC Jr, Diethrich EB, Crawford HW, et al: Surgical management of penetrating cardiac injuries. Am J Surg 1966;112:686-692.

Beall AC Jr, Diethrich EB, Morris GC Jr, DeBakey ME: Surgical management of vascular trauma. Surg Clin North Am 1966;46:1001-1011.

Beall AC Jr, Gasior RM, Bricker DL: Gunshot wounds of the heart: Changing patterns of surgical management. Ann Thorac Surg 1971;11:523-531.

Beall AC Jr, Harrington OB, Crawford ES, DeBakey ME: Surgical management of traumatic arteriovenous aneurysms. Am J Surg 1963;106:610-618.

Beall AC Jr, Morris GC Jr, Cooley DA: Temporary cardiopulmonary bypass in the management of penetrating wounds of the heart. Surgery 1962;52:330-337.

Beall AC Jr, Ochsner JL, Morris GC Jr, et al: Penetrating wounds to the heart. J Trauma 1961;1:195-207.

Beall AC Jr, Patrick TA, Okies JE, et al: Penetrating wounds of the heart: Changing patterns of surgical management. J Trauma 1972;12:468-473.

Beall AC Jr, Roof WR, DeBakey ME: Successful surgical management of through and through stab wound of the aortic arch. Ann Surg 1962;156:283-286.

Beall AC Jr, Shirkey AL, DeBakey ME: Penetrating wounds of the carotid arteries. J Trauma 1963;3:276-287.

Beattie EJ Jr, Greer D: Laceration of the aorta: Case report of successful repair forty-eight hours after injury. J Thorac Surg 1952;23:293-298.

Beattie EJ Jr, Oldham JB, Ross JA: Superior thyroid arteriovenous aneurysm. Br J Surg 1961;48:456-457.

Beatty RA: Dissecting hematoma of the internal carotid artery following chiropractic cervical manipulation. J Trauma 1977;17:248-249.

Beck CS: Wounds of the heart: The technique of suture. Arch Surg 1926;13:205-227.

Beck CS: Further observations on stab wounds of the heart. Ann Surg 1942;115:698-704.

Beck DE, Robison JG, Hallett JE Jr: Popliteal artery pseudoaneurysm following arthroscopy. J Trauma 1986;26:87-89.

Becker G, Palmaz J, Rees C: Angioplasty-induced dissections in human iliac arteries: Management with Palmaz-balloon–expandable intraluminal stents. Radiology 1990;176:31.

Becker HM, Ramirez J, Echave V, Heberer G: Traumatic aneurysms of the descending thoracic aorta. Ann Vasc Surg 1986;1:196-200.

Becker HM, Wexler J, Frater RW: False aneurysm of aorta secondary to partial occlusion clamp injury diagnosis by nuclear flow study. Chest 1981;80:331-333.

Bednarski JJ, Nayduch DA: Thoracic aorta rupture as a cause of paraplegia: A diagnostic dilemma (case report). J Trauma 1989;29:531-533.

Beebe GW, Bergan JJ, Bergqvist D, et al: Classification and grading of chronic venous disease in the lower limbs. A consensus statement. Eur Vasc Endovasc Surg 1996;12:487-492.

Beebe HG: Complications in Vascular Surgery. Philadelphia, JB Lippincott Co, 1973.

Beel T, Harwood AL: Traumatic rupture of the thoracic aorta. Ann Emerg Med 1980;9:483-486.

Begg JW: Recanalization of autogenous vein graft. Southern Med J 1988;81:1446-1447.

Beggs CW, Helling TS, Evans LL, et al: Evaluation of cardiac injury by two-dimensional echocardiography in patients suffering blunt chest trauma. Ann Emerg Med 1987;16:542-545.

Belcaro G, Nicolaides AN: Pressure index in hypotensive of hypertensive patients. J Cardiovasc Surg 1989;30:614-617.

Beless DJ, Muller DS, Perez H: Aortoiliac occlusion secondary to atherosclerotic plaque rapture as the result of blunt trauma. Ann Emerg Med 1990;19:922-924.

Belkin M, Dunton R, Crombie HD Jr, Lowe R: Preoperative percutaneous intraluminal balloon catheter control of major arterial hemorrhage. J Trauma 1988;28:548-550.

Bell D, Cockshott WP: Angiography of traumatic arterio-venous fistulae. Clin Radiol 1965;16:241-247.

Bell J: Principles of surgery. Discourse 1801;9:4.

Bell KA, Simon BK: Aneurysm of popliteal artery after medial meniscectomy: An unusual complication. South Med J 1979;72:1126-1134.

Bellamy RF: The causes of death in conventional land warfare: Implications for combat casualty care research. Mil Med 1984;149:55-62.

Belley G, Gallix BP, Derossis AM, et al: Profound hypotension in blunt trauma associated with superior gluteal artery rupture without pelvic fracture. J Trauma 1997;43:703-705.

Ben-Menachem Y: Vascular injuries of the extremities: Hazards of unnecessary delays in diagnosis. Orthopedics 1986;9:333-338.

Ben-Menachem Y: Avulsion of the innominate artery associated with fracture of the sternum. Am J Cardiol 1988;150:621-622.

Ben-Menachem Y: Rupture of the thoracic aorta by broadside impacts in road traffic and other collisions: Further angiographic observations. J Trauma 1993;36:363-367.

Ben Hur N, Gemer M, Milwidsky H: Perforating injury of the heart caused by nail fired from a studgun. J Trauma 1964;84:850-853.

Benckart DH, Magovern GJ, Lievler GA, et al: Traumatic aortic transection: Repair using left arterial to femoral bypass. J Cardiac Surg 1989;4:43-49.

Benitez PR, Newell MA: Vascular trauma in drug abuse: Patterns of injury. Ann Vasc Surg 1986;1:175-180.

Benito MC, Garcia F, Fernandez-Quero L, et al: Lesion of the internal carotid artery caused by a car safety belt. J Trauma 1990;30:116-117.

Bennett DE, Cherry JK: The natural history of traumatic aneurysms of the aorta. Surgery 1967;61:516.

Bennett JE: Expanding forearm hematoma after apparent minor injury. Plastic Reconstr Surg 1965;36:622-625.

Benvenuto R, Rodman FS, Glimour J, et al: Composite venous grafts for replacement of the superior vena cava. Arch Surg 1962;84:570-573.

Berendes JN, Bredee JJ, Schipperheyn JJ, Mashhour YAS: Mechanisms of spinal cord injury after cross-clamping of the descending thoracic aorta. Circulation 1982;66:112-116.

Bergan F: Traumatic intimal rupture of the popliteal artery with acute ischemia of the limb in cases with supracondylar fractures of the femur. J Cardiac Surg 1963;4:300-302.

Bergan JJ, Conn J Jr, Trippel OH: Severe ischemia of the hand. Ann Surg 1971;173:301-307.

Bergan JJ, Dean RH, Yao JST: Vascular injuries in pelvic cancer surgery. Am J Obstet Gynecol 1976;124:562-566.

Bergan JJ, Yao JST: Symposium on Venous Problems in Honor of Geza de Takats. Chicago, Year Book Medical Publishers, 1978.

Bergan JJ, Yao JST: Surgery of the Veins. Orlando, Grune & Stratton, 1985.

Bergentz SE, Bergqvist D: Iatrogenic Vascular Injuries. New York: Springer-Verlag, 1989.

Bergentz SE, Hansson LO, Norbäck B: Surgical management of complications to arterial puncture. Ann Surg 1966;164:1021-1026.

Bergin PJ: Aortic thrombosis and peripheral embolization after thoracic gunshot wound by transesophageal echocardiography. Am Heart 1990;119:688-690.

Berglund B, Swanbeck G, Hedin H: Low molecular weight dextran therapy for digital ischemia due to collagen vascular disease. Dermatologica 1981;163:353-357.

Bergman K, Spence L, Wesson D, Dykes E: Thoracic vascular injuries: A post mortem study. J Trauma 1990;30:604-606.

Bergquist D, Takolander R: Aortic occlusion following blunt trauma of the abdomen. J Trauma 1981;21:319-322.

Bergquist D, Carlsson AS, Ericsson BF: Vascular complications after total hip arthroplasty. Acta Orthop Scand 1983;54:157-163.

Berguer R, Feldman AJ, Wilner HI, Lazo A: Arteriovenous vertebral fistulae: Cure by combination of operation and detachable intravascular balloon. Ann Surg 1982;196:65-68.

Berkoff HA, Carpenter EW, Frey CF: Evaluation of balloon tamponade of the abdominal aorta. J Surgery 1971;11:496-500.

Bernheim BM: Surgery of the vascular system. Philadelphia, JB Lippincott Co, 1913.

Bernheim BM: Blood vessel surgery in the war. Surg Gynecol Obstet 1920;30:564-567.

Bertini JE Jr, Flechner SM, Miller P, et al: The natural history of traumatic branch renal artery injury. J Urol 1986;135:228-230.

Bezreh AA: Injuries resulting from hostile action against army aircrew members in flight over Vietnam. Aerospace Med 1970;41:763.

Bhatnagar MK, Smith GS: Trauma in the Afghan Guerilla War: Effects of lack of access to care. Surgery 1989;105:699.

Bickell WH, Shaftan GW, Mattox KL: Intravenous fluid administration and uncontrolled hemorrhage. J Trauma 1989;29:409.

Bickell WH, Wall MJ Jr, Pepe PE, et al: Immediate versus delayed fluid resuscitation for hypotensive patients with penetrating thoracoabdominal trauma. N Engl J Med 1994;331:1105-1109.

Bickham WS: Arteriovenous aneurysm. Ann Surg 1904;39:767-775.

Bigger IA: Heart wounds: A report of seventeen patients operated upon in the Medical College of Virginia Hospitals and discussion of the treatment and prognosis. J Thorac Surg 1939;8:239-253.

Billings KJ, Nasca RJ, Griffin HA: Traumatic arteriovenous fistula with spontaneous closure. J Trauma 1973;13:741-743.

Billroth T: The surgery of the heart (Bradshaw Lecture). Lancet 1920;1-1:73-134.

Billroth T: Wounds of the heart: The technique of suture. Arch Surg 1926;13:205-227.

Billroth T: Historical studies on the nature and treatment of gunshot wounds from the 15th century to the present time. Yale J Biol Med 1931;4:16-36.

Billy LJ, Amato JJ, Rich NM: Aortic injuries in Vietnam. Surgery 1971;70:385-391.

Binet JP, Langlois J, Cormier JM, Saint Florent GD: A case of recent traumatic avulsion of the innominate artery at its origin from the aortic arch: Successful surgical repair with deep hypothermia. J Thorac Cardiovasc Surg 1962;43:670-676.

Binkley FM, Wylie EJ: A new technique for obliteration of cerebrovascular arteriovenous fistulae. Arch Surg 1973;106:524-527.

Birchall D, Fields JM, Chalmers N, Walker MG: Case report: Delayed superficial femoral artery pseudoaneurysm rupture following successful compression therapy. Clin Radial 1997;52:629-630.

Birchard JD, Pichara DR, Brown PM: External iliac artery and lumbosacral plexus injury secondary to an open book fracture of the pelvis: Report of a case. J Trauma 1990;30:906-908.

Birkeland IW, Taylor TK: Major vascular injuries in lumbar disc surgery. J Bone Joint Surg 1969;51B:4-19.

Birnholz JC: Radionuclide angiography in the diagnosis of aortocaval fistula. J Thorac Cardiovasc Surg 1973;65:292-295.

Bisenkov LN, Isamukhamedov T, Panin SM: Heart wound with migration of a bullet into the abdominal aorta. Vestn Khir 1983;131:97-98.

Bishara RA, Pasch AR, Lim LT, et al: Improved results in the treatment of civilian vascular injuries associated with fractures and dislocations. J Vasc Surg 1986;3:707-711.

Bizer L: Peripheral vascular injuries in the Vietnam War. Arch Surg 1969;98:165-166.

Blackford JM, McLaughlin JS: Pseudoaneurysm of the carotid artery. Am Surg 1973;39:257-260.

Blacklay PF, Duggan E, Wood RFM: Vascular trauma. Br J Surg 1987;74:1077-1083.

Blackmore TL, Whelan TJ: Arteriovenous fistula as a complication of gastrectomy. Am J Surg 1965;109:197.

Bladergroen M, Brockman R, Luna G, et al: A twelve-year survey of cervicothoracic vascular injuries. Am J Surg 1989;157:483-486.

Blaisdell FW: Discussion in Buscaglia: Penetrating abdominal vascular injuries. Arch Surg 1969;109:197.

Blaisdell FW, Cooley DA: The mechanism of paraplegia after temporary thoracic aortic occlusion and its relationship to spinal fluid pressure. Surgery 1962;51:351-355.

Blaisdell FW, Hall AD, Lim RC: Aortoiliac arterial substitution utilizing subcutaneous grafts. Ann Surg 1970;172:775-780.

Blake HA, Inmon TW, Spencer FC: Emergency use of antegrade aortography in diagnosis of acute aortic rupture. Ann Surg 1960;152:954-956.

Blakemore AH: Restorative endoaneurysmorrhaphy by vein graft inlay. Ann Surg 1947;126:841-849.

Blakemore AH, Lord JE Jr: A non-suture method of blood vessel anastomosis: Review of experimental study and report of clinical cases. Ann Surg 1945;121:435-453.

Blakemore AH, Lord JW, Stefko PL: The severed primary artery in the war wounded; a non suture method of bridging arterial defects. Surgery 1942;12:488-508.

Blalock A: A successful suture of a wound of the ascending aorta. JAMA 1934;103:1617-1618.

Blalock A, Ravitch MM: Consideration of the non-operative treatment of cardiac tamponade resulting from wounds to the heart. Surgery 1943;14:157-162.

Blanchard DG, Kimura BJ, Dittrich HC, DeMaria AN: Transesophageal echocardiography of the aorta. JAMA 1994;272:546-551.

Bland-Sutton J: A lecture on missiles as emboli. Lancet 1919;1:773-775.

Bland EF, Beebe GW: Missiles in the heart. A twenty-year follow-up report of World War II cases. New Engl J Med 1966;274:1039-1046.

Blatchford JW III, Anderson RW: The evolution of the management of penetrating wounds of the heart. Ann Surg 1985;202:615-623.

Blegvad S, Lippert H, Lund O, et al: Acute delayed surgical treatment of traumatic rupture of the descending aorta. J Cardiovasc Surg 1989;30:559-564.

Blickenstaff KL, Weaver FA, Yellin AE, et al: Trends in management of traumatic vertebral artery injuries. Am J Surg 1989;158:101-106.

Blohmè I, Brynger H: Emergency ligation of the external iliac artery. Ann Surg 1985;201:505-510.

Bloom AI, Sasson T, Ravkind A, Pikarski B-ZJ: Diagnosis of traumatic rupture of the thoracic aorta using dynamic rapid sequence axial computerized tomography. Isr J Med Sci 1995;31:314-320.

Bloom JD, Mozersky DJ, Buckley CG, Hagood CO Jr: Defective limb growth as a complication of catheterization of the femoral artery. Surg Gynecol Obstet 1974;138:524-526.

Blumoff RL, Powell T, Johnson G Jr: Femoral venous trauma in a university referral center. J Trauma 1982;22:703-705.

Blumoff RL, Proctor HJ, Johnson G Jr: Recanalization of a saphenous vein interposition venous graft. J Trauma 1981;21:407-408.

Bodai BI, Smith P, Ward RE: Emergency thoracotomy in the management of trauma: A review. JAMA 1983;249:1891.

Bodily K, Perry JF, Strate R, Fischer RP: The salvageability of patients with posttraumatic rupture of the descending thoracic aorta in a primary trauma center. J Trauma 1977;17:754-760.

Boerhaave H: Cited in Elkin 1941. Aphorismi de Cognoscendis et Curandis Morbis (aphorism 170). 1709.

Bogaert AM, DeScheerder I, Calardyn F: Successful treatment of aortic rupture presenting as a syncope: The role of echocardiography in diagnosis. Int J Cardiology 1987;16:212-214.

Bolanowki PJP, Swaminatham AP, Neville WE: Aggressive surgical management of penetrating cardiac injuries. J Thorac Cardiovasc Surg 1973;66:52-57.

Bolasny BL, Killen DA: Surgical management of arterial injuries secondary to angiography. Ann Surg 1971;174:962-964.

Bole P, Andronaco JT, Purdy R: Superior mesenteric arteriovenous fistula secondary to a gunshot wound. J Cardiac Surg 1973;14:456.

Bole PV, Cortes LE, Munda RT, et al: Repair of false aneurysm of the abdominal aorta. J Trauma 1975;15:255-259.

Bole PV, Katz M, Cohen NH, Clauss RH: Carotid crossover bypass: Cerebral revascularization after ligation of common carotid artery. Cardiovasc Surg 1977;18:533-538.

Bole PV, Munda R, Purdy RT: Traumatic pseudoaneurysms: A review of 32 cases. J Trauma 1976;16:63-70.

Bole PV, Purdy RT, Munda RT, et al: Civilian arterial injuries. Ann Surg 1976;183:13-23.

Bollett AJ: Wounded presidents: 1981 almost repeats the events of 1881. Mil Med 1981;109:19-23.

Bongard F, Dubrow T, Klein S: Vascular injuries in the urban battleground: Experience at a metropolitan trauma center. Ann Vasc Surg 1990;4:415.

Bongard F, Johs SM, Leighton TA, Klein SR: Peripheral arterial shotgun missile emboli: Diagnostic and therapeutic management case reports. J Trauma 1991;31:1426-1431.

Bongard FS, White GH, Klein SR: Management strategy of complex extremity injuries. Am J Surg 1989;158:151-155.

Bongard FS, Wilson SE, Perry MO: Vascular injuries in surgical practice. In Bongard FS, Wilson SE, Perry MO (eds): Norwalk, Conn, Appleton & Lange, 1991.

Boontje AH: Iatrogenic vascular trauma. J Cardiac Surg 1978;19:335-340.

Boontje AH: True aneurysm of the abdominal aorta due to blunt trauma. J Cardiac Surg 1978;19:359-363.

Bordeaux J, Guys JM, Magnan PE: Multiple aneurysms in a seven-year-old child. Ann Vasc Surg 1990;4:26-28.

Borja AR, Lansing AM: Thrombosis of the abdominal aorta caused by blunt trauma. J Trauma 1970;10:499-501.

Borja AR, Lansing AM: Traumatic rupture of the heart: A case successfully treated. J Vasc Surg 1970;171:438-440.

Borlase BC, Metcalf RK, Moora EE: Penetrating wounds to the anterior chest. Analysis of thoracotomy and laparotomy. Am J Surg 1986;6:649.

Borlase BC, Moore EE, Moore FA: The abdominal trauma index: A critical reassessment and validation. J Trauma 1990;30:1340-1344.

Borman KR, Aurbakken CM, Weigelt JA: Treatment priorities in combined blunt abdominal and aortic trauma. Am J Surg 1982;144:728-732.

Borman KR, Jones GH, Snyder WH Jr: A decade of lower extremity venous trauma: Patency and outcome. Am J Surg 1987;154:608-612.

Borman KR, Snyder WH III, Weigelt JA: Civilian arterial trauma of the upper extremity: 11-year experience in 267 patients. Am J Surg 1984;148:796-799.

Boruchow IB, Iyengar R, Jude JR: Injury to ascending aorta root trauma. J Thorac Cardiovasc Surg 1977;73:303-305.

Boruchow IB: Delayed death from aortic root trauma. Ann Thorac Surg 1991;51:317-319.

Bosher LH, Freed TA: The surgical treatment of traumatic rupture of avulsion of the innominate artery. J Thorac Cardiovasc Surg 1967;54:732-739.

Bouchard JF, Lamontagne D: Protection afforded by preconditioning to the diabetic heart against ischaemic injury. Cardiovasc Res 1998;37:82-90.

Bourland WA, Kispert JF, Hyde GL, Kazmers A: Trauma to the proximal superior mesenteric artery: A case report and review of the literature. J Vasc Surg 1992;15:669-674.

Bower TC, Murray MJ, Gloviczki P: Effects of thoracic aortic occlusion and cerebrospinal fluid drainage on regional spinal cord blood flow in dogs: Correlation with neurologic outcome. J Vasc Surg 1989;9:135-144.

Boyd DP, Farha GJ: Arteriovenous fistula and isolated vascular injuries secondary to intervertebral disk surgery: Report of four cases and review of the literature. Ann Surg 1965;161:524-531.

Boyd TF, Strieder JW: Immediate surgery for traumatic heart disease. J Thorac Cardiovasc Surg 1965;50:305-315.

Boyden AM: Personal communication, 1970.

Boyle EM Jr, Canty T Jr, Morgan E, et al: Treating myocardial ischemia-reperfusion injury by targeting endothelial cell transcription. Ann Thor Surg 1999;68:1949-1953.

Bradham GB, Nunn D, Brailsford LE: Successful repair of a bullet wound of the abdominal aorta. Ann Surg 1962;155:86-89.

Bradham RR, Buxton J, Stallworth J: Arterial injury of the lower extremity. Surg Gynecol Obstet 1964;118:995-1000.

Bradham WG, Lewis J, Sewell D, Garrett A: Bullet embolus to the ascending aorta following a gunshot wound to the chest. J Tenn Med Assoc 1991;84:592-593.

Bradley EL III: Management of penetrating carotid injuries: An alternative approach. J Trauma 1973;13:248-255.

Branday JM, Kumar E, Spencer H: Intrapericardial heart and great vessel injuries. West Indian Med J 1984;33:176-119.

Branham HH: Aneurysmal varix of the femoral artery and vein following a gunshot wound. Int J Surg 1890;3:250.

Brantigan CO: Delayed major vessel hemorrhage following tracheostomy. J Trauma 1973;13:235-237.

Brathwaite CE, Rodriguez: Injuries of the abdominal aorta from blunt trauma. Am Surg 1992;58:350-352.

Brathwaite CE, Cilley J, O'Connor W, et al: The pivotal role of transesophageal echocardiography in the management of traumatic thoracic aortic rupture with associated intra-abdominal hemorrhage. Chest 1994;105:1899.

Brawley RK, Murray G, Crisler C, Cameron J: Management of wounds of the innominate, subclavian and axillary blood vessels. Surg Gynecol Obstet 1970;131:1130-1140.

Breaux EP, Dupont J Jr, Alvert HM, et al: Cardiac tamponade following penetrating mediastinal injuries: Improved survival with early pericardiocentesis. J Trauma 1979;19:461-466.

Brener BJ, Couch N: Peripheral arterial complications of left heart catheterization and their management. Am J Surg 1973;125:521-526.

Brengman ML, O'Donnell S, Mullenix P, et al: The fate of a patent carotid artery contralateral to an occlusion. Ann Vasc Surg 2000;14:77-81.

Brentlinger A, Hunter J: Perforation of the external iliac artery and ureter presenting as acute hemorrhagic cystitis after total hip replacement. J Bone Joint Surg 1987;69:620-622.

Brewer LA III: Wounds of the chest in war and peace, 1943–1968. Ann Thorac Surg 1969;7:387-408.

Brewer LA III: The contributions of the Second Auxiliary Surgical Group to military surgery during World War II with special reference to thoracic surgery. Ann Surg 1983;197:318-326.

Brewer LA III, Carter R: Wounds of the great vessels of the thorax: Diagnosis and surgical approach in twenty-four cases. Am J Surg 1967;114:340-350.

Brewer LA III, Carter R: Elective cardiac arrest for the management of massively bleeding heart wounds. JAMA 1967;200:1023-1025.

Brewer LA III, Carter R: A rational treatment of small and large wounds of the heart. Surg Gynecol Obstet 1968;126:977-985.

Brewer PL, Schramel R, Menendez C, Creech O Jr: Injuries of the popliteal artery: A report of sixteen cases. Am J Surg 1969;118:36-42.

Brewster D, May A, Darling RC: Variable manifestations of vascular injury during lumbar disk surgery. Arch Surg 1979;114:1026-1030.

Brewster SA, Thirlby R, Synder WH: Subxiphoid pericardial window and penetrating cardiac trauma. 1988.

Bricker D, Hallman GL: Complete transection of the thoracic aorta: Management of a case associated with massive total body injury. J Trauma 1970;10:420-426.

Bricker DL, Beall AC Jr, DeBakey ME: The differential response to infection of autogenous vein versus Dacron arterial prosthesis. Chest 1970;58:566-570.

Bricker DL, Morton JR, Okies JE, Beall AC Jr: Surgical management of injuries the vena cava: Changing patterns of injury and newer techniques of repair. J Trauma 1971;11:725-735.

Bricker DL, Noon G, Beall AC Jr: Vascular injuries of the thoracic outlet. J Trauma 1970;10:1-15.

Bricker DL, Waltz T, Telford R, Beall AC Jr: Major abdominal and thoracic trauma associated with spinal cord injury: Problems in management. J Trauma 1971;11:63-75.

Brigham RA, Eddleman W, Clagett GP, Rich NM: Isolated venous injury produced by penetrating trauma to the lower extremity. J Trauma 1983;23:255-257.

Brigham RA, Salander J, Rich NM: Abdominal venous trauma. In Scribner RG, Brown WH, Tawes RL (eds): Decision Making in Vascular Surgery. Toronto, BC Decker, 1988.

Brigham RA, Salander JM, Rich NM: Extremity venous trauma. In Scribner RG, Brown WH, Tawes RL (eds): Decision Making in Vascular Surgery. Toronto, BC Decker, 1988.

Bright EF, Beck CS: Nonpenetrating wounds of the heart. Am Chest J 1935; 10:293-320.

Brink BE: Vascular trauma. Surg Clin North Am 1977;57:189-196.

Brinton M, Miller S, Lim RC Jr, Trunkey DD: Acute abdominal aortic injuries. J Trauma 1982;22:481-486.

Brisbin RL, Geib PO, Eiseman B: Secondary disruption of vascular repair following war wounds. Arch Surg 1969;99:787-791.

Brittain RS, Marchioro TL, Hermann G, et al: Accidental hepatic artery ligation in humans. Am J Surg 1964;107:822-832.

Bromley LL, Hobbs JT, Robinson RE: Early repair of traumatic rupture of the aorta. Br Med J 1965;2:17-19.

Brooks AL, Fowler SB: Axillary artery thrombosis after prolonged use of crutches. J Bone Joint Surg 1964;46-A:863-864.

Brooks AP, Olson LK, Shackford SR: Computed tomography in the diagnosis of traumatic rupture of the thoracic aorta. Clinical Radiology 1989;40:133-138.

Brooks SW, Cmolik BL, Young JC, et al: Transesophageal echocardiographic examination of a patient with traumatic aortic transection from blunt chest trauma: A case report. J Trauma 1991;31:841-845.

Brooks SW, Young JC, Cmolik BL, et al: The use of transesophageal echocardiography in the evaluation of chest trauma. J Trauma 1992;23:761-765.

Brophy DP, Sheiman RG, Amatulle P, Akbari CM: Iatrogenic femoral pseudoaneurysms: Thrombin injection after failed US-guided compression. Radiology 2001;214:278-282.

Bross W: Injuries of the thoracic aorta. J Cardiac Surg 1971;12:95-103.

Brotman S, Browner B, Cox E: MAST trousers improperly applied causing compartmental syndrome in lower extremity trauma. J Trauma 1982;22:598-599.

Brown AJ: Old masterpieces in Surgery: The surgery of Hieronymus Brunschwig. Surg Gynecol Obstet 1924;38:133.

Brown C: Inadvertent prolonged cannulation of the carotid artery. Anesth Analg 1982;61:150-152.

Brown JJ, Greene FL, McMillan RD: Vascular injuries associated with pelvic fractures. Am J Surg 1984;140:802-806.

Brown MF, Graham JM, Feliciano DV, et al: Carotid artery injuries. Am J Surg 1982;144:748-753.

Brown OW, Kerstein MD: Injuries to the peripheral vasculature: In Management of Vascular Trauma. Baltimore, University Park Press, 1985.

Brown PS Jr, Nath R, Votapka T, et al: Traumatic ventricular septal defect and disruption of the descending thoracic aorta. Ann Thorac Surg 1991;52:143-144.

Brown RS, Boyd DR, Masuda T, Lowe R: Temporary internal vascular shunt for retrohepatic vena cava injury. J Trauma 1971;11:736-737.

Brunner JH, Stanley RJ: Superior mesenteric arteriovenous fistula. JAMA 1973;223:316.

Brunsting LA, Ouriel K: Traumatic fracture of the abdominal aorta: Rupture of a calcified abdominal aorta with minimal trauma. J Vasc Surg 1988;8:184-186.

Bryant MF Jr, Lazenby WD, Howard JM: Experimental replacement of short segment of veins. Arch Surg 1958;76:289-293.

Brzowski BK, Mills JL, Beckett M, Beckett WC: Iatrogenic subclavian artery pseudoaneurysms: Case reports. J Trauma 1990;30:1-3.

Buchbinder D, Karmody A, Leather R, Shah D: Hypertonic mannitol: Its use in prevention of revascularization syndrome after acute arterial ischemia. Arch Surg 1981;116:414-421.

Buchman RJ, Thomas PAJ, Park B: Carotid artery injuries: Follow-up of fifteen patients treated in Vietnam. Angiology 1972;23:97-102.

Buchmaster MJ, Kearney PA, Johnson SB, et al: Further experience with trans-esophageal echocardiography in the evaluation of thoracic aortic injury. J Trauma 1994;37:989-995.

Buchness MP, Lo Gerfo FW, Mason GR: Gunshot wounds of the suprarenal abdominal aorta. Am Surg 1976;42:1-7.

Buckman RF, Badellino MM, Mauro LH, Asensio JA: Penetrating cardiac wounds: Prospective study of factors influencing initial resuscitation. J Trauma 1993;34:717-727.

Buckner F, Lyons C, Perkins R: Management of lacerations of the great vessels of the upper thorax and base of the neck. Surg Gynecol Obstet 1958;107:135-142.

Buechter KH, Gomez GA, Zeppa R: A new technique for exposure of injuries at the confluence of the retrohepatic veins and the retrohepatic vena cava. J Trauma 1990;30:328-331.

Buechter KJ, Sereda D, Gomez G, Zeppa R: Retrohepatic vein injuries: Experience with twenty cases. J Trauma 1989;29:1698-1704.

Bunt TJ: Iatrogenic vascular injury: A discourse on surgical technique. Mt. Kisco, Futura Publishing, 1990.

Bunt TJ, Malone JM, Moody M, et al: Frequency of vascular injury with blunt trauma-induced extremity injury. Am J Surg 1190;160:226.

Bunt TJ, Manship L, Moore W: Iatrogenic vascular injury during peripheral revascularization. J Vasc Surg 1985;2:491-498.

Burch JM, Brock JC, Gevirtzman L, et al: The injured colon. Ann Surg 1986;203:701-711.

Burch JM, Feliciano DV, Mattox KL: The atriocaval shunt: Facts and fiction. Ann Surg 1988;207:555-568.

Burch JM, Feliciano DV, Mattox KL: Colostomy and drainage for civilian rectal injuries: Is that all? Ann Surg 1989;209:600-611.

Burch JM, Feliciano DV, Mattox KL, Edelman M: Injuries of the inferior vena cava. Am J Surg 1988;156:548-552.

Burch JM, Richardson RJ, Martin RR, Mattox KL: Penetrating iliac vascular injuries: Recent experience with 233 consecutive patients. J Trauma 1990;30:1450-1459.

Burihan I, Pepe EVA, Miranda R: Bullet embolism following gunshot wound of the chest. J Cardiovasc Surg 1980;21:711-716.

Burnett HF, Parnell CL, Williams GD, Campbell GS: Peripheral arterial injuries: A reassessment. Ann Surg 1976;183:701-709.

Burney RE, Gundry SR, MacKenzie JR, et al: Comparison of mediastinal width, mediastinal-thoracic and cardioratios, and "mediastinal widening" in detection of traumatic aortic rupture. Ann Emerg Med 1983;12:668-671.

Burney RE, Gundry SR, MacKenzie JR, et al: Chest roentgenograms in diagnosis of traumatic rupture of the aorta. Chest 1984;85:605-609.

Burns GR, Sherman RT: Trauma of the abdominal aorta and inferior vena cava. Am Surg 1972;38:303-306.

Burnsed DW, Weiss JB, Campbell GS, William GD: The relative merits of the heparin-bonded shunt vs. femoral bypass of aortic arch injury. Surgery 1975;78:176-180.

Burrell HL: Ligature of the innominate artery with a report of a case. Am Soc A 1895;13:291.

Burrows PE, Tubman DE: Multiple extracranial arterial lesions following closed cranial facial trauma. J Trauma 1981;21:497-498.

Buscaglia LC, Blaisdell FW, Lim RC Jr: Penetrating abdominal vascular injuries. Arch Surg 1969;99:764-769.

Buscaglia LC, Matolo N, Macbeth A: Common iliac artery injury from blunt trauma: Case reports. J Trauma 1989;29:697-699.

Busuttil RW, Kitahama A, Cerise E, et al: Management of blunt and penetrating injuries to the porta hepatis. Ann Surg 1980;191:641-648.

Byrne DE, Pass HI, Crawford FA Jr: Traumatic vena caval injuries. Am J Surg 1980;140:600-602.

Cabrera A, Palomar S, Pastor E: Aortic rupture in a child diagnosed by cross sectional echocardiography. Int J Cardiol 1987;15:249-252.

Caes LF, Cham B, Sacre J, et al: A patient with two chronic posttraumatic aneurysms of the thoracic aorta. Thorac Cardiovasc Surg 1989;37:105-106.

Caldeira CCB, Velmahos GC, Modrall JG: Acute suprarenal aortogastric fistulae caused by gunshot wounds: The importance of early recognition in directing surgical strategy. J Trauma 1996;40:838-839.

Calhoon JH, Hoffmann TH, Trinkle JK, et al: Management of blunt rupture of the heart. J Trauma 1986;26:495-502.

Callander CL: Study of arteriovenous fistula with an analysis of 447 cases. Ann Surg 1920;19:428-459.

Cameron HS, Laird JJ, Carroll SE: False aneurysms complicating closed fractures. J Trauma 1972;12:67-74.

Cammack K, Rapport R, Paul J, Baird WC: Deceleration injuries of the thoracic aorta. Arch Surg 1959;79:244-251.

Campbell DK, Austin RF: Seat belt injury: Injury of the abdominal aorta. Radiology 1969;92:123-124.

Campt PC, Rogers FB, Shackford SR, et al: Blunt traumatic thoracic aortic lacerations in the elderly: An analysis of outcome. J Trauma 1994;37:418-425.

Capone AC, Safar P, Stezoski W, et al: Improved outcome with fluid restriction in treatment of uncontrolled hemorrhagic shock. J Am Coll Surg 1995;180:49-56.

Cappelen A: Vulnus cordis, sutur of hjrtet. Nor Mag f Laegevidensk 1896;11:285-288.

Carden DL, Granger DN: Pathophysiology of ischaemia-reperfusion injury. J Pathol 2000;190:255-266.

Cargile JS III, Hunt JL, Purdue GF: Femoral vascular trauma: A review of 218 cases. J Trauma 1991;31:1025.

Cargile JS III, Hunt JL, Purdue GF: Acute trauma of the femoral artery and vein. J Trauma 1992;32:364-371.

Carlsson E, Silander T: Rupture of the subclavian and innominate artery due to nonpenetrating trauma of the chest. Acta Chir Scand 1963;125:294-300.

Carrasquilla C, Weaver AW: Aneurysm of the saphenous graft to the common carotid artery. Vasc Surg 1972;6:66-68.

Carrasquilla C, Wilson RF, Walt AJ, Arbulu A: Gunshot wounds of the heart. Ann Thorac Surg 1972;13:208-213.

Carrel A: La technique opératories des anastomoses vasculaires et la transplantation des viscéres. Lyon Medical 1902;98:859.

Carrel A: The surgery of blood vessels. Bull Johns Hopkins Hosp 1907;18:18.

Carrel A: Results of transplantation of blood vessels, organs and limbs. JAMA 1908;51:1662-1667.

Carrel A, Guthrie CC: Uniterminal and biterminal venous transplantations. Surg Gynecol Obstet 1906;2:266-286.

Carroll PR, McAninch JW, Klosterman P, Greenblatt M: Renovascular trauma: Risk assessment, surgical management, and outcome. J Trauma 1990;30:547-554.

Carter BN, DeBakey ME: Current observations on war wounds of the chest. J Thorac Surg 1944;13:271-293.

Carter SL, McKenzie JG, Hess DR: Blunt trauma to the common femoral artery. J Trauma 1981;21:178-179.

Cass AS, Luxemberg M: Management of renal artery injuries from external trauma. J Urol 1987;138:266-268.

Cass AS, Luxemberg M: Traumatic thrombosis of a segmental branch of the renal artery. J Urol 1987;137:1115-1116.

Catinella FP, De Laria GA, De Wald RL: False aneurysm of the superior gluteal artery: A complication of iliac crest bone grafting. Spine 1990;15:1360.

Catoire P, Bonnet F, Delaunay L, et al: Traumatic laceration of the ascending aorta detected by transesophageal echocardiography. Ann Emerg Med 1994;23:356-359.

Catoire P, Orliaguet G, Liu N, et al: Systematic transesophageal echocardiography for detection of mediastinal lesions in patients with multiple injuries. J Trauma 1995;38:96-102.

Caudros CL, Hutchinson JE, Mogtader AH: Laceration of a mitral papillary muscle and the aortic root as a result of blunt trauma to the chest. J Thorac Cardiovasc Surg 1984;88:134-140.

Cerino M, McGraw JY, Luke JC: Autogenous vein graft replacement of thrombosed deep veins: Experimental approach to the treatment of the post phlebitic syndrome. Surgery 1964;55:123-134.

Cernaianu AC, Cilley JH Jr, Baldino WA, et al: Determinants of outcome in lesions of the thoracic aorta in patients with multiorgan system trauma. Chest 1992;101:331-335.

Cernaianu AC, Olah A, Cilley JH Jr, et al: Effect of sodium nitroprusside on paraplegia during cross-clamping of the thoracic aorta. Ann Thorac Surg 1993;56:1035-1037.

Chaikof EL, Shamberger RC, Brewster DC: Traumatic pseudoaneurysms of the abdominal aorta. J Trauma 1985;25:169-173.

Champion HR, Sacco WJ, Carnazzo AJ, et al: Trauma score. Crit Care Med 1981;9:672-676.

Champion MC, Sullivan SN, Coles JC, et al: Aortoenteric fistula: Incidence, presentation, recognition and management. Ann Surg 1982;195:314-317.

Chan EL, Bardin JA, Bernstein EF: Inferior vena cava bypass. J Vasc Surg 1984;1:675-680.

Chandler JG, Knapp RW: Early definitive treatment of vascular injuries in the Vietnam conflict. JAMA 1967;202:960-966.

Chang FC, Harrison PB, Beech RR, Helmer SD: PASG: Does it help in the management of traumatic shock? J Trauma 1995;39:453-456.

Chang H, Chu SH, Lee YT: Traumatic aorto-right arterial fistula blunt chest injury. Ann Thorac Surg 1989;47:778-779.

Chapman AJ, McClain J: Wandering missiles: Autopsy study. J Trauma 1984;24:634-637.

Charles KP, Davidson KG, Miller H, Caves PK: Traumatic rupture of the ascending aorta and aortic valve following blunt chest trauma. J Thorac Cardiovasc Surg 1977;73:208-211.

Chase CW, Layman TS, Barker DE, Clements JB: Traumatic abdominal aortic pseudoaneurysm causing biliary obstruction: A case report and review of the literature. J Vasc Surg 1997;25:936-940.

Chase MD, Schwartz SI: Suture anastomosis of small arteries. Surg Gynecol Obstet 1963;117:44-46.

Chaudry IH: Cellular mechanisms in shock and ischemia and their correction. Am J Physiol 1983;245:R117–R134.

Chaudry IH: ATP-MgCl2 and liver blood flow following shock and ischemia. Prog Clin Biol Res 1989;299:19-31.

Chaudry IH: The use of ATP following shock and ischemia. In Dubyak BR, Fedan JS (eds): Biological Actions of Extracellular ATP. Ann NY Acad Sci, 1990: 130-141.

Chaudry IH, Ohkawa M, Clemens MG: Improved mitochondrial function following ischemia and reflow by ATP-MgCl$_2$. Am J Physiol 1984;246:R799–R804.

Chaudry IH, Ohkawa M, Clemens MG, Baue AE: Alterations in electron transport and cellular metabolism with shock and trauma. Prog Clin Biol Res 1983;111:67-88.

Chedid MK, Deeb ZL, Rothfus WE, et al: Major cerebral vessel injury caused by a seatbelt strap: Case report. J Trauma 1989;29:1601-1603.

Cheek RC, Pope JC, Smith HF, et al: Diagnosis and management of major vascular injuries: A review of 200 operative cases. Am Surg 1975;41:755-760.

Cherng WJ, Bullard MJ, Chang HJ, Lin FC: Diagnosis of coronary artery dissection following blunt chest trauma by transesophageal echocardiography. J Trauma 1995;39:772-774.

Cherry JK, Bennett DE: False aneurysm of the aorta following penetrating trauma: Report of a case with secondary infection and delayed rupture. Arch Surg 1966;93:404-408.

Chervu A, Quinones-Baldrich WJ: Vascular complications in orthopaedic surgery. Clin Orthop 1988;235:275-288.

Chew FS, Panicek DM, Heitzman ER: Late discovery of a posttraumatic right aortic arch aneurysm. AJR Am J Roentgenol 1985;145:1001-1002.

Childs D, Wilkes RG: Puncture of the ascending aorta. A complication of subclavian venous cannulation. Anesthesia 1986;41:331-332.

Chitwood W, Austin E: Cardiac trauma: Penetrating and blunt. In Trauma Surgery. Philadelphia, JB Lippincott Co, 1988.

Chiu CL, Roelofs JD, Go RT: Coronary angiographic and scintigraphic findings in experimental cardiac contusion. Radiology 1975;116:679-683.

Choo MH, Chia BL, Chia FK: Penetrating cardiac injury evaluated by two-dimensional echocardiography. Am Heart J 1984;108:417-420.

Ciaravella JM, Ochsner JL, Mills NL: Traumatic avulsion of the innominate artery: A case report and literature review. J Trauma 1976;16:751-754.

Cikrit DF, Dalsing MC, Bryant BJ, Lalka SG: An experience with upper-extremity vascular trauma. Am J Surg 1990;160:229.

Cioffi WG Jr, Pruitt BA Jr: Vascular abnormalities associated with thermal and electrical trauma. In Flanigan DP (ed): Civilian Vascular Trauma. Philadelphia, Lea & Febiger, 1992, pp 255-264.

Clark DE, Georgia JW, Ray FS: Renal arterial injuries caused by blunt trauma. Surgery 1981;90:87-96.

Clark DE, Zeiger MA, Wallace KL, et al: Blunt aortic trauma: Signs of high risk. J Trauma 1990;30:701-705.

Clarke CP, Brandt PW, Cole DS, Barratt-Boyes BG: Traumatic rupture of the thoracic aorta: Diagnosis and treatment. Br J Surg 1967;54:353-358.

Clarke P, Whittaker M: Traumatic aneurysm of the internal carotid artery and rupture of the duodenum following seatbelt injury. Injury 1980;12:158-160.

Clemens MG, McDonagh PF, Chaudry IH, Baue AE: Hepatic microcirculatory failure after ischemia and reperfusion: improvement with ATP-MgCl$_2$ treatment. Am J Physiol 1985;248:H804–H811.

Clermont G: Suture laterale et circulaire des veines. Presse Med 1901;1:229.

Cleveland JC, Cleveland RJ: Successful repair of aortic root and aortic valve injury caused by blunt chest trauma in a patient with prior aortic dissection. Chest 1974;66:447-450.

Cleveland JC, Ellis J, Dague J: Complete disruption of axillary artery caused by severe atherosclerosis and trivial non-penetrating trauma. J Trauma 1979;19:635-636.

Clyne CAC, Ashbrooke EA: Seat-belt aorta: Isolated abdominal aortic injury following blunt injury. Br J Surg 1985;72:239.

Coelho JC, Siegel B, Flanigan DP, et al: Arteriographic and ultrasonic evaluation of vascular clamp injury using an in vitro human experimental model. Surg Gynecol Obstet 1982;155:506-512.

Cogbill TH, Moora EE, Jurkovich GJ, et al: Severe hepatic trauma: A multicenter experience with 1,335 liver injuries. J Trauma 1988;28:1433-1438.

Cogbill TH, Moore EE, Milikan JS, Cleveland HC: Rationale for selective application of emergency department thoracotomy in trauma. J Trauma 1983;23:453-460.

Cohen A, Baldwin JN, Grant RN: Problems in the management of battlefield vascular injuries. Am J Surg 1969;118:526-530.

Cohen A, Brief D, Mathewson C Jr: Carotid artery injuries: An analysis of 85 cases. Am J Surg 1970;120:210-214.

Cohen AM, Crass JR, Thomas HA, et al: CT evidence for the "osseous pinch" mechanism for traumatic aortic injury. AJR Am J Roentgenol 1992;159:271-274.

Cohn SM, Burns GA, Jaffe C, Milner KA: Exclusion of aortic tear in the unstable trauma patient: The utility of transesophageal echocardiography. J Trauma 1995;39:1087-1090.

Coimbra R, Pinto MC, Razuk A: Penetrating cardiac wounds: Predictive value of trauma indices and the necessity of terminology of standardization. Am Surg 1995;61:448-452.

Coin D, Crighton J, Schorn L: Successful management of hepatic vein injury from blunt trauma in children. Am J Surg 1980;140:858.

Coley RW. Case of rupture of the carotid artery and wound of several of its branches successfully treated by tying off the common trunk of the carotid itself. Med Chir J (Lond) 1817;3:2.

Collicott PE: Initial assessment of the trauma patient. In Mattox KL, Moore EE, Feliciano DV (eds): Trauma. East Norwalk, Conn, Appleton & Lange, 1988, pp 107-124.

Collins HA, Jacobs JK: Acute arterial injuries due to blunt trauma. J Bone Joint Surg 1961;43-A:193-197.

Collins JA: Recent developments in the area of massive transfusion. World J Surg 1987;11:75-81.

Collins PS, Golocvsky M, Salander JM, et al: Intra-abdominal vascular injury secondary to penetrating trauma. J Trauma 1988;28:S165–S168.

Collins RE, Douglass FM: Small vein anastomosis with and without operative microscope: A comparative study. Arch Surg 1964;88:740-742.

Colon R, Frazier OH, Cooley DA, McAllistr HA: Hypothermic regional perfusion for protection of the spinal cord during periods of ischemia. Ann Thorac Surg 1987;43:639-643.

Cone JB: Vascular injury associated with fracture-dislocations of the lower extremity. Clin Orthop 1989:30.

Conkle DM, Richie RE: Surgical treatment of popliteal artery injuries. Arch Surg 1975;110:1351-1353.

Conn J, Trippel OH, Bergan JJ: A new atraumatic aortic occluder. Surgery 1968;64:1158.

Conn JH, Hardy JD, Chavez CM, Fain WR: Challenging arterial injuries. J Trauma 1971;11:167-177.

Connelly JE, Brownell DA, Levine EF: Complications of renal dialysis access procedures. Arch Surg 1984;119:1325-1328.

Connery C, Geller E, Dulchavsky S, Kreis DJ: Paraparesis following emergency room thoracotomy: Case report. J Trauma 1990;30:362-363.

Connolly J, Williams E, Whittaker D: The influence of fracture stabilization on the outcome of arterial repair in combined fracture-arterial injuries. Surg Forum 1969;20:450-452.

Connolly J: Management of fractures associated with arterial injuries. Am J Surg 1970;120:331.

Connolly JE: Prevention of paraplegia secondary to operations on the aorta. J Cardiovasc Surg 1986;27:410-417.

Connolly JE, Kwaan JHM, McCart PM: Complications after percutaneous transluminal angioplasty. Am J Surg 1981;142:60-66.

Connolly JF, Whittaker D, Williams E: Femoral and tibial fractures combined with injuries to the femoral or popliteal artery. J Bone Joint Surg 1971;53-A:56-67.

Conti VR, Calverley J, Safley WL, et al: Arterial spinal artery syndrome with chronic traumatic thoracic aortic aneurysm. Ann Thorac Surg 1982;33:81-85.

Contino JP, Follette DM, Berkoff HA, et al: Use of Carmeda-coated femoral-femoral bypass repair of traumatic aortic pseudoaneurysm. Arch Surg 1994;129:933-937.

Cook FW, Haller JA Jr: Penetrating injuries of the subclavian vessels associated with venous complications. Ann Surg 1962;155:370-372.

Cook P, Erdoes L, Selzer P: Dissection of the external iliac artery in highly trained athletes. J Vasc Surg 1995;22:173.

Cook TA, Jones AJ, Webb AK, Baird RN: Traumatic abdominal aortic aneurysm. Eur J Vasc Surg 1994;8:364-365.

Cooley DA, Dunn JR, Brockman HL, DeBakey ME: Treatment of penetrating wounds of the heart: Experimental and clinical observations. Surgery 1955;37:882.

Cooper B: Wounds in arteries and traumatic aneurysms. Guys Hosp Rep 1852;8:195.

Cope C, Zeit R: Coagulation of aneurysms by direct percutaneous thrombin injection. AJR Am J Roentgenol 1986;147:383-387.

Copper ES: Aneurysm of the right carotid and subclavian arteries. Am J Med Sci 1859;38:395.

Cornwell EE, Kennedy F, Berne TV, et al: Gunshot wounds to the thoracic aorta in the '90s: Only prevention will make a difference. Am Surg 1995;61:721-723.

Cosby RL, Miller PD, Schirir RW: Traumatic renal artery thrombosis. Am J Med 1986;81:890-894.

Coselli JS, Crawford ES: Surgical treatment of aneurysms of the intrathoracic segment of the subclavian artery. Chest 1987;91:704-708.

Costa M, Robbs JV: Management of retroperitoneal haematoma following penetrating trauma. Br J Surg 1985;72:662-664.

Costa MC, Robbs JV: Nonpenetrating subclavian artery trauma. J Vasc Surg 1988;8:71-75.

Couch NP, Cerundolo D: A clip for the rapid control of the vascular injuries. Surg Gynecol Obstet 1981;153:408-409.

Courcy PA, Brotman S, Oster-Granite ML, et al: Superior mesenteric artery and vein injury from blunt abdominal trauma. J Trauma 1984;24:843-845.

Couves CM, Lumpkin MB, Howard JM: Arterial injuries due to blunt-nonpenetrating trauma: Experiences with 15 patients. Can J Surg 1958; 1:197-200.

Cowgill LD, Campbell DN, Clarke DR, et al: Ventricular septal defect due to non-penetrating chest trauma: Use of the intra-aortic balloon pump. J Trauma 1987;27:1087-1090.

Cranley JJ, Krause RJ: Injury to the axillary artery following anterior dislocation of the shoulder. Am J Surg 1958;95:524-526.

Crawford ES, Fenstermacher JM, Richardson W, Frank S: Reappraisal of adjuncts to avoid ischemia in the treatment thoracic aortic aneurysms. Surgery 1970;67:182-196.

Crawford ES, Mizrahi EM, Hess KR, et al: The impact of distal aortic perfusion and somatosensory evoked potential monitoring on prevention of paraplegia after aortic aneurysm operation. J Thorac Cardiovasc Surg 1988;95:357-367.

Crawford ES, Morris GC Jr, Myhre HO, Roehm JO: Celiac axis, superior mesenteric artery and inferior mesenteric artery occlusion: considerations. Surgery 1977;82:856-866.

Crawford ES, Svensson LG, Hess KR, et al: A prospective randomized study of cerebrospinal fluid drainage to prevent paraplegia after high-risk surgery on the thoracoabdominal aorta. J Vasc Surg 1991;13:36-46.

Creagh TA, Broe PJ, Grace PA, Bouchier-Hayes DJ: Blunt trauma induced upper extremity vascular injuries. J R Coll Surg Edinb 1991;36:158.

Creech O Jr: Acute arterial injuries. Postgrad Med 1961;29:581.

Creech O Jr, Gantt J, Wren H: Traumatic arteriovenous fistula at unusual sites. Ann Surg 1965;161:908-920.

Crepps JT Jr, Rodriguez A: Combined abdominal aortic and visceral artery injury secondary to blunt trauma. Injury 1989;20:176-177.

Crissey MM, Bernstein EF: Delayed presentation of carotid intimal tear following blunt craniocervical trauma. Surgery 1974;75:543-549.

Cronenwett JL, Walsh DB, Garrett HE: Tibial artery pseudoaneurysms: delayed complication of balloon catheter embolectomy. J Vasc Surg 1988;8:483-488.

Cronenwett JL, McDaniel M, Zwolak R, et al: Limb salvage despite extensive tissue loss: Free tissue transfer combined with distal revascularization. Arch Surg 1989;124:609-615.

Cryer HM, Miller FB, Evers M, et al: Pelvic fracture classification: Correlation with hemorrhage. J Trauma 1988;28:973-980.

Cterctko G, Mok CK: Aorto-esophageal fistula induced by a foreign body: The first recorded survival. J Thorac Cardiovasc Surg 1980;80:233-235.

Curley SA, Demarest G, Hauswald M: Pericardial tamponade and hemothorax after penetrating injury to the internal mammary artery. J Trauma 1987;27:957-958.

Currarino G, Engle ME: The effects of ligation of the subclavian artery on the bones and soft tissues of the arms. J Pediatr 1965;67:808-811.

Curtin JJ, Goodman LR, Thorsen MK: Aortic traumatic lesion: Has tomodensitometry a role? J Radiol 1993;74:523-530.

Cusick JF, Daniels D: Spontaneous reversal of internal carotid artery occlusion: Case report. J Neurosurg 1981;54:811-813.

Dainko EA: Complications of the use of the Fogarty balloon catheter. Arch Surg 1972;105:79-82.

Dajani OM, Haddad FF, Hajj HA, et al: Injury to the femoral vessels: The Lebanese War experience. Eur J Vasc Surg 1988;2:293-296.

Dajee H, Richardson IW, Iype MO: Seatbelt aorta: Acute dissection and thrombosis of the abdominal aorta. Surgery 1979;85:263-267.

Dale WA: Chronic iliofemoral venous occlusion including seven cases of cross-over vein grafting. Surgery 1966;59:117-132.

Dale WA: Management of arterial occlusive disease (national conference on management of arterial occlusive disease, Naashville, 1970). In Dale WA (ed): Chicago, Year Book Publisher Inc, 1971.

Dale WA: The beginnings of vascular surgery. Surgery 1974;76:849-866.

Dale WA, Harris J, Terry RB: Polytetrafluoroethylene reconstruction of the inferior vena cava. Surgery 1984;95:625-630.

Dalton HC: Report of a case of stab wound of the pericardium, terminating in recovery after resection of a rib and suture of the pericardium. Ann Surg 1895;21:147-152.

Dameron TB Jr: False aneurysm of femoral profundus artery resulting from internal-fixation device (screw). J Bone Joint Surg 1964;46A:577-580.

Damron T, McBeath A: Diagnosis and management of vascular injuries associated with skeletal trauma. Orthop Rev 1990;19:1063.

Dana A, Skarli M, Papakrivopoulou J, Yellon DM: Adenosine A(1) receptor induced delayed preconditioning in rabbits: Induction of p38 mitogen-activated protein kinase. Circ Res 2000;86:989-997.

Danielson GK, Wood R, Holloway JB: Traumatic avulsion of the innominate artery from the aorta. Ann Thorac Surg 1968;5:451-458.

Danto LA, Wolfman EF Jr: Linear abdominal trauma. J Trauma 1976;16:179-183.

Danza R, Mauro L, Arias J: Reconstruction of the femoro-popliteal vessels with a double graft (arterial and venous) in severe injury of the limb. J Cardiac Surg 1970;11:60-64.

Dart CH Jr, Braitman HE: Traumatic rupture of the thoracic aorta: diagnosis and management. Arch Surg 1976;111:697-702.

Dart CH Jr, Braitman HE: Popliteal artery injury following fracture or dislocation at the knee: Diagnosis and management. Arch Surg 1977;112:969-973.

David D, Blumenberg RM: Subintimal aortic dissection with occlusion after blunt abdominal trauma. Arch Surg 1970;100:302-304.

Davie JC, Coxe W: Occlusive disease of the carotid artery in children. Arch Neurol 1967;17:313-323.

Davies MG, Hagen PO: The vascular endothelium: A new horizon. Ann Surg 1993;218:593-609.

Davis. 1834. Cited in: Straus R. Pulmonary embolism caused by lead bullet following gunshot wound of abdomen. Arch Path 1942;33:63-68.

Davis JM, Zimmerman RA: Injury of the carotid and vertebral arteries. Neuroradiology 1983;25:55-69.

Davis TP, Feliciano DV, Rozycki GS: Results with abdominal vascular trauma in the modern era. Am Surg 2001;67:565-571.

Dawson D, Johanse K, Jurkovich G: Injuries to the portal triad. Am J Surg 1991;161:545.

Daxini BV, Desai AG, Sharma S: Echo-Doppler diagnosis of aortocaval fistula following blunt trauma to abdomen. Am Heart J 1989;118:843-844.

de Guzman E, Shankar MN, Mattox KL: Limited volume resuscitation in penetrating thoracoabdominal trauma. AACN Clin Issues 1999;10:61-68.

De Nayer P, Jaumin P, Linard D: Lesions osteo-articulaires des membres compliquees de traumatismes vasculaires. Acta Chir Belg 1973;72:427.

De Takats G: Vascular surgery in the war. War Med 1943;3:291-296.

De Takats G: Vascular Surgery. Philadelphia, WB Saunders, 1959.

De Takats G: Symptoms and signs of peripheral arterial disease. Med Clin North Am 1962;46:647-657.

De Takats G: Trauma to the arteriosclerotic limb. J Trauma 1963;4:47.

De Takats G, Pirani C: Aneurysms: General considerations. Angiology 1954;5:173-208.

De Wet Lubbe JJ, Janson PM: Penetrating wounds of the heart and great vessels: Experience with cases including three with intracardiac defects. South Afr Med J 1975;29:512-516.

Dean RH: Management of renal artery trauma. J Vasc Surg 1988;8:89-90.

DeBakey ME, Simeone FA: Battle injuries of the arteries in World War II: An analysis of 2,471 cases. Ann Surg 1946;123:534-579.

DeBakey ME, Cooley DA, Morris GC Jr, Collins H: Arteriovenous fistula involving the abdominal aorta: Report of four cases with successful repair. Ann Surg 1958;147:646-658.

DeBakey ME, Beall AC Jr, Wukasch DC: Recent developments in vascular surgery with particular reference to orthopaedics. Am J Surg 1965;109:134-142.

DeBakey ME: The development of vascular surgery. Am J Surg 1979;137:697-738.

Defore WW Jr, Mattox KL, Jordan GL Jr: Management of 1590 consecutive cases of liver trauma. Arch Surg 1976;111:493-497.

Degianni E, Levy RD, Sofianos C, et al: Arterial gunshot injuries of the extremities: A South African experience. J Trauma 1995;39:570-575.

DelRossi AJ, Cernaianu AC, Cilley JH Jr, et al: Multiple traumatic disruptions of the thoracic aorta. Chest 1990;97:1307-1309.

DelRossi AJ, Cernaianu AC, Madden LD, et al: Traumatic disruptions of the thoracic aorta: Treatment and outcome. Surgery 1990;108:864-870.

DeLucia A III, Fromm D: Retropancreatic control of the suprarenal aorta. Surg Gynecol Obstet 1988;166:475-476.

Demetriades D: Cardiac wounds. Ann Surg 1986;203:315-317.

Demetriades D, Rabinowitz B, Pezikis A, et al: Subclavian vascular injuries. Br J Surg 1987;74:1001-1003.

Demetriades D, Skalkides J, Safianos C: Carotid artery injuries: Experience with 124 cases. J Trauma 1989;29:91-94.
Corrected

Demetriades D, Charalambides L, Sareli P: Later sequelae of penetrating cardiac injuries. Br J Surg 1990;77:813-814.

Demetriades D, Theodorou D, Murray J, et al: Mortality and prognostic factors in penetrating injuries of the aorta. J Trauma 1996;40:761-763.

Demetriades D, Chan L, Cornwell E, et al: Paramedic vs. private transportation of trauma patients. Arch Surg 1996;131:133-138.

DeMeules JE, Cramer G, Perry JF Jr: Rupture of aorta and great vessels due to blunt thoracic trauma. J Thorac Cardiovasc Surg 1971;61:438-442.

DeMuth WE: Bullet velocity makes the difference. J Trauma 1969;9:642-643.

DeMuth WE Jr, Baue AE, Odom JA Jr: Contusions of the heart. J Trauma 1967;7:443-445.

DeMuth WE Jr, Roe H, Hobbie W: Immediate repair of traumatic rupture of the aorta. Arch Surg 1965;91:602-603.

Dennis JW, Frykberg ER, Crump JM, et al: New perspectives on the management of penetrating trauma in proximity to major limb arteries. J Vasc Surg 1990;11:85-93.

Dent RI, Jena GP: Missile injuries of the abdomen in Zimbabwe-Rhodesia. Br J Surg 1980;67:305-310.

DePriest W, Barish R, Almquist T, Groleau G: Echocardiographic diagnosis of acute pericardial effusion in penetrating chest trauma. Am J Emerg Med 1988;6:21-23.

DeSa'Neto A, Padnick MB, Desser KB, Steinhoff NG: Right sinus of Valsalva-right atrial fistula secondary to nonpenetrating chest trauma. Circulation 1979;60:205-209.

Desai SB, Modhe JM, Aulakh BG: Percutaneous transcatheter steel-coil embolization of a large proximal post-traumatic superior mesenteric arteriovenous fistula. J Trauma 1987;27:1091.

DeSaussure RL: Vascular injury coincident to disc surgery. J Neurosurg 1959;16:222-228.

DesChamps GT, Morano JU: Intracranial bullet migration: A sign of brain abscess: Case report. J Trauma 1991;31:293-295.

DesForges G, Ridder WP, Lenoci RJ: Successful suture of ruptured myocardium after nonpenetrating injury. N Engl J Med 1955;252:567-569.

Detwiler K, Godersky JC, Gentry L: Pseudoaneurysm of the extracranial vertebral artery. J Neurosurg 1987;67:935-939.

DeWeese JA, Mattox KL, Seltzer SE, Bukley JM: Symposium on traumatic thoracic aortic rupture. Contemp Surg 1984;24:109-131.

Dharker SR, Dharker RS: Traumatic occlusion of internal carotid artery in an infant. Surg Neurol 1978;9:77-78.

Dichtel WJ, Miller RH, Woodson GE, et al: Lateral mandibulotomy: A technique of exposure for penetrating injuries of the internal carotid artery at the base of the skull. Laryngoscope 1984;94:1140-1144.

Dickerman RM, Gewertz BL, Foley DW, Fry WJ: Selective intra-arterial tolazoline infusion in peripheral arterial trauma. Surgery 1977;81:605-609.

Diebel LN, Wilson RF, Bennder J, Paules B: A comparison of passive and active shunting for bypass of retrohepatic IVC. J Trauma 1991;31:987-990.

Dieter RA, Asselmeier GH, Hamouda F, et al: Traumatic disruption of the thoracic aorta: A community hospital experience. Mil Med 1983;148:502-506.

Dieux JJ, Milani H, Maillet P, Brahy R: A case of 2-stage traumatic rupture of the abdominal aorta. Acta Chir Belg 1985;85:367-370.

Dillard BM, Nelson DL, Norman HG: Review of 85 major traumatic arterial injuries. Surgery 1968;63:391-395.

Dillard BM, Staple TW: Bullet embolism from the aortic arch to the popliteal artery. Arch Surg 1969;98:326-328.

Dillman RO, Crumb CK, Lidsky MJ: Lead poisoning from a gunshot wound. Am J Med 1979;66:509-514.

DiMaio VJ, DiMaio DJ: Bullet embolism: Six cases and a review of the literature. J Forens Sci 1972;17:394-398.

Dimond FC Jr, Rich NM: M-16 wounds in Vietnam. J Trauma 1967;7:618-625.

Dingeldein GP, Proctor HJ, Jaques PF: Traumatic aorto-caval-portal-duodenal fistula: Case report. J Trauma 1977;17:474-476.

Diveley WL, Daniel RA Jr, Scott HW Jr: Surgical management of penetrating injuries of the ascending aorta arch. J Thorac Cardiovasc Surg 1961;41:23-33.

DiVincenti FC, Weber BB: Traumatic carotid artery injuries in civilian practice. Am Surg 1974;40:277-280.

Dixon RG, McEwan P: Notes on a case of penetrating wound of the heart. Br Med J 1916;1:755.

Doan E, Gorton ME: Traumatic disruption of the innominate and right pulmonary arteries: Case report. J Trauma 19;43:701-702.

Dobell ARC, MacNaughton EA, Crutchlow EF: Successful early treatment of subadventitial rupture of the thoracic aorta. N Engl J Med 1964;270:410-412.

Dobrin PB: Mechanisms and prevention of arterial injuries caused by balloon embolectomy. Surgery 1989;106:457-466.

Donahue TK, Strauch GO: Ligation as definitive management of injury to the superior mesenteric vein. J Trauma 1988;28:541-543.

Donchin Y, Rivkind AI, Bar-Ziv J, et al: Utility of postmortem computed tomography in trauma victims. J Trauma 1994;37:552-556.

Donell ST, Hudson MJK: Iatrogenic superior mesenteric arteriovenous fistula: Report of a case. J Vasc Surg 1988;8:335.

Donovan DL, Sharp WV: Blunt trauma to the axillary artery. J Vasc Surg 1984;1:681-683.

Dorfman GS, Cronan JJ: Bayesian analysis of chest plain film finding in traumatic rupture of the aorta. Invest Radiol 1987;22:S4.

Dorion RP, Hamati HF, Landis B: Risk and clinical significance of developing antibodies induced by topical thrombin preparations. Arch Pathol Lab Med 1998;122:887-894.

Dosios TJ, Magoven GJ, Gay TC, Joyner CR: Cardiac tamponade complicating percutaneous catheterization of subclavian vein. Surgery 1975;78:261-263.

Doty DB, Baker WH: Bypass of superior vena cava with spiral vein graft. Ann Thorac Surg 1976;22:490-493.

Doty DB, Treiman RL, Rothschild PD, Gaspar MR: Prevention of gangrene due to fractures. Surg Gynecol Obstet 1967;125:284-288.

Downs AR, MacDonald P: Popliteal artery injuries: Civilian experience with sixty-three patients during a twenty-four year period. J Vasc Surg 1986;4:55-62.

Dörfler J: Uber arteriennaht. Beitr Klin Chir 1889;25:781.

Dragojevic D, Hetzer R, Oelert H: Surgery for traumatic rupture of the thoracic aorta. Thorac Cardiovasc Surg 1980;28:436-440.

Dragon R, Saranchak H, Lakin P, Strauch G: Blunt injuries to the carotid vertebral arteries. Am J Surg 1981;141:497-500.

Drapanas T, Hewitt RL, Weichert RF III, Smith AD: Civilian vascular injuries: A critical appraisal of three decades of management. Ann Surg 1970;172:351-360.

Dronen SC, Stern SA, Wang X, Stanley M: A comparison of the response of near fatal acute hemorrhage mode with and with out a vascular injury to rapid volume expansion. Am J Emerg Med 1993;11:331-335.

Drost TF, Rosemurgy AS, Proctor D, Kearney RE: Outcome of treatment of combined orthopedic and arterial trauma to the lower extremity. J Trauma 1989;29:1331-1334.

Drury JK, Scullion JE: Vascular complications of anterior dislocation of the shoulder. Br J Surg 1980;67:579-581.

Dshanelidze II. Manuskript petrograd. 1922. Cited in: Lilianthal H: 1926.

Du Toit DF, Greeff M: Low-velocity gunshot injury of the abdominal aorta managed by debridement and re-anastomosis. S Afr Med J 1986;18:139-140.

Du Toit DF, Rademan F: Traumatic superior mesenteric arteriovenous fistula: A case report. S Afr Med J 1987;71:587.

Dube P: Control of massive carotid hemorrhage by balloon catheter. Thorax 1973;28:399-400.

Dubinskiy MB: Suture of the abdominal aorta. Khirurgiya 1944;4:71.

Duhaylongsod FG, Glower DD, Wolfe WG: Acute traumatic aortic aneurysm: The Duke experience from 1970 to 1990. J Vasc Surg 1992;15:331-343.

Dula DJ, Hughes HG, Majernick T: Traumatic disruption of the brachiocephalic artery. Ann Emerg Med 1983;12:639-641.

Dulchavsky SA, Geller ER, Iorio DA: Analysis of injuries following the crash of Avianca flight 52. J Trauma 1993;34:282-284.

Duncan A, Scalea T, Sclafani SJ: Evaluation of occult cardiac injuries using subxiphoid pericardial window. J Trauma 1989;29:955-960.

Durham LA, Richardson RJ, Wall MJ: Emergency center thoracotomy impact of prehospital resuscitation. J Trauma 1992;32:775.

Earle AS, Horsley JS, Villavicencio JL, Warren R: Replacement of venous defects by venous autografts. Arch Surg 1960;80:119-124.

Eastcott HH: The management of arterial injuries. J Bone Joint Surg 1965;47B:394-398.

Eastcott HHG: Arterial Surgery. Philadelphia, JB Lippincott Co, 1969.

Eaves CC: Traumatic rupture of the thoracic aorta presenting as transient paraplegia. J Emerg Med 1990;8:429-431.

Eck NV: K. voprosu o perevyazkie vorotnois veni. Predvaritelnoye soobshtshjenye (Ligature of the portal vein). Voen Med J 2001;130:1-2.

Eddy AC, Misbach GA, Luna GK: Traumatic rupture of the thoracic aorta in the pediatric patient. Pediatr Emerg Care 1989;8:429-431.

Eddy AC, Nance DR, Goldman MA, et al: Rapid diagnosis of thoracic aortic transection using intravenous digital subtraction angiography. Am J Surg 1990;159:500-503.

Eddy AC, Rusch VW, Fligner CL, et al: The epidemiology of traumatic rupture of the thoracic aorta in children: A 13-year review. J Trauma 1990;30:989-992.

Eddy AC, Rusch VW, Marchioro T, et al: Treatment of traumatic rupture of the thoracic aorta. Arch Surg 1990;125:1351-1356.

Edmundson K: Transfixion of the aorta. Br J Surg 1963;23:869-870.

Edwards WS, Lyons C: Traumatic arterial spasm and thrombosis. Ann Surg 1957;140:318-323.

Egan TJ, Neiman RJ, Malave SR, Sanders JH: Computed tomography in the diagnosis of aortic aneurysm dissection or traumatic injury. Radiology 1980;136:141-146.

Eger M, Glocman L, Goldstein A, Hirsch M: The use of temporary shunt in the management of arterial vascular injuries. Surg Gynecol Obstet 1971;132:67-70.

Eger M, Glocman L, Torok G, Hirsch M: Inadvertent arterial stripping in the lower limb: Problems of management. Surgery 1973;73:23-27.

Eger M, Glocman L, Schmidt D, Hirsch M: Problems in the management of popliteal artery injuries. Surg Gynecol Obstet 1973;134:921-926.

Eger M, Schmidt B, Torok G: Replantation of the upper extremities. Am J Surg 1974;4:47-50.

Ehrenfeld WK, Wilber BG, Olcott CN, Stoney RJ: Autogenous tissue reconstruction in the management of infected prosthetic grafts. Surgery 1979;85:82-91.

Eifert S, Villavicencio JL, Kao TC, et al: Prevalence of deep venous anomalies in congenital vascular malformations of venous predominance. J Vasc Surg 2000;31:462-471.

Eiseman B, Rainer WG: Clinical management of post traumatic rupture of the thoracic aorta. J Thorac Cardiovasc Surg 1958;35:347-358.

Eisenbrey AB: Arteriovenous aneurysm of the superficial femoral vessels. JAMA 1913;61:2155-2157.

Ekbom B, Towne JB, Majewski JT, Woods JH: Intra-abdominal vascular trauma: A need for prompt operation. J Trauma 1981;21:1040-1044.

Eklof B, Gjores JE, Thulesius O, Bergqvist D: Controversies in the Management of Venous Disorders. Stoneham, Butterworths, 1989.

Elderding SC, Manart FD, Moore EE: A reappraisal of penetrating neck injury management. J Trauma 1980;20:695-697.

Elford J, Burrell C, Roobottom C: Ultrasound guided percutaneous thrombin injection for the treatment of iatrogenic pseudoaneurysms. Heart 1999;82:526-527.

Elkin DC: Diagnosis and treatment of cardiac trauma. Ann Surg 1941;114:169-185.

Elkin DC: Vascular injuries of warfare. Ann Surg 1944;120:284-310.

Elkin DC: Wounds of the heart. Ann Surg 1944;120:817-821.

Elkin DC: Arteriovenous aneurysm. Surg Gynecol Obstet 1945;80:217-224.

Elkin DC: Traumatic aneurysm: The Matas Operation 57 years after. Surg Gynecol Obstet 1946;82:1-12.

Elkin DC, Banner EA: Arteriovenous aneurysms following surgical operations. JAMA 1946;131:1117-1119.

Elkin DC, Campbell RE: Cardiac tamponade: Treatment by aspiration. Ann Surg 1941;133:623-630.

Elkin DC, DeBakey ME: Vascular surgery in World War II. Washington, DC, US Government Printing Office, 1955.

Elkin DC, Harris MH: Arteriovenous aneurysm of the vertebral vessels. Ann Surg 1946;124:934-951.

Elkin DC, Shumacker HB Jr: In Elkin DC, DeBakey ME (eds): Vascular Surgery in World War II. Washington, DC, US Government Printing Office, 1944.

Elkin DC, Woodhall B: Combined vascular and nerve injuries of warfare. Ann Surg 1944;119:411-431.

Elkins RC, DeMeester TR, Brawley RK: Surgical exposure of the upper abdominal aorta and its branches. Surgery 1971;70:622-627.

Eller JL, Ziter FMH: Avulsion of the innominate artery from the aortic arch. Radiology 1970;94:75-78.

Elliot JA: Acute arterial occlusion: An unusual cause. Surgery 1956;39:825-827.

Ellis F: Surgical repair of a traumatic rupture of the thoracic aorta. Br J Surg 1959;46:495-499.

Ellis J: Case of gunshot wound, attended with secondary hemorrhage in which both carotid arteries were tied at an interval of four and a half days. N Y J Med 1845;5:187.

Ellis J: A case of probable lead poisoning, resulting fatally from a bullet lodged in the knee joint twelve years previously. Boston Med Surg J 1874;91:472.

Ellison RG, Meares CH: Traumatically injured aortic arch repaired under profound hypothermia and circulatory arrest. Am Surg 1977;43:298-302.

Elmore JR, Gloviczki P, Harper CM Jr, et al: Spinal cord injury in experimental thoracic aortic occlusion: Investigation of combined methods of protection. J Vasc Surg 1992;15:789-799.

Enderson BL, Reath DB, Meadors J, Dallas W: The tertiary trauma survey: A prospective study of missed injury. J Trauma 1990;30:666.

Enge I, Aakhus T, Evensen A: Angiography in vascular injuries of the extremities. Acta Radiol Diag 1975;16:193-199.

Engleman RM, Clements JM, Herrmann JB: Stab wounds and traumatic false aneurysms in the extremities. J Trauma 1969;9:77-87.

Epstein BM, Bocchiola FC, Andrews JC, Bester L: Traumatic arteriovenous fistula involving the portal venous system. Clin Radiol 1987;38:91-93.

Ergin MA, O'Connor JV, Blanche C, Griepp RB: Use of stapling instruments in surgery for aneurysms of the aorta. Ann Thorac Surg 1983;36:161-166.

Ernst CB, Daugherty ME, Bristow DL: Supraceliac pseudoaneurysm of abdominal aorta. Arch Surg 1975;110:211-225.

Ernst CB, Kaufer F: Fibulectomy-fasciotomy: An important adjunct in the management of lower extremity arterial trauma. J Trauma 1971;11:365.

Erskine JM: Case report: A true traumatic aneurysm of the radial artery at the wrist successfully treated by resection and arterial repair. J Trauma 1964;4:530-534.

Escobar GA, Escobar SC, Marquez L, et al: Vascular trauma: Late sequelae and treatment. J Cardiac Surg 1980;21:35-40.

Eshaghy B, Loeb HS, Miller SE, et al: Mediastinal and retropharyngeal hemorrhage. A complication of cardiac catheterization. JAMA 1973;226:427-431.

Esmarch F: The Surgeons Handbook of the Treatment of the Wounded in War. New York, LW Schmidt, 1878.

Espada R, Wisennand HH, Mattox KL, Beall AC Jr: Surgical management of penetrating injuries to the coronary arteries. Surgery 1975;78:755-760.

Espinoza R, Sonneborn R: Contusion of the abdominal aorta and massive embolization from the use of a seat belt. Rev Med Chil 1990;118:1376-1379.

Esposito TJ, Jurkovich G, Rice CL: Reappraisal of emergency room thoracotomy in a changing environment. J Trauma 1991;31:881-887.

Esterera AS, Pass LJ, Platt MR: Systemic arterial air embolism in penetrating lung injury. Ann Thorac Surg 1990;2:257.

Ettien JT: Crutch-induced aneurysms of the axillary artery. Am Surg 1980;46:267-269.

Evans J, Gray LA, Rayner A, Fulton RL: Principles for the management of penetrating cardiac wounds. Ann Surg 1979;189:777-784.

Evans WE, Bernhard VM: Tibial artery bypass for ischemia resulting from fractures. J Trauma 1971;11:999-1007.

Fabian TC, Turkleson ML, Connelly TL, Stone HH: Injury to the popliteal artery. Am J Surg 1982;143:225-228.

Fabian TC, Mangiante EC, Patterson CR, et al: Myocardial contusion in blunt trauma: Clinical characteristics, means of diagnosis and implications for patient management. J Trauma 1988;28:50-57.

Fabian TC, George SM Jr, Croce MA, et al: Carotid artery trauma: Management based on mechanism of injury. J Trauma 1990;30:953-963.

Fabian TC, Richardson JD, Croce MA, et al: Prospective study of blunt aortic injury: Multicenter trial of the American Association for the Surgery of Trauma. J Trauma 1997;42:748-755.

Fabian TC, Richardson JD, Croce MA, et al: Perspective study of blunt aortic injury: Multicenter trial of the American Association for Surgery of Trauma. J Trauma 1997;42:374-387.

Fakhry BM, Jaques FF, Proctor HJ: Cervical vessel injury after blunt trauma. J Vasc Surg 1988;8:501-508.

Falkmer L, Eriksson A, Arnerlov C, Domellof L: Arterial bullet embolism with radiologic demonstration of vessel entrance site. World J Surg 1987;11:548-558.

Fallahnejad M, Kutty ACK, Menut H: The importance of intra-aortic balloon pumping in the management of coronary artery laceration. J Cardiac Surg 1983;23:426-428.

Fallahnejad M, Kutty ACK, Wallace HW: Secondary lesions of penetrating cardiac injuries: A frequent complication. Ann Surg 1980;191:228-233.

Fallahnejad M, Wallace HW, Su CC, et al: Unusual manifestations of penetrating cardiac injuries. Arch Surg 1975;110:1357-1362.

Fallon G, Thomford NR: False aneurysm of the superficial femoral artery associated with fracture of the femur. Angiology 1970;21:120-123.

Falor WH, Hansel JR, Williams GB: Gangrene of the hand: A complication of radial artery cannulation. J Trauma 1976;16:713-716.

Fargally M, Christenson JT: Combined aortic and inferior vena cava injury during laminectomy. Vasa 1988;17:288-292.

Farhood A, McGuire GM, Manning AM, et al: Intercellular adhesion molecule 1 (ICAM-1) expression and its role in neutrophil induced ischemia-reperfusion injury in rat liver. J Leukoc Biol 1995;57:368-374.

Farina C, Cavallaro A, Schultz RD, et al: Popliteal aneurysms. Surg Gynecol Obstet 1989;169:7-13.

Faro RS, Monson DO, Weinberg M, Javid H: Disruption of aortic arch branches due to nonpenetrating chest trauma. Arch Surg 1983;118:1333-1336.

Farret A, Da Ros CT, Fischer CA, et al: Suprarenal aorta reconstruction using a saphenous spiral graft: A case relate? J Trauma 1994;37:114-118.

Fasol R, Irvine S, Zilla P: Vascular injuries caused by anti-personnel mines. J Cardiac Surg 1989;30:467.

Fay R, Brosman S, Lidstrom R: Renal artery thrombosis: A successful revascularization by autotransplantation. J Urol 1974;111:572.

Feczko JD, Lynch L, Pless JE, et al: An autopsy case review of 142 nonpenetrating (blunt) injuries of the aorta. J Trauma 1992;33:846-849.

Fee JF, Cavoy JM, Dainko EA: Pseudoaneurysm of the axillary artery following a modified Bristow operation: A report of a case and review. Cardiovasc Surg 1978;19:65-68.

Feigenbaum H, Waldhausen JA, Hyde LP: Ultrasonic diagnosis of pericardial effusion. JAMA 1965;191:107.

Feigenbaum H, Zaky A, Waldhausen JA: Use of ultrasound in diagnosis of pericardial effusion. Intern Med 1966;65:443.

Feliciano DV: Managing peripheral vascular trauma. Infect Surg 1986;5:659-669.

Feliciano DV: Pitfalls in the management of peripheral vascular injuries. In Roses D (ed): Problems in General Surgery. Philadelphia, JB Lippincott Co, 1986, pp 101-113.

Feliciano DV: Vascular injuries. Adv Trauma 1987;179:206.

Feliciano DV: Abdominal gunshot wounds. Ann Surg 1988;208:362-370.

Feliciano DV: Approach to major abdominal vascular injury. J Vasc Surg 1988;7:730-736.

Feliciano DV: Counterpoint. J Trauma 1992;32:553-554.

Feliciano DV: Abdominal vessels. In Ivatury R, Cayten C (eds): The Textbook of Penetrating Trauma. Baltimore, Williams & Wilkins, 1996, pp 702-716.

Feliciano DV: Abdominal vascular injuries. Surg Clin North Am 2001;68:741.

Feliciano DV, Accola KD, Burch JM, Spjut-Patrinely V: Extra-anatomic bypass for peripheral arterial injuries. Am J Surg 1989;158:505.

Feliciano DV, Bitondo CG, Mattox KL, et al: Civilian trauma in 1980s: A one-year experience with 456 vascular and cardiac injuries. Ann Surg 1984;199:717-724.

Feliciano DV, Bitondo CG, Mattox KL, et al: Combined tracheoesophageal injuries. Am J Surg 1985;150:710-715.

Feliciano DV, Burch JM, Graham JM: Abdominal vascular injury. In Mattox KL, Feliciano DV, Moore EE (eds): Trauma. New York, McGraw-Hill, 1999, pp 783-805.

Feliciano DV, Burch JM, Mattox KL, et al: Balloon catheter tamponade in cardiovascular wounds. Am J Surg 1990;160:583-587.

Feliciano DV, Cosseli JS, Bitondo CG: Bilateral external iliac artery injury from a single missile. J Cardiac Surg 1986;27:46.

Feliciano DV, Cruse PA, Burch JM, Bitondo CF: Delayed diagnosis of arterial injuries. Am J Surg 1987;154:579-584.

Feliciano DV, Cruse PA, Spjvi-Patrinely V, et al: Fasciotomy after trauma to the extremities. Am J Surg 1988;156:533-536.

Feliciano DV, Gentry LO, Bitondo CG, et al: Single agent cephalosporin prophylaxis for penetrating abdominal trauma. Am J Surg 1986;152:674-681.

Feliciano DV, Herskowitz K, O'Gorman RB: Management of vascular injuries in lower extremities. J Trauma 1988;28:319-328.

Feliciano DV, Mattox KL: Major complications of percutaneous subclavian vein catheters. Am J Surg 1979;138:869-874.

Feliciano DV, Mattox KL, Graham JM, Bitondo CG: Five-year experience with PTFE grafts in vascular wounds. J Trauma 1985;25:71-82.

Feller I: Surgical anatomy of the abdominal aorta. Ann Surg 1961;154:239.

Fellmeth BD, Roberts AC, Bookstein JJ: Postangiographic femoral artery injuries: Nonsurgical repair with US-guided compression. Radiology 1991;178:671-675.

Fenner MN, Fisher KS, Sergel NL, et al: Evaluation of possible traumatic thoracic aortic injury using aortography. Am Surg 1990;56:497-499.

Ferguson IA, Byrd WM, McAfee DK: Experiences in the management of arterial injuries. Ann Surg 1961;153:980-986.

Ferguson WM: Arteriovenous aneurysm following osteotomy for genu valgum. Lancet 1914;1:532.

Fernandez LG, Lain KY, Messersmith RN, et al: Transesophageal echocardiography for diagnosing aortic injury: A case report and summary of current imaging techniques. J Trauma 1994;36:877-880.

Fernandez LG, Radhakrishnan J, Gordon RT, et al: Thoracic injuries in pediatric patients. J Trauma 1995;38:384-388.

Ferriter P, Hirschy J, Kesseler H, Scott WN: Popliteal pseudoaneurysm: A case report. J Bone Joint Surg 1983;65-A:695-697.

Finkelmeier BA, Mentzer RM Jr, Kaiseer DL, et al: Chronic traumatic thoracic aneurysm: Influence of operative treatment on natural history: An analysis of reported cases. J Thorac Cardiovasc Surg 1982;84:257-266.

Fish GD Jr, Hockhauser M: Laceration of the popliteal artery due to blunt trauma. Am J Surg 1957;94:651.

Fisher GW: Acute arterial injuries treated by the United States Army Medical Service in Vietnam, 1965-1966. J Trauma 1967;7:844-855.

Fisher RD, Rienhoff WF III: Subclavian artery laceration resulting from fracture first rib. J Trauma 1966;6:579.

Fisher RG, Ben-Manachem Y: Penetrating injuries of the thoracic aorta and brachiocephalic arteries: Angiographic finding in 18 cases. AJR Am J Roentgenol 1987;149:607-611.

Fisher RG, Chasen MH, Lamki N: Diagnosis of injuries of the aorta and brachiocephalic arteries caused by blunt chest trauma: CT vs aortography. AJR Am J Roentgenol 1994;162:1047-1052.

Fisher RG, Oria RA, Mattox KL, et al: Conservative management of aortic lacerations due to blunt trauma. J Trauma 1990;30:1562-1566.

Fisher RG, Ward RE, Ben-Manachem Y, et al: Arteriography and the fractured first rib: Too much or too little? AJR Am J Roentgenol 1982;117:657-661.

Fitchett VH, Pomerantz M, Butsch DW, et al: Penetrating wounds of the neck. Arch Surg 1969;99:307-314.

Fitts CT, Barnett LT, Webb CM, et al: Perforating wounds of the heart caused by central venous catheters. J Trauma 1970;10:764-769.

Fitzgerald EJ, Brumsler WG, Ruttley ST: False aneurysm of the femoral artery: Computed tomography and ultrasound appearance. Clin Radiat 1986;37:585-588.

Fitzgerald JB, Crawford ES, DeBakey ME: Surgical consideration of non penetrating abdominal injuries. Am J Surg 1960;100:22-29.

Fitzgerald JF, Keates J: False aneurysm as a late complication of anterior dislocation of the shoulder. Ann Surg 1975;181:785-786.

Fitzsimons LE, Garvey FK: Inferior vena caval injury: Case report. J Urol 1959;83:258-259.

Flanigan DP: Civilian Vascular Trauma. Philadelphia, Lea & Febiger, 1992.

Flanigan DP, Keifer TJ, Schuler JJ, et al: Experience with iatrogenic pediatric vascular injuries: Incidence, etiology, management, and results. Ann Surg 1983;198:430-442.

Fleckenstein JL, Schultz SM, Miller RH: Serial aortography assesses stability of "atypical" aortic arch ruptures. Cardiovasc Intervent Radiol 1987;10:194-197.

Fleming A, Bishop M, Shoemaker W, et al: Prospective trial of supranormal values as goals of resuscitation in severe trauma. Arch Surg 1992;127:1175-1181.

Fleming AW, Green DC: Traumatic aneurysms of the thoracic aorta: A report of 43 patients. Ann Thorac Surg 1974;18:91-101.

Fleming JI: Case of rupture of the carotid artery and wound of several of its branches successfully treated by tying off the common trunk of the carotid itself. (Translated by Coley RW). Med Chir J (Lond) 1817;3:2.

Fleming JFR, Petrie D: Traumatic thrombosis of the internal carotid artery with delayed hemiplegia. Can J Surg 1968;11:166-172.

Fleming WB: A case of attempted repair of the superior mesenteric vessels. Aust N Z J Surg 1961;31:151-154.

Fletcher JP, Little JM: Injuries of branches of the aortic arch. Aust N Z J Surg 1988;58:217-219.

Flint LM: Arterial injuries with lower extremity fracture. Surgery 1983;93: 5-8.

Flint LM, Synder WH, Perry MO, Shires GT: Management of major vascular injuries in the base of the neck: An 11-year experience with 146 cases. Arch Surg 1973;106:407-413.

Fogarty TJ: Catheter technique for arterial embolectomy. Ann Surg 1965;161:325-330.

Fogarty TJ, Cranley JJ, Strasser ES, Hafner CD: A method for extraction of arterial emboli and thrombi. Surg Gynecol Obstet 1963;116:241-244.

Fogelman MJ, Stewart RD: Penetrating wounds of the neck. Am J Surg 1965;91:581-596.

Fomon JJ, Warren WD: Complications of peripheral arterial injuries. Arch Surg 1965;91:610-616.

Foramitti KI: Wien Klin Wschr 1910;25:46-55. (Cited in Foramitti.H)

Forbes AD, Ashbaugh DG: Mechanical circulatory support during repair of thoracic aortic injuries improves morbidity and prevents spinal cord injury. Arch Surg 1994;129:497-498.

Forbes HW, Thompson CQ, Smith JW: Mesenteric arteriovenous fistula after a gunshot wound. J Trauma 1969;9:806.

Forrest CR, Pang CY, Zhong AG, Kreidstein ML: Efficacy of intravenous infusion of prostacyclin (PG12) or prostaglandin E_1 (PGE_1) in augmentation of skin flap blood flow and viability in the pig. Prostaglandins 1991;225:518-527.

Forster DA: Letter to editor. J Trauma 1985;25:1115.

Foster JH, Carter JW, Grahamm CP Jr, Edwards WH: Arterial injury secondary to the use of the Fogarty catheter. Ann Surg 1970;171:971-978.

Foster RD, Albright JA: Acute compartment syndrome of the thigh: A case report. J Trauma 1990;30:108-110.

Fouin A: Sur la sutre des vaisseaux. Presse Med 1908;16:233-236.

Fox S, Pierce WS, Waldhausen JA: Acute hypertension: Its significance in traumatic aortic rupture. J Thorac Cardiovasc Surg 1979;77:622-625.

Fradet G, Nelems B, Meuller NL: Penetrating injury of the torso with impalement of the thoracic aorta: Preoperative value of the computed tomographic scan. Ann Thorac Surg 1988;45:680-681.

Frame SB, Timberlake GA, Rush DS, et al: Penetrating injuries of the abdominal aorta. Am Surg 1990;56:651-654.

Francis H III, Thal ER, Weigelt JA, Redman HC: Vascular proximity: Is it a valid indication for arteriography in asymptomatic patients? J Trauma 1991; 31:512-514.

Frank MJ, Nadimi M, Lesniak LJ: Effects of cardiac tamponade on myocardial performance blood flow and metabolism. Am J Physiol 1971;220:179-185.

Franz JL, Simpson CR, Penny RM, et al: Avulsion of the innominate artery after blunt chest trauma. J Thorac Cardiovasc Surg 1974;67:478-480.

Fraser GA: Closed traumatic rupture of common femoral artery. Ann Surg 1965;161:539-544.

Freeark RJ: Role of angiography in the management of multiple injuries. Surg Gynecol Obstet 1969;128:761-771.

Freeman NE: Secondary hemorrhage arising from gunshot wounds of the peripheral blood vessels. Ann Surg 1945;122:631-640.

Freeman NE: Arterial repair in the treatment of aneurysms and arteriovenous fistulae: A report of 18 successful restorations. Ann Surg 1946;124:888-919.

Freeman NE, Shumacker HB Jr: Vascular surgery. In Elkin DC, DeBakey ME (eds): Washington, DC, US Government Printing Office, 1955.

Freidman AL, Gertler JP: Thoracoabdominal repair of post-traumatic aorta-renal vein fistula following a previous transabdominal approach: A case report. J Trauma 1991;31:287-289.

French BG, Hughes CF: Post-traumatic chromic false aneurysm of the ascending aorta with long-term survival. Aust N Z J Surg 1994;64:284-285.

Freshman SP, Wisner DH, Weber CJ: 2D echocardiography: Eemergent use in the evaluation of penetrating precordial trauma. J Trauma 1991;31:902-906.

Fried G, Salerno T, Burke D, et al: Management of the extremity with combined neurovascular and musculoskeletal trauma. J Trauma 1978;18:481-484.

Friedman SG: A History of Vascular Surgery. Mt. Kisco, NY, Futura Publishing, 1989.

Fromm SH, Lucas CE: Obturator bypass for mycotic aneurysm in the drug addict. Arch Surg 1970;100:82-83.

Fromm SH, Carrasquilla C, Lucas C: The management of gunshot wounds of the aorta: The use of Dacron grafts to replace the injured aorta. Arch Surg 1970;101:388-390.

Fry RE, Fry WJ: Extracranial carotid artery injuries. Surgery 1980;88:581-587.

Frydenberg M, Royle JP, Hoare M: Blunt abdominal aortic trauma. Aust N Z J Surg 1990;60:347-350.

Frykberg ER: Arteriography of the injured extremity: Are we in proximity to an answer. J Trauma 1992;32:551-552.

Frykberg ER, Crump JM, Dennis JW, et al: Nonoperative observation of clinically occult arterial injuries: A prospective evaluation. Surgery 1991;109:85-96.

Frykberg ER, Crump JM, Vines FS, et al: A reassessment of the role of arteriography in assessing acute vascular injuries. J Trauma 1989;29:1041-1052.

Frykberg ER, Crump JM, Vines FS, McLellan GL: A reassessment of the role of arteriography in penetrating proximity extremity: A prospective study. J Trauma 1989;29:1041-1052.

Frykberg ER, Dennis JW, Bishop K, et al: The reliability of physical examination in the evaluation of penetrating extremity trauma for vascular injury: Results at one year. J Trauma 1991;31:502-511.

Frykberg ER, Vines FS, Alexander RH: The natural history of clinically occult arterial injuries: A prospective evaluation. J Trauma 1989;29:577-583.

Fu WR: Angiography of Trauma. Springfield, Ill, Charles C Thomas, 1972.

Fulda G, Rodriguez A, Turney SZ, Cowley RA: Blunt traumatic pericardial rupture: A ten-year experience 1979-89. J Cardiac Surg 1990;31:525-530.

Fullen WD, Hunt J, Altemeier WA: The clinical spectrum of penetrating injury to the superior mesenteric arterial circulation. J Trauma 1972;12:656-664.

Furman S, Vijaynagar R, McMullen M, Scher DJW: Lethal sequelae of intra-aortic balloon rupture surgery. Surgery 1971;69:121-129.

Furnas DW, Saliblan AH, Achauer BM: Genesis of a replantation program. Am J Surg 1978;136:21-25.

Gaddard P, Jones AG, Wisheart JD: Self-inflicted stab wound causing aorto-right ventricular fistula. Am Heart J 1981;46:101-103.

Gage M: Traumatic injuries to the peripheral vessels in both civil and military practice. Surgery 1942;11:983-986.

Gainor BJ, Metzler M: Humeral shaft fracture with brachial artery injury. Clin Orthop Relat Res 1986;204:154-161.

Gale SS, Scissons RP, Jones L, Salles-Cunha SX: Femoral pseudoaneurysm thrombinjection. Am J Surg 2001;181:379-383.

Gallen J, Wiss DA, Cantelmo N, Menzoian JO: Traumatic pseudoaneurysm of the axillary artery: Report of three cases and literature review. J Trauma 1984;24:350-354.

Gammie JS, Katz WE, Swanson ER, Peitsman AB: Acute aortic dissection after blunt chest trauma. J Trauma 1996;40:126-127.

Garamella JJ, Schmidt WR, Jensen NK, Lynch MF: Traumatic aneurysms of the thoracic aorta. Report of four cases, including one of spontaneous rupture into the esophagus. N Engl J Med 1962;266:1341-1348.

Garcia-Rinaldi R, Defore WW, Mattox KL, Beall AC Jr: Unimpaired renal myocardial and neurologic function after cross clamping of the thoracic aorta. Surg Gynecol Obstet 1976;143:249-252.

Gardner C: Traumatic vasospasm and its complications. Am J Surg 1952;83:468-470.

Gardner WJ, Storer J: The use of the G Suit in control of intra-abdominal bleeding. Surg Gynecol Obstet 1966;123:792.

Garrison RN, Richardson JD, Fry DE: Diagnostic transdiaphragmatic pericardiotomy in thoracoabdominal trauma. J Trauma 1982;22:147-149.

Garzon A, Gleidman ML: Peripheral embolization of bullet following perforation of the thoracic aorta. Am Surg 1964;160:901.

Gaspar MR: Vascular injury secondary to drug abuse. In Ernst CB, Stanley JC (eds): Current Therapy in Vascular Surgery. Philadelphia, BC Decker, 1987.

Gaspar MR, Hare RR: Gangrene due to intraarterial injection of drugs by drug addicts. Surgery 1987;72:573-577.

Gaspar MR, Treiman RL: The management of injuries to major veins. Am J Surg 1960;100:171-175.

Gaspar MR, Treiman RL, Payne JH, et al: Principles of treatment and special problems in vascular trauma. Surg Clin North Am 1968;48:1355.

Gaspard DJ, Gaspar MR: Arteriovenous fistula after Fogarty catheter thrombectomy. Arch Surg 1972;105:90-92.

Gasparini D, Lovaria A, Saccheri S: Percutaneous treatment of iliac aneurysms and pseudoaneurysms with Cragg Endopro System 1 stent-grafts. Cardiovasc Intervent Radiol 1997;20:348-352.

Gates JD, Clair DG, Hechtman DH: Thoracic aortic dissection with renal artery involvement following blunt thoracic trauma: Case report. J Trauma 1994;36:430-432.

Gates JD, Knox JB: Axillary artery injuries secondary to anterior dislocation of the shoulder. J Trauma 1995;39:581-583.

Gauderer MW, Wolkoff JS, Izant RJ: Traumatic aneurysm of the suprarenal abdominal aorta: Surgical reconstruction in a 7-year-old patient. J Pediatr Surg 1982;17:940-945.

Gaudio KM, Taylor MR, Chaudry IH, et al: Accelerated recovery of single nephron function by the postischemic infusion of ATP-MgCl2. Kidney Int 1982;22:13-20.

Gavant ML, Gold RE, Fabian TC, Tonkin LI: Vascular trauma to the extremities and lower neck: Initial assessment with intravenous digital subtraction angiography. Radiology 1986;158:755-760.

Gay W: Blunt trauma to the heart and great vessels. Surgery 1982;91:507-509.

Gazzanaga AB, IKhuri EI, Mir-Sepasi HM, Bartlett RH: Rupture of the thoracic aorta following blunt trauma. Arch Surg 1975;110:1119-1123.

Geer TM, Rich NM: Cardiac trauma in Vietnam: Unpublished data in the Vietnam Vascular Registry. 1972.

Geer TM: Personal communication, 1972.

Geiran O, Solheim K: Cardiac and aortic injuries. Scand J Thorac Cardiovasc Surg 1974;8:27-33.

Geis WP, Johnson CF, Zajtchuk R, Kittle CF: Extrapericardial (mediastinal) cardiac tamponade. Arch Surg 1970;100:305-306.

Gelberman RH, Blasingame JP, Arnost F, et al: Forearm arterial injuries. J Hand Surg 1979;4:401-408.

Gelberman RH, Menon J, Fronek A: The peripheral pulse following arterial injury. J Trauma 1980;20:948-950.

Gelberman RH, Nunley JA, Koman LA, et al: The results of radial and ulnar arterial repair in the forearm. J Bone Joint Surg 1982;64:383-387.

Geller DA, Chia SH, Takahashi Y, et al: Protective role of the L-arginine-nitric oxide synthase pathway on preservation injury after rat-liver transplantation. J Parenter Enter Nutr 2001;25:142-147.

Gensoul: Note sur les Bless és reçus á l'Hôtel Dieu de Lyon, pendant les troubles de 1831. Gaz Méd Paris 1883;297.

Gensoul: 1883 Cited in Simeone, et al. On the question of ligation of the concomitant vein when a major artery is interrupted. Surgery 1951;29:932-951.

Gentry LO, Feliciano DV, Lea AS, et al: Perioperative antibiotic therapy for penetrating injuries of the abdomen. Ann Surg 1984;200:561-566.

George SM Jr, Croce MA, Fabian TC: Cervicothoracic arterial injuries: Recommendations for diagnosis and management. World J Surg 1991;15:134-140.

Ger R: The coverage of vascular repairs by muscle transposition. J Trauma 1976;16:974-978.

Gerbode F, Holman E, Dickenson EH, Spencer FC: Arteriovenous fistulas and arterial aneurysms: The repair of major arteries injured in warfare, and the treatment of an arterial aneurysm with a vein graft inlay. Surgery 1952;32:259-274.

Gerbode F, Braimbridge M, Osborn JJ, et al: Traumatic thoracic aneurysms: Treatment by resection and grafting with the use of an extracorporeal bypass. Surgery 1957;42:975-985.

Gerlock AJ Jr: The use of pedal venous pressure (PVP) as a guide in evaluating the patency of venous repairs. J Trauma 1977;17:108-110.

Gerlock AJ Jr, Mathis J, Goncharenko V, Maravilla A: Angiography of intimal and intramural arterial injuries. Radiology 1978;129:357-361.

Gerlock AJ Jr, Muhletaler CA: Venography of peripheral venous injuries. Radiology 1979;133:77-80.

Gerlock AJ Jr, Thal ER, Snyder WH III: Venography in penetrating injuries of the extremities. AJR Am J Roentgenol 1976;126:1023-1027.

German DS, Shapiro MJ, Willman VL: Acute aortic valvular incompetence following blunt thoracic deceleration injury: Case report. J Trauma 1990;30:1411-1412.

Gertsch P: Lesions vasculaires des blesses de guerre Afghans Traitees a l'Hospital du CICR a Peshawar. Med Milit 1986;2:46.

Gervin AS, Fischer CA: The importance of prompt transport in salvage of patients with penetrating heart wounds. J Trauma 1982;22:443-448.

Getzen LC, Bellinger SB, Kendall LW: Should all neck, axillary, groin or popliteal wounds be explored for possible vascular or visceral injuries. J Trauma 1972;12:906.

Geuder JW, Hobson RW II, Padberg FT Jr, et al: The role of contrast arteriography in suspected arterial injuries of the extremities. Am Surg 1985;51:89-93.

Gewertz B, O'Brien C, Kirsh MM: Use of the intra-aortic balloon support of refractory low cardiac output in myocardial contusion. J Trauma 1977;17:325-327.

Gewertz BL, Samson DS, Ditmore QM, Bone GE: Management of penetrating injuries of the internal carotid artery at the base of the skull utilizing extracranial-intracranial bypass. J Trauma 1980;20:365-369.

Gibbons JR: Treatment of missile injuries of the chest: Belfast experience. J Cardiothorac Surg 1989;4:297.

Gibson JMC: Rupture of axillary artery. J Bone Joint Surg 1962;44B:114-115.

Gielchinsky I, McNamara JJ: Cardiac wounds at a military evacuation hospital in Vietnam: A review of one-year's experience. J Thorac Cardiovasc Surg 1970;60:603-606.

Gielchinsky I, McNamara JJ: Fléchette wounds of the heart. Surgery 1971;69:229-231.

Giglia JS, Zelenock GB, D'Alecy L: Prevention of paraplegia during thoracic aortic cross-clamping: Importance of patent internal mammary arteries. J Vasc Surg 1994;19:1044-1051.

Gill SS, Eggleston FC, Singh CM: Arterial injuries of the extremities. J Trauma 1976;16:766-772.

Gingrass RP, Cunningham DS, Paletta FX: Skin grafting of exposed arterial grafts: A clinical and experimental study. J Trauma 1973;13:951-957.

Giraud RM: Arteriovenous fistula of the aortic arch complicating stab wound of the neck. S Afr Med J 1965;12:474-476.

Glaser RL, McKellar D, Scher KS: Arteriovenous fistulas after cardiac catheterization. Arch Surg 1989;124:1313-1315.

Glück T: Uber zwei fälle von aortenaneurysmen nebst bemerkungen uber die naht der blutgefässe. Arch Klin Chir 1883;28:548.

Gnanadev DA, Fandrich BL: Popliteal artery trauma: Update and recent advances in management. Ann Vasc Surg 1988;2:332-335.

Goff JB, Gillespie DL, Rich NM: Long-term follow-up of a superficial femoral vein injury: A case report from the Vietnam Vascular Registry. J Trauma 1998;44:209-211.

Goff J, Gillespie D, Rich NM: Long-Term Follow-up of Military Superficial Femoral Vein Injury: A Case Report from Vietnam Vascular Registry. 1996 February 23-25, San Diego. San Diego, American Venous Forum, 1996.

Gold AH, Lee GW: Upper extremity replantation: Current concepts and patient. J Trauma 1981;21:551-557.

Goldberg BB, Ostrium BJ, Isard JJ: Ultrasonic determination of pericardial effusion. JAMA 1967;202:103.

Goldberger M: Clinical experience with intra-aortic balloon counter pulsation in 112 consecutive patients. Am Heart 1986;111:497-502.

Goldman BS, Firor WB, Key JA: The recognition and management of peripheral arterial injuries. Can Med Assoc J 1965;92:1154-1160.

Goldman LI, Maier WP, Drezner AD: Another complication of subclavian puncture: Arterial laceration. JAMA 1971;217:78.

Goldman MH, Kent S, Schaumburg E: Brachial artery injuries associated with posterior elbow dislocation. Surg Gynecol Obstet 1987;164:95-97.

Goletti O, Ghiselli G, Lippolis PV, et al: The role of ultrasonography in blunt abdominal trauma: Results in 250 consecutive cases. J Trauma 1994;36:178-181.

Golman BS, Firor WB, Key JA: The recognition and management of peripheral arterial injuries. Can Med Assoc J 1965;92:1154-1160.

Golueke PJ, Goldstein AS, Sclanfani SJA, et al: Routine versus selective exploration of penetrating neck injuries: A randomized, prospective study. J Trauma 1984;24:1010-1014.

Golueke PJ, Sclanfani S, Phillips T, et al: Vertebral artery injury: Diagnosis and management. J Trauma 1987;27:856-865.

Gomes MMR, Gernatz PE: Arteriovenous fistulas: A review and 10-year experience at the Mayo Clinc. Mayo Clin Proc 1970;45:81-102.

Gomez GA, Kreis DJ Jr, Ratner L, et al: Suspected vascular trauma of the extremities: The role of arteriography in proximity injuries. J Trauma 1986;26:1005-1008.

Gomez RL, Bole PV, Lande A, et al: Successful repair of two false aneurysms of the abdominal aorta. Arch Surg 1973;107:91-94.

Goodman C: Suture of blood vessel from projectiles of war. Surg Gynecol Obstet 1918;27:528.

Goodman P, Jeffrey R, Brant-Zawadki M: Digital subtraction angiography in extremity trauma. Radiology 1984;153:61-64.

Gordon RL, Landau RH, Shifrin E, Romanoff H: The use of a balloon catheter in the treatment of an iatrogenic pseudoaneurysm of the subclavian artery. J Cardiovasc Surg 1983;24:178-180.

Gorman JF: Combat wounds of the popliteal artery. Ann Surg 1968;24:178-180.

Gorman JF: Combat arterial trauma: Analysis of 106 limb-threatening injuries. Arch Surg 1969;98:160-164.

Gosselin RA, Yukka Siegberg CJ, Coupland R, Agerskov K: Outcome of arterial repairs in 23 consecutive patients at the ICRC-Peshawar hospital for war wounded. J Trauma 1993;34:373-376.

Gott VL: Heparinized shunts for thoracic vascular operations. Ann Thorac Surg 1972;14:219-220.

Goyanes J: Neuvos trabajos de chirurgial vascular: Substitution plastica de las the arterias por las venas, o arterio-plastia venosa, aplicado, como neuvo metodo, al traitamiento de los aneurismas. El Siglo Med 1906;53:546-561.

Grablowsky OM, Weichert RF III, Goff JB, Schlegel JU: Renal artery thrombosis following blunt trauma: Report of four cases. Surgery 1970;67:895.

Graeber GM, Clagett GP, Wolf RE, et al: Alteration in serum creatine kinase and lactate dehydrogenase: Association with abdominal aortic surgery, myocardial infarction and bowel necrosis. Chest 1990;97:521-527.

Graham JM, Feliciano DV, Mattox KL: Combined brachial, axillary and subclavian artery injuries of the same extremity: A case report. J Trauma 1980;20:899-901.

Graham JM, Feliciano DV, Mattox KL, Beall AC Jr: Innominate vascular injury. J Trauma 1982;22:647-655.

Graham JM, Feliciano DV, Mattox KL, et al: Management of subclavian vascular injuries. J Trauma 1980;20:537-544.

Graham JM, Mattox KL: Right ventricular bullet embolectomy without cardiopulmonary bypass. J Thorac Cardiovasc Surg 1981;82:310-313.

Graham JM, Mattox KL, Beall AC Jr: Portal venous system injuries. J Trauma 1978;18:419-422.

Graham JM, Mattox KL, Beall AC Jr, DeBakey ME: Traumatic injuries of the inferior vena cava. Arch Surg 1978;113:413-418.

Graham JM, Mattox KL, Beall AC Jr, DeBakey ME: Injuries to the visceral arteries. Surgery 1978;84:835-839.

Graham JM, Mattox KL, Feliciano DV, DeBakey ME: Vascular injuries of the axilla. Ann Surg 1982;195:232-238.

Gray WA: Prehospital resuscitation: The good, the bad, and futile. JAMA 1993;22:1471-1472.

Green NE, Allen BL: Vascular injuries associated with dislocation of the knee. J Bone Joint Surg 1977;59-A:236-239.

Greenfield LJ, Ebert PA: Technical considerations in the management of axillobrachial arterial injuries. J Trauma 1967;7:606-612.

Greenfield LJ: Perforation of the inferior vena cava with aortic and vertebral penetration by a suprarenal Greenfield filter. Radiology 1990;175:287.

Greenholz SK, Moore EE, Peterson NE, Moore GE: Traumatic bilateral renal artery occlusion: Successful outcome without surgical intervention. J Trauma 1986;26:941-944.

Greenough J: Operations on innominate artery: Report of a successful ligation. Arch Surg 1929;19:1484-1544.

Griffen WO, Belin RP, Walder AL: Traumatic aneurysm of the abdominal aorta. Surgery 1966;60:813-816.

Griffiths SJH: Traumatic rupture of the aorta. Br J Surg 1931;18:664-665.

Grimley RP, Ashton F, Slaney G, Batten RL: Popliteal artery injuries associated with civilian knee trauma. Injury 1981;13:1-6.

Griswold RA, Maguire CH: Penetrating wounds of the heart in pericardium. Surg Gynecol Obstet 1942;74:406-418.

Griswold RA, Drye JC: Cardiac wounds. Ann Surg 1954;139:783-785.

Groms GA, Flint LT: Repair of two traumatic aneurysms of the supraceliac abdominal aneurysm in a single patient. Surgery 1972;72:371-377.

Gross WS, Flanigan P, Kraft RO, Stanley JC: Chronic upper extremity arterial insufficiency. Arch Surg 1978;113:419-423.

Grossi EA, Krieger KH, Cunningham JN Jr, et al: Venoarterial bypass: A technique for spinal cord protection. J Thorac Cardiovasc Surg 1985;89:228-234.

Grosso MA, Simson MA, Kobayaski K: Myocardial ischemia pattern determines predisposition to ventricular arrhythmias. Surg Forum 1984;34:239-240.

Groves LK: Traumatic aneurysm of the thoracic aorta. N Engl J Med 1964;270:220-224.

Gruber HE, Weisman WH: Aortic thrombosis during sigmoidoscopy in Behçet's syndrome. Arch Intern Med 1983;143:343-345.

Gryska PF: Major vascular injuries: Principles of management in selected cases of arterial and venous injuries. N Engl J Med 1962;266:381-385.

Gschaedler R, Dollfus P, Loeb JP, et al: Traumatic rupture of the aorta and paraplegia. Paraplegia 1978;16:123-127.

Gubler KD, Wisner DH, Blaisdell FW: Multiple vessel injury to branches of the aortic arch: Case report. J Trauma 1991;31:1566-1568.

Guerriero WG, Carlton CE Jr, Scott R, Beall AC Jr: Renal pedical injuries. J Trauma 1971;11:53-62.

Gugenheim S, Sanders RJ: Axillary artery rupture caused by shoulder dislocation. Surgery 1984;95:55.

Guilfoil PH, Christiansen T: An unusual vascular complication of fractured clavicle. JAMA 1967;200:72-73.

Gundry SR, Willimams S, Burney RE, et al: Indications for aortography in blunt thoracic trauma: A reassessment. J Trauma 1982;22:664-671.

Gundry SR, Burney RE, MacKenzie JR, et al: Clinical contact with the trauma patient enhances accuracy of chest roentgenogram interpretation in predicting traumatic rupture of the aorta. J Cardiovasc Surg 1985;26:332-336.

Gunnlaugnson GH, Hallgrimsson JG, Sigurdsson JL, et al: Complete traumatic avulsion of the innominate artery from the aortic arch with a unique mechanism of injury. J Thorac Cardiovasc Surg 1973;66:235-240.

Gupta BK, Khaneja SC, Flores L, et al: The role of intra-aortic balloon occlusion in penetrating abdominal trauma. J Trauma 1989;29:861-865.

Gupta SK, Veith FJ: Management of juxtarenal aortic occlusion: Technique for suprarenal clamp placement. Ann Vasc Surg 1992;6:306-310.

Gurdjian ES, Hardy WG, Lindner DW, Thomas LM: Closed cervical cranial trauma, associated with involvement of carotid and vertebral arteries. Neurosurgery 1963;20:418.

Gurri JA, Johnson G Jr: Management of brachial artery occlusion after cardiac catheterization. Am Surg 1980;46:233-235.

Guthrie CC: Blood Vessel Surgery. London, Edward Arnold & Company, 1912.

Guthrie CC: Blood Vessel Surgery and Its Application. New York, Longmans, Green and Co, 1912.

Guthrie GJ: Disease and injuries of arteries. 1830.

Guvendik L, Davis NR, Starr A: Repair of traumatic aortic transection: A management protocol and review of 21 patients. J Thorac Cardiovasc Surg 1988;36:198-201.

Gwathmey O, Byrd CW: Clinical experience with acute traumatic rupture of the thoracic aorta in a general hospital. Ann Surg 1964;159:846-857.

Hafez HM, Woolgar J, Robbs JV: Lower extremity artery injury: Results of 550 cases and review of risk factors associated with limb loss. J Vasc Surg 2001;33:1212-1219.

Haimovici H: History of arterial grafting. J Cardiac Surg 1963;4:152-174.

Haimovici H: Iatrogenic acute arterial thrombosis: In Vascular Emergencies. New York, Appleton-Century-Crofts, 1982, pp 225-232.

Haimovici H, Hoffert PW, Zinicola N, Steinman C: An experimental and clinical evaluation of grafts in the venous system. Surg Gynecol Obstet 1970;131:1173-1186.

Hall RL, Anderson CA, Bickerstaff LK: Isolated vertebral artery injuries. Contemp Surg 1986;29:57-62.

Haller JA: Bullet transection of both carotid arteries: Immediate repair with recovery. Am J Surg 1962;103:532-535.

Hallowell. Extract of a letter from Mr. Lambert, surgeon at Newcastle upon Tyne, to Dr. Hunter, giving an account of new method of treating an aneurysm. Med Obser Inq 1762;30:360.

Halpern AA, Nagel DA: Anterior compartment pressures in patients with tibial fractures. J Trauma 1980;20:786-790.

Halpern NB, Aldrete JS: Factors influencing mortality and morbidity from injuries to the abdominal aorta and inferior vena cava. Am J Surg 1979;137:384-388.

Halsted W: Ligation of the first portion of the left subclavian artery and excision of subclavico-axillary aneurysm. Bull Johns Hopkins Hosp 1892;3:93.

Halsted W: Discussion in Bernheim, BM. Bull Johns Hopkins Hosp 1916;27:93.

Halsted WS: The effect of ligation of the common iliac artery on the circulation and function of lower extremity. Report of a cure of iliofemoral aneurysm by their application of an aluminum band to the vessel. Bull Johns Hopkins Hosp 1912;23:191-220.

Halsted WS: Ligation of the left subclavian artery in its first portion. Bull Johns Hopkins Hosp 1924;21:1.

Hamerlijnck RP, Rutsaert RR, De Geest R, et al: Surgical correction of descending thoracic aortic aneurysms under simple aortic cross-clamping. J Vasc Surg 1989;9:568-573.

Hammond SL, Gomez ER, Coffey JA, et al: Involvement of the lymphatic system in chronic venous insufficiency. In Bergan JJ, Yao JST (eds): Venous Disorders. Philadelphia, WB Saunders, 1991.

Hamza N, Marath A, Al-Fakhry MR: The management of aneurysms and arteriovenous fistulae of the popliteal artery arising from war trauma: Emphasis on sigmoid operative approach. J Cardiovasc Surg 1990;31:457-461.

Hanobrugh JF, Narrod JA: Arteriovenous fistulas following central venous catheterization. Care Med 1983;9:287-289.

Hansaker G: An ordeal in a snowdrift. The Evening Star 14 June 1971.

Harbison SP: Major vascular complications of intervertebral disc surgery. Ann Surg 1954;140:342-348.

Hardin WD Jr, Adinolfi MF, O'Connell RC, Kerstein MD: Management of traumatic peripheral vein injuries: Primary repair or vein ligation. Am J Surg 1982;144:235-238.

Hardin CA: Bypass saphenous grafts for the relief of venous obstruction of the extremity. Surg Gynecol Obstet 1962;115:709-712.

Hardin WD, O'Connell RC, Adinolfi MF, Kerstein MD: Traumatic arterial injuries of the upper extremity: Determinants of disability. Am J Surg 1985;150:266-270.

Hardy JD, Raju S, Neely WA, Berry DW: Aortic and other arterial injuries. Ann Surg 1975;181:640-653.

Hardy JD, Timmis HH: Repair of intracardiac gunshot injuries: Report of three cases. Ann Surg 1969;169:906-913.

Hardy JD, Williams RD: Penetrating heart wounds: Analysis of 12 consecutive cases without morality. Ann Surg 1967;166:228-231.

Hare RR, Gaspar MR: The intimal flap. Arch Surg 1971;102:552-555.

Harken DE: Foreign bodies in, and in relation to, the thoracic blood vessels and heart: Techniques for approaching and removing foreign bodies from the chambers of the heart. Surg Gynecol Obstet 1946;83:117-125.

Harken DE, Williams AC: Foreign bodies in and in relation to the thoracic blood vessels and heart: Migratory foreign bodies within the blood vascular system. Am J Surg 1946;72:80-90.

Harken DE, Zoll PM: Foreign bodies in and in relation to the thoracic blood vessels and heart: Indications for the removal of intracardiac foreign bodies and the behavior of the heart during manipulation. Am Heart J 1946;32:1-19.

Harley DP, Mena I: Cardiac and vascular sequelae of sternal fractures. J Trauma 1986;26:553-555.

Harrington DP, Barth KH, Whit RI Jr, Brawley RK: Traumatic pseudoaneurysm of the thoracic aorta in close proximity ot the anterior spinal artery: A therapeutic dilemma. Surgery 1980;87:153-156.

Harrington EB, Schwartz M, Jacobson JH II, et al: Aortocaval fistula: A clinical spectrum. J Cardiovasc Surg 1989;30:579-583.

Harris JD: A case of arteriovenous fistula following closed fracture of tibia and fibula. Br J Surg 1963;50:774-776.

Hart RJ Jr, Gregoratos G: Ventricular septal defects caused by stab wounds: Report of two cases. Milit Med 1974;139:289-292.

Hartford JM, Fayer RL, Shaver TE, et al: Transection of the thoracic aorta: Assessment of a trauma system. Am J Surg 1986;151:224-229.

Hartling RP, McGahan JP, Lindfors KK: Letter. Radiology 1987;165:291-292.

Hartling RP, McGahan JP, Blaisdell FW, Lindfors KK: Stab wounds to the extremities: Indications for arteriography. Radiology 1987;162:465-467.

Hartsuck JM, Moreland HJ, Williams GR: Surgical management of vascular trauma distal to the popliteal artery. Arch Surg 1972;105:937-940.

Harvey EN, Butler EG, McMillen JH, Puckett WO: Mechanism of wounding. War Med 1945;8:91-104.

Harvey EN, Korr IM, Oster G, McMillen JH: Secondary damage in wounding due to pressure changes accompanying the passage of high velocity missiles. Surgery 1947;21:218-239.

Harvey EN, McMillen JH: An experimental study of shock waves resulting from the impact of high velocity missiles on animal tissues. J Exp Med 1947;85:321-328.

Hashizume M, Yang Y, Galt S: Intimal response of saphenous vein to intraluminal trauma simulated angioscopic insertion. J Vasc Surg 1987;5:862-868.

Hashmonai M, Schramek KA, Abrahamson J, et al: Acute vascular injuries of the upper extremity. Isr J Med Sci 1974;10:599.

Haskell RJ, French WJ, Harley DP: Traumatic aorto-right ventricular fistula presenting with a diastolic murmur. Am Heart J 1985;109:1110-1112.

Hass GM: Types of internal injuries of personnel involved in aircraft accidents. J Aviat Med 1944;15:77.

Hass L, Staple T: Arterial injures associated with fractures of the proximal tibia following blunt trauma. South Med J 1969;62:1439.

Hassantash SA, Mock C, Maier RV: Traumatic visceral artery aneurysm: Presentation as massive hemorrhage from perforation into an adjacent hollow viscus. J Trauma 1995;38:357-360.

Hasselgren PO, Eriksson B, Lukes P, Seeman T: False popliteal aneurysm caused by exostosis of the femur. J Cardiovasc Surg 1983;24:540-542.

Hassett A, Moran J, Sabiston DC, Kisslo J: Utility of echocardiography in the management of patients with penetrating missile wounds of the heart. Am J Cardiol 1987;7:1151-1156.

Hawkes SZ: Traumatic rupture of the heart and intrapericardial structures. Am J Surg 1935;27:503-507.

Hawkins ML, Carraway RP, Ross SE: Pulmonary artery disruption from blunt thoracic trauma. Am Surg 1988;54:148-152.

Hayes JM, Vanwickle GN: Axillary artery injury with minimally displaced fracture of the neck of the humerus. J Trauma 1983;23:431-433.

Heaton LD, Hughes CW, Rosegay H, et al: Military surgical practices of the United States Army in Vietnam. In Current Problems in Surgery. Chicago, Year Book Medical Publishers, 1966.

Heberer G: Ruptures and aneurysms of the thoracic aorta after blunt chest trauma. J Cardiac Surg 1971;12:115-120.

Heberer G, Becker HM, Stelter WJ: Vascular injuries in polytrauma. World J Surg 1983;7:68-79.

Hebra A, Roison JG, Elliott BM: Traumatic aneurysm associated with fibrointimal proliferation of the common carotid artery following blunt trauma: Case report. J Trauma 1993;34:297-299.

Hegarty MM, Angorn IB, Gollogy J, Baker LW: Traumatic arteriovenous fistulae. Injury 1975;7:20-28.

Heggtveit HA, Campbell JS, Hooper GD: Innominate arterial aneurysms occurring after blunt trauma. Am J Clin Pathol 1974;42:69-74.

Heiberg E, Wolverson MK, Sundaram M, Shields JB: CT in aortic trauma. AJR Am J Roentgenol 1983;140:1119-1124.

Heidenhain L: Über naht von arterienwunden. Centralbl Chir 1895;22:1113-1115.

Helfet DL, Howey T, Sanders R, Johansen K: Limb salvage versus amputation. Preliminary results of the Mangled Extremity Severity Score. Clin Orthop 1990;256:80.

Helvie MA, Rubin JM, Silver TM, Kresowik TF: The distinction between femoral artery pseudoaneurysms and other causes of groin masses: Value of duplex doppler sonography. AJR 1988;150:1177-1180.

Henderson V, Nambisan R, Smith ME, et al: Angiographic yield in penetrating extremity trauma. Wes J Med 1991;155:253.

Hennessy OF, Gibson RN, Allison DJ: Use of giant steel coils in the therapeutic embolization of a superior mesenteric artery-portal vein fistula. Cardiovasc Intervent Radiol 1986;9:42.

Henroteaux D, Thoorens P, Trotteur G: Rupture of the external iliac artery after total hip replacement. J Belge Radiol 1989;72:518-519.

Heppenstall RB, Sapega AA, Izant T, et al: Compartment syndrome: A quantitative study of high-energy phosphorus compounds using 31P-magnetic resonance spectroscopy. J Trauma 1989;29:1113-1119.

Herget CH: Wound ballistics. In Bowers WB (ed): Surgery of Trauma. Philadelphia, JB Lippincott Co, 1956.

Herlyn KE: Erfahrungen auf dem gebiete von aneurysmen und arteriovenosen fisteln. Atti della prima Riunione Internacionale de Angio-cardio-Chirurgia. Milano: Casa Edetrice "Mellon," 1951.

Hermreck AS, Sifers TM, Reckling FW, et al: Traumatic vascular injuries: Methods and results of repair. Am J Surg 1974;128:813-817.

Hershey FB. Secondary repair of arterial injuries. Am Surg 1961;27:33-41.

Hershey FB, Spencer AD: Surgical repair of civilian arterial injuries. Arch Surg 1960;80:953-962.

Hershey FB, Spencer AD: Autogenous vein grafts for repairs of arterial injuries. Arch Surg 1963;86:836-845.

Herskowitz K, Sclafani S: Acute traumatic dissection of the common iliac arteries with spontaneous healing: Case report. Cardiovasc Intervent Radiol 1990;13:364.

Hertzer NR: Peripheral atheromatous embolization following blunt abdominal trauma. Surgery 1977;82:244-247.

Hess PJ, Howe HR, Robicsek F, et al: Traumatic tears of the thoracic aorta: Improved results using the Bio-Medicus pump. Ann Thorac Surg 1989;48:6-9.

Hessel SJ, Adams DF: Complication of angiography. Radiology 1981;138:273-281.

Hewes RC, Smith DC, Lavine MH: Iatrogenic hydromediastinum simulating aortic laceration. AJR Am J Roentgenol 1979;133:817-820.

Hewitt RL: Technical considerations in acute military vascular injuries of the extremities. Milit Med 1969;134:617-621.

Hewitt RL, Collins DJ: Acute arteriovenous fistulas in war injuries. Ann Surg 1969;169:447-449.

Hewitt RL, Collins DJ, Hamit HF: Arterial injuries at a surgical hospital in Vietnam. Arch Surg 1969;98:313-316.

Hewitt RL, Grablowsky OM: Acute traumatic dissecting aneurysm of the abdominal aorta. Ann Surg 1970;171:160-164.

Hewitt RL, Smith AD, Becker ML, et al: Penetrating injuries of the thoracic outlet. Surgery 1974;76:715-722.

Hewitt RL, Smith AD, Drapanas T: Acute traumatic arteriovenous fistulas. J Trauma 1973;13:901-906.

Hewitt RL, Smith AD Jr, Weichert RF, Drapanas T: Penetrating cardiac injuries: Current trends in management. Arch Surg 1970;101:683-688.

Heyes FLP, Aukland A: Occlusion of the common femoral artery complicating total hip arthroplasty. J Bone Joint Surg 1985;67:533-535.

Hiatt JR, Busuttil RW, Wilson SE: Impact of routine arteriography on management of penetrating neck injuries. J Vasc Surg 1984;1:860-866.

Hiatt JR, Yeatman LA, Child JB: The value of echocardiography in blunt chest trauma. J Trauma 1988;28:914-922.

Hiatt JR, Martin NA, Machleder HI: The natural history of a traumatic vertebral artery aneurysm: Case report. J Trauma 1989;29:1592-1603.

Hiebert CA, Gregory FJ: Bullet embolism from the head to the heart. JAMA 1974;229:442-443.

Hierholzer C, Harbercht BG, Billiar TR, Tweardy DJ: Hypoxia-inducible factor-1 activation and cyclo-oxygenase-2 induction are early reperfusion independent inflammatory events in hemorrhagic shock. Arch Orthop Trauma Surg 2001;121:219-222.

Hiertonn T, Lindberg K, Rob CG: Cystic degeneration of the popliteal artery. Br J Surg 1957;44:348.

Hiertonn T, Rybeck B: Traumatic Arterial Lesions. Stockholm, Försvarets Forskningsanstalt, 1968.

Higgins RSD, Sanchez JA, DeGuidis L: Mechanical circulatory support decreases neurologic complications in the treatment of traumatic injuries of the thoracic aorta. Arch Surg 1992;127:516-519.

Highbloom RY, Koolpe H, Morris MC: Traumatic occlusion of two radiocephalic fistulas: Case report and their management. J Trauma 1990;30:364-365.

Hilgenberg AD, Logan DL, Adkins CW, et al: Blunt injuries of the thoracic aorta. Ann Thorac Surg 1992;53:233-239.

Hill LL: A report of a case of successful suturing of the heart, and a table of 37 other cases of suturing by different operators with various terminations and conclusions drawn. Med Rec N Y 2001;62:846.

Hillborn M, Downey D: Deep venous thrombosis complicating sonographically guided compression repair of pseudoaneurysm of the common femoral artery. AJR Am J Roentgenol 1993;161:1334-1335.

Hills MW, Delprado AM, Deane SA: Sternal fractures: Associated injuries and management. J Trauma 1993;35:55-60.

Hills MW, Thomas SG, McDougall PA, et al: Traumatic thoracic aortic rupture: Investigation determines outcome. Aust N Z J Surg 1994;64:312-318.

Hiratzka LF, Wright CB: Experimental and clinical results of grafts in the venous system: A current review. J Surg Res 1978;25:542-561.

Hirsch B: Blood Vessel Surgery. London, Edward Arnold & Company, 1912.

Hirsch EF: Internal versus external fixation of fractures with concomitant vascular injuries in Vietnam. J Trauma 1971;11:463-473.

Hirshberg A, Wall MJ, Allen MK: Double jeopardy: Thoracoabdominal injuries requiring surgical intervention in both chest and abdomen. J Trauma 1995;39:225-231.

Hix WR, Mills M: Management of esophageal wounds. Ann Surg 1970;172:1002-1006.

Ho RM, Freed MM: Persistent hypertension in young spinal cord injured individuals resulting from aortic repair. Arch Phys Med Rehabil 1991;72:743-746.

Hobson RW II, Croom RD III, Rich NM: Influence of heparin and low molecular weight dextran on the patency of autogenous vein grafts: Vein grafts in the venous system. Ann Surg 1973;178:773-776.

Hobson RW II, Croom RD III, Swan KG: Hemodynamics of the distal arteriovenous fistula in venous reconstruction. J Surg Res 1973;14:483-489.

Hobson RW II, Israel MR, Lynch TG: Axillosubclavian arterial aneurysms. New York, Grune & Stratton, 1982.

Hobson RW II, Lee BC, Lynch TG, et al: Use of intermittent pneumatic compression of the calf in femoral venous reconstruction. Surg Gynecol Obstet 1984;159:284-286.

Hobson RW II, Rich NM: Traumatismes veineux des membres inférieurs. In Kieffer E (ed): Traumatismes Artériels. Paris, AERCV, 1995.

Hobson RW II, Rich NM, Wright CB: Venous Trauma: Pathophysiology, Diagnosis and Surgical Management. Mt. Kisco, NY, Futura Publishing, 1983.

Hobson RW II, Rich NM, Wright CB: Complications of direct venous reconstruction. In Complications of Vascular Surgery. Orlando, Grune & Stratton, 1985, pp 351-367.

Hobson RW II, Howard EW, Wright CB, et al: Pathophysiology of venous ligation: Significance in arterial/venous injuries. Surgery 1972;74:824.

Hobson RW II, Howard EW, Wright CB, et al: Hemodynamics of canine femoral venous ligation: Significance in combined arterial and venous injuries. Surgery 1973;74:824-829.

Hobson RW II, Wright CB: Peripheral side to side arteriovenous fistula: Hemodynamics and application in venous reconstruction. Am J Surg 1973;126:411-414.

Hobson RW II, Wright CB, Rich NM, Collins GJ Jr: Assessment of colonic ischemia during aortic surgery by Doppler ultrasound. J Surg Res 1976;20:231-235.

Hobson RW II, Wright CB, Swan KG, et al: Current status of venous injury and reconstruction in the lower extremities. In Bergan JJ, Yao JST (eds): Venous Problems. Chicago, Year Book Medical Publishers, 1978, pp 469-484.

Hobson RW II, Yeager RA, Lynch TG, et al: Femoral venous trauma: Techniques for surgical management and early results. Am J Surg 1983;146:220-224.

Hoff SJ, Reilly MK, Merrill WH, et al: Analysis of blunt and penetrating injury of the innominate and subclavian arteries. Am Surg 1994;60:151-154.

Hohf RP: Arterial injuries occurring during orthopaedic operations. Clin Orthop 1963;28:21.

Holcomb GW, Meacham PW, Dean RH: Penetrating popliteal artery injuries in children. J Pediatr Surg 1988;23:859-861.

Holleman JH, Killebrew LH: Tibial artery injuries. Am J Surg 1982;144:362-364.

Hollerman JH, Killebrew LH: Injury to the popliteal artery. Surg Gynecol Obstet 1981;153:392-394.

Hollier LH: Protecting the brain and spinal cord. J Vasc Surg 1987;5:524-528.

Hollingsworth RK, Johnston WW, McCooey JF: Traumatic saccular aneurysm of the thoracic aorta. J Thorac Surg 1952;24:325-345.

Holman E: Arteriovenous Aneurysms: Abnormal Communication between the Arterial and Venous Circulations. New York, Macmillan, 1937.

Holman E: Clinical and experimental observations on arteriovenous fistulae. Ann Surg 1940;112:840-875.

Holman E: War injuries to arteries and their treatment. Surg Gynecol Obstet 1942;75:183-192.

Holman E: Contributions to cardiovascular physiology gleaned from clinical and experimental observations of abnormal arteriovenous communications. J Cardiovasc Surg 1962;3:48-63.

Holman E: Abnormal arteriovenous communications: Great variability of effects with particular reference to delayed development of cardiac failure. Circulation 1965;32:1001-1009.

Holman E: Abnormal Arteriovenous Communications: Peripheral and Intracardiac, Acquired and Congenital, 2nd ed. Springfield, Ill, Charles C Thomas, 1968.

Holman E, Sir William Osler, Halsted WS: Two contrasting personalities. Pharos AOA 1971;34:134.

Holman EF: Physiology of an arteriovenous fistula. Arch Surg 1971;7:64-82.

Holmes TW Jr, Netterville RE: Complications of first rib fracture including one case each of tracheoesophageal fistula and aortic arch aneurysm. J Thoracic Surg 1956;32:74-91.

Holzer CE Jr: Gunshot wound involving the abdominal aorta. Surgery 1948;23:645-652.

Honigman B: Mast increase mortality 7 times with heart injury. JAMA 1991;266.

Hoover NW: Injuries of the popliteal artery associated with fractures and dislocations. Surg Clin North Am 1961;41:1099-1112.

Horowitz MD, Schultz CS, Stinson EB: Sensitivity and specificity of echocardiogram diagnosis of pericardial effusion. Circulation 1974;50:239-247.

Horsely V: The destructive effects of small projectiles. Nature 1894;1:104-108.

Horsley JS: Surgery of the Blood Vessels. St. Louis, Mosby, 1915.

Horwitz JR, Black CT, Lally KP, Andrassy RJ: Venous bypass as an adjunct for the management of a retrohepatic venous injury in a child. J Trauma 1995;39:584-585.

Hoshida S, Yamashita N, Otsu K, et al: Cholesterol feeding exacerbates myocardial injury in Zucker diabetic fatty rats. Am J Physiol Heart Circ Physiol 2000;278:H256-H262.

Houck WS: Blunt trauma to the popliteal artery: Review and presentation of four cases. Am Surg 1977;43:434-437.

Howanitz EP, Murray KD, Galbraith TA, Myerowitz PD: Peripheral venous bullet embolization to the heart: Case report and review of the literature. J Vasc Surg 1988;8:55-58.

Howanitz EP, Buckley D, Galbraith TA, et al: Combine blunt traumatic rupture of the heart and aorta: Two case reports and review of the literature. J Trauma 1990;30:506-508.

Howard C, Thal ER, Redman HC, Gibson P: Intra-arterial digital subtraction angiography in the evaluation of peripheral vascular trauma. Ann Surg 1989;210:108-111.

Howe HR Jr, Poole GV Jr, Hansen KJ, et al: Salvage of lower extremities following combined orthopaedic and vascular trauma: A predictive salvage index. Am Surg 1987;53:205-208.

Howe HR, Pennell PC: A superior temporary shunt for management of vascular trauma of extremity. Arch Surg 1986;121:1212.

Hoyt DB, Shackford SR, Davis JW, et al: Thoracotomy during trauma resuscitations: An appraisal by board certified general surgeons. J Trauma 1989;29:1318-1321.

Huang MS, Liu M, Wu J, et al: Ultrasonography for the evaluation of hemoperitoneum during resuscitation: A simple scoring system. J Trauma 1994;36:173-177.

Huang P, Fong C, Radmaker A: Prediction of traumatic aortic rupture from plain chest film findings using stepwise logistic regression. Ann Emerg Med 1987;16:1330-1333.

Hudson HM II, Woodson J, Hirsch E: The management of traumatic aortic tear in the multiply-injured patient. Ann Vasc Surg 1991;5:445-448.

Hughes CW: Acute vascular trauma in Korean War casualties: An analysis of 180 cases. Surg Gynec Obstet 1954;99:91-100.

Hughes CW: Use of intra-aortic balloon catheter tamponade for controlling intra-abdominal hemorrhage in man. Surgery 1954;36:65-68.

Hughes CW: The primary repair of wounds of major arteries: An analysis of experience in Korea in 1953. Ann Surg 1955;141:297-303.

Hughes CW: Arterial repair during the Korean War. Ann Surg 1958;147:555-561.

Hughes CW: Vascular injuries in the orthopaedic patient. J Bone Joint Surg 1958;40A:1271.

Hughes CW: Vascular surgery in the armed forces. Milit Med 1959;124:30-46.

Hughes CW: Acute vascular injuries: Civilian and military. J Trauma 1971;11:189-190.

Hughes CW, Bowers WF: Traumatic Lesions of Peripheral Vessels. Springfield, Ill, Charles C Thomas, 1961.

Hughes CW, Cohen A: The repair of injured blood vessels. Surg Clin North Am 1958;38:1529-1543.

Hughes CW, Jahnke EJ Jr: The surgery of traumatic arteriovenous fistulas and aneurysms: A five-year follow up study of 215 lesions. Surg Clin North Am 1958;148:790-797.

Hughes CW, Rich NM. The management of vascular injuries. South Med Bull 1969;57:36.

Hugier: Anévrisme ratérioso-veineux de l'artère fémorale gauche. BullSoc Chir Paris 1852;2:106.

Hugier (1848). Cited by Horsely. The destructive effects of small projectiles. Nature 1894;1:104-108.

Huk I, Brovkovych V, Nanobashvili J, et al: Prostaglandin E_1 reduces ischemia/reperfusion injury by normalizing nitric oxide and superoxide release. Shock 2000;14:234-242.

Hull DA, Hyde CL: Arterial injuries in civilian practice. J Kentucky Med Assoc 1967;65:975-978.

Hunink MG, Bos JJ: Triage of patients to angiography for detection of aortic rupture after blunt chest trauma: Cost-effectiveness analysis of using CT. AJR 1995;165:27-36.

Hunt JP, Baker CC, Lentrz CW, et al: Thoracic aorta injuries: Management and outcome of 144 patients. J Trauma 1996;40:547-556.

Hunt TK, Blaisdell FW, Okimoto J: Vascular injuries of the base of the neck. Arch Surg 1969;98:586-590.

Hunt TK, Leeds FH, Wanebo HJ, Blaisdell FW: Arteriovenous fistulas of major vessels of the abdomen. J Trauma 1971;11:483-493.

Hunter J: A Treatise on the Blood, Inflammation and Gunshot Wounds. London, George Nicol, 1974.

Hunter JI: Cited in Power, D-Arcy. Hunter's operation for the cure of aneurysm. Br J Surg 1929;17:193-196.

Hunter W: The history of an aneurysm of the aorta, with some remarks on aneurysms in general. Med Obs Soc Phys Lond 1757;1:323.

Hunter W: Further observations upon a particular species of aneurysm. Med Obs Soc Phys Lond 1762;2:390.

Hurwitt ES, Seidenberg B: The nonoperative management of two cases of catheter perforation of the aorta. Am J Surg 1965;110:452-455.

Hurwitt E, Seidenberg B: Rupture of the heart during cardiac massage. Ann Surg 1953;137:115-119.

Hutton JE Jr, Rich NM: Pathophysiology of wounding. In McAninch JW (ed): Traumatic and Reconstructive Urology. Philadelphia, WB Saunders, 1995.

Iannettoni MD, McCurry KR, Rodriguez JL, et al: Simultaneous traumatic ascending and descending thoracic aortic rupture. Ann Thoracic Surg 1994;57:481-484.

Ikard R, Merendino KA: Accidental excision of the superior mesenteric artery: Technical and physiological considerations. Surg Clin North Am 1970; 50:1075-1085.

Ikeda Y, Young LH, Scalia R, Lefer AM: Cardioprotective effects of citrulline in ischemia/reperfusion injury via a non-nitric oxide–mediated mechanism. Methods Find Exp Clin Pharmacol 2000;22:563-571.

Imamoglou K, Read RC, Heubl HC: Cervicomediastinal vascular surgery. Surgery 1967;61:274-80.

Inahara T: Arterial injuries of the upper extremity. Surgery 1962;51:605-610.

Inberg MC, Laaksonen V, Scheinin TM, et al: Early repair of traumatic rupture of the thoracic aorta: Report of two cases. Scand J Thorac Cardiovasc Surg 1972;6:287.

Inoue T, Kawada K, Tanaka S, et al: Clinical application of the temporary long external bypass method for cross-clamping of the descending thoracic aorta. J Thorac Cardiovasc Surg 1972;63:787-793.

Inui FK, Shannon J, Howard JM: Arterial injuries in the Korean conflict: Experiences with 111 consecutive injuries. Surgery 1955;37:850-857.

Isaacs JP: Sixty penetrating wounds of the heart: Clinical and experimental observations. In Blalock A (ed): Recent Advances in Surgery. 1959, p 696.

Isaacs JP, Swanson HS, Smith RA: Transient childhood strokes from internal carotid stenosis. JAMA 1969;207:1859-1862.

Iskecelli OK: Bullet embolus of left femoral artery: Report of a case which occurred after abdominal gunshot wound. Arch Surg 1962;85:184-185.

Iskersky V, Reines HD, Vujic I: Left-sided vena cava mimicking traumatic ruptured thoracic aorta. J Trauma 1987;27:797-799.

Israel. Cited in Murphy JB: Resection of arteries and veins injured in continuity—end-to-end suture: Experimental clinical research. Med Rec 1897;51:73.

Itani KM, Burch JM, Spjut-Patrinely V, et al: Emergency center arteriography. J Trauma 1992;32:302-307.

Ivatury RR, Shah PM, Ho K, et al: Emergency room thoracotomy for the resuscitation of patients with fatal penetrating injuries of the heart. Ann Thorac Surg 1981;32:377-385.

Ivatury RR, Rohman M, Lankin DH, Stahl WM: Ultrasonography in the diagnosis and management of post-venorrhaphy thrombosis of the protal vein. J Trauma 1985;25:362-365.

Ivatury RR, Nallanthambi M, Roberge RJ: Penetrating thoracic injuries: Stabilization vs. prompt transport. J Trauma 1987;27:1066.

Ivatury RR, Nallanthambi M, Lankin DH, et al: Portal vein injuries: Noninvasive follow-up of venorrhaphy. Ann Surg 1987;206:733-737.

Jackson FE, Mazur J: Traumatic aortic aneurysms in neurological patients. Milit Med 1965;130:878-886.

Jackson MR, Olson DW, Beckett WC Jr, et al: Abdominal vascular trauma: A review of 106 injuries. Am Surg 1992;58:622-626.

Jackson MR, Brengman ML, Rich NM: Delayed presentation of 50 years after a World War II vascular injury with intraoperative localization by duplex ultrasound of a traumatic false aneurysm. J Trauma 1997;43:159-161.

Jacobs JP, Horowitz MD, Ladden DA: Intra-aortic balloon counterpulsation in penetrating cardiac trauma. J Cardiovasc Surg 1992;33:38-40.

Jacobson JH, Haimov J: Venous revascularization of the arm: Report of three cases. Surgery 1977;81:599-604.

Jaeschke H: Mechanisms of reperfusion injury after warm ischemia of the liver. Hepatobiliary Pancreat Surg 1998;5:402-408.

Jaggers RC, Feliciano DV, Mattox KL, et al: Injury to popliteal vessels. Arch Surg 1982;117:657-661.

Jahnke EJ Jr: The surgery of acute vascular injuries: A report of 77 cases. Milit Surg 1953;112:249-251.

Jahnke EJ Jr: Late structural and functional results of arterial injuries primarily repaired. Surgery 1958;43:175-183.

Jahnke EJ Jr, Fisher GW, Jones C: Acute traumatic rupture of the thoracic aorta: Report of six consecutive cases of successful early repair. J Thorac Cardiovasc Surg 1964;48:63-77.

Jahnke EJ Jr, Howard JM: Primary repair of major arterial wounds: Report of 58 battle casualties. Arch Surg 1953;66:646-649.

Jahnke EJ Jr, Hughes CW, Howard JM: The rationale of arterial repair on the battlefield. Am J Surg 1954;87:396-401.

Jahnke EJ Jr, Seeley SF: Acute vascular injuries in the Korean War: An analysis of 77 consecutive cases. Ann Surg 1953;138:158-177.

Jain SP, Roubin GS, Iyer SS: Closure of an iatrogenic femoral artery pseudoaneurysm by transcutaneous coil embolization. Cathet Cardiovasc Diagn 1996;39:317-319.

Jamieson NV, Watson CJ, Dunn DC: Dissection of the abdominal aorta associated with traumatic aneurysms of the iliac vessels. Case report. Acta Chir Scand 1986;152:473-475.

Jamous MA, Silver JR, Baker JHE: Paraplegia and traumatic rupture of the aorta: A disease process or surgical complication. Injury 1992;23:475-478.

Jarrar D, Chaudry IH, Wang P: Organ dysfunction following hemorrhage and sepsis: Mechanisms and therapeutic approaches. Int J Mol Med 1999;57:368-374.

Jarrar D, Wang P, Chaudry IH: Hepatocellular dysfunction: Basic considerations. In Holzheimer RG, Mannick JA (eds): Surgical Treatment Evidence-based and Problem-oriented. Munich, Zuckschwerdt, 2001, pp 763-767.

Jarrar D, Wang P, Song GY, et al: Inhibition of tyrosine kinase signaling after trauma-hemorrhage: A novel approach for improving organ function and decreasing susceptibility to subsequent sepsis. Ann Surg 2000;231:399-407.

Jarstfer BS, Rich NM: The challenge of arteriovenous fistula formation following disk surgery: A collective review. J Trauma 1976;16:726-733.

Jassinowsky A: Die arteriennhat: Eine experimentelle studie. Inaug Diss Dorpat 1889.

Javid H: Vascular injuries of the neck. Clin Orthop 1963;28:70.

Jay JB, French SW III: Traumatic rupture of the thoracic aorta: Review of literature and case report. Arch Surg 1954;68:657-662.

Jensen: Ueber circulare gefassutur. Arch Klin Chir 1903;69:938-998.

Jensen AR: Bullet wound of the abdominal aorta with survival. J Fla Med Assoc 1963;49:656-657.

Jensen BT: Fourteen years' survival with an untreated traumatic rupture of the thoracal aorta. Am J Forens Med Pathol 1988;9:58-59.

Jeresaty RM, Liss JP: Effects of brachial artery catheterization on arterial pulse and blood pressure in 203 patients. Am Heart J 1968;76:481-485.

Jernigan WR, Gardner WC: Carotid artery injuries due to closed cervical trauma. J Trauma 1971;11:429-435.

Jimenez E, Martin M, Krukenkamp I, Barrett J: Subxiphoid pericardiotomy versus echocardiography: A prospective evaluation of the diagnosis of occult penetrating cardiac injuries. Surgery 1990;108:676-680.

Jimenez F, Utrilla A, Cuesta C, et al: Popliteal artery and venous aneurysm as a complication of arthroscopic meniscectomy. J Trauma 1988;28:1404-1405.

Johansen K, Bandyk D, Thiele B, Hansen ST Jr: Temporary intraluminal shunts: Resolution of a management dilemma in complex vascular injuries. J Trauma 1982;22:395-402.

Johansen K, Daines M, Howey T, et al: Objective criteria accurately predict amputation following lower extremity trauma. J Trauma 1990;30:568-573.

Johansen K, Lynch K, Paun M, Copass M: Non-invasive vascular tests reliably exclude occult arterial trauma in injured extremities. J Trauma 1991;31:515-522.

Johns TNP: A comparison of suture and non-suture methods for the anastomosis of veins. Surg Gynecol Obstet 1947;84:939-942.

Johnson G Jr, Peters RM, Dart CH Jr: A study of cardiac vein negative pressure in arterio-venous fistula. Surg Gynecol Obstet 1967;124:82-86.

Johnson G Jr, Blythe WB: Hemodynamic effects of arteriovenous shunts used for hemodialysis. Ann Surg 1970;171:715-723.

Johnson B, Thursby P: Subclavian artery injury caused by a screw in a clavicular compression plate. Cardiovasc Surg 1996;4:414-415.

Johnson GW, Lowry JH: Rupture of the axillary artery complicating anterior dislocation of the shoulder. J Bone Joint Surg 1962;44B:116.

Johnson RH, Wall MJ, Mattox KL: Innominate artery trauma: A thirty-year experience. J Vasc Surg 1993;17:134-140.

Johnson SB, Kearney PA, Smith MD: Echocardiography in the evaluation of thoracic aorta. Surg Clin North Am 1995;75:193-205.

Johnson V, Eiseman B: Evaluation of arteriovenous shunts to maintain patency of venous autograft. Am J Surg 1969;118:915.

Johnston R, Wall M, Mattox K: Innominate artery trauma: A 30-year experience. J Vasc Surg 1993;17:134-139.

Jones AM, Graham NJ, Looney JR: Arterial embolism of a high-velocity rifle bullet after a hunting accident: Case report and literature review. Am J Forsensic Med Pathol 1983;4:259-264.

Jones EW, Helmsworth J: Penetrating wounds of the heart: Thirty years' experience. Arch Surg 1968;96:671-682.

Jones JC: Traumatic rupture of ascending aorta and left main bronchus. Ann Thorac Surg 1989;47:484.

Jones JW, Hewitt RL, Drapanas T: Cardiac contusion: A capricious syndrome. Ann Surg 1975;181:567-574.

Jones RE, Smith EC, Bone GE: Vascular and orthopaedic complications of knee dislocation. Surg Gynecol Obstet 1979;149:554-558.

Jones RF, Terrell JC, Walyer FE: Penetrating wounds of the neck: An analysis of 274 cases. J Trauma 1967;7:228-234.

Jousi M, Leppäninemi A: Management and outcome of traumatic aortic injuries. Ann Chirurgiae Gynaecol 2000:89.

Jurkovich GJ, Zingarelli W, Wallace J, Curreri PW: Penetrating neck trauma: Diagnostic studies in the asymptomatic patients. J Trauma 1985;25:819-822.

Jurkovich GJ, Hoyt DB, Moore FA, et al: Portal triad injuries. J Trauma 1995; 39:426-434.

Kadambi A, Skalak TC: Role of leukocytes and tissue-derived oxidants in short-term skeletal muscle ischemia reperfusion injury. Am J Physiol Heart Circ Physiol 2000;278:H435–H443.

Kaeffer N, Richard V, Thuillez C: Delayed coronary endothelial protection 24 hours after preconditioning: Role of free radicals. Circulation 1997;96:2311-2316.

Kahn AM, Joseph WL, Hughes RK: Traumatic aneurysms of the thoracic aorta: Excision and repair without graft. Ann Thorac Surg 1967;4:175-181.

Kakkar VV: The cephalic vein as a peripheral vascular graft. Surg Gynecol Obstet 1969;128:551-556.

Kakos GS, Williams TE Jr, Kilman JW, Kalssen KP: Traumatic left ventricular aneurysms after penetrating chest injury. Ann Surg 1971;174:202-206.

Kalmar P, Otto CB, Rodewald G: Selection of proper time of operation of traumatic thoracic aortic aneurysms (TTA). J Thorac Cardiovasc Surg 1982;36-37.

Kam J, Jackson H, Ben-Menachem Y: Vascular injuries in blunt pelvic trauma. Radiol Clin North Am 1981;19:171-186.

Kamiya H, Hanaki Y, Kojima S: Fistula between noncoronary sinus of Valsalva and right atrium after blunt chest trauma. Am Heart J 1987;114:429-431.

Kang SS, Labropoulos N, Mansour MA, Baker WH: Percutaneous ultrasound guided thrombin injection: A new method for treating postcatheterization femoral pseudoaneurysms. J Vasc Surg 1998;27:1032-1038.

Kang SS, Labropoulos N: Postcatheterization femoral pseudoaneurysms: Treatment with ultrasound-guided thrombin injection. Vasc Ultrasound Today 1998;3:125-140.

Kang SS, Labropoulos N, Mansour MA: Expanded indications for ultrasound-guided thrombin injection of pseudoaneurysms. J Vasc Surg 2000;31:289-298.

Kapp JP, Gielchinsky I, Jelsma R: Metallic fragment embolization to the cerebral circulation. J Trauma 1973;13:256-261.

Kappes S, Towne J, Adams M: Perforation of the superior vena cava: A complication of subclavian dialysis. JAMA 1983;249:2232-2233.

Karalis DE, Victor MF, Davis GA, et al: The role of echocardiography in blunt chest trauma: A transthoracic and transesophageal echocardiographic study. J Trauma 1994;36:53-58.

Karmody AM, Lempert N, Jarmolych J: The pathology of post-catheterization brachial artery occlusion. J Surg Res 1976;20:601-606.

Karrell R, Shaffer MA, Franaszek JB: Emergency diagnosis, resuscitation, and treatment of acute penetrating cardiac trauma. Ann Emerg Med 1982;11:504-517.

Kashuk JL, Moore EE, Millikan JS, Moore JB: Major abdominal vascular trauma: A unified approach. J Trauma 1982;22:672-679.

Kassel BA, Pugkhem T, Schechter LS, Chassin JL: Traumatic rupture of distal thoracic aorta. N Y State J Med 1980;80:1615-1617.

Kato M, Matsuda T, Kaneko M: Experimental assessment of newly devised transcatheter stent-graft for aortic dissection. Ann Thorac Surg 1995;59:908-915.

Katz NM, Blackstone EH, Kirklin JW, Karp RM: Incremental risk factors for spinal cord injury following operation for acute traumatic aortic transection. J Thorac Cardiovasc Surg 1981;81:669-674.

Katz S, Mullin R, Berger RL: Traumatic transection associated with retrograde dissection and rupture of the aorta: Recognition and management. Ann Thorac Surg 1974;17:273-276.

Kaufman JL, Dinerstein CR, Shah DM, et al: Renal artery intimal flaps after blunt trauma: Indications for non-operative therapy. J Vasc Surg 1988;8:33-37.

Kaushik VS, Mandel AK, Awariefe OA, et al: Early thoracotomy for stab wounds of the heart. J Cardiovasc Surg 1979;20:423-426.

Kavic SM, Atweh N, Ivy ME, et al: Celiac axis ligation after gunshot wound to the abdomen: Case report and literature review. J Trauma 2001;50:738-739.

Kawada T, Mieda T, Abe H, et al: Surgical experience with traumatic rupture of the thoracic aorta. J Cardiovasc Surg 1990;31:359-363.

Kay JK, Dykstra PC, Tsuji HK: Retrograde ilioaortic dissection: A complication of common femoral artery perfusion during open-heart surgery. Am J Surgery 1966;111:464-468.

Kazui T, Komatsu S, Yokoyama H: Surgical treatment of aneurysms of the thoracic aorta with the aid of partial cardiopulmonary bypass: An analysis of 95 patients. Ann Thorac Surg 1987;43:622-627.

Kearney P, Smith D, Johnson S, et al: Use of transesophageal echocardiography in the evaluation of traumatic aortic injury. J Trauma 1993;34:696-703.

Keeley JL: A bullet embolus to the left femoral artery following a thoracic gunshot wound: Probable entrance through thoracic aorta: Case report and resume of peripheral arterial bullet emboli. J Thorac Surg 1951;21:608-620.

Keeley SB, Snyder WH III, Weigelt JA: Arterial injuries below the knee: Fifty-one patients with eighty-two injuries. J Trauma 1983;23:285-290.

Kelly GL, Eiseman B: Civilian vascular injuries. J Trauma 1975;15:507-514.

Kelly GL, Eiseman B: Management of small arterial injuries: Clinical and experimental studies. J Trauma 1976;16:681-685.

Kelly JJ, Reuter KL, Waite RJ: Vascular injury complicating lumbar diskectomy: CT diagnosis. AJR Am J Roentgenol 1989;153:1233-1234.

Kemmerer WT, Eckert WG, Gathright JB, et al: Patterns of thoracic injuries in fatal traffic accidents. J Trauma 1961;1:595-599.

Kennedy FR, Cornwell EE, Camel J: Aortoesophageal fistula due to gunshot wounds: Report of two cases with one survivor. J Trauma 1995;38:971-974.

Kennedy JC: Complete dislocations of the knee. J Bone Joint Surg 1959;41:878.

Kennedy JC: Complete dislocation of the knee joint. J Bone Joint Surg 1963;45:889-904.

Keynes G: The Apologie and Treatise of Ambroise Paré. Chicago, University of Chicago, 1952.

Khalil IM, Livingston DH: Intravascular shunts in complex lower limb trauma. J Vasc Surg 1986;4:582-587.

Khoury G, Sfeir R, Khalifeh M, et al: Penetrating trauma to the abdominal vessels. Cardiovasc Surg 1996;4:405-407.

Kieny R, Charpentier A: Traumatic lesions of the thoracic aorta: A report of 73 cases. J Cardiovasc Surg 1991;32:613-619.

Kikta MJ, Meyer JP, Bishara RA, et al: Crush syndrome due to limb compression. Arch Surg 1987;122:1078-1081.

Kilburn P, Sweeney JG, Silk FF: Three cases of compound posterior dislocation of the elbow with rupture of the brachial artery. J Bone Joint Surg 1962;44:119-121.

Killen DA: Injury of the superior mesenteric vessel secondary to non-penetrating abdominal trauma. Am Surg 1964;30:306-312.

Killewich LA, Bedford GR, Beach KW, Strandness DE: Diagnosis of deep venous thrombosis: A prospective study comparing duplex scanning to contrast venography. Circulation 1989;79:810-814.

Kim H, Hwan KK: Role of nitric oxide and mucus in ischemia/reperfusion-induced gastric mucosal injury in rats. Pharmacology 2001;62:200-207.

Kinmonth JB: A report on the physiology and relief of traumatic arterial spasm. Br Med J 1952;1:59.

Kipfer B, Leupi F, Schuepbach P, et al: Acute traumatic rupture of the thoracic aorta: Immediate or delayed surgical repair? Eur J Cardiothorac Surg 1994;8:30-33.

Kirkup JR: Major arterial injury complicating fracture of the femoral shaft. J Bone Joint Surg 1963;45:337-343.

Kirsh MM, Behrendt DM, Orringer MB, et al: The treatment of acute traumatic rupture of the aorta: A 10-year experience. Ann Surg 1976;184:308.

Kirsh MM, Crane J, Kahn DG, et al: Roentgenographic evaluation of trauma rupture of the aorta. Surg Gynecol Obstet 1970;131:900-904.

Kirsh MM, Kahn DR, Crane JD, et al: Repair of acute traumatic rupture of the aorta without extracorporeal circulation. Ann Thorac Surg 1970;10:227-236.

Kirshner R, Seltzer S, D'Orsi C, DeWeese JA: Upper rib fractures and mediastinal widening: Indications for aortography. Ann Thorac Surg 1983;35:450-454.

Kitzmiller JW, Hertzer NR, Beven EG: Routine surgical management of brachial artery occlusion after cardiac catheterization. Arch Surg 1982;117:1066-1071.

Kizer KW, Boone HA, Heneveld E, Orozco JR: Nail gun injury to the heart. J Trauma 1995;38:382-383.

Kjellstrom T, Risberg B: Vascular trauma: Review of 10 years' experience. Acta Chir Scand 1980;146:261.

Klein MD, Coran AG, Whitehouse WM Jr, et al: Management of iatrogenic arterial injuries in infants and children. J Pediatr Surg 1982;17:933-939.

Klein SR, Bongard FS, White RA: Neurovascular injuries of the thoracic outlet and axilla. Am J Surg 1988;156:115-118.

Klein SR, Baumgartner FJ, Bongard FS: Contemporary management strategy of major inferior vena caval injuries. J Trauma 1991;31:1032.

Kleinert HE: Homograft patch repair of bullet wounds of the aorta: Experimental study and report of a case. Arch Surg 1958;76:811-820.

Kleinert HE, Romero J: Blunt abdominal trauma. J Trauma 1961;1:226-240.

Kleinert HE, Kasdan ML: Restoration of blood flow in upper extremity injuries. J Trauma 1963;3:461.

Kleinert HE, Kasdan ML, Romero JL: Small blood vessel anastomosis for salvage of severely injured upper extremity. J Bone Joint Surg 1963;45:788-796.

Kleinert HE, Volianitis GJ: Thrombosis of the Palmar Arch and its tributaries: Etiology and newer concepts in treatment. J Trauma 1965;5:447-457.

Kleinert HE: Vascular diseases. 1972 (unpublished paper).

Kleinert HE, Burget GC, Morgan JA, et al: Aneurysms of the hand. Arch Surg 1973;106:554-557.

Kleinsasser LJ: The removal of a wire lodged in the interventricular septum of the heart. Surgery 1961;50:500-503.

Kline DG, Hackett ER: Reappraisal of timing for exploration of civilian peripheral nerve injuries. Surgery 1975;78:54-65.

Kline RM, Hertzer NR, Beven EG, et al: Surgical treatment of brachial artery injuries after cardiac catheterization. J Vasc Surg 1990;12:20-24.

Klingensmith W, Oles P, Martinez H: Arterial injuries associated with dislocation of the knee or fracture of the lower femur. Surg Gynecol Obstet 1965;120:961-964.

Klingensmith W, Oles P, Martinez H: Fractures with associated blood vessel injury. Am J Surg 1965;110:849-852.

Kluger Y, Sagie B, Soffer D, et al: The use of hemorrhage occluder pins for controlling paravertebral intercostal artery bleeding: Case report. J Trauma 1997;43:687.

Knott-Craig CJ, Przybojewski JZ, Barnard PM: Penetrating wounds of the heart and great vessels: A new therapeutic approach. S Afr Med J 1982;62:316-320.

Knott LH, Crawford FA, Grogan JB: Comparison of autogenous vein, Dacron and Gore-Tex in infected wounds. J Surg Res 1978;24:288-293.

Knudson MM, Lewis FR, Atkinson K, Neuhaus A: The role of duplex ultrasound arterial imaging in patients with penetrating extremity trauma. Arch Surg 1993;128:1033.

Kollmeyer KR, Hunt JL: Aortoazygous fistula from gunshot wounds to the suprarenal abdominal aorta. J Trauma 1985;25:257-259.

Kootstra G, Schipper JJ, Klasen HJ, Binnendijk B: Femoral shaft fracture with injury of the superficial femoral artery in civilian accidents. Surg Gynecol Obstet 1976;142:399-403.

Kornblith BA: Gunshot wound through the abdominal aorta. Ann Surg 1941;113:637-640.

Kowalenko T, Stern S, Wang X, Dronen S: Improved outcome with "hypotensive" resuscitation of uncontrolled hemorrhagic shock in the swine model. J Trauma 1991;31:1032.

Kozloff L, Rich NM, Brott WH, et al: Vascular trauma secondary to diagnostic and therapeutic procedures: Cardiopulmonary bypass and intra-aortic balloon assist. Am J Surg 1980;140:302-305.

Kozlov AV, Sobhian B, Duvigneau C, et al: Organ specific formation of nitrosyl complexes under intestinal ischemia/reperfusion in rats involves NOS-independent mechanism(s). Shock 2001;15:366-371.

Krajewski LP, Hertzer NR: Blunt carotid artery trauma. Ann Surg 1980;191:341-346.

Kram HB, Appel PL, Shoemaker WC: Increased incidence of cardiac contusion in patients with traumatic thoracic aortic rupture. Ann Surg 1988;208:615-618.

Kram HB, Appel PL, Wohlmuth DA, Shoemaker WC: Diagnosis of traumatic thoracic aortic rupture: A ten-year retrospective analysis. Ann Thorac Surg 1989;47:282-286.

Kram HB, Wohlmuth DA, Appel PL, Shoemaker WC: Clinical and radiographic indications for aortography in blunt chest trauma. J Vasc Surg 1987;6:168-176.

Kraus TW, Paetz B, Richter GM, Allenberg JR: The isolated posttraumatic aneurysm of the brachiocephalic artery after blunt thoracic contusion. Ann Vasc Surg 1993;7:275-281.

Krauss M: Studies in wound ballistics: Temporary cavity effects in soft tissues. Milit Med 1957;120:221.

Krige JEJ, Spence RAJ: Popliteal artery trauma: A high risk injury. Br J Surg 1987;74:91-94.

Krishnasastry KV, Friedman SG, Deckoff SL, Doscher W: Traumatic juxtarenal aortocaval fistula and pseudoaneurysm. Ann Vasc Surg 1990;4:378-380.

Kronzon I: Diagnosis and treatment of iatrogenic femoral artery pseudoaneurysm: A review. J Am Soc Echocardiogr 1997;10:236-245.

Kropilak M, Satiani B: Combined superficial femoral artery and vein injury with deep venous thrombosis: Elements of proper management. Contemp Surg 1988;32:24-28.

Krosnick A: Death due to migration of the ball from an aortic-valve prosthesis. JAMA 1965;191:1083-1084.

Kruse-Andersen S, Lorentzen JE, Rohr N: Arterial injuries of the upper extremities. Acta Chir Scand 1983;149:473-477.

Kudok KA, Bongard F: Determinants of survival after vena caval injury. Arch Surg 1984;119:1009-1012.

Kudsk K, Sheldon G, Lim R: Atrial-caval shunting (ACS) after trauma. J Trauma 1982;22:81-85.

Kudsk KA, Bongard F, Lim RC Jr: Determinants of survival after vena caval injury: Analysis of a 14-year experience. Arch Surg 1984;119:1009-1012.

Kuiper DH: Cardiac tamponade and death in a patient receiving total parenteral nutrition. JAMA 1974;230:877.

Kulick DL, Kotlewski A, Hurvitz RJ, et al: Aortic rupture following percutaneous catheter balloon coarctoplasty in an adult. Am Heart J 1990;119:190-193.

Kulshrestha P, Iyer KS, Das B, et al: Chest injuries: A clinical and autopsy profile. J Trauma 1988;28:844-847.

Kurtoglu M, Ertekin C, Bulut T, et al: Management of vascular injuries of the extremities. One hundred and fifteen cases. Int Angiol 1991;10:95.

Kurzel RB, Edinger DD: Injury to the great vessels: A hazard of transabdominal endoscopy. South Med J 1983;76:656-657.

Kurzweg FT: Vascular injuries associated with penetrating wounds of the groin. J Trauma 1980;20:214-217.

Kuzman M, Tomic B, Stevanovic R, et al: Fatalities in the war in Croatia, 1991 and 1992: Underlying and external causes of death. JAMA 1993;270:626-628.

Kümmel: Über circuläre naht der gefässe. Munch Med Wschr 1899;46:1398.

Kwaan JHM, Connolly JE: Successful management of prosthetic graft infection with continuous povidone-iodine irrigation. Arch Surg 1981;116:716-720.

Kyosola K, Jarvinen A: Abdominal aortic aneurysm and dissection after blunt trauma. J Cardiovasc Surg 1987;28:737-739.

La Berge JM, Jeffrey RB: Aortic lacerations: Fatal complications of thoracic aortography. Radiology 1987;165:367-369.

La Garde LA: Report of the Surgeon General of the Army to the Secretary of War. Washington, DC, Government Printing Office, 1893.

La Garde LA: Gunshot Injuries (How They Are Inflicted, Their Complications and Treatment). New York, William Wood & Company, 1916.

Lacy JH, Box JM, Connors D, et al: Pseudoaneurysm: Diagnosis with color Doppler ultrasound. J Cardiovasc Surg 1990;31:727-730.

Lafani SJA, Shatzkes D, Scalea T: The removal of intravascular bullets by interventional radiology: The prevention of central migration by balloon occlusion—Case report. J Trauma 1991;31:1423-1425.

Lagerstrom CF, Reed RL, Rowlands BJ, Fisher R: Early fasciotomy for acute clinically evident posttraumatic compartment syndrome. Am J Surg 1989;158:36-39.

Lai MD, Hoffman HB, Adamkiewicz JJ: Dissecting aneurysm of internal carotid artery after non-penetrating neck injury. Acta Radiol Diag 1966;5:290-295.

Lain KC, Williams GR: Arteriography in acute peripheral arterial injuries: An experimental study. Surg Forum 1970;21:179-181.

Lam CR, McIntyre R: Air-pistol injury of pulmonary artery and aorta. Report of a case with peripheral embolization of pellet and residual aorticopulmonary fistula. J Thorac Cardiovasc Surg 1970;59:729-732.

Lamb RK, Pawade A, Prior AL: Intravascular missile: Apparent retrograde course from the left ventricle. Thorax 1988;43:499-500.

Lancey RA, Davliakos GP, Vander Salm TJ: Simultaneous repair of multiple traumatic aortic tears. Ann Thorac Surg 1995;60:1120-1121.

Landreneau R, Mitchum P, Fry W: Iliac arterial transposition. Arch Surg 1989;124:978-981.

Lange R, Bach A, Hansen S, Johansen K: Open tibial fractures with associated vascular injuries: Prognosis of limb salvage. J Trauma 1985;25:203-207.

Lange R: Limb reconstruction versus amputation decision making in massive lower extremity trauma. Clin Orthop 1989;243:92-99.

Langenbeck B: Beitrage zur chirurgischen pathologie der venen. Arch Klin Chir 1861;1:1.

Langley G: Gunshot wound of the innominate artery. Br Med J 1943;2:711-712.

LaRoque G: Penetrating bullet wound of the thoracic aorta followed by lodgment of the bullet in the femoral artery. Ann Surg 1931;4:16.

Larrey D: Sur une blessure du pericorde suivie d'hydropericarde. Bull Sci Med 1810;6:1.

Larrey D: Clin Chir Paris 1829;2:284.

Lassonde J, Laurendeau F: Blunt injury of the abdominal aorta. Am Surg 1981;194:745-748.

Lassonde J, Morin M, Laurendeau F: Arterial injuries. Can J Surg 1984;27:343-345.

Lau J, Mattox KL, Beall AC Jr, DeBakey ME: Use of substitute conduits in traumatic vascular injury. J Trauma 1977;17:541-546.

Launois B, Chateaubriant P, Rosat P, Kiroff G: Repair of suprahepatic caval lesions under extracorporeal circulation in major trauma. J Trauma 1989;29:127-128.

Lavenson GJ, Rich NM, Baugh JH: Value of ultrasonic flow detector in the management of peripheral vascular disease. Am J Surg 1970;120:522.

Lavenson GJ, Rich NM, Strandness DE Jr: Ultrasonic flow detector value in combat vascular injuries. Arch Surg 1971;103:644-647.

Laverick MD, D'sa Barros, Kirk SJ, Mollan RAB: Management of blunt injuries of the axillary and the neck of the humerus: Case report. J Trauma 1990;30:360-361.

Lawrence K, Shefts L, McDaniel J: Wounds of common carotid arteries: Report of 17 cases from World War II. Am J Surg 1948;76:29-37.

Lawton R, Rossi N, Funk D: Intracardiac perforation. Arch Surg 1969;98:213-216.

Layton T, Stroh A, Villella E: Missile embolus of the portal vein. J Trauma 1985;25:1111-1112.

Le Bret F, Ruel P, Rosier H, et al: Diagnosis of traumatic mediastinal hematoma with transesophageal echocardiography. Chest 1994;105:373-376.

Learmonth J: Combined neuro-vascular lesions. Acta Chir Scand 1952;104:93-99.

Learmonth J: An unusual type arteriovenous communication. Br J Surg 1945;32:321-323.

Learmonth J: Vascular injuries in war. Royal Soc Med 1946;39:488.

Leavitt B, Meyer J, Morton JR, et al: Survival following nonpenetrating traumatic rupture of cardiac chambers. Ann Thorac Surg 1987;44:532-535.

Leblanc J, Wood A, O'Shea M, Williams W: Peripheral arterial trauma in children. J Cardiovasc Surg 1985;26:325-331.

Ledgerwood A, Lucas C: Survival following superior mesenteric artery occlusion from trauma. J Trauma 1974;14:622-626.

Ledgerwood A, Lucas C: Biological dressings for exposed vascular grafts: A reasonable alternative. J Trauma 1975;15:567-574.

Ledgerwood A, Kazmers M, Lucas C: The role of thoracic aortic occlusion for massive hemoperitoneum. J Trauma 1976;16:610-615.

Ledgerwood A: The wandering bullet. Surg Clin North Am 1977;57:97-109.

Ledgerwood A, Mullins R, Lucas C: Primary repair vs ligation for carotid artery injuries. Arch Surg 1980;115:488-493.

Lee F, Katzberg R, Gutierrez O, et al: Reevaluation of plain radiographic findings in the diagnosis of aortic rupture: The role of inspiration and positioning on mediastinal width. J Emerg Med 1993;11:289-296.

Lee H, Beale LS: On the repair of arteries and veins after injury. Trans Med Chir Soc 1865;50:477.

Lee R, Stahlman G, Sharp K: Treatment priorities in patients with traumatic rupture of the thoracic aorta. Am Surg 1992;58:37-43.

Lefer A, Lefer D: Pharmacology of the endothelium in ischemia-reperfusion and circulatory shock. Ann Rev Pharmacol Toxicol 1993;33:71-90.

Lefer A: Endotoxin, Cytokines, and nitric oxide in shock. Shock 1994;1:79-80.

Lefer A: Role of the beta2-integrins and immunoglobulin superfamily members in myocardial ischemia-reperfusion. Ann Thorac Surg 1999;68:1920-1923.

Lehr HA, Guhlmann A, Nolte D, et al: Leukotrienes as mediators in ischemia-reperfusion injury in a microcirculation model in the hamster. J Clin Invest 1991;87:2036-2041.

Lemaire J, Dondelinger R: Percutaneous coil embolization of iatrogenic femoral arteriovenous fistula or pseudo-aneurysm. Eur J Radiol 1994;18:96-100.

Lemos P, Okumura M, Azevedo AC, et al: Cardiac wounds: Experience based on a series of 121 operated cases. J Cardiovasc Surg 1976;17:1-8.

Lennox A, Griffin M, Nicolaides A, Mansfield A: Percutaneous ultrasound guided thrombin injection: A new method for treating postcatheterization femoral pseudoaneurysms. J Vasc Surg 1998;28:1120-1121.

Lennox.AF, Griffin M, Cheshire N: Treatment of an iatrogenic femoral artery pseudoaneurysm with percutaneous duplex-guided injection of thrombin. Circulation 1999;100:39-41.

Lennox.AF, Delis K, Szendro G: Duplex-guided thrombin injection for iatrogenic femoral artery pseudoaneurysm is effective even in anticoagulated patients. Br J Surg 2001;87:796-801.

Leppäniemi A, Wherry D, Pikoulis E, et al: Arterial and venous repair with vascular clips: Comparison with suture closure. J Vasc Surg 1997;26:24-28.

Leppäniemi A, Wherry D, Pikoulis E, et al: Common bile duct repair with titanium staples: Comparison with suture closure. Surg Endosc 1997;11:714-717.

Leppäniemi AK, Salo J, Haapiainen R: Civilian low velocity gunshot wounds of the liver. Eur J Surg 1994;160:663-668.

Leppäniemi AK, Savolainen H, Salo J: Traumatic inferior vena caval injuries. Scand J Thorac Cardiovasc Surg 1994;28:103-108.

Leppäniemi AK, Rich NM, Pikoulis E, et al: Sutureless vascular reconstruction with titanium clips. Int Angiol 2000;19:69-74.

Lester J: Arteriovenous fistula after percutaneous vertebral angiography. Acta Radiol Diag 1966;5:337-340.

Letsou G, Gertler J, Baker CC, Hammond G: Blunt innominate injury: A report of three cases. J Trauma 1989;29:104-108.

Letsou G, Gusberg R: Isolated bilateral renal artery thrombosis: An unusual consequence of blunt abdominal trauma—Case report. J Trauma 1990;30:509-511.

Lev El A, Adar R, Rubinstein Z: Axillary artery injury in erect dislocation of the shoulder. J Trauma 1981;21:323-324.

LeVeen H, Cerruti M: Surgery of large inaccessible arteriovenous fistulas. Ann Surg 1963;158:285-289.

Levin A, Gover P, Nance F: Surgical restraint in the management of hepatic injury: A review of the Charity Hospital experience. J Trauma 1978;18:399-404.

Levin L, Goldner R, Urbaniak J, et al: Management of severe musculoskeletal injuries of the upper extremity. J Orthop Trauma 1990;4:432.

Levin P, Rich NM, Hutton JE Jr, et al: Role of arteriovenous shunts in venous reconstruction. Am J Surg 1971;122:183-191.

Levin P, Rich NM, Hutton JE Jr: The role of collateral circulation in arterial injuries. Arch Surg 1971;102:392-398.

Levin P, Rich NM, Hutton JE Jr: Patency of venous grafts in the venous system. J Cardiovasc Surg (Torino) 1972;13:421-427.

Levine E, Alverdy JC: Carotid-esophageal fistula following a penetrating neck injury: Case report. J Trauma 1990;30:1588-1590.

Levitsky S, James P, Anderson RW, Hardeway RI: Vascular trauma in Vietnam battle casualties: An analysis of 55 consecutive cases. Ann Surg 1968;168:831-836.

Lewis D, Davies A, Irvine C: Compression ultrasonography for false femoral artery aneurysms: Hypocoagulability is a cause of failure. Eur J Vasc Surg 1998;16:427-428.

Lewis T: The adjustment of blood flow to the affected limb in arteriovenous fistula. Clin Sci 1940;4:277-285.

Lewtas J: Traumatic subclavian aneurysm: Ligature of innominate and carotid arteries: Recovery. Br Med J 1889;2:312.

Lexer E: Die ideale operation des arteriellen und des arteriell-venosen aneurysma. Arch Klin Chir 1907;83:459-477.

Liau C, Ho F, Chen M, Lee Y: Treatment of iatrogenic femoral artery pseudoaneurysm with percutaneous thrombin injection. J Vasc Surg 1997;26:18-23.

Lichtenstein M: Acute injuries involving the large blood vessels in the neck. Surg Gynecol Obstet 1947;85:165-175.

Lichti E, Erickson T: Traumatic arteriovenous fistula: Clinical evaluation and intraoperative monitoring with the Doppler ultrasonic flowmeter. Am J Surg 1974;127:333-335.

Liddicoat J, Bekassy SM, Daniell M, DeBakey ME: Inadvertent femoral artery "stripping": Surgical management. Surgery 1975;77:318-320.

Liekweg W, Greenfield L: Management of penetrating carotid arterial injuries. Ann Surg 1966;188:587-592.

Lilienthal H: Thoracic surgery: The surgical treatment of thoracic disease. Philadelphia: WB Saunders Company, 1926.

Lillehei K, Robinson M: A critical analysis of the fatal injuries resulting from the Continental flight 1713 airline disaster: Evidence in favor of improved passenger restraint system. J Trauma 1994;37:826-830.

Lim LT, Michuda M, Flanigan DP, Pankovich A: Popliteal artery trauma: 31 consecutive cases without amputation. Arch Surg 1980;115:1307-1313.

Lim LT, Saletta J, Flanigan DP: Subclavian and innominate artery trauma. Surgery 1979;86:890-897.

Lim RC, Glickman M, Hunt TK: Angiography in patients with bunt trauma to the chest and abdomen. Surg Clin North Am 1972;52:551-565.

Lim RC, Miller S: Management of acute civilian vascular injuries. Surg Clin North Am 1982;62:113-119.

Lim RC, Trunkey DD, Blaisdell FW: Acute abdominal aortic injury: An analysis of operative and post-operative management. Arch Surg 1974;109:706-712.

Linberg E: Bullet wound of the thoracic aorta with survival. Maryland State Med J 1959;8:285-286.

Linden J: Molecular approach to adenosine receptors: Receptor-mediated mechanisms of tissue protection. Ann Rev Pharmacol Toxicol 2001;41:775-787.

Lindenauer S, Thompson N, Kraft R: Late complications of traumatic arteriovenous fistulas. Surg Gynecol Obstet 1969;129:525-532.

Lindenbaum B: Complications of knee joint arthroscopy. Clin Orthop Rel Res 1981;160:157.

Lindenbaum G, Jacobs L, Morris M: Perioperative surface and transesophageal color-flow Doppler evaluation of posttraumatic intracardiac shunt. Am Heart J 1990;119:193-196.

Lindskog G: The surgery of the innominate artery. N Engl J Med 1946;235:71-76.

Lindskog G, Liebow A, Glenn W: Thoracic and Cardiovascular Surgery with Related Pathology. New York, Appleton-Century-Crofts, 1962.

Linker R, Crawford F Jr, Rittenbury M, Barton M: Traumatic aortocaval fistula: case report. J Trauma 1989;29:255-257.

Linson M: Axillary artery thrombosis after fracture of the humerus. J Bone Joint Surg 1980;62-A:1214-1215.

Linton R: Injuries to major arteries and their treatment. N YJ Med 1949;49:2039.

Linton R: Arterial injuries associated with fractures of the extremity. J Bone Joint Surg 1964;46:575-576.

Lipscomb P, Burleson R: Vascular and neural complications in the supracondylar fractures of the humerus in children. J Bone Joint Surg 1955;37:487-497.

Litchford B, Okies JE, Sugimura S, Starr A: Acute aortic dissection from cross clamp injury. J Thorac Cardiovasc Surg 1976;72:709-713.

Little J, Ferguson D: The incidence of hypothenar hammer syndrome. Arch Surg 1972;105:684.

Lizama V, Zerbini M, Gagliardi R, Howell L: Popliteal vein thrombosis and popliteal artery pseudoaneurysm complicating osteochondroma of the femur. AJR Am J Roentgenol 1987;148:783-784.

Lloyd J: Traumatic peripheral aneurysms. Am J Surg 1987;93:755-764.

Lock J, Huffman A, Johnson R: Blunt trauma to the abdominal aorta. J Trauma 1987;27:674-677.

Loello F, Nunn D: False aneurysm of the inferior epigastric artery as a complication of abdominal retention sutures. Surgery 1973;74:460.

Lohse J, Botham RJ, Waters R: Traumatic bilateral renal artery thrombosis. J Urol 1982;127:522.

Loose H, Haslam P: The management of peripheral arterial aneurysms using percutaneous injection of fibrin adhesive. Br J Radial 1998;17:1255-1259.

Lopez-Viegro M, Synder WH, Clagett GP: Penetrating abdominal aortic trauma: A review of 129 patients. J Vasc Surg 1992;15:247-248.

Lord JW, Stone P, Clouthier W, Breidenbach L: Major blood vessel injury during elective surgery. Arch Surg 1958;77:282.

Lord R, Ehrenfeld W, Wylie EJ: Arterial injury from the Fogarty catheter. Med J Aust 1968;2:70-71.

Lord R, Irana C: Assessment of arterial injury in limb trauma. J Trauma 1974;14:1042-1053.

Lorenz P, Steinmetz B, Lieberman J: Emergency thoracotomy: Survival correlates with physiologic status. J Trauma 1992;32:780.

Louridas G, Perry MO: Basic data related to vascular trauma. Ann Vasc Surg 1989;3:397.

Love C, Evans S: Gunshot wound of the abdominal aorta and anoxic cardiac arrest: Report of a survival. Ann Surg 1963;158:131-132.

Love L, Braun T: Arteriography of peripheral vascular trauma. AJR Am J Roentgenol 1968;102:431-440.

Lovric Z: Reconstruction of major arteries of extremities after war injuries. J Cardiovasc Surg (Turin) 1993;34:33-37.

Lovric Z, Wertheimer B, Candric K, et al: Reconstruction of the popliteal artery after war injury. Unfallchirurg 1993;97:375-377.

Lovric Z, Wertheimer B, Candric K, et al: War injuries of major extremity vessels. J Trauma 1994;36:248-251.

Lowen H, Fink S, Helpern M: Transfixion of the heart by embedded ice pick blade with eight months' survival. Circulation 1950;2:426-433.

Lozman H, Beaufils AT, Rossi G, et al: Vascular trauma observed at an urban hospital center. Surg Gynecol Obstet 1978;146:237-240.

Lozman H, Robbins H: Injury to the superior gluteal artery as a complication of total hip replacement arthroplasty: A case report. J Bone Joint Surg 1983;65:268-269.

Lucas A, Richardson JD, Flint LM, Polk H: Traumatic injury of the proximal superior mesenteric artery. Ann Surg 1981;193:30-34.

Lucas R, Tumacder O, Wilson G: Hepatic artery occlusion following hepatic artery catheterization. Ann Surg 1971;173:238-243.

Ludewig RM, Wangensteen S: Aortic bleeding and the effect of external counter pressure. Surg Gynecol Obstet 1969;128:252-258.

Luetic V, Sosa T, Tonkovic I, et al: Military vascular injuries in Croatia. Cardiovasc Surg 1993;1:3-6.

Luke J: Arterial trauma. J Cardiovasc Surg 1962;3:165-168.

Lumpkin M, Logan W, Couves C, Howard JM: Arteriography as an aid in the diagnosis and localization of acute arterial injuries. Ann Surg 1958;147:353-358.

Lumsden A, Miller J, Kosinski A: A prospective evaluation of surgically treated groin complications following percutaneous cardiac procedures. Am Surg 1994;60:132-137.

Lundell C, Quinn M, Finck E: Traumatic laceration of the ascending aorta: Angiographic assessment. AJR Am J Roentgenol 1985;145:715-719.

Lupetin A, Beckman I, Daffner R: CT diagnosis of traumatic abdominal aortic rupture. J Comput Assist Tomogr 1990;14:313-314.

Lynch K, Johansen K: Can Doppler pressure measurement replace "exclusion" arteriography in extremity trauma? Ann Surg 1991;214:737-741.

Lynch K, Johansen K: Can non-invasive vascular tests replace screening arteriography in extremity trauma? J Vasc Surg 9999.

Lyons C, Perkins R: Cardiac stab wounds. Am Surg 1957;23:507.

Macbeth A, Malone J, Norton L, Peltier L: Paralysis and aortic thrombosis following blunt abdominal trauma. J Trauma 1982;22:591-594.

MacDonell J: Traumatic aortic aneurysm. Can Med Assoc J 1956;75:581-584.

MacGowan W: Acute ischemia complicating limb trauma. J Bone Joint Surg 1968;50-B:472-484.

Machiedo G, Jain K, Swan KG, et al: Traumatic aortocaval fistula. J Trauma 1983;23:243-247.

Machle W: Lead absorption from bullets lodged in tissues: Report of two cases. JAMA 1940;115:1536.

Machleder HI, Sweeney J, Barker WF: Pulseless arm after brachial artery catheterization. Lancet 1972;1:407.

MacLachlin A, Carroll S, Meades G, Amacher AL: Valve replacement in the recanalized incompetent superficial femoral vein in dogs. Ann Surg 1965;162:446.

MacLean L: The diagnosis and treatment of arterial injuries. Can Med Assoc J 1963;88:1091-1101.

MacLean L, Flam R, Petersen D: Diagnosis and treatment of arterial injuries. Minn Med 1961;44:133-142.

Maggisano R, Nathans A, Alexandrova NA, et al: Traumatic rupture of the thoracic aorta: Should one always operate immediately? Ann Vasc Surg 1995;9: 44-52.

Magilligan D, Davila J: Innominate artery disruption due to blunt trauma. Arch Surg 1979;114:307-309.

Mahoney B, Gerdes D, Roller B, Ruiz E: Aortic compressor for aortic occlusion in hemorrhagic shock. Ann Emerg Med 1984;13:11-16.

Majeski JA, Gants A: A management of peripheral arterial vascular injuries with Javid shunt. Am J Surg 1979;138:324-345.

Makins G: Blessures des vaisseaux. Comptes-endus conférence Chirurgicale Interalliée pour l'etude des Plaies de Guerre. Arch Med Pharm Mil 1917;68:341.

Makins G: Influence exerted by military experience of John Hunter himself and the military surgeon of today. Lancet 1917;1:249-254.

Makins G: Gunshot injuries to the blood vessels. Bristol, England, John Wright and Sons, 1919.

Makins G: Injuries to the blood vessels. Official History of the Great War Medical Service. Surgery of the War, vol 2. London, His Majesty's Stationary Office, 1922, pp 170-296.

Makins G: Specimen showing the effects of gunshot injury on the heart and blood vessels. Now on exhibit in the museum of the Royal College of Surgeons of England. Br J Surg 1977;18:141-146.

Makins G, Howard JM, Green R: Arterial injuries complicating fractures and dislocations: The necessity for a more aggressive approach. Surgery 1966;59:203-209.

Maleux G, Soula P, Otal P, et al: Traumatic aortobiliac dissection treated by kissing-stent placement. J Trauma 1997;43:706-708.

Malt R, McKhann C: A report on replantation of severed arms. JAMA 1964;189:716-722.

Man B, Kraus L, Shachor D: Self-inflicted stab wound of the abdominal aorta. J Cardiovasc Surg 1978;19:503-505.

Mandal A, Boitano MA: Reappraisal of low-velocity gunshot wounds of the aorta and inferior vena cava in civilian practice. J Trauma 1978;18:580-585.

Mandal A, Oparah S: Unusually low mortality of penetrating wounds of the chest: Twelve years experience. J Thorac Cardiovasc Surg 1989;1: 119.

Mandelbaum I, Kalsbeck J: Extrinsic compression of internal carotid artery. Ann Surg 1970;171:434-437.

Manlove G, Quattlebaum F, Flom R, LaFave J: Gunshot wounds of the abdominal aorta. Am J Surg 1960;99:941-944.

Mansberger A, Linberg E: First rib resection for distal exposure of subclavian vessels. Surg Gynecol Obstet 1965;120:579.

Mansour MA, Moore FA, Moore EE: Hypogastric arterial embolization in pelvic fracture hemorrhage: Case report. J Trauma 1990;30:1417-1418.

Marcove R, Lindeque B, Silane M: Pseudoaneurysm of the popliteal artery with an unusual arteriographic presentation. Clin Orthop Related Res 1988;234:142-144.

Margolies M, Ring E, Waltman A: Arteriography in the management of hemorrhage from pelvic fractures. N Engl J Med 1972;287:317-321.

Marin M, Veith F, Cynamon J, et al: Initial experience with transluminally placed endovascular grafts for the treatment of complex vascular lesions. J Vasc Surg 1995;222:449-465.

Marin M, Veith F, Panetta T: Transluminally placed endovascular stented graft repair for arterial trauma. J Vasc Surg 1994;20:466-473.

Marin M, Veith F, Panetta T, et al: Percutaneous transfemoral insertion of a stented graft to repair a traumatic femoral arteriovenous fistula. J Vasc Surg 1993;18:299-302.

Markey JJ, Hines J, Nance C: Penetrating neck wounds: A review of 218 cases. Am Surg 1975;41:77-83.

Marnocha K, Maglinte D: Plain-film criteria for excluding aortic rupture in blunt chest trauma. AJR Am J Roentgenol 1985;144:19-21.

Marnocha K, Maglinte D, Woods J, et al: Blunt chest trauma and suspected aortic rupture: Reliability of chest radiographs finds. Ann Emerg Med 1985;14:644-649.

Marsh C, Moore R: Deceleration trauma. Am J Surg 1957;93:623.

Marsh D, Sturm J: Traumatic aortic rupture: Roentgenographic indications for angiography. Ann Thorac Surg 1976;21:337-340.

Martin L, McKenney M, Sosa J, et al: Management of lower extremity arterial trauma. J Trauma 1994;37:591-599.

Martin RR, Mattox KL, Burch JM, Richardson R: Advances in treatment of vascular injuries from blunt and penetrating limb trauma. World J Surg 1992;16:930-937.

Martin R, Flynn T, Rowlands G: Blunt cardiac rupture. J Trauma 1984;24:287-290.

Marts B, Durham R, Shapiro M, et al: Computed tomography in the diagnosis of blunt thoracic injury. Am J Surg 1994;168:688-692.

Marty-Ané C, Alric P, Prudhomme M, et al: Intravascular stenting of traumatic abdominal dissection. J Vasc Surg 1996;23:156-161.

Marty-Ané C, Serres-Cousiné O, Laborde J, et al: Endovascular stent for use in acute aortic dissection: An experimental study. Ann Vasc Surg 1994;8:434-442.

Marvasti M, Meyer J, Ford B, Parker FJ: Spinal cord ischemia following operation for traumatic aortic transection. Ann Thorac Surg 1986;42:425-428.

Marvasti M, Parker FJ, Bredenberg CE: Injury to arterial branches of aortic arch. J Thorac Cardiovasc Surg 1984;32:293-298.

Marymont J, Cotler H, Harris JJ, et al: Posterior hip dislocation associated with acute traumatic injury of the thoracic aorta: A previously unrecognized injury complex. J Orthop Trauma 1990;4:383-387.

Marzelle J, Nottin R, Dartevelle P, et al: Combined ascending aorta rupture and left main bronchus disruption from blunt chest trauma. Ann Thorac Surg 1989;1989:769-771.

Massberg S, Enders G, Matos F, et al: Fibrinogen deposition at the postischemic vessel wall promotes platelet adhesion during ischemia–reperfusion in vivo. Blood 1999;94:3829-838.

Massberg S, Messmer K: The nature of ischemia/reperfusion injury. Transplant Proc 1998;30:4217-4223.

Massberg S, Sausbier M, Klatt P, et al: Increased adhesion and aggregation of platelets lacking cyclic guanosine 3′,5′–monophosphate kinase I. J Exp Med 1999;189:1255-1264.

Matas R: Traumatic aneurysm of the left brachial artery—Incision and partial excision of sac: Recovery. Phil Med News 1888;53:462-466.

Matas R: Traumatisms and traumatic aneurysms of the vertebral artery and their surgical treatment. Ann Surg 1893;18:477-521.

Matas R: Traumatic arteriovenous aneurysms of the subclavian vessels, with an analytical study of fifteen reported cases, including one operated. Trans Am Surg Assoc 1901;19:237.

Matas R: An operation for radical cure of aneurysm based on arteriography. Ann Surg 1903;37:161-196.

Matas R: Recent advances in the technique of thoracotomy and pericardiotomy for wounds of the heart. South Med J 1908;1:75-81.

Matas R: Surgery of the vascular system. In Keen WW, DaCosta JC (eds): Philadelphia, WB Saunders, 1909, p 67.

Matas R: Testing the efficiency of the collateral circulation as a preliminary to the occlusion of the great surgical arteries. Ann Surg 1911;53:1-43.

Matas R: Testing the efficiency of the collateral circulation as a preliminary to the occlusion of the great surgical arteries. JAMA 1914;68:1441-1447.

Matas R: Endoaneurysmorrhaphy, I: Statistics of operation of endoaneurysmorrhaphy, II: Personal experiences and observations on the treatment of arteriovenous aneurysms by the intravascular method of suture: With special references to the transvenous route. Surg Gynecol Obstet 1920;30:456-458.

Matas R: Military Surgery of the Vascular System. Philadelphia, WB Saunders, 1921.

Mathieu D, Wattel F, Bouachour G, et al: Post-traumatic limb ischemia: Prediction of final outcome by transcutaneous oxygen measurements in hyperbaric oxygen. J Trauma 1990;30:307-314.

Mathur A, Pochaczevsky R, Levotitz B, Feraru F: Fogarty balloon catheter for removal of catheter fragment in subclavian vein. JAMA 1971;217:481.

Matloff D, Morton J: Acute trauma to the subclavian arteries. Am J Surg 1968;115:675-680.

Matolo M, Danto L, Wolfman E. Traumatic aneurysm of the abdominal aorta: Report of two cases and review of the literature. Arch Surg 1974;108:867-869.

Matsubara J, Seko T, Ohta T, et al: Traumatic aneurysm of the abdominal aorta with acute thrombosis of bilateral iliac arteries. Arch Surg 1983;118:1337-1339.

Mattox KL: Comparison of techniques of autotransfusion. Surgery 1978;84:700-702.

Mattox KL: Emergency department thoracotomy. JACEP 1978;7:455.

Mattox KL: Abdominal venous injuries. Surgery 1982;91:497-501.

Mattox KL: CPR: Not for everyone. Emerg Med 1983;15:147-150.

Mattox KL: Thoracic great vessel injury. Surg Clin North Am 1988;68:693-703.

Mattox KL: Thoracic vascular trauma. J Vasc Surg 1988;7:725-729.

Mattox KL: Approaches to trauma involving the major vessels of the thorax. Surg Clin North Am 1989;69:77-92.

Mattox KL: Fact and Fiction about management of aortic transection. Ann Thorac Surg 1989;48:1-3.

Mattox KL: Indications for thoracotomy: Deciding to operate. Surg Clin North Am 1989;1:47.

Mattox KL: Invited editorial comment: What drives the need for new technology? J Trauma 1992;32:761-768.

Mattox KL: The abbreviated injury scale, 1985 revision: A condensed chart for clinical use. J Trauma 1997;42:353-368.

Mattox KL, Allen MK: Penetrating wounds of the thorax. Injury 1986;174:313-317.

Mattox KL, Beall AC Jr, Ennix C, DeBakey ME: Intravascular migratory bullets. Am J Surg 1979;137:192-195.

Mattox KL, Beall AC Jr, Jordan GL Jr, DeBakey ME: Cardiorrhaphy in the emergency center. J Thorac Cardiovasc Surg 1974;68:886-895.

Mattox KL, Bickell W, Pepe PE, et al: Prospective MAST study in 911 patients. J Trauma 1989;20:1104.

Mattox KL, Bickell WH, Pepe PE, Mangelsdorff A: Prospective randomized evaluation of antishock MAST in posttraumatic hypotension. J Trauma 1986;26:779-786.

Mattox KL, Burch JM, Richardson R, Martin RR: Retroperitoneal vascular injury. Surg Clin North Am 1990;70:635-653.

Mattox KL, Espada R, Beall AC Jr: Performing thoracotomy in the emergency center. J Am Coll Emerg Phys 1974;3:13-17.

Mattox KL, Espada R, Beall AC Jr: Traumatic injury to the portal vein. Ann Surg 1975;181:519-522.

Mattox KL, Feliciano DV: Role of external cardiac compression in truncal trauma. J Trauma 1982;22:934-935.

Mattox KL, Feliciano DV, Burch J, et al: Five thousand seven hundred sixty cardiovascular injuries in 4459 patients: Epidemiologic evolution 1958 to 1987. Ann Surg 1989;209:698-707.

Mattox KL, Holzman M, Pickard LR, et al: Clamp/repair: A safe technique for treatment of blunt injury to the descending thoracic aorta. Ann Thorac Surg 1985;40:456-465.

Mattox KL, Limacher M, Feliciano D: Cardiac evaluation following heart injury. J Trauma 1985;25:758-765.

Mattox KL, Maningas P, Moore EE, et al: Prehospital hypertonic saline/dextran infusion for post-traumatic hypotension. The USA multicenter trial. Ann Surg 1991;213:482-491.

Mattox KL, McCollum W, Beall AC Jr, et al: Management of penetrating injuries of the suprarenal aorta. J Trauma 1975;15:808-815.

Mattox KL, McCollum W, Jordan GL Jr, et al: Management of upper abdominal vascular trauma. Am Surg 1974;128:823-828.

Mattox KL, Moore EE, Feliciano DV: Trauma. East Norwalk, Conn, Appleton & Lange, 1988, pp 519-536.

Mattox KL, Pickard L, Allen MK: Emergency thoracotomy for injury. Injury 1986;17:327-331.

Mattox KL, Pickard L, Allen MK, Garcia-Rinaldi R: Suspecting thoracic aortic transection. JACEP 1978;7:12-15.

Mattox KL, Rea J, Ennix C, et al: Penetrating injuries to the iliac arteries. Am J Surg 1978;136:663-667.

Mattox KL, Von Koch L, Beall AC Jr, DeBakey ME: Logistic and technical considerations in the treatment of the wounded heart. Circulation 1975;51(suppl I) and 52:210-214.

Mattox KL, Whisennand H, Espada R, Beall AC Jr: Management of acute combined injuries to the aorta and inferior vena cava. Am J Surg 1975;130:720-724.

Maughon J: An inquiry into the nature of wounds resulting in killed in action in Vietnam. Milit Med 1970;135:8-13.

Mavroudis C, Roon A, Baker CC, Thomas AN: Management of acute cervicothoracic vascular injuries. J Thorac Cardiovasc Surg 1980;80:342-349.

May A, Lipchik E, DeWeese JA: Repair of hepatic and superior mesenteric artery injury: Patency demonstrated by aortography. Ann Surg 1965;162:869-872.

McBride L, Tidik S, Stothert J, et al: Primary repair of traumatic aortic disruption. Ann Thorac Surg 1987;43:65-67.

McBurney R, Vaughn R: Rupture of the aorta due to nonpenetrating trauma. Ann Surg 1961;153:670-679.

McBurney R, Gegan E: Blunt trauma to the aorta and major arteries. JAMA 1962;180:330.

McCabe C, Ferguson C, Ottinger L: Improved limb salvage in popliteal artery injuries. J Trauma 1983;23:982-985.

McCann W: Successful wound repair of a stab wound of the ascending aorta. N Y State J Med 1958;58:3177-3178.

McCarthy W, Yao JST, Schafer M, et al: Upper extremity arterial injury in athletes. J Vasc Surg 1989;9:317-327.

McCollum C, Mavor E: Brachial artery injury after cardiac catheterization. J Vasc Surg 1986;4:355-359.

McCord J: Oxygen-derived free radicals in postischemic tissue injury. N Engl J Med 1985;312:159-163.

McCorkell S, Harley J, Morishima M, Cummings D: Indications for angiography in extremity trauma. AJR 1985;145:1245-1247.

McCormack L, Cauldwell E, Anson BJ: Brachial and antebrachial arterial patterns: a study of 750 extremities. Surg Gynecol Obstet 1953;96:43-54.

McCormick T, Burch B: Routine angiographic evaluation of neck and extremity injuries. J Trauma 1979;19:384-387.

McCready R: Upper extremity vascular injuries. Surg Clin North Am 1988;68:725-740.

McCready R, Logan N, Daugherty M: Long-term results with autogenous tissue repair of traumatic extremity vascular injuries. Ann Surg 1987;206:804-808.

McCready R, Procter C, Hyde GL: Subclavian-axillary vascular trauma. J Vasc Surg 1986;3:24-31.

McCroskey B, Moore EE, Moore FA, Abernathy CM: A unified approach to the torn thoracic aorta. Am J Surg 1991;162:473-476.

McCroskey B, Moore EE, Pearce W, et al: Traumatic arterial injuries of the upper extremity: Determinants of disability. Am J Surg 1988;156:553-555.

McCroskey B, Moore EE, Rutherford R: Vascular Trauma. The Surgical Clinics of North America. Philadelphia, WB Saunders, 1988.

McCullough J, Hollier L, Nugent M: Paraplegia after thoracic aorta occlusion: Influence of cerebrospinal fluid drainage. Experimental and early clinical results. J Vasc Surg 1988;7:153-160.

McCutchan J, Gillham N: Injury to the popliteal artery associated with dislocation of the knee: Palpable distal pulses do not negate the requirement for arteriography. Injury 1989;20:307-310.

McDonald E, Goodman P, Weinstock D: Clinical indications for arteriography in trauma to the extremity: A review of 114 cases. Radiology 1975;166:45-47.

McDonald M, Mota-Filipe H, Paul A, et al: Calpain inhibitor I reduces the activation of nuclear factor-kappaB and organ injury/dysfunction in hemorrhagic shock. FASEB J 2001;15:171-186.

McDonough J, Altemeier WA: Subclavian venous thrombosis secondary to indwelling catheters. Surg Gynecol Obstet 1971;133:397-400.

McFadden P, Jones J, Ochsner JL: The fuzzy foreign body fragment: A subtle roentgenographic clue to mediastinal vascular injury. Am J Surg 1985; 149:809-811.

McFadden D, Lawelor B, Ali I: Portal vein injury. Can J Surg 1987;30:91.

McGough E, Helfrich L, Hughes R: Traumatic intimal prolapse of the common carotid artery. Am J Surg 1972;123:724-75.

McIlduff J, Foster E, Alley RD: Traumatic aortic rupture: An additional roentgenographic sign. Ann Thorac Surg 1977;24:77-79.

McIntyre RJ, Moore EE, Read R, et al: Transesophageal echocardiography in the evolution of a transmediastinal gunshot wound: Case report. J Trauma 1994;36:125-127.

McKenzie A, Sinclair A: Axillary artery occlusion complicating shoulder dislocation: A report of two cases. Ann Surg 1958;148:139-144.

McKnight J, Meyer J, Neville JJ: Nonpenetrating traumatic rupture of the thoracic aorta. Ann Surg 1964;160:1069-1072.

McLaughlin JS, Suherlis H, Yeager G: Sterile pericarditis from foreign body: Acute tamponade one month following gunshot wound. Ann Thorac Surg 1967;3:52-56.

McLean T, McManus R: Penetrating trauma involving the innominate artery. Ann Thorac Surg 1991;51:113-115.

McMillan R, Landreneau M, McCormic G, McDonald J: Major vascular injuries of the torso. South Med J 1992;85:375-377.

McNab A, Fabinyi G, Miline P: Blunt trauma to the carotid artery. Aust N Z J Surg 1988;58:651-656.

McNally W: Lead poisoning caused by a bullet embedded for twenty-seven years. Indust Med 1949;18:77.

McNalley M, Sugg W: Traumatic communication between the aorta, right atrium, and left atrium. J Thorac Cardiovasc Surg 1967;54:150-152.

McNamara JJ, Brief DK, Beasley W, Wright J: Vascular injury in Vietnam combat casualties: Results of treatment at the 24th Evacuation Hospital, 1 July 1967 to 12 August 1969. Ann Surg 1973;178:143-147.

McNamara JJ, Brief DK, Stremple J, Wright J: Management of fractures with associated arterial injury in combat casualties. J Trauma 1973;13:17-19.

McNutt R, Seabrook G, Schmitt D, Aprahamian C: Blunt tibial artery trauma: predicting the irretrievable extremity. J Trauma 1989;29:1624.

McQuillan W, Nolan B: Ischaemia complicating injury: A report of thirty-seven cases. J Bone Joint Surg 1968;50-B:482-492.

McSwain NE Jr: Pneumatic trousers and the management of shock. J Trauma 1977;17:719-724.

McSwain NE Jr: PASG–Holding on for dear life. Emergency 1990.

Meagher DJ, Defore W, Mattox KL, Harberg F: Vascular trauma in infants and children. J Trauma 1979;19:532-536.

Meek A, Robbs J: Vascular injury with associated bone and joint trauma. Br J Surg 1984;71:341-344.

Meissner M, Paun M, Johansen K: Duplex sonography for arterial trauma. Am J Surg 1991;161:552.

Melki J, Tabley A, Bessou JP, Soyer R: Chronic false aneurysm of the sub-renal abdominal aorta after abdominal contusion (French). J Maladies Vasculaires 1990;15:377-379.

Melton S, Croce MA, Patton JJ, et al: Popliteal artery trauma: Systemic anticoagulation and intraoperative thrombolysis improve limb salvage. Ann Surg 1997;225:518-527.

Menger MD, Kerger H, Geisweid A, et al: Leukocyte-endothelium interaction in the microvasculature of postischemic striated muscle. Adv Exp Med Biol 1994;361:541-545.

Menger MD, Pelikan S, Steiner D, Messmer K: Microvascular ischemia-reperfusion injury in striated muscle: Significance of "reflow paradox." Am J Physiol 1992;263:H1901-H1906.

Menger MD, Rucker M, Vollmar B: Capillary dysfunction in striated muscle ischemia/reperfusion: On the mechanisms of capillary "no reflow." Shock 1997;8:2-7.

Menger MD, Vollmar B: In vivo analysis of microvascular reperfusion injury in striated muscle and skin. Microsurgery 1994;15:383-389.

Mengoli L: Aneurysmorrhaphy of the internal carotid artery utilizing intralu-minal distal control. Am J Surg 1969;117:397-399.

Menzoian J, Doyle J, Cantelmo N, et al: A comprehensive approach to extrem-ity vascular trauma. Arch Surg 1985;120:801-805.

Menzoian J, Doyle J, Logerfo F, et al: Evaluation and management of vascular injuries of the extremities. Arch Surg 1983;118:93-95.

Menzoian J, Logerfo F, Doyle J, et al: Management of vascular injuries to the leg. Am J Surg 1981;144:231-234.

Meredith J, O'Neil E, Snow D, Hansen K: Femoral vein catheter related deep venous thrombosis: A perspective evaluation with venous duplex sonog-raphy. J Trauma 1991;31:1034.

Merin G, Bitran D, Donchin Y, et al: Traumatic rupture of the thoracic aorta during pregnancy. Surgical considerations. Chest 1981;79:99-100.

Merine D, Brody W: Role of CT in excluding major arterial injury after blunt thoracic trauma. Invest Radiol 1989;24:733-734.

Merrill W, Lee R, Hammon JJ, et al: Surgical treatment of acute traumatic tear of the thoracic aorta. Ann Surg 1988;207:699-706.

Messina L, Brothers T, Wakefield T: Clinical characteristics and surgical man-agement of vascular complications in patients undergoing cardiac catheter-ization: Interventional versus diagnostic procedures. J Vasc Surg 1991; 13:593-600.

Metzdroff M, Hill J, Matar A, et al: Use of sutureless intraluminal aortic pros-theses in traumatic rupture of the aorta. J Trauma 1986;26:691-694.

Metzger D, Hamilton R, Stephenson D: Mesenteric arteriovenous fistula: Unusual cause of distal gastrointestinal bleeding. Am J Surg 1972;124: 767.

Meyer D, Jessen M, Grayburn P: Use of echocardiography to detect occult cardiac injury after penetrating thoracic trauma: A prospective study. J Trauma 1995;39:902-909.

Meyer JP, Lim LT, Schuler J, et al: Peripheral vascular trauma from close-range shotgun injuries. Arch Surg 1985;120:1126-1131.

Meyer JP, Walsh J, Barrett J, et al: Analysis of 18 recent cases of penetrating injuries to common and internal carotid arteries. Am J Surg 1988;156:96-99.

Meyer JP, Walsh J, Schuler J: The early fate of venous repair following civilian vascular trauma: A clinical hemodynamic and venographic assessment. Ann Surg 1987;206:458-464.

Meyer JP, Goldfaden D, Barrett J, et al: Subclavian and innominate artery trauma: A recent experience with nine patients. J Cardiovasc Surg 1988;29:283-289.

Meyer J, Neville JJ, Hansen W: Traumatic rupture of the aorta in a child. JAMA 1969;208:527-529.

Meyer TJ, Slager R: False aneurysm following subtrochanteric osteotomy. J Bone Joint Surg 1964;46:581-582.

Michaels A, Gerndt S, Taheri P, et al: Blunt force injury to the abdominal aorta. J Trauma 1996;41:105-109.

Michaels J: Choice of material for above-knee femoropopliteal bypass graft. Br J Surg 1989;76:7-14.

Michaud P, Chassignolle J, Termet H, et al: Traumatic aneurysms of the aorta. Analysis of 11 observations. J Cardiovasc Surg 1971;12:121-130.

Michelassi F, Pietrabissa A, Ferrari M, et al: Bullet emboli to the systemic and venous circulation. Surgery 1990;107:239-245.

Midgley F, Behrendt DM: Surgical repair of chronic post-traumatic aneurysm of the aortic arch. J Thorac Cardiovasc Surg 1974;67:229-232.

Mikulin T, Walker E: False aneurysm following blunt trauma. Injury 1984;15:309-310.

Miller D: Gangrene from arterial injuries associated with fractures and dislocations of the leg in the young and in adults with normal circulation. Am J Surg 1957;93:367-375.

Miller D, Freeark R: Injuries to the popliteal artery among the young. Am J Surg 1962;104:633-639.

Miller F, Bond SJ, Shumate C: Diagnostic pericardial window: A safe alternative to exploratory thoracotomy for suspected heart injuries. Arch Surg 1987;122:605-609.

Miller F, Richardson JD, Thomas H, et al: Role of CT in diagnosis of major arterial injury after blunt thoracic trauma. Surgery 1988;106:596-602.

Miller F, Seward J, Gersh B, Tajik A: Two-dimensional echocardiographic findings in cardiac trauma. Am J Cardiol 1982;50:1022-1027.

Miller F, Shumate C, Richardson JD: Myocardial contusion: when can the diagnosis be eliminated? Arch Surg 1989;124:805-808.

Miller H, Welch C: Quantitative studies on time factor in arterial injuries. Ann Surg 1949;130:428-438.

Millham F, Grindlinger G: Survival determinants in patients undergoing emergency room thoracotomy for penetrating chest injury. J Trauma 1993;34:332-336.

Millikan JS, Moore EE, Cogbill TH: Inferior vena cava injuries: A continuing challenge. J Trauma 1983;23:207-212.

Millikan JS, Moore EE, Van Way G, Kelly GL: Vascular trauma in the groin: Contrast between iliac and femoral injuries. Am J Surg 1981;142:695-698.

Millikan JS, Moore EE: Outcome of resuscitative thoracotomy and descending aortic occlusion. J Trauma 1984;24:387-392.

Millikan JS, Moore EE: Critical factors in determining mortality from abdominal aortic trauma. Surg Gynecol Obstet 1985;160:313-316.

Mills J, Wiedeman J, Robison JG, Hallett JJ: Minimizing mortality and morbidity from iatrogenic arterial injuries: The need for early recognition and prompt repair. J Vasc Surg 1986;4:22-27.

Mirvis S, Kostrubiak I, Whitley N, et al: Role of CT in excluding major arterial injury after blunt thoracic trauma. AJR Am J Roentgenol 1987;149:601-605.

Mitchell D, Needlemon L, Bezzi M, et al: Femoral artery pseudoaneurysm: Diagnosis with conventional duplex and color Doppler. Radiology 1987;165:687-690.

Mitchell FI, Thal E: Results of venous interposition grafts in arterial injuries. J Trauma 1990;30:336-339.

Mitchell R, Enright L: The surgical management of acute and chronic injuries of the thoracic aorta. Surg Gynecol Obstet 1983;157:1-4.

Mittal A, May I, Samson P: Traumatic aneurysm of the aortic arch. Ann Thorac Surg 1972;13:494-498.

Corrected

Monson D, Saletta J, Freeark R: Carotid vertebral trauma. J Trauma 1969;9:987-999.

Montales E, Yao S, Silva Y: Management of traumatic peripheral arteriovenous fistulas. J Trauma 1973;13:161-165.

Montgomery M: Effect of therapeutic venous ligation on blood flow in cases of arterial occlusion. Proc Soc Exp Biol Med 1929;27:178.

Montgomery M: Therapeutic venous occlusion: Its effect on blood flow in the extremity in acute obstruction. Arch Surg 1932;24:1016-1027.

Moon M, Dake M, Pelc L, et al: Intravascular stenting of acute experimental type B dissections. J Surg Res 1993;54:381-388.

Moore C, Cohen A: Combined arterial, venous and ureteral injury complicating lumbar disc surgery. Am J Surg 1968;115:574-577.

Moore C, Wolma F, Brown R, Derrick J: Vascular trauma: A review of 250 cases. Am J Surg 1971;122:576-578.

Moore EE, Burch JM, Franciose RJ, et al: Staged physiologic restoration and damage control surgery. World J Surg 1998;22:1184.

Moore EE, Cogbill TH, Jurkovich GJ: Organ injury scaling III: Chest wall, abdominal vascular, ureter, bladder and urethra. J Trauma 1992;33:337-339.

Moore EE, Cogbill TH, Malangoni M, et al: Organ injury scaling. Surg Clin North Am 1995;75:293-303.

Moore EE, Malangoni M, Cogbill TH: Organ Injury Scaling IV: Thoracic, vascular, lung, cardiac, and diaphragm. J Trauma 1994;36:229-300.

Moore E, Webb W, Verrier E, et al: MRI of chronic posttraumatic aneurysms of the thoracic aorta. AJR Am J Roentgenol 1984;143:1195-1196.

Moore HJ, Nyhus L, Kanar E, Harkins H: Gunshot wounds of the major arteries: An experimental study with clinical implications. Surg Gynecol Obstet 1954;98:129-147.

Moore T: Acute arterial obstruction due to the traumatic circumferential intimal fracture. Ann Surg 1958;148:111-114.

Moore T, Peters M: Thru-and-thru gunshot penetration of the abdominal aorta in a 4-year-old child managed by aortic transection, debridement and reanastomosis with survival. J Trauma 1979;19:537-539.

Moore W: Vascular Surgery. Orlando, Grune & Stratton, 1986.

Morano J, Burkhalter J, Daniel C Jr: Bilateral popliteal arteriovenous fistulas. J Trauma 1987;27:577-578.

Moreno C, Moore EE, Majune J: Pericardial tamponade. A critical determinant for survival following penetrating cardiac wounds. J Trauma 1986;26:821.

Moreno C, Moore EE, Rosenberger A, Cleveland H: Hemorrhage associated with major pelvic fracture: A multispecialty challenge. J Trauma 1986;26:987-994.

Morgan P, Goodman L, Aprahamian C, et al: Evaluation of traumatic aortic injury: Does dynamic contrast-enhanced CT ply a role? Radiology 1992;182:661-666.

Morin J, Provan J, Jewett M, Ameli FM: Vascular injury and repair associated with retroperitoneal lymphadenectomy for nonseminomatous germinal cell tumours of the testis. Can J Surg 1992;35:253-256.

Morin R, Wright CB, Dunn E, et al: Vascular trauma. In James E, Corry R, Perry JF Jr (eds): Basic Surgical practice. St. Louis, Hanley & Belfus, 1987, pp 521-523.

Morris GC Jr, Beall AC Jr, Berry WB, et al: Anatomical studies of the distal popliteal artery and its branches. Surg Forum 1960;10:498-502.

Morris GC Jr, Beall AC Jr, Roof WR, DeBakey ME: Surgical experience with 220 acute arterial injuries in civilian practice. Am J Surg 1960;99:775-781.

Morris GC Jr, Creech O Jr, DeBakey ME: Acute arterial injuries in civilian practice. Am J Surg 1957;93:565-572.

Morton J, Southgate W, DeWeese JA: Arterial injuries of the extremities. Surg Gynecol Obstet 1966;123:611-627.

Morton JR, Crawford ES: Bilateral traumatic renal artery thrombosis. Ann Surg 1972;176:62-67.

Morton JR, Reul GJ, Arbegast NR, et al: Bullet embolus to the right ventricle: Report of three cases. Am J Surg 1971;122:584-590.

Moss A, Bruhn F: The echocardiogram. An ultrasound technic for the detection of pericardial effusion. N Engl J Med 1996;274:380.

Moss C, Veith F, Jason R, Rudavsky A: Screening isotope angiography in arterial trauma. Surgery 1969;86:881-889.

Motsay G, Manlove C, Perry JF: Major venous injury with pelvic fracture. J Trauma 1969;9:343-346.

Mott V: Reflections on securing in a ligature the arteria innominata. Med Surg 1918;1:9.

Moure P: Les Greffes Vasculaires. Paris, Doin, 1914.

Moya J, de Pablo C, Sanchez M, et al: Diagnosis by Doppler echocardiography. Chest 1990;98:1016-1017.

Mozingo J, Denton I: The neurologic deficit associated with sudden occlusion of the abdominal aorta due to blunt trauma. Surgery 1975;77:118-125.

Mubarak S, Owen C: Double-incision fasciotomy of the leg for decompression in compartment syndromes. J Bone Joint Surg 1977;59A:184.

Mucha PJ, Olivier HJ, Pairolero P, Farnell M: Blunt thoracic aortic injury: A reappraisal. J Trauma 1983;23:652.

Mucha PJ, Schaff H, Pairolero P: Clamp/repair of traumatic transection of descending aorta. Ann Thorac Surg 1987;43:351-352.

Mufti M, LaGuerre J, Pochaczevsky R, et al: Diagnostic value of hematoma in penetrating arterial wounds of the extremities. Arch Surg 1970;101:562-569.

Mulder D, Grollman JJ: Traumatic disruption of the thoracic aorta. Am J Surg 1969;118:311-316.

Muller WJ, Goodwin W: Renal arteriovenous fistula following nephrectomy. Ann Surg 1956;144:240-244.

Mullins R, Lucas C, Ledgerwood A: The natural history following venous ligation for civilian injuries. J Trauma 1980;20:737-743.

Munda R, Bole PV, Lande A, Clauss RH: The use of an external Dacron shunt in repair of a supraceliac abdominal aortic traumatic aneurysm. J Cardiovasc Surg 1977;18:141-146.

Murdock C: Traumatic rupture of the thoracic aorta. Arch Surg 1957;74:589-592.

Murphy J: Resection of arteries and veins injured in continuity end-to-end suture. Exp Clin Res Med Rec 1897;51:73-104.

Murphy J: Myositis; ischemic myositis; infiltration myositis; cicatricial muscular or tendon fixation in forearm; internal, external and combined compression myositis, with subsequent musculo-tendinous shortening. JAMA 1914; 63:1249-1255.

Murphy T, Dorfman G, Segall M: Iatrogenic arterial dissection: Treatment by percutaneous transluminal angioplasty. Cardiovasc Intervent Radiol 1991;14:302.

Murphy T, Piper C, Anderson CL: Complications of left heart catheterization. Am Surg 1971;37:472-475.

Murray D: Posttraumatic thrombosis of the internal carotid and vertebral arteries after non-penetrating injuries of the neck. Br J Surg 1957;44: 556.

Murray E, Minami K, Kortke H, et al: Traumatic sinus of Valsalva fistula and aortic valve rupture. Ann Thorac Surg 1993;55:760-761.

Murray G: Heparin in thrombosis and embolism. Br J Surg 1940;27:567-598.

Murray G: Surgical repair of injuries to main arteries. Am J Surg 1952;83:480.

Murray G, Brawley RK, Gott V: Reconstruction of the innominate artery by means of a temporary heparin-coated shunt bypass. J Thorac Cardiovasc Surg 1971;62:34-41.

Murray G, Janes J: Prevention of acute failure of circulation following injuries to large arteries: Experiments with glass cannulae kept patent by administration of heparin. Br Med J 1940;2:6-7.

Mustard W, Bull C: A reliable method for relief of traumatic vascular spasm. Ann Surg 1962;155:339-344.

Myers S, Reed M, Black CT, et al: Noniatrogenic pediatric vascular trauma. J Vasc Surg 1989;10:258-265.

Myers S, Harward T, Cagle L: Isolated subclavian artery dissection after blunt trauma. Surgery 1991;109:336.

Myers SI, Harward TRS, Maher DP, et al: Complex upper extremity vascular trauma in an urban population. J Vasc Surg 1990;12:305-309.

Myers W, Lawton B, Sautter R: An operation for tracheal-innominate artery fistula. Arch Surg 1972;105:269-274.

Myles R, Yellin AE: Traumatic injuries of the abdominal aorta. Am J Surg 1979;138:273-277.

Nabatoff R, Blum L, Touroff A: Long-term sequelae of common femoral vein ligation in the treatment of thromboembolic disease. Surgery 1970;67:272-276.

Nachbur B, Meyer R, Verkkala K, Zurcher R: The mechanisms of severe arterial injury in surgery of the hip joint. Clin Orthop 1979;141:122-133.

Naclerio E: Penetrating wounds of the heart: Experience with 249 patients. Dis Chest 1964;46:1-22.

Nakano J, DeSchryver C: Effects of arteriovenous fistula on systemic and pulmonary circulations. Am J Physiol 1964;207:1319.

Napoli P, Meade P, Adams CW: Primary aortoenteric fistula from a post traumatic pseudoaneurysm. J Trauma 1996;41:149-152.

Nashef S, Talwalkar N, Janieson M: Aortic arch rupture in a child following minor blunt trauma. J Thorac Cardiovasc Surg 1987;35:240-241.

Natali J, Lacombe M, Bruchou P, Vinardi G: Les traumatismes artériels vus tardivement conduite à tenir en leur présence. Presse Med 1964;72:2273.

Natali J, Maraval M, Kieffer E, Petrovic P: Fractures of a clavicle and injuries of the subclavian artery: Report of 10 cases. J Cardiovasc Surg 1975;16:541.

Natali J, Benhemori AC: Iatrogenic vascular injuries. J Cardiovasc Surg 1979;20:169-176.

Naude G, Back M, Perry MO, Bongard FS: Blunt disruption of the abdominal aorta: Report of a case and review of the literature. J Vasc Surg 1997;25:931-935.

Navarre J, Cardillo P: Vascular trauma in children and adolescents. Am J Surg 1982;143:229-231.

Neagu S: Abdomino-thoracic shooting wound with multivisceral involvement including injury of abdominal aorta in the supra-mesocolic segment. Acta Chir Belg 1993;93:107-109.

Neel S: Army aeromedical evacuation procedures in Vietnam. JAMA 1968;204:99-103.

Neely W, Hardy JD, Artz CP: Arterial injuries in civilian practice: A current reappraisal with analysis of 43 cases. J Trauma 1961;1:424-439.

Neville R, Franco C, Anderson RJ, et al: Popliteal artery agenesis: a new anatomic variant. J Vasc Surg 1990;12:573-576.

Neville R, Hobson R, Wantanabe B: A prospective evaluation of arterial intimal injuries in an experimental model. J Trauma 1991;31:669-675.

Neville R, Yasuhara H, Watanabe B: Endovascular management of arterial intimal defects: An experimental comparison by arteriography, angioscopy, and intravascular ultrasonography. J Vasc Surg 1991;13:496-502.

Nghiem D, Boland JP: Four-compartment fasciotomy of the lower extremity without fibulectomy: A new approach. Am Surg 1980;46:414-417.

Ngu V, Konstam PG: Traumatic dissecting aneurysm of the abdominal aorta. Br J Surg 1965;52:981-982.

Nguyen L, Lewin J: Angiographic demonstration of fistula between abdominal aorta and thoracic duct. JAMA 1970;211:499-500.

Nicholas G, Lane F: Traumatic superior mesenteric artery–superior mesenteric vein fistula. J Trauma 1974;14:344.

Nicholas G, DeMuth WE Jr: Long-term results of brachial thrombectomy following cardiac catheterization. Ann Surg 1976;183:436-438.

Nichols J, Svoboda J, Parks S: Use of temporary intravascular shunts in selected peripheral arterial injuries. J Trauma 1986;26:1094-1096.

Nichols J, Lillehei K: Nerve injury associated with acute vascular trauma. Surg Clin North Am 1988;68:837-852.

Nicholson J, Foster R, Heath R: Bryant's traction: A provocative cause of circulatory complication. JAMA 1955;157:415-418.

Nicoladoni C: Phlebarteriectasie der rechten oberen extremitat. Arch Klin Chir 1875;18:252.

Nizzero A, Miles J: Blunt trauma of the abdominal aorta. Can Med Assoc J 1986;135:219-220.

Nolan B, McQuillan N: A study of acute traumatic limb ischaemia. Br J Surg 1965;52:559-565.

Nolan B: Vascular injuries. J Royal Coll Surg 1968;13:72.

Nolte D, Lehr HA, Messmer K: Adenosine inhibits postischemic leukocyte-endothelium interaction in postcapillary venules of the hamster. Am J Physiol 1991;261:H651-H655.

Nolte D, Hecht R, Schmid P, et al: Role of Mac-1 and ICAM-1 in ischemia-reperfusion injury in a microcirculation model of BALB/C mice. Am J Physiol 1994;267:H295-H930.

Noon G, Boulafendis D, Beall AC Jr: Rupture of the heart secondary to blunt trauma. J Trauma 1971;11:122-128.

Nordestgaard A, Bodily KC, Osborne RJ, Buttorff J: Major vascular injuries during laparoscopic procedures. Am J Surg 1995;169:543-545.

Norotsky M, Rogers F, Shackford S: Delayed presentation of splenic artery pseudoaneurysms following blunt abdominal trauma: Case reports. J Trauma 1995;38:444-447.

Norris C, Zlotnick R, Silva W, Wheeler H: Traumatic pseudoaneurysm following blunt trauma. J Trauma 1986;28:480-482.

Norris G: Varicose aneurysm at the bend of the arm: Ligature of the artery above and below the sac; Secondary hemorrhages with a return of the aneurysm thrill on the tenth day; Cure. Am J Med Sci 1843;5:17.

North C, Ahmadi J, Segall H, Zee C: Penetrating vascular injuries of the face and neck: Clinical and angiographic correlation. AJR Am J Roentgenol 1986;147:995-999.

Norton L, Spencer FC: Long-term comparison of vein patch with direct suture. Arch Surg 1964;89:1083.

Noth P: Electrocardiographic patterns in penetrating wounds of the heart. Am Heart J 1946;32:713.

Nunley D: Radiographic diagnosis of aortic injury. Ann Thorac Surg 1984;38:424-425.

Nunley J, Koman L, Urbaniak J: Arterial shunting as an adjunct to major limb revascularization. Ann Surg 1981;193:271-273.

Nunn D: Abdominal aortic dissection following non-penetrating abdominal trauma. Am Surg 1973;39:117-179.

Nypaver T, Schuler J, McDonnell P: Long-term results of venous reconstruction after trauma in civilian practice. J Vasc Surg 1992;16:762-768.

O'Donnell V, Atik M, Pick R: Evaluation and management of penetrating wounds of the neck. Am J Surg 1979;138:309-314.

O'Donnell TJ, Brewster DC, Darling RC, et al: Arterial injuries associated with fractures and/or dislocations of the knee. J Trauma 1977;17:775-784.

O'Gorman R, Feliciano DV: Arteriography performed in the emergency center. Am J Surg 1986;152:323-325.

O'Gorman R, Feliciano DV, Bitondo CG, et al: Emergency center arteriography in the evaluation of suspected peripheral vascular injuries. Arch Surg 1984;119:568-573.

O'Neill JJ: Traumatic vascular lesions in infants and children. In Dean RH, O'Neill JJ (eds): Vascular Disorders of Childhood. Philadelphia, Lea & Febiger, 1983, pp 181-193.

O'Neill JJ, Killen DA: Autogenous vein graft for repair of acute tibial artery injury. Ann Surg 1965;162:218-220.

O'Neill MJ, Myers J, Brown G, et al: Avulsion of the innominate artery from the aortic arch associated with a posterior tracheal tear. J Trauma 1982;22:56-59.

O'Reilly M, Hood J, Livingston RH, Irwin J: Penetrating injuries of the popliteal vein: A report on 34 cases. Br J Surg 1980;67:337-340.

O'Sullivan M, Folkerth T, Morgan J, Fosburg R: Posttraumatic thoracic aortic aneurysm: Recognition and treatment. Arch Surg 1972;105:14-18.

Ochsner JL, Crawford ES, DeBakey ME: Injuries of the vena cava caused by external trauma. Surgery 1961;49:397-405.

Ochsner M, Harviel J, Stafford P, et al: Development and organization for casualty management on a 1,000-bed hospital ship in the Persian Gulf. J Trauma 1992;32:501-513.

Ochsner M, Hoffman A, DiPasquale D, et al: Associated aortic rupture-pelvic fracture: An alert for orthopaedic and general surgeons. J Trauma 1992;33:429-434.

Ochsner MJ, Champion HR, Chambers R, Harviel J: Pelvic fracture as an indicator of increased risk of thoracic rupture. J Trauma 1980;29:1376-1379.

Odekwu P, Oller D: Hematemesis as initial presentation of traumatic paraceliac pseudoaneurysm of the abdominal aorta. Cardiovasc Surg 1994;2:781-782.

Odom C: Causes of amputations of battle injuries with emphasis on vascular injuries. Surgery 1946;19:562.

Ogilvie W: War surgery in Africa. Br J Surg 1944;31:313.

Ohkawa M, Clemens M, Chaudry IH: Studies on the mechanism of beneficial effects of ATP-MgCl2 following hepatic ischemia. Am J Physiol 1983;244:R695-R702.

Ohkawa M, Chaudry IH, Clemens M, Baue AE: ATP-MgCl$_2$ produces sustained improvement in hepatic mitochondrial function and blood flow after hepatic ischemia. J Surg Res 1984;37:226-234.

Okubo S, Bernardo NL, Elliot G, et al: Tyrosine kinase signaling in action potential shortening and expression of HSP72 in late preconditioning. Physiol Heart Circ Physiol 2000;279:H2269-H2276.

Olinde A: Letters to the editors: Traumatic subclavian-axillary aneurysm. J Vasc Surg 1990;11:848-849.

Oller D, Rutledge R, Thomason M, et al: Vascular injuries in a rural state: A review of 940 patients from state trauma registry. J Trauma 1991;31:1036.

Oller D, Rutledge R, Clancey T, et al: Vascular injuries in a rural state: A review of 978 patients from a state trauma registry. J Trauma 1992;32:740-746.

Orcutt M, Levine B, Gaskill H III, Sirinek K: Iatrogenic vascular injury: A reducible problem. Arch Surg 1985;120:384-385.

Orcutt M, Levine B, Gaskill H III, Sirinek K: Civilian vascular trauma of the upper extremity. J Trauma 1986;26:63-67.

Orcutt M, Levine B, Root H, Sirinek K: The continuing challenge of popliteal vascular injuries. Am J Surg 1983;146:758-761.

Ordog G, Albin D, Wasserberger J, Balasubramanium S: Shotgun "birdshot" wounds to the neck. J Trauma 1988;28:491-497.

Orringer M, Kirsh MM: Primary repair of acute traumatic aortic disruption. Ann Thorac Surg 1983;35:672-675.

Ortner A, Berg HF, Ledbendiger A: Limb salvage through small-vessel surgery. Arch Surg 1961;83:414-421.

Osler T, Baker SP, Long W: A modification of the injury severity score that both improves accuracy and simplifies scoring. J Trauma 1997;43:922-926.

Osler W: Case of arteriovenous aneurysm of the axillary artery and vein of 14 years duration. Ann Surg 1893;17:37-40.

Osler W: Report of a case of arteriovenous aneurysm of the thigh. Johns Hopkins Hosp Bull 1905;16:119.

Osler W: An arteriovenous aneurysm of the axillary vessels of 30 years duration. Lancet 1913;2:1248.

Osler W: Remarks on arteriovenous aneurysm. Lancet 1915;1:949.

Ottolenghi C: Vascular complications in injuries about the knee joint. Clin Orthop 1982;165:148-156.

Ouchi H, Ohara I, Kijima M: Intraluminal protrusion of completely disrupted intima: An unusual form of acute arterial injury. Surgery 1965;57:220-224.

Overbeck W, Gruenagel N, Krauss H: Eisensplitterverletzung der intraprikardialen aorta. Thoraxchirurgie 1968;16:274.

Oweida S, Roubin G, Smith RI, Salam A: Postcatheterization vascular complications associated with percutaneous transluminal coronary angioplasty. J Vasc Surg 1990;12:310-315.

Owen D, Hodgson P: Control of hemorrhage following missile wound to the pelvis. J Trauma 1980;20:906-908.

Owens J: The management of arterial trauma. Surg Clin North Am 1963;43:371-385.

Owens T, Watson W, Prough D, et al: Limiting initial resuscitation of uncontrolled hemorrhage reduces internal bleeding and subsequent volume requirements. J Trauma 1995;39:200-207.

Pachter H, Spencer F, Hofsetter S: Experience with the finger fracture technique to achieve intra-hepatic hemostasis in 75 patients with severe injuries of the liver. Ann Surg 1978;197:771-777.

Pachter H, Spencer FC, Hofsetter S, et al: The management of juxtahepatic venous injuries without an atriocaval shunt: Preliminary clinical observations. Surgery 1986;99:569-575.

Padar S: Air gun pellet embolizing the intracranial internal carotid artery: Case report. J Neurosurg 1975;43:222-224.

Padberg FT, Rubelowsky J, Hernandez-Maldonado J, et al: Infrapopliteal arterial injury: Prompt revascularization affords optimal limb salvage. J Vasc Surg 1992;16:877-886.

Page C, Hagood C, Kremmerer W: Management of catheterization brachial artery thrombosis. Surgery 1982;72:619-623.

Paget S: The Surgery of the Chest. London, John Wright and Company, 1896.

Pairolero P, Walls J, Payne W, et al: Subclavian-axillary artery aneurysms. Surgery 1981;90:757-763.

Palma E, Esperon R: Vein transplants and graft in the surgical treatment of the post-phlebitic syndrome. J Cardiovasc Surg 1960;1:94-107.

Pan M, Medina A, Suarez de Lezo J: Obliteration of femoral pseudoaneurysm complicating coronary intervention by direct puncture and permanent or removable coil insertion. Am J Cardiol 1997;80:786-788.

Panes J, Kurose I, Rodriguez-Vaca D, et al: Diabetes exacerbates inflammatory responses to ischemia-reperfusion. Circulation 1996;93:161-167.

Panetta T, Sclafani S, Goldstein A, et al: Percutaneous transcatheter embolization for massive bleeding from pelvic fractures. J Trauma 1985;25:1021-1029.

Panetta T, Bottiurai VS, Batson RC: Nonreversed translocated saphenous vein bypass for arterial trauma. J Trauma 1988;28:1065-1070.

Panetta T, Hunt J, Buechter K: A blind, randomized canine study of duplex scanning and arteriography for the diagnosis of arterial injury. J Trauma 9999.

Panetta TF, Hunt JP, Buechter KJ, et al: Duplex ultrasonography versus arteriography in the diagnosis of arterial injury: An experimental study. J Trauma 1992;33:627-636.

Panetta T, Hunt J, Buechter K, et al: Duplex ultrasonography versus arteriography in the diagnosis of arterial injury: An experimental study. J Trauma 1992;33:627-636.

Pappas P, Haser P, Teehan E, et al: Outcome of Complex Venous Reconstructions in Trauma Patients: Proceedings of the Eight American Venous Forum, 1996 February 23-25: San Diego. San Diego, American Venous Forum, 1996.

Parkinson D, West M: Traumatic intracranial aneurysms. J Neurosurg 1980;52:11-20.

Parks T: Surgical management of gunshot injures of the large intestine. J R Soc Med 1979;72:412-416.

Parmley L, Mattingly T, Manion W, Jahnke EJ Jr: Non-penetrating traumatic injury of the aorta. Circulation 1958;17:1086-1101.

Parmley L, Mattingly T, Manion W: Penetrating wounds of the heart and aorta. Circulation 1958;17:953-973.

Parmley LJ, Orbison J, Hughes CW, Mattingly T: Acquired arteriovenous fistulas complicated by endarteritis and endocarditis lenta due to streptococcus faecalis. N Engl J Med 1954;250:305-309.

Parodi J: Endovascular repair of abdominal aortic aneurysms and other arterial lesions. J Vasc Surg 1995;21:556-557.

Parodi J: Endovascular repair of aortic aneurysms, arteriovenous fistulas, and false aneurysms. World J Surg 1996;20:655-663.

Partap V, Cassoff J: Ultrasound-guided percutaneous thrombin injection for treatment of femoral pseudoaneurysms: Technical note. Can Assoc Radiol J 1999;50:182-184.

Pasch AR, Bishara RA, Lim LT, et al: Optimal limb salvage in penetrating civilian vascular trauma. J Vasc Surg 1986;3:189-195.

Pasch AR, Rashad A, Bishara RA, et al: Results of venous reconstruction after civilian vascular trauma. Arch Surg 1986;121:607-611.

Passaro EJ, Pace W: Traumatic rupture of the aorta. Surgery 1959;46:787-791.

Pate J: Traumatic rupture of the aorta: Emergency operation. Ann Thorac Surg 1985;39:531-537.

Pate J, Butterick O, Richardson R: Traumatic rupture of the thoracic aorta. JAMA 1968;203:1022-1024.

Pate J, Cole F, Walker W, Fabian TC: Penetrating injuries of the aorta arch and its branches. Ann Thorac Surg 1993;55:586-592.

Pate J, Fabian TC, Walker W: Acute traumatic rupture of the aortic isthmus: Repair with cardiopulmonary bypass. Ann Thorac Surg 1995;59:90-99.

Pate J, Fabian TC, Walker W: Traumatic rupture of the aortic isthmus: An emergency? World J Surg 1995;19:119-125.

Pate J, Richardson RJ: Penetrating wounds of cardiac valves. JAMA 1969;207:309-311.

Pate J, Sherman R, Jackson T, Wilson H: Cardiac failure following traumatic arteriovenous fistula: A report of 14 cases. J Trauma 1965;5:398-403.

Pate J, Wilson H: Arterial injuries of the base of the neck. Arch Surg 1964;89:1106-1110.

Patel A, Marin M, Veith F, et al: Endovascular graft repair of penetrating subclavian artery injuries. J Endovasc Surg 1996;3:383-388.

Patel K, Kulkarni S, Babu S, Clauss RH: Abdominal vascular trauma. Dis Chest 1987;30:13-23.

Patel K, Cortes LE, Semel L, et al: Bullet embolism. J Cardiovasc Surg 1989;30:584-590.

Patel N, Mann F, Jurkovich GJ: Penetrating ulcer of the descending aorta mimicking a traumatic aortic laceration. AJR Am J Roentgenol 1996;166:20.

Pathria M, Zlatkin M, Sartoris D, et al: Ultrasonography of the popliteal fossa and lower extremities. Radiol Clin North Am 1988;26:77-85.

Patman R, Poulos E, Shires G: The management of civilian arterial injuries. Surg Gynecol Obstet 1964;118:725-738.

Patman R, Thompson J: Fasciotomy in peripheral vascular surgery: Report of 164 patients. Arch Surg 1970;101:633-672.

Patman R: Indications and technique. In Rutherford R (ed): Vascular Surgery. Philadelphia, WB Saunders, 1984.

Paton B, Elliot D, Taubman J, Owens J: Acute treatment of traumatic aortic rupture. J Trauma 1971;11:1-14.

Patt A, McCroskey B, Moore EE: Hypothermia-induced coagulopathies in trauma. Surg Clin North Am 1988;64:775-785.

Patterson F, Morton K: The cause of death on fractures of the pelvis: With a note on treatment by ligation of the hypogastric (internal iliac) artery. J Trauma 1973;13:849-856.

Patterson R, Burns W, Jannotta F: Rupture of the thoracic aorta: Complication of resuscitation. JAMA 1973;226:197.

Patton A, Guyton S, Lawson D: Treatment of severe arterial injuries. Am J Surg 1981;141:465-471.

Payne S, Snell M: Traumatic renal artery dissection. Urology 1988;16:335-337.

Peacock J, Proctor HJ: Factors limiting extremity function following vascular injury. J Trauma 1977;17:532-534.

Pearlman A: Transesophageal echocardiography: Sound diagnostic technique or two edged sword? N Engl J Med 1991;324:841-843.

Peck C: The operative treatment of heart wounds. Ann Surg 1909;50:100-134.

Peck J, Eastmen A, Bergan JJ, Sedwitz M: Popliteal vascular trauma: A community experience. Arch Surg 1990;120:1339-1344.

Pecunia R, Raves J: A technique for evaluation of the injured extremity with a single film exclusion arteriography. Surg Gynecol Obstet 1990;170:448.

Peiper H: Significance of traumatology in abdominal and vascular surgery. Jpn J Surg 1985;15:93-102.

Pemberton J, Seefeld P, Barker NW: Traumatic arteriovenous fistula involving the abdominal aorta and the inferior vena cava. Ann Surg 1946;123:580-586.

Penn I: The vascular complications of fractures of the clavicle. J Trauma 1964;4:819-831.

Pennington D, Dranpanas T: Acute post-traumatic coarctation of the abdominal aorta. Surgery 1975;78:538-542.

Pepe PE, Bass RR, Mattox KL: Clinical trail of the pneumatic antishock garment in the urban prehospital setting. Ann Emerg Med 1986;15:1407-1410.

Perchinsky M, Long WB, Hill J, et al: Extracorporeal cardiopulmonary life support with heparin-bonded circuitry in the resuscitation of massively injured trauma patients. Am J Surg 1995;169:488-491.

Perdue GJ, Smith RI: Intra-abdominal vascular injury. Surgery 1968;64:562-568.

Perkins R, Elchos T: Stab wound of the aortic arch. Ann Surg 1958;147:83-86.

Perler B, McCabe C, Abbott WM, Buckley MJ: Vascular complications of intra-aortic balloon counterpulsation. Arch Surg 1983;118:957-9562.

Perry MO: The Management of Acute Vascular Injuries. Baltimore, Williams & Wilkins, 1981.

Perry M: Metabolic consequences of vascular trauma. Contemp Surg 1981;18:39-46.

Perry MO: Iatrogenic injuries of arteries in infants. Surg Gynecol Obstet 1983;157:415-418.

Perry MO: Compartment syndromes and reperfusion injury. Surg Clin North Am 1988;68:853-864.

Perry MO, Synder W, Thal E: Carotid artery injuries caused by blunt trauma. Ann Surg 1980;192:74-77.

Perry MO, Thal E, Shires G: Management of arterial injuries. Ann Surg 1971;173:403-408.

Peterson A, Williams D, Rodriguez J, Francis I: Percutaneous treatment of a traumatic aortic dissection by balloon fenestration and stent placement. AJR Am J Roentgenol 1996;164:1274-1276.

Peterson H, Greenspan J, Ory H: Death following puncture of the aorta during laparoscopic sterilization. Obstet Gynecol 1982;59:133-134.

Peterson N: Traumatic bilateral renal infraction. J Trauma 1989;29:158-161.

Petit-Dutaillis D, Janet H, Thiébaut F, Guillaumat L: Effets d'une inversion circulatoire par anastomose carotido-jugulaire sure une hémiplégie droit avec aphasie due à una thrombose de la carotide interne d'Origine inconnue chez un adolescent de 13 ans. Rev Neurol 1949;81:75.

Petrovsky B, Milinov O: "Arterialization" and "venization" of vessels involved in traumatic arteriovenous fistulae: Aetiology and pathogenesis (an experimental study). J Cardiovasc Surg 1967;8:396-407.

Petty S, Parker L, Mauro M, et al: Chronic posttraumatic aortic pseudoaneurysm: Recognition before rupture. Postgrad Med 1991;89:177-178.

Pezzella A, Todd E, Dillon M, et al: Early diagnosis and individualized treatment of blunt thoracic aortic trauma. Am Surg 1978;44:699-703.

Pezzella A, Griffen W, Ernst CB: Superior mesenteric artery injury following blunt abdominal trauma: Case report with successful primary repair. J Trauma 1978;18:472-474.

Phifer T, Gerlock A, Vekovius W, et al: Amputation risk factors in concomitant superficial femoral artery and vein injuries. Ann Surg 1984;199:241-243.

Phifer T, Gerlock A, Rich NM, McDonald J: Long-term patency of venous repairs demonstrated by venography. J Trauma 1985;25:342-346.

Phillips C, Jacobsen D, Brayton DF, Bloch JH: Central vessel trauma. Am Surg 1979;45:517-530.

Phillips E, Rogers W, Gaspar MR: First rib fractures: Incidence of vascular injury and indications for angiography. Surgery 1981;89:42-47.

Pick T: On partial rupture of arteries from external violence. St George's Hosp Rep (Lond) 1873;6:161.

Pick T: A clinical lecture of a case of arteriovenous aneurysm. Lond Med Times Gaz 1883;2:677.

Pickard L, Mattox KL, Espada R, et al: Transection of the descending thoracic aorta secondary to blunt trauma. J Trauma 1977;17:749-754.

Pickelmann S, Nolte D, Leiderer R, et al: Attenuation of postischemic reperfusion injury in striated skin muscle by diaspirin-cross-linked Hb. Am J Physiol 1998;275:H361-H368.

Pietri P, Alagni G, Settembrini P: Iatrogenic vascular lesions. Int Surg 1981;66:213-216.

Pikoulis E, Rhee P, Nishibe T, et al: Arterial repair with synthetic patch by using titanium clips. J Trauma 2000;48:292-295.

Pisters P, Heslin M, Riles T: Abdominal aortic pseudoaneurysm after blunt trauma. J Vasc Surg 1993;18:307-309.

Pitner S: Carotid thrombosis due to intraoral trauma: An unusual complication of a common childhood accident. N Engl J Med 1966;274:764-767.

Piwnica A, Chetochine F, Soyer R, Winckler C: Traumatic rupture of the aortic arch with disinsertion of the innominate artery. J Thorac Cardiovasc Surg 1971;61:246-252.

Plume S, DeWeese JA: Traumatic rupture of the thoracic aorta. Arch Surg 1979;114:240-243.

Plummer D, Bunette D, Asinger R, Ruiz E: Emergency department echocardiography improves outcome in penetrating cardiac injury. Ann Emerg Med 1992;21:709-712.

Pochaczevsky R, Mufti M, LaGuerre J: Arteriography of penetrating wound of the extremities: Help or hindrance? J Canad Assoc Radiol 1973;24:354-361.

Pomerantz M, Hutchison D: Traumatic wounds of the heart. J Trauma 1969;9:135-139.

Pontius G, Kilbourne B, Paul E: Non-penetrating abdominal trauma. Arch Surg 1957;72:800.

Pool E: Treatment of heart wounds. Ann Surg 1912;55:485-512.

Poole G: Fracture of the upper ribs and injury to the great vessels. Surg Gynecol Obstet 1989;169:275-282.

Pope M, Johnston K: Anaphylaxis after thrombin injection of a femoral pseudoaneurysm: Recommendations for prevention. J Vasc Surg 2000;32:190-191.

Porter W, Bigger IA: Stab wounds of the heart and great vessels: A study of seventeen cases. Trans Am Clin Climatol Asoc 1939;54:96-104.

Posner M, Moore EE, Greenholz S, et al: Natural history of untreated inferior vena cava injury and assessment of venous access. J Trauma 1986;26:698-701.

Postempski P: La sutura dei vasi sanguigni. Arch Soc Ital Chir Roma 1886;3:391.

Potts R, Alguire PC: Pseudoaneurysm of the abdominal aorta: A case report and review of the literature. Am J Med Sci 1991;301:265-268.

Pouyanne H, Arne L, Loiseau P, Mouton L: Considerations sur deux cas de thrombose de la carotide interne chez l'enfant. Rev Neurol 1957;97:525.

Power D-A: Hunter's operation for the cure of aneurysm. Br J Surg 1929;17:193.

Pradham D, Juanteguy J, Wilder R: Arterial injuries of extremities associated with fractures. Arch Surg 1972;105:582-585.

Prat A, Warembourg HJ, Watel A, et al: Chronic traumatic aneurysm of the descending thoracic aorta (19 cases). J Cardiovasc Surg 1986;27:268-272.

Pratt G: Importance of a knowledge of vascular surgery in World War II. Am J Surg 1942;56:335.

Prean G, Aragon GE: Arterial embolism from a bullet: A case report. Am Surg 1976;42:863-865.

Preston A: Arterial injuries of warfare: Complications and management. Surgery 1946;20:786.

Pretre R, Kursteiner K, Khatchatourian G, Faidutti B: Traumatic occlusion of the left anterior descending artery and rupture of the aortic isthmus. J Trauma 1995;39:388-390.

Pretre R, LaHarpe R, Cheretakis A: Blunt injury to the ascending aorta: Three patterns of presentation. Surgery 1996;119:603-610.

Pridgen W, Jacobs J: Postoperative arteriovenous fistula. Surgery 1962;51:205.

Pritchard D, Maloney J, Barnhorst DA, Spittel JJ: Traumatic popliteal arteriovenous fistulas. Arch Surg 1977;112:849-852.

Proudfoot R, Harris M, Victor D, Bennett S: Arterial bullet embolism. J Ky Med Assoc 1989;87:17-18.

Puckett W: The wounding effect of small high velocity fragments as revealed by high speed radiography. J Elisha Mitchell Sci Soc 1946;62:59.

Puijlaert C: Roentgen diagnosis of traumatic rupture of the aorta. Radiol Clin North Am 1976;45:217-235.

Puri R, Clark J, Corkey P: Axillary artery damage following a closed fracture of the neck of the humerus: A case report. Injury 1985;16:426-427.

Qinyao W, Weijin S, Youren Z: New concepts in severe presacral hemorrhage during proctectomy. Arch Surg 1982;19:1013-1020.

Quast D, Shirkey AL, Fitzgerald J, et al: Surgical correction of injuries to the vena cava: An analysis of sixty-one cases. J Trauma 1965;5:1-10.

Queral L, Flinn W, Yao JST, Bergan JJ: Management of peripheral arterial aneurysms. Surg Clin North Am 1979;59:693-706.

Quigley M, Bret PM: Occult pseudoaneurysm of the abdominal aorta following gunshot wound: The importance of plain film findings. J Trauma 1995;38:269-273.

Rabhan N, Guillebeau J, Brackney EL: Arteriovenous fistula of the superior mesenteric vessels after a gunshot wound. N Engl J Med 1962;266:603.

Rabinowitz R, Goldfarb D: Surgical treatment of axillosubclavian venous thrombosis: A case report. Surgery 1971;70:703.

Rabinsky I, Sidhu G, Wagner R: Mid-descending aortic traumatic aneurysms. Ann Thorac Surg 1990;50:155-160.

Raffa H, Sorefan A: Repair of torn aortic root with the left atrial appendage. Jpn Heart J 1992;33:265-269.

Rahat M, Lahat N, Smollar J, et al: Divergent effects of ischemia/reperfusion and nitric oxide donor on TNF-alpha mRNA accumulation in rat organs. Shock 2001;15:312-317.

Ramakantan R, Shah P: False aneurysm secondary to aortic cannulation: Rupture into lung with fatal hemoptysis during aortography. J Thorac Cardiovasc Surg 1989;37:322-323.

Ramanathan T, Somasundaram K, Yong N: Successful repair of penetrating wound of the thoracic aorta. Thorax 1975;30:348-351.

Rana M, Singh G, Wang P, et al: Protective effects of preheparinization on the microvasculature during and after hemorrhagic shock. J Trauma 1992;32:420-426.

Randhawa MJ, Menzoian J: Seat belt aorta. Ann Vasc Surg 1990;4:370-377.

Ransdell H, Glass HJ: Gunshot wounds of the heart: A review of 20 cases. Am J Surg 1960;999:788-797.

Ranshoff J: Arteriovenous aneurysm of the superior thyroid artery and vein. Surg Gynecol Obstet 1935;61:816.

Rapoport S, Sniderman U, Morse S, et al: Pseudoaneurysm: A complication of faulty technique in femoral artery puncture. Radiology 1985;154:529-530.

Rau S, Carner D: Brachial plexus compression. Arch Surg 1981;116:175-178.

Rautio J, Paavolainen P: Afghan war wounded: Experience with 200 cases. J Trauma 1988;28:523.

Ravikumar S, Stahl WM: Intraluminal balloon catheter occlusion for major vena cava injuries. J Trauma 1985;25:458-460.

Razek M, Mnaymneh W, Yacoubian HD: Injuries of peripheral arteries with associated bone and soft tissue injuries. J Trauma 1973;13:907.

Razzouk A, Gundry S, Wang N, et al: Pseudoaneurysms of the aorta after cardiac surgery or chest trauma. Am Surg 1993;59:818-823.

Rea W, Sugg W, Wilson L, et al: Coronary artery lacerations: An analysis of 22 patients. Ann Thorac Surg 1969;7:518-528.

Read R, Moore EE, Moore FA, et al: Intravascular ultrasound for the diagnosis of traumatic aortic disruption: A case report. Surgery 1993;114:624-628.

Read R, Moore EE, Moore FA, Haenel J: Partial left heart bypass for thoracic aorta repair. Arch Surg 1993;128:746-752.

Reckling F, Peltier L: Acute knee dislocations and their complications. J Trauma 1969;9:181-191.

Redman H: Thoracic, abdominal, and peripheral trauma: Evaluation with angiography. JAMA 1977;237:2415-2418.

Reed J, McGinn R, Gorman JF: Traumatic mesenteric arteriovenous fistula presenting as the superior mesenteric artery syndrome. Arch Surg 1986;121:1209.

Rees R, Bonneval M, Batson R, Hollier L: Angiography in extremity trauma: A prospective study. Am Surg 1978;44:661-663.

Rehn L: Ueber penetrirende herzwunden und hernalt. Arch Klin Chir 1897;55:56-60.

Rehr R, Mack M, Firth B: Aortic regurgitation and sinus of Valsalva-right atrial fistula after blunt thoracic trauma. Br Heart J 1982;48:410-412.

Reichle F, Golsorkhi M: Diagnosis and management of penetrating arterial and venous injuries in the extremities. Am J Surg 1980;140:365-367.

Reid C, Kawanishi D, Rahimtoola SH, Chandraratna P: Chest trauma: Evaluation by two-dimensional echocardiography. Am Heart J 1987;113:971-976.

Reid J, Redman H, Weigelt JA, et al: Wounds of the extremities in proximity to major arteries: Value of angiography in the detection of arterial injury. AJR 1988;151:1053-1059.

Reid J, Weigelt JA: Forty-three cases of vertebral trauma. J Trauma 1988;28:1007-1012.

Reid J, Weigelt JA, Thal E, Francis H III: Assessment of proximity of a wound to major vascular structures as an indication for arteriography. Arch Surg 1988;123:942-946.

Reid M: The effect of arteriovenous fistula upon the heart and blood vessels: An experiment and clinical study. Bull Johns Hopkins Hosp 1920;31:43-50.

Reid M: Abnormal arteriovenous communications. Acquired and congenital, II. The origin and nature of arteriovenous aneurysms, cirsoid aneurysms and simple angiomas. Arch Surg (Chicago) 1925;10:996-1009.

Reid M, McGuire J: Arteriovenous aneurysm. Ann Surg 1938;108:643-693.

Reiley M, Bond D, Branick RI, Wilson E: Vascular complications following total hip arthroplasty: A review of the literature and a report of two cases. Clin Orthop 1984;186:23-28.

Reilly PM, Rotondo MF, Carpenter JP, et al: Temporary vascular continuity during damage control: Intraluminal shunting for proximal superior mesenteric artery injury. J Trauma 1996;39:757-760.

Reilly L, Ramos T, Murray S, et al: Optimal exposure of the proximal abdominal aorta: A critical appraisal of transabdominal medial visceral rotation. J Vasc Surg 1994;19:375-389.

Reines HD, Dill L, Saad S: Neurogenic pulmonary edema and missile emboli. J Trauma 1980;20:698-701.

Reisman J, Morgan A: Analysis of 46 intra-abdominal aortic injuries from blunt trauma: Case reports and literature review. J Trauma 1990;30:1294-1297.

Reissman P, Rivkind A, Jurim O, Simon D: Case report: The management of penetrating cardiac trauma with major coronary artery injury—Is cardiopulmonary bypass essential? J Trauma 1992;33:773-775.

Requena R, Cherukuri R, Lerner R: A logical approach in the management of intraabdominal vascular trauma. Contemp Surg 1983;23:31.

Reul GJ, Beall AC Jr, Jordan GL Jr, Mattox KL: The early operative management of injuries to the great vessels. Surgery 1973;74:862-873.

Reul GJ, Mattox KL, Beall AC Jr, Jordan GL Jr: Recent advances in the operative management of massive chest trauma. Ann Thorac Surg 1973;16:521-662.

Reul GJ, Rubio P, Beall AC Jr: The surgical management of acute injury to the thoracic aorta. J Thorac Cardiovasc Surg 1974;67:272-281.

Reyes L, Rubio P, Korompai F, Guinn G: Successful treatment of transection of aortic arch and innominate artery. Ann Thorac Surg 1975;19:468-471.

Reynolds B, Balsano NA: Venography in pelvic fractures: A clinical evaluation. Ann Surg 1971;173:104-106.

Reynolds R, McDowell H, Diethelm A: The surgical treatment of blunt and penetrating injuries of the popliteal artery. Am Surg 1983;49:405-410.

Reynolds R, McDowell H, Diethelm A: The surgical treatment of arterial injuries in the civilian population. Am Surg 1979;189:700-708.

Rhee PM, Acosta J, Bridgeman A, et al: Survival after emergency department thoracotomy: Review of published data from the past 25 years. J Am Coll Surg 2000;190:288-298.

Rhee P, Talon E, Eifert S, et al: Induced hypothermia during emergency department thoracotomy: An animal model. J Trauma 2000;48:439-447.

Rhodes G, Cox C, Silver D: Arteriovenous fistula and false aneurysm as the cause of consumption coagulopathy. Surgery 1973;73:535-540.

Riccen E, Dickens P: Traumatic aneurysm of the abdominal aorta of 27 years duration: Case report. US Nav Med Bull 1942;40:692-694.

Rice W, Wittstruck K: Acute hypertension and delayed traumatic rupture of the aorta. JAMA 1951;147:915-917.

Rich NM: Vietnam missile wounds evaluated in 750 patients. Milit Med 1968;133:9-22.

Rich NM: Wounding power of various ammunition. Resident Physician 1968;14:72.

Rich NM: Missile wound evaluation at the 2nd Surgical Hospital in Vietnam. In Georjiade N (ed): Plastic and Maxillofacial Trauma Symposium. St. Louis, CV Mosby, 1969.

Rich NM: Vascular trauma in Vietnam. J Cardiovasc Surg 1970;11:368-377.

Rich NM: Surgery for arterial trauma. In Dale WA (ed): Management of Arterial Occlusive Disease. Chicago, Year Book Medical Publishers, 1971.

Rich NM: Complications of operations for vascular trauma. In Beebe HG (ed): Complications in Vascular Surgery. Philadelphia, JB Lippincott Co, 1973.

Rich NM: Vascular trauma. Surg Clin North Am 1973;53:1367-1392.

Rich NM: Vascular injuries. In Whelan TJ (ed): Emergency War Surgery: NATO Handbook. Washington, DC, Government Printing Office, 1975.

Rich NM: Weapons and wounds. J Trauma 1975;15:464-465.

Rich NM: Bullets and blood vessels. Surg Clin North Am 1978;58:995-1003.

Rich NM: Principles and indications for primary venous repair. Surgery 1982;91:492-496.

Rich NM: Vascular injuries. In Cameron J (ed): Current Surgical Therapy. Philadelphia, BC Decker, 1984.

Rich NM: The management of trauma to the carotid-vertebral system. In Robicsek F (ed): Extracranial Cerebrovascular Disease Diagnosis and Management. New York, Macmillan Publishing, 1986.

Rich NM: Venous injuries. In Sabiston DJ (ed): Textbook of Surgery. Philadelphia, WB Saunders, 1986, pp 2009-2018.

Rich NM: Arterial injuries associated with fracture, dislocation, and extensive soft tissue trauma. In Ernst CB, Stanley JC (eds): Current Therapy in Vascular Surgery. Philadelphia, BC Decker, 1987.

Rich NM: Management of venous trauma. Surg Clin North Am 1988;68:809-821.

Rich NM: Gunshot wound to the groin. In Brewster DC (ed): Common Problems in Vascular Surgery. Chicago, Year Book Medical Publishers, 1989, pp 305-308.

Rich NM: Mechanism and reversibility of proximal arterial dilatation with large arteriovenous fistulas. In Veith F (ed): Current Critical Problems in Vascular Surgery. St. Louis, Quality Medical Publishing, 1989.

Rich NM: Current status of lower extremity venous repair. In Veith F (ed): Current Critical Problems in Vascular Surgery. St. Louis, Quality Medical Publishing, 1990.

Rich NM: Trauma: Responsibility, resources, and responsiveness (Scudder Oration). ACS Bull 1990;76:6-13.

Rich NM: Brief history of vascular trauma. Trauma Q 1991;7:1-5.

Rich NM: Vascular trauma: A brief military perspective. World J Surg 1992;16:938-939.

Rich NM: History of vascular trauma. In Flanigan DP, Schuler J, Meyer JP (eds): Civilian Vascular Trauma. Philadelphia, Lea & Febiger, 1992, pp 3-7.

Rich NM: Military vascular injuries in Croatia. Cardiovasc Surg 1993;1:2.

Rich NM: Surgeon's response to battlefield vascular trauma (Hume Memorial Lecture). Am J Surg 1993;166:91-96.

Rich NM: Venous injuries. In Sabiston DJ (ed): Textbook of Surgery. Philadelphia, WB Saunders, 1995.

Rich NM: Commentary. In Ivatury RR, Cayten C (eds): The Textbook of Penetrating Trauma. Philadelphia, Williams & Wilkins, 1996.

Rich NM, Amato JJ, Billy LJ: Arterial thrombosis secondary to temporary cavitation. Surg Dig 1971;6:12.

Rich NM, Andersen CA, Ricotta J, et al: Arterial trauma: A remaining problem of increasing magnitude. Milit Med 1977;141:847-852.

Rich NM, Baugh JH, Hughes CW: Popliteal artery injuries in Vietnam. Am J Surg 1969;118:531-534.

Rich NM, Baugh JH, Hughes CW: Acute arterial injuries in Vietnam: 1,000 cases. J Trauma 1970;10:359-369.

Rich NM, Baugh JH, Hughes CW: Significance of complications associated with vascular repairs performed in Vietnam. Arch Surg 1970;100:646-651.

Rich NM, Clagett GP, Salander J, Piscevic S: The Matas/Soubbotitch connection. Surgery 1983;93:17-19.

Rich NM, Clarke J, Baugh JH: Successful repair of a traumatic aneurysm of the abdominal aorta. Surgery 1969;66:492-496.

Rich NM, Collins GJ Jr, Andersen CA, et al: Venous trauma: Successful venous reconstruction remains an interesting challenge. Am J Surg 1977;134:226-230.

Rich NM, Collins GJ Jr, Andersen CA, et al: Missile emboli. J Trauma 1978;18:236-239.

Rich NM, Collins GJ, Andersen CA, McDonald P: Autogenous venous interposition grafts in repair of major venous injuries. J Trauma 1977;17:512-520.

Rich NM, Collins GJ Jr, Hobson RW II, et al: Carotid-axillary bypass: Clinical and experimental evaluation. Am J Surg 1977;134:805-808.

Rich NM, Collins GJ Jr, Youkey JR: Cervical and Thoracic Outlet Venous Injuries. Surgery of the Veins. New York, Grune & Stratton, 1985.

Rich NM, Gomez ER, Coffey JA, et al: Long-term follow-up of venous reconstruction following trauma. In Bergan JJ, Yao JST (eds): Venous Disorders. Philadelphia, WB Saunders, 1991.

Rich NM, Gomez ER, Jackson MR: Pulsating hematomas and pseudoaneurysms: Should they be managed by noninvasive compression under duplex control? In Veith F (ed): Current Critical Problems in Vascular Surgery. St. Louis, Quality Medical Publishing, 1994, pp 319-323.

Rich NM, Hobson RW II: Historical background of repair venous injuries. In Witkin E (ed): Venous Diseases, Medical and Surgical Management. Hague, the Netherlands, Mouton, 1974.

Rich NM, Hobson RW II: Trauma to the venous system. In Swan KG, Hobson RW II, Reynolds D, et al (eds): Symposium on Venous Surgery in the Lower Extremities. St. Louis, Green Publishers, 1975.

Rich NM, Hobson RW II: Venous trauma: Emphasis for repair is indicated. J Cardiovasc Surg 1975; special issue:571.

Rich NM, Hobson RW II, Collins GJ Jr: Traumatic arteriovenous fistulas and false aneurysms: A review of 558 lesions. Surgery 1975;78:817-828.

Rich NM, Hobson RW II, Collins GJ Jr: Elective vascular reconstruction after trauma. Am J Surg 1975;130:712-719.

Rich NM, Hobson RW II, Collins GJ Jr, Anderson CA: The effect of acute popliteal venous interruption. Ann Surg 1976;183:365-368.

Rich NM, Hobson RW II, Fedde C: Vascular trauma secondary to diagnostic and therapeutic procedures. Am J Surg 1974;128:715-721.

Rich NM, Hobson RW II, Fedde C, Collins GJ Jr: Acute common femoral arterial trauma. J Trauma 1975;15:628-637.

Rich NM, Hobson R II, Hutton JE Jr: Arterial trauma: Lessons of the Vietnam war. Paper presented at: Annual International Vascular Meeting, Paris, France, 1995.

Rich NM, Hobson RW II, Hutton JE Jr: Traumatismes artériels: les lecons de la guerre du Vietnam. In Kieffer E (ed): Traumatismes Artériels. Paris, AERCV, 1995.

Rich NM, Hobson RW II, Jarstfer B, Geer TM: Subclavian artery trauma. J Trauma 1973;13:485-496.

Rich NM, Hobson RW II, Wright CB: Historical aspects of direct venous reconstruction. In Bergan JJ, Yao JST (eds): Symposium on Venous Problems in Honor of Geza de Takats. Chicago: Year Book Medical Publishers, 1978.

Rich NM, Hobson RW II, Wright CB, Fedde C: Repair of lower extremity venous trauma: A more aggressive approach required. J Trauma 1974;14:639-652.

Rich NM, Hobson RW II, Wright CB, Swan KG: Techniques of venous repair. In Swan KG, Hobson RW II, Reynolds D, et al (eds): Symposium on Venous Surgery in the Lower Extremities. St. Louis, Warren H Green Publishers, 1975.

Rich NM, Hughes CW: Vietnam Vascular Registry: A preliminary report. Surgery 1969;65:218-226.

Rich NM, Hughes CW: Stistiques sur les plaies vasculaires au Vietnam (4500 Cas). Social Med Chir 1970;9:805-809.

Rich NM, Hughes CW: Rapport sur les plais vasculaires au Vietnam (Translation, D. Rignault). Revue des corps de Sante 1971;12:673.

Rich NM, Hughes CW: Fifty years' progress in vascular surgery. Bull Am Coll Surg 1972;57:35.

Rich NM, Hughes CW: The fate of prosthetic material used to repair vascular injuries in contaminated wounds. J Trauma 1972;12:459-467.

Rich NM, Hughes CW, Baugh JH: Management of venous injuries. Ann Surg 1970;171:724-730.

Rich NM, Jarstfer B, Geer TM: Popliteal artery repair failure: Causes and possible prevention. J Cardiovasc Surg 1974;15:340-351.

Rich NM, Jarstfer B, Geer TM: Concomitant popliteal arterial and venous trauma. In Swan KG, Hobson RW II, Reynolds D, et al (eds): Symposium on venous surgery in the lower extremities. St. Louis, Warren H Green Publishers, 1975, pp 29-40.

Rich NM, Johnson E, Dimond F Jr: Wounding power of missiles used in the Republic of Vietnam. JAMA 1967;199:157.

Rich NM, Levin P, Hutton JE Jr: Effect of distal arteriovenous fistulas on venous graft patency. In Swan KG, Hobson RW II, Reynolds D, et al (eds): Symposium on Venous Surgery in the Lower Extremities. St. Louis, Warren H Green Publishers, 1975.

Rich NM, Manion W, Hughes CW: Surgical and pathological evaluation of vascular injuries in Vietnam. J Trauma 1969;9:279-291.

Rich NM, Metz CJ, Hutton JE Jr, et al: Internal versus external fixation of fractures with concomitant vascular injuries in Vietnam. J Trauma 1971;11:463-473.

Rich NM, Rhee P: An historical tour of vascular injury management: From its inception to the new millennium. Surg Clin North Am 2001;81:1199-1215.

Rich NM, Rob CG: Ischemia-induced myonecrosis, myoglobinuria and secondary renal failure. In Ernst CB, Stanley JC (eds): Current Therapy in Vascular Surgery. Philadelphia, BC Decker, 1990.

Rich NM, Salander J, Orecchia P, et al: Venous injuries. In Bergan JJ, Yao JST (eds): Vascular Surgical Emergencies. Orlando, Grune & Stratton, 1987, pp 275-282.

Rich NM, Shumacker HB Jr: Cold injury. In Ernst CB, Stanley JC (eds): Current Therapy in Vascular Surgery. Philadelphia, BC Decker, 1990.

Rich NM, Spencer FC: Vascular Trauma. Philadelphia, WB Saunders, 1978.

Rich NM, Sullivan W: Clinical recanalization of an autogenous vein graft in the popliteal vein. J Trauma 1972;12:919-920.

Richards AJ, Lamis PJ, Rogers JJ, Bradham GB: Laceration of abdominal aorta and study of intact abdominal wall as tamponade: Report of survival and literature review. Ann Surg 1966;164:321-324.

Richardson D, Shina M, Miller F, Bergamini TM: Peripheral vascular complications of coronary angioplasty. Am Surg 1989;55:675-680.

Richardson JD: Indications for thoracotomy in thoracic trauma. Curr Surg 1985;42:361-364.

Richardson JD, Fallat M, Nagaraj H, et al: Arterial injuries in children. Arch Surg 1981;116:685-690.

Richardson JD, Simpson C, Miller F: Management of carotid artery trauma. Surgery 1988;104:673-680.

Richardson JD, Vitale G, Flint LM: Penetrating arterial trauma: Analysis of missed vascular injuries. Arch Surg 1987;122:678-683.

Richardson JJ, Jurkovich GJ, Walker G, et al: A temporary arteriovenous shunt in the management of traumatic venous injuries of the lower extremity (Scribner). J Trauma 1986;26:503-509.

Richardson R, Khandeadar A, Moseley P: Traumatic rupture of the thoracic aorta. South Med J 1979;72:300-302.

Ricketts R, Finck E, Yellin AE: Management of major arteriovenous fistulas by arteriographic techniques. Arch Surg 1978;113:1153.

Ricks R, Howell J, Beall AC Jr, DeBakey ME: Gunshot wounds of the heart: A review of 31 cases. Surgery 1965;57:787-790.

Rielly J, Brandt ML, Mattox KL, Pokorny W: Thoracic trauma in children. J Trauma 1993;34:329-331.

Risely T, McClerkin W: Bullet transection of both carotid arteries: Delayed repair with recovery. Am J Surg 1971;121:385-386.

Rittenhouse E, Dillard D, Winterscheid L, Merendino K: Traumatic rupture of the thoracic aorta: A review of the literature and a report of five cases with attention to special problems in early management. Ann Surg 1969;170:87-100.

Ritter D, Chang F: Delayed hemothorax resulting form stab wounds to the internal mammary artery. J Trauma 1995;39:586-589.

Rob CG: Diagnosis of abdominal trauma in warfare. Surg Gynecol Obstet 1947;85:147-154.

Rob CG: Reconstruction of a stenosed internal carotid artery. Br Med J 1956;2:1265.

Rob CG: Die indikationstellung zur operativen widerherstellung der aorta und der groesseren arterien. Arch and Deutschen Zt J Chir 1957;287:305.

Rob CG: Obliterations of the aortic bifurcation (Leriche's syndrome). Cardioangiologica 1957;5:1.

Rob CG: Arterial wounds, acute ischemia of the limbs. J Cardiovasc Surg 1963;4:249-252.

Rob CG: A history of arterial surgery. Arch Surg 1972;105:821-823.

Rob CG: Military surgery, our debt to our patients and predecessors. J R Army Med Corps 1986;132:11-15.

Rob CG, Battle S: Arteriovenous fistula following the use of the Fogarty balloon catheter. Arch Surg 1971;102:144-145.

Rob CG, Standeven A: Closed traumatic lesions of the axillary and brachial arteries. Lancet 1956;1:597-599.

Robbs J, Baker LW: Subclavian and axillary artery injury. S Afr Med J 1977;51:227-231.

Robbs J, Baker LW: Arterial trauma involving the lower limb. J Trauma 1978;18:324-328.

Robbs J, Baker LW: Major arterial trauma: Review of experience with 267 injuries. Br J Surg 1978;65:532-538.

Robbs J, Baker LW: Cardiovascular trauma. Curr Prob Surg 1984;21:7-87.

Robbs J, Baker LW, Human R, et al: Cervicomediastinal arterial injuries. Arch Surg 1981;116:663-668.

Robbs J, Naidoo K: Nerve compression injuries due to traumatic false aneurysm. Ann Surg 1984;200:80-82.

Robbs J, Reddy E: Management options for penetrating injuries to the great veins of the neck and superior mediastinum. Surg Gynecol Obstet 1987;165:323-326.

Roberson G: Combined stab wounds of the aorta and vena cava of the abdomen. Arch Surg 1967;95:12-15.

Roberts R, String T: Arterial injuries in extremity shotgun wounds: Requisite factors for successful management. Surgery 1984;96:902-907.

Roberts S, Main D, Pinderton J: Surgical therapy of femoral artery pseudoaneurysm after angioplasty. Am J Surg 1987;10:676-680.

Robinson J, Moyer C: Comparison of late sequelae of common and superficial femoral vein ligations. Surgery 1954;35:690-697.

Robinson N, Flotte C: Traumatic aneurysm of the carotid arteries. Am Surg 1974;40:121-124.

Robison R, Brown J, Caldwell R, Stone K: Management of asymptomatic intracardiac missiles using echocardiography. J Trauma 1988;28:1402-1403.

Roche K, Genieser N, Berger DK, Ambrosino MM: Traumatic abdominal pseudoaneurysm secondary to child abuse. Pediatr Radiol 1995;25:S247–S248.

Roe B: Cardiac trauma including injury of great vessels. Surg Clin North Am 1972;52:573-583.

Rohman M, Ivatury RR, Steichen F, et al: Emergency room thoracotomy for penetrating cardiac injuries. J Trauma 1983;23:570-576.

Rohrer M, Cardullo P, Pappas A, et al: Axillary artery compression and thrombosis in throwing athletes. J Vasc Surg 1990;11:761-769.

Rojas R, Levitsky S, Stansel HC Jr: Acute traumatic subclavian Steal Syndrome. J Thorac Cardiovasc Surg 1966;51:113-115.

Rollins D, Bernhard VM, Towne JB: Fasciotomy: An appraisal of controversial issues. Arch Surg 1981;116:1474-1481.

Romanoff H, Goldberger S: Major peripheral vein injuries. Vasc Surg 1976;10:157-163.

Roostar L: Indications for surgery in penetrating chest injuries. Ann Chirurgiae Gynaecol 1993;82:177-181.

Roper B, Provan J: Late thrombosis of the femoral artery complicating fracture of the femur. J Bone Joint Surg 1965;47:510-513.

Roques X, Bourdeaudhui A, Collet D, et al: Traumatic rupture and aneurysm of the aortic isthmus: Late results of repair by direct suture. Ann Vasc Surg 1989;3:47-51.

Rose S, Moore EE: Angiography in patients with arterial trauma: Correlations between angiographic abnormalities, operative findings and clinical outcome. AJR Am J Roentgenol 1987;149:613-619.

Rose S, Moore EE: Emergency trauma angiography: Accuracy, safety, and pitfalls. AJR Am J Roentgenol 1987;148:1243-1246.

Rose S, Moore EE: Trauma angiography: The use of clinical findings to improve patient selection and case preparation. J Trauma 1988;28:240-245.

Rosemurgy AS, Norris P, Olson S, et al: Prehospital traumatic cardiac arrest: The cost of futility. J Trauma 1993;35:468-474.

Rosenberg J, Bredenberg CE, Marvasti M, et al: Blunt injuries to the aortic arch vessels. Ann Thorac Surg 1989;48:508-513.

Rosenblatt M, Lemer J, Best LA: Thoracic wounds in Israeli battle casualties during the 1982 evacuation of wounded from Lebanon. J Trauma 1985;4:350.

Rosenbloom M, Fellows B: Chronic pseudoaneurysm of the popliteal artery after blunt trauma. J Vasc Surg 1989;10:187-189.

Rosensweig J, Simon MA: Traumatic aneurysm of the axillary artery: A golf hazard. Can Med Assoc J 1965;93:165-167.

Rosenthal D, Ellison R, Luke J: Traumatic superior mesenteric arteriovenous fistula: Report of a case and review of the literature. J Vasc Surg 1987;5:486-491.

Rosenthal J, Gaspar MR, Gjerdrum T, Newman J: Vascular injuries associated with fractures of the femur. Arch Surg 1975;110:494-499.

Ross S, Ransom K, Shatney C: The management of venous injuries in blunt extremity trauma. J Trauma 1985;25:150-153.

Roth S, Wheeler J, Gregory R, et al: Blunt injury of the abdominal aorta: A review. J Trauma 1997;42:748-755.

Rothlin M, Naf R, Amgwerd M, et al: Ultrasound in blunt abdominal and thoracic trauma. J Trauma 1993;34:488-495.

Rotondo M, Schwab CW, McGonigal MD, et al: "Damage control": An approach for improved survival in exsanguinating penetrating abdominal injury. J Trauma 1993;35:375-383.

Rovito P: Arterial caval shunting in blunt hepatic vascular injury. Ann Surg 1987;205:318-321.

Roy-Shapira A, Levi I, Khoda J: Sternal fractures: A red flag or a red herring? J Trauma 1994;37:59-61.

Rozin L, Perper J: Spontaneous fatal perforation of aorta and vena cava by Mobin-Uddin umbrella. Am J Forensic Med Pathol 1989;10:149-151.

Rozycki G, Ochsner M, Schmidt J, et al: A prospective study of surgeon-performed ultrasound as the primary adjuvant modality for injured patient assessment. J Trauma 1995;39:492-500.

Rozycki G, Kraut E: Isolated blunt rupture of the infrarenal inferior vena cava: The role of ultrasound and computed tomography in an occult injury. J Trauma 1995;38:402-405.

Rpatopoulos V, Sheiman R, Phillips D, et al: Traumatic aortic tear: Screening with chest CT. Radiology 1992;182:667-673.

Ruberti U, Odero A, Arpesani A, et al: Acute ruptures of the thoracic aorta. Personal experience. J Cardiovasc Surg 1987;28:81-84.

Ruberti U, Odero A, Arperani A, et al: Surgical treatment of thoracic aortic aneurysms: Personal experience. J Cardiovasc Surg 1988;29:245-256.

Rubio P, Reul GJ, Beall AC Jr, et al: Acute carotid artery injury: 25 years' experience. J Trauma 1974;14:967-973.

Rubio P, Reul GJ: Penetrating cardiac injury by wire thrown from a lawn mower. Int Surg 1979;64:9-10.

Rudich M, Rowland M, Seibel R, Border J: Survival following a gunshot wound of the abdominal aorta and inferior vena cava. J Trauma 1978;18:548-549.

Rush D, Frame S, Bell RM, Berg EE: Does open fasciotomy contribute to morbidity and mortality after acute lower extremity ischemia and revascularization? J Vasc Surg 1989;10:343.

Ruskey J, Lieberman M, Shaikh K, Talucci R: Unusual subclavian artery lacerations resulting from lap-shoulder seatbelt trauma: Case reports. J Trauma 1989;29:1598-1600.

Russell W, Sailors D, Whittle T, et al: Limb salvage versus traumatic amputation: A decision based on a seven part predictive index. Ann Surg 1991;213:473.

Russo P, Orszulak T, Arnold PG, et al: Concomitant repair of a chronic traumatic aortic aneurysm with tracheal erosion. Ann Thorac Surg 1987;43:559-560.

Rutherford R: Diagnostic evaluation of extremity vascular injuries. Surg Clin North Am 1988;68:683-691.

Rutherford R, Baue AE: Extraanatomic bypass. In Rutherford R (ed): Vascular Surgery. Philadelphia, WB Saunders, 1989, pp 705-716.

Rutsaert R, Van Schil P, Martens C, et al: Occlusion of the left common femoral artery after total hip replacement. Report of a case and review of the literature. J Cardiovasc Surg 1988;29:216-218.

Ryan J, Cooper G, Haywood I, Milner S: Field surgery on a future conventional battlefield: Strategy and wound management. Ann R Coll Surg Engl 1991;73:13.

Ryan W, Snyder WH III, Bell T, Hunt J: Penetrating injuries of the iliac vessels: Early recognition and management. Am J Surg 1982;144:642-645.

Rybeck B: Missile wounding and hemodynamic effects of energy absorption. Acta Chir Scand 1974;450:1.

Rybuck J, Thomford N: Acute occlusion of the infrarenal aorta from blunt trauma. Am Surg 1969;36:444-447.

Saaman H: The hazards of radial artery pressure monitoring. J Cardiovasc Surg 1971;12:342.

Sachtello C, Ernst CB, Griffen WJ: The acute ischemic upper extremity: Selected management. Surgery 1974;76:1002.

Sadow S, Murray C, Wilson R, et al: Traumatic rupture of ascending aorta and left main bronchus. Ann Thorac Surg 1988;45:682-683.

Sagalowski A, McConnell J, Peters P: Renal trauma requiring surgery: An analysis of 185 cases. J Trauma 1983;23:128-131.

Sahler O, Jaretzki AI: Thrombosis of the abdominal aorta: Its production by ureteral compression during intravenous pyelography. Arch Surg 1968;96:76-77.

Sako Y, Varco R: Arteriovenous fistula: Results of management of congenital and acquired forms, blood flow measurements and observations on proximal arterial degeneration. Surgery 1970;67:40-61.

Salam A, Stewart M: New approach to wounds of the aortic bifurcation and inferior vena cava. Surgery 1985;98:105-108.

Salander J, Youkey J, Rich NM, et al: Vascular injury related to lumbar disk surgery. J Trauma 1984;24:628-631.

Salas A, Panes J, Rosenbloom C, et al: Differential effects of a nitric oxide donor on reperfusion-induced microvascular dysfunction in diabetic and non-diabetic rats. Diabetologia 1999;42:1350-1358.

Saletta J, Freeark R: The partially severed artery. Arch Surg 1968;97:198-205.

Saletta J, Freeark R: Vascular injuries associated with fractures. Orthop Clin North Am 1970;1:93.

Saletta J, Freeark R: Injuries to the profunda femoris artery. J Trauma 1972;12:778.

Saletta J, Lowe RLL: Penetrating trauma of the neck. J Trauma 1976;16:579-587.

Saletta S, Lederman E, Fein S, et al: Transesophageal echocardiography for the initial evaluation of the widened mediastinum in trauma patients. J Trauma 1995;39:137-141.

Samaan H: Vascular injuries of the upper thorax and the root of the neck. Br J Surg 1971;58:881-886.

Samson P: Two unusual cases of war wounds of the heart. Surgery 1946;20:373.

Samson P: Battle wounds and injuries of the heart and pericardium: Experiences in forward hospitals. Ann Surg 1948;127:1127.

Samson R, Pasternak B: Traumatic arterial spasm: Rarity or nonentity. J Trauma 1980;20:607-609.

Samson R, Sprayregen S, Veith F, et al: Management of angioplasty complications, unsuccessful procedures and early and late failures. Ann Surg 1984;199:234-240.

Santanello S, Barnes S, Price J, Falcone R: Below the belt: Seat belt related injuries. Contemp Surg 1991;39:29-32.

Sato O, Tada Y, Sudo K, et al: Arteriovenous fistula following central venous catheterization. Arch Surg 1986;121:729-731.

Saueracker A, McCroskey B, Moore EE: Intraoperative hypogastric artery embolization for life-threatening pelvic hemorrhage: A preliminary report. J Trauma 1987;27:1127-1129.

Sauerbruch: Uber die Verwendbarkeit der pneumatischen Kammer fur die Herschirurgie. Centralbl Chir 1907;34:44.

Saunders M, Riberi A, Massullo E: Delayed traumatic superior mesenteric arteriovenous fistula after a stab wound: Case report. J Trauma 1992;32:101-106.

Savage R: Popliteal artery injury associated with knee dislocation: Improved outlook? Am Surg 1980;46:627-632.

Saylam A, Melo J, Ahmad A, et al: Early surgical repair in traumatic rupture of the thoracic aorta. (Report of 9 cases and review of the current concepts). J Cardiovasc Surg 1980;21:295-302.

Scalea T, Sclafani S: Angiographically placed balloons for arterial control: A description of a technique. J Trauma 1991;31:1671-1677.

Schaff H, Brawley RK: Operative management of penetrating vascular injuries of the thoracic outlet. Surgery 1977;82:182-191.

Schede M: Zur frage von der jodoformvergiftung. Zentralb Chir Beil 1882;9:33-38.

Scheerlinck T, Van den Brande P: Post-traumatic intima dissection and thrombosis of the external iliac artery in a sportsman. Surg J Vasc Surg 1994;8:645.

Schenk WJ, Bahn RA, Cordell A, Stephens J: The regional hemodynamics of acute experimental arteriovenous fistulas. Surg Gynecol Obstet 1957;105:733.

Schenk WJ, Martin J, Leslie M, Portin B: The regional hemodynamics of chronic arteriovenous fistulas. Surg Gynecol Obstet 1960;110:44-50.

Schlosser W, Spillner G, Breymann T, Urbayni B: Vascular injuries in orthopaedic surgery. J Cardiovasc Surg 1982;23:323-327.

Schmidt C, Jacobson J: Thoracic aortic injury: A ten-year experience. Arch Surg 1984;119:1244-1246.

Schmitt H, Armstrong RC: Wounds causing loss of limb. Surg Gynecol Obstet 1970;130:682-684.

Schoenfeld H: Heart Injuries with suture. Ann Surg 2001;87:823-828.

Schonholtz G, Jahnke EJ Jr: Occult injury of the thoracic aorta associated with orthopaedic trauma. J Bone Joint Surg 1964;46A:1421.

Schorn B, Reitmeier F, Falk V, et al: True aneurysm of the superior gluteal artery: Case report and review of the literature. J Vasc Surg 1995;21:851.

Schott U, Lindbom L, Sjostrand U: Hemodynamic effects of colloid concentration in experimental hemorrhage: A comparison of Ringer's acetate, 3% dextran-60 and 6% dextran-70. Crit Care Med 1998;16:346-352.

Schramek A, Hashmonai M: Distal arteriovenous fistula for the prevention of occlusion of venous interposition grafts to veins. J Cardiovasc Surg 1974;15:392-395.

Schramek A, Hashmonai M, Farbstein J, Adler O: Reconstructive surgery in major vein injuries in the extremities. J Trauma 1975;15:816-822.

Schramek A, Hashmonai M: Vascular injuries in the extremities in battle casualties. Br J Surg 1977;64:644-648.

Schwab C, Lawson R, Lind J, Garland L: Aortic injury: Comparison of supine and upright portable chest films to evaluate the widened mediastinum. Ann Emerg Med 1984;13:896-899.

Schwab C, Adcock OT, Max H: Emergency department thoracotomy (EDT): A 26-month experience using an "agonal" protocol. Am Surg 1986;52:20-28.

Schwab C, McMahan D, Phillips G, Pentecost M: Aortic balloon control of a traumatic aortoenteric fistula after damage control laparotomy: A case report. J Trauma 1996;40:1021-1023.

Schwartz A: The historical development of methods of hemostasis. Surgery 1958;44:604.

Schwartz D, Haller JA Jr: Open anterior hip dislocation with femoral vessel transection in a child. J Trauma 1974;14:1054.

Schwartz L, McCann R: Traumatic false aneurysm of the common carotid artery presenting as a mediastinal mass: A case report. J Vasc Surg 1989;10:281-284.

Schwartz ML, Fisher R, Sako Y, et al: Posttraumatic aneurysms of the thoracic aorta. Surgery 1975;78:589-593.

Sclafani SJ, Panetta T, Goldstein A, et al: The management of arterial injuries caused by penetration of Zone III of the neck. J Trauma 1985;25:878-881.

Sclafani S, Cooper R, Shaftan GW, et al: Arterial trauma: Diagnostic and therapeutic angiography. Radiology 1986;161:165-172.

Sclafani S, Cavaliere G, Atweh N, et al: The role of angiography in penetrating neck trauma. J Trauma 1991;31:557-563.

Scott C, Pinson W, Inahara T: Common femoral artery injury by blunt trauma: A case report. Surgery 1984;96:122-125.

Scott R. Aspects of military surgery. Injury 1970;2:116.

Scultetus AH, Villavicencio JL, Rich NM: Historical review: Facts and fiction surrounding the discovery of the venous valves. J Vasc Surg 2001;33:435-441.

Sechas M, Fotiadis C, Baramily B, Skalkeas G: Plaie des vaisseaux mésentériques supérieurs à propos d'un cas. Ann Chir 1988;42:423-425.

Seeley S: Vascular surgery at Walter Reed Army Hospital. US Armed Forces Med J 1954;8.

Seeley S, Hughes CW, Cooke F, Elkin DC: Traumatic arteriovenous fistulas and aneurysms in war wounded. Am J Surg 1952;83:471-479.

Seeley S, Hughes CW, Jahnke EJ Jr: Surgery of the popliteal artery. Ann Surg 1953;138:712-717.

Seeley S, Hughes CW, Jahnke EJ Jr: Major vessel damage in lumbar disc operation. Surgery 1954;35:421-429.

Sefczek D, Sefczek RJ, Deeb Z. Radiographic signs of acute traumatic rupture of the thoracic aorta. AJR Am J Roentgenol 1983;141:1259-1262.

Segar R, Palmisano D: Repair of gunshot wounds of the aorta and vena cava. Ohio State Med J 1969;65:501-505.

Seguin J, Bouillon P, Aubry P, et al: Aorto-right ventricular shunt and associated aortic valve injury resulting from a penetrating wound of the heart. Thorac Cardiovasc Surg 1984;32:386-388.

Seidenberg B, Hurwitt E: Retrograde femoral-Seldinger-aortography: Surgical complications in twenty-six cases. Ann Surg 1966;163:221-226.

Seiler JI, Richardson JD: Amputation after extremity injury. Am J Surg 1986;152:260-264.

Seltzer S, D'Orsi C, Kirshner R, DeWeese JA: Traumatic aortic rupture: Plain radiographic findings. AJR 1981;137:1011-1014.

Sencert L: Les Blessures des Vaisseaux. Paris, Masson & Cie, 1917.

Sethi G, Scott S, Takaro T: False aneurysm of the abdominal aorta due to blunt trauma. Ann Surg 1975;182:33-36.

Sethi G, Scott S, Bhayana J, Takaro T: Traumatic avulsion of the innominate artery: Report of a case and review of literature. J Cardiovasc Surg 1975;16:171-175.

Sethi G, Scott S: Subclavian artery laceration due to migration of a Hagie Pin. Surgery 1976;80:644.

Shackford SR, Sise MJ: Renal and mesenteric vascular trauma: In Vascular Injuries in Surgical Practice. In Bongard FS, Wilson SE, Perry MO (eds): Norwalk, Conn, San Mateo, Appleton & Lange, 1991, pp 173-184.

Shadow S, Murray CI, Wilson R, et al: Traumatic rupture of ascending aorta and left main bronchus. Ann Thorac Surg 1988;45:682-683.

Shaftan GW, Chiu C, Dennis C, Harris B: Fundamentals of physiologic control of arterial hemorrhage. Surgery 1965;58:851-856.

Shah D, Leather R, Corson J, Karmody A: Polytetrafluoraethylene grafts in the rapid reconstruction of acute contaminated peripheral vascular injuries. Am J Surg 1984;148:229-233.

Shah D, Naraynsingh V, Leather R, et al: Advances in the management of acute popliteal vascular blunt injuries. J Trauma 1985;25:793-797.

Shah D, Corson J, Karmody A, et al: Optimal management of tibial arterial trauma. J Trauma 1988;28:228-234.

Shah PM, Ito K, Clauss RH, et al: Expanded microporous polytetrafluoroethylene (PTFE) grafts in contaminated wounds: Experimental and clinical study. J Trauma 1983;23:1030-1033.

Shah PM, Mackey R, Babu SC, et al: Pseudoaneurysm of anterior tibial artery after occlusion from blunt trauma: Nonoperative management. J Trauma 1985;25:656-658.

Shah PM, Agarwal N, Babu SC, et al: Causes of limb loss in civilian arterial injuries. J Cardiovasc Surg 1986;27:278-281.

Shah PM, Ivatury RR, Babu SC, et al: Is limb loss avoidable in civilian vascular injuries? Am J Surg 1987;154:202-205.

Shaker I, White J, Signer R, et al: Special problems of vascular injuries in children. J Trauma 1976;16:863-867.

Shamoun J, Barraza KR, Jurkovich GJ, Salley R: In extreme use of staples for cardiorrhaphy in penetrating cardiac trauma: Case report. J Trauma 1989;29:1589-1591.

Shandall A, Leopold P, Shah D, et al: Visceral aortic aneurysm in 4 1/2 year old child: An unusual complication of umbilical artery catheterization. Surgery 1986;100:928-931.

Shannon J, Vo N, Stanton P: Peripheral arterial missile embolization. J Vasc Surg 1987;5:773-778.

Shanthakumar RE, Zwaveling JH, Waterbolk TW, Girbes ARJ: Aorto-esophageal fistula: An "early" complication following rupture of the thoracic aorta. 2001.

Sharar S, Winn R, Murry C, et al: A CD18 monoclonal antibody increases the incidence and severity of subcutaneous abscess formation after high-dose Staphylococcus aureus injection in rabbits. Surgery 1991;110:213-220.

Sharma P, Babu SC, Shah PM, Clauss RH: Changing patterns in civilian arterial injuries. J Cardiovasc Surg 1985;26:7-11.

Sharma P, Ivatury RR, Simon R, Vinzons A: Central and regional hemodynamics determine optimal management of major venous injuries. J Vasc Surg 1992;16:887-894.

Sharma P, Shah PM, Vinzons A, et al: Meticulously restored lumina of injured veins remain patent. Surgery 1992;112:928-932.

Shauna R, Main D, Pinkerton J: Surgical therapy of femoral artery pseudoaneurysm after angiography. Am J Surg 1987;154:676-680.

Sheikh A, Culbertson C: Emergency department thoracotomy in children: Rationale for selective application. J Trauma 1993;34:323-328.

Sheiman R, Brophy D, Perry L, Akbari C: Thrombin injection for the repair of brachal artery pseudoaneurysms. AJR Am J Roentgenol 1999;173:1029-1030.

Sheldon G, Lim RC, Yee E, Petersen S: Management of injuries to the porta hepatis. Ann Surg 1985;202:539-542.

Sheldon P, Oglevie S, Kaplan L: Prolonged generalized urticarial reaction after percutaneous thrombin injection for treatment of a femoral artery pseudoaneurysm. JVIR 2000;11:759-761.

Shepard G, Rich NM, Dimond F Jr: Punji stick wounds: Experience with 342 wounds in 324 patients in Vietnam. Ann Surg 1967;166:902-907.

Sher M: Principles in the management of arterial injuries associated with fracture/dislocations. Ann Surg 1975;182:630-636.

Sherman M, Saini V, Yarnox M, et al: Management of penetrating heart wounds. Am J Surg 1978;135:553-558.

Shield CI, Richardson JD, Buckley C, Hagood C: Pseudyaneurysm of the brachiocephalic arteries: A complication of percutaneous internal jugular vein catheterization. Surgery 1975;78:190-194.

Shih F, Wang S, Dang K, et al: Successful management of traumatic mesenteric arteriovenous fistula after failure of steel coil embolization: Case report. J Trauma 1994;37:682-686.

Shin D, Wall MJ Jr, Mattox KL: Combined penetrating injury of the innominate artery, left common carotid artery, trachea, and esophagus. J Trauma 2000;49:780-783.

Shirkey AL, Quast DC, Jordan GL: Superior mesenteric artery division and intestinal function. J Trauma 1967;7:7-24.

Shoemaker WC, Carey J, Yao S: Hemodynamic alterations in acute cardiac tamponade after penetrating injuries of the heart. Surgery 1970;67:754-764.

Shoemaker WC, Carey J, Yao S: Hemodynamic monitoring for physiologic evaluation, diagnosis, and therapy of acute hemopericardial tamponade from penetrating wounds. J Trauma 1973;13:36-44.

Shoenfeld N, Stuchin S, Pearl R, Haveson S: The management of vascular injuries associated with total hip arthroplasty. J Vasc Surg 1990;11:549-555.

Shorr R, Crittenden M, Indeck M, et al: Blunt thoracic trauma. Analysis of 515 patients. Ann Surg 1987;206:200-205.

Shrock T, Blaisdell FW, Mathewson CJ: Management of blunt trauma to the liver and hepatic veins. Arch Surg 1968;96:698-704.

Shuck J, Trump D: Nonpenetrating abdominal trauma with injuries to blood vessels. Am Surg 1961;27:693-697.

Shuck J, Omer GJLCJ: Arterial obstruction due to intimal disruption in extremity fractures. J Trauma 1972;12:481-489.

Shumacker HB Jr: Incisions in surgery of aneurysm: With special reference to explorations in the antecubital and popliteal fossae. Ann Surg 1946;124:586-598.

Shumacker HB Jr: Resection of the clavicle with particular reference to the use of bone chips in the periosteal bed. Surg Gynecol Obstet 1947;84:245-248.

Shumacker HB Jr: Surgical cure of innominate aneurysm: Report of a case with comments on applicability of surgical measures. Surgery 1947;22:729-739.

Shumacker HB Jr: Operative exposure of the blood vessels in the superior anterior mediastinum. Am Surg 1948;127:464-475.

Shumacker HB Jr: Problem of maintaining the continuity of artery in surgery of aneurysms and arteriovenous fistulae: Notes on the development and clinical application of methods of arterial suture. Ann Surg 1948;127:207-230.

Shumacker HB Jr: Arterial aneurysms and arterialvenous fistulas. Spontaneous problems. Cures in Surgery. In Elkin DC, DeBakey ME (eds): World War II, Vascular Surgery. Washington, DC: US Government Printing Office, OTSG, Department of the Army, 1955: 361-374.

Shumacker HB Jr: Arterial suture techniques and grafts: Past, present and future. Surgery 1969;66:419-433.

Shumacker HB Jr: Book review: Vascular disorders of the upper extremity. Ann Surg 1984;199:249.

Shumacker HB Jr: Ramuald Weglowski: Neglected pioneer in vascular surgery. J Vasc Surg 2001;6:95-97.

Shumacker HB Jr, Carter K: Arteriovenous fistulas and false aneurysms in military personnel. Surgery 1946;20:9-25.

Shumacker HB Jr, Stahl N: A study of the cardiac frontal area in patients with arteriovenous fistulas. Surgery 1949;26:928-944.

Shumacker HB Jr, Stokes G: Studies of combined vascular and neurologic injuries. Ann Surg 1950;132:386-393.

Shumacker HB Jr, Wayson E: Spontaneous cure of aneurysms and arteriovenous fistulas, with some notes on intrasaccular thrombosis. Am J Surg 1950;79:532-544.

Siavelis H, Marsan R, Marshall W, Maull K: Aortoventricular fistula secondary to blunt trauma: A case report and review of the literature. J Trauma 1997;43:713-715.

Sibbitt R, Palmaz J, Garcia F, Reuter S: Trauma to the extremities: Prospective comparison of digital and conventional angiography. Radiology 1986;160:179-182.

Siegel R: Galen on surgery of the pericardium: An early record of therapy based on anatomical and experimental studies. Am J Cardiol 1970;26:524-527.

Siegmeth A, Gaebler C, Sandbach G, Vécsei V: A rare case of a traumatic aneurysm of the inferior thyroid artery. J Vasc Surg 1995;22:812-813.

Sigel B, Popky G, Wagner D, et al: Comparison of clinical and Doppler ultrasound evaluation of confirmed lower extremity venous disease. Surgery 1968;64:332-338.

Sigler L, Gutiérrez-Carreño R, Martinez-López, et al: Aortocaval fistula: Experience with five patients. Vasc Surg 2001;35:207-212.

Silen W, Spieker D: Fatal hemorrhage from the innominate artery after tracheostomy. Ann Surg 1965;162:1005-1012.

Simeone F, Grillo H, Rundle F: On the question of ligation of the concomitant vein when a major artery is interrupted. Surgery 1951;29:932-951.

Simmons K: Defense against free radicals has therapeutic implications. JAMA 1984;251:2187-2192.

Simstein N, Poole GV Jr, Nelson L: Perforation of the intrapericardial aorta during subclavian catheterization. South Med J 1984;77:1605.

Sinclair T, Stephenson HJ: Survival following abdominal aortic rupture from blunt trauma: Case report. Mo Med 1972;69:271-272.

Singh I, Gorman JF: Vascular injuries in closed fractures near junction of middle and lower thirds of the tibia. J Trauma 1972;12:592-598.

Sinkler W, Spencer A: The importance of early exploration of vascular injuries. Surg Gynecol Obstet 1958;107:228-234.

Sinkler W, Spencer A: The value of peripheral arteriography in assessing acute vascular injuries. Arch Surg 1960;80:300-304.

Sirinek KR, Levine BA: Trauma injury to the proximal superior mesenteric vessels. Surgery 1985;98:831-835.

Sirinek K, Levine B, Gaskill H III, Root H: Reassessment of the role of routine operative exploration in vascular trauma. J Trauma 1981;21:339-344.

Sirinek K, Gaskill H, Root H: Visceral vascular injury: Factors influencing survival. J Trauma 1982;22:641.

Sirinek K, Gaskill H III, Dittman W, Levine B: Exclusion angiography for patients with possible vascular injuries of the extremities: A better use of trauma center resources. Surgery 1983;94:598-603.

Sirinek K, Gaskill H III, Root H, Levine B: Truncal vascular injury: Factors influencing survival. J Trauma 1983;23:372-377.

Sitzmann J, Ernst CB: Management of arm arterial injuries. Surgery 1984;96:895-901.

Skillman J, Ducksoo K, Bain DS: Vascular complications of percutaneous femoral cardiac interventions: Incidence and operative repair. Arch Surg 1988;123:1207-1212.

Skinner D: Traumatic renal artery thrombosis: A successful thrombectomy and revascularization. Ann Surg 1973;177:264-267.

Skipper R, Debski R: Intramyocardial shotgun pellets diagnosed on initial emergency room chest x-ray: Case report. J Trauma 1990;30:1609-1610.

Skyhar M, Hargens A, Strauss M, et al: Hyperbaric oxygen reduces edema and necrosis of skeletal muscle in compartment syndromes associated with hemorrhagic hypotension. J Bone Joint Surg 1986;68:1218-1224.

Slaney G, Ashton F, Abrams LD: Traumatic rupture of the aorta. Br J Surg 1966;53:361-364.

Slater R, Edge A, Salman A: Delayed arterial injury after hip replacement. J Bone Joint Surg 1989;71:699.

Sloop R, Robertson K: Non-penetrating traumas of the abdominal aorta due to blunt trauma. Ann Surg 1975;182:33-36.

Sloop R, Robertson K: Nonpenetrating trauma of the abdominal aorta with partial vessel occlusion: Report of two cases. Am Surg 1975;41:555-559.

Smejkal R, Izaznt T, Born C, et al: Pelvic crush injuries with occlusion of the iliac artery. J Trauma 1988;28:1479-1482.

Smith C, Green R: Pediatric vascular injuries. Surgery 1981;90:20-31.

Smith G, Northrop C: Stab wound causing mesenteric-portal arteriovenous fistula: An unusual case with a spontaneous closure. J Trauma 1976;16:408.

Smith K, Ben-Menachem B, Duke J, Hill G: The superior gluteal: An artery at risk in blunt pelvic trauma. J Trauma 1976;16:273-279.

Smith L, Foran R, Gaspar MR: Acute arterial injuries of the upper extremity. Am J Surg 1963;106:144-151.

Smith M, Cassidy J, Souther S, et al: Transesophageal echocardiography in the diagnosis of traumatic rupture of the aorta. N Engl Med J 1995;332:356-362.

Smith P, Lim W, Ferris E, Casali R: Emergency arteriography in extremity trauma: Assessment of indications. AJR Am J Roentgenol 1981;137:803-807.

Smith R, Perdue GJ, Walker LJ, Israel P: Posttraumatic aneurysm of the abdominal aorta with recurrent emboli of the superior mesenteric artery: A case report. Surgery 1968;64:736-742.

Smith RI, Stone H: Traumatic fistulas involving the portal venous system. Am J Surg 1970;119:570.

Smith R, Szilagyi D, Pfeifer J: A study of arterial trauma. Arch Surg 1963;86:825-835.

Smith R, Szilagyi D, Elliott J Jr: Fracture of long bones with arterial injury due to blunt trauma. Arch Surg 1969;99:315-324.

Smith R, Elliot J, Hageman J: Acute penetrating arterial injuries of the neck and limbs. Arch Surg 1974;109:198-205.

Smith R, Chang F: Traumatic rupture of the aorta: Still a lethal injury. Am J Surg 1986;152:660-663.

Smith V, Hughes CW, Sapp O, et al: High-output circulatory failure due to arteriovenous fistula: complication of intervertebral-disk surgery. AMA Arch Int Med 1957;100:833-841.

Smith W: Cardiorraphy in acute injuries. Ann Surg 1923;78:696-710.

Smyth E: Major arterial injury in closed fracture of the neck of the humerus: Report of a case. J Bone Joint Surg 1969;51:B:508.

Snyder WH III: Vascular injuries near the knee: An updated series and overview of the problem. Surgery 1982;91:502-506.

Snyder III WH: Popliteal and shank arterial injury. Surg Clin North Am 1988;68:787-807.

Snyder WH III, Thal E, Bridges RA, et al: The validity of normal arteriography in penetrating trauma: A review of 114 cases. Arch Surg 1978;113:424-428.

Snyder III WH, Thal E, Perry MO. Vascular injuries of the extremities. In Vascular Surgery. In Rutherford R (ed): Philadelphia, PA: WB Saunders, 1989: 613-637.

Snyder WH III, Watkins W, Whiddon L: Civilian popliteal artery trauma: An 11-year experience with 83 injuries. Surgery 1979;85:101-108.

Soldano S, Rich NM, Collins GJ, et al: Long-term follow-up of penetrating abdominal aortic injuries after 15 years. J Trauma 1988;28:1358-1362.

Solovei G, Alame A, Bardoux JL: Paraplegia and dissection of the abdominal aorta after closed trauma: A proposal of a case. Current review of the literature (1982-1993) [in French]. J Chirurgie 1994;131:236-244.

Sondenaa K, Tveit B, Kordt K, et al: Traumatic rupture of the thoracic aorta: A clinicopathological study. Acta Chir Scand 1990;156:137-143.

Soots G, Warembourg HJ, Pratt A, Roux J: Acute traumatic rupture of the thoracic aorta: Place of delayed surgical repair. J Cardiovasc Surg 1989;30:173-177.

Sotta R: Vascular problems in the proximal upper extremity. Clin Sports Med 1990;9:379.

Soubbotitch V: Military experiences of traumatic aneurysms. Lancet 1913;2:720-721.

Soyer R, Brunet A, Piwnica A, et al: Traumatic rupture of the thoracic aorta with reference to 34 operated cases. J Cardiovasc Surg 1981;22:103-108.

Soyer R, Bessou JP, Bouchart F, et al: Long-term results of surgical treatment of traumatic rupture of the thoracic aorta: 47 cases. J Cardiovasc Surg 1990;31(suppl):102.

Speechly-Dick M, Grover G, Yellon D: Does ischemic preconditioning in the human involve protein kinase C and the ATP dependent K+ channel? Circ Res 1995;77:1030-1035.

Spellman M, Mandal A, Freeman HP: Successful repair of an arteriovenous fistula between the superior mesenteric vessels secondary to a gunshot wound. Ann Surg 1967;165:458.

Spence R, DelRossi AJ, Cilley J, Civil I: Exsanguinating upper extremity vascular injury: Is an initial approach by clavicular resection adequate? J Cardiovasc Surg 1989;30:450.

Spencer A: The reliability of signs of peripheral vascular injury. Surg Gynec Obstet 1962;114:490-494.

Spencer FC: The use of optical magnification in coronary bypass grafting. J Thorac Cardiovasc Surg 1970.

Spencer FC, Grewe R: The management of acute arterial injuries in battle casualties. Ann Surg 1955;141:304-313.

Spencer FC, Tompkins R: Management of acute arterial injuries. Postgrad Med 1960;28:476-481.

Spencer FC, Guerin P, Blake HA, Bahnson HT: A report of fifteen patients with traumatic rupture of the thoracic aorta. J Thorac Cardiovasc Surg 1961;41:1-22.

Spirnak J, Resnick M: Revascularization of traumatic thrombosis of the renal artery. Surg Gynec Obstet 1987;164:22-26.

Sponge A, Borrows PE, Armstrong D, Daneman A: Traumatic aortic rupture in the pediatric population: Role of plain film, CT, and angiography in the diagnosis. Pediatr Radiat 1991;21:324-328.

Stables D, Fouche R, de Villiers van Niekerek J, et al: Traumatic renal artery occlusion: 21 cases. J Urol 1976;115:229.

Stafford G, O'Brien M: Traumatic rupture of the thoracic aorta. Aust N Z J Surg 1977;47:175-179.

Stain SC, Yellin AE, Weaver FA, Pentecost M: Selective management of nonocclusive arterial injuries. Arch Surg 1989;124:1136-1141.

Stain SC, Weaver FA, Yellin AE: Extra-anatomic bypass of failed traumatic arterial repairs. J Trauma 1991;31:575-578.

Starnes BW, O'Donnell SD, Gillespie DL, et al: Endovascular management of renal ischemia in a patient with acute aortic dissection and renovascular hypertension. Ann Vasc Surg 2002.

Starzl T, Kaupp HJ, Beheler EM: The treatment of penetrating wounds to the inferior vena cava. Surgery 1962;51:195-204.

Stavens B, Hasim S, Hammond G, et al: Optimal methods of repair of descending thoracic aortic transections and aneurysms. Am J Surg 1983;145:508-513.

Steenburg R, Ravitch MM: Cervico-thoracic approach for subclavian vessel injury from compound fracture of the clavicle: Consideration of subclavian-axillary exposure. Ann Surg 1963;15j7:839-846.

Steichen F, Dargan E, Efron G, et al: A graded approach to the management of penetrating wounds of the heart. Arch Surg 1971;103:574-580.

Stein AJ: Arterial injury in orthopaedic surgery. J Bone Joint Surg 1956;38:669.

Stein L, Shubin H, Weil M: Recognition in management of pericardial tamponade. JAMA 1973;225:503.

Stein M, Mirvis S, Wiles CI: Delayed embolization of a shotgun pellet from the chest to the middle cerebral artery. J Trauma 1995;39:1006-1009.

Stein R, Bono J, Korn J, Wolff W: Axillary artery injury in closed fracture of the neck of the scapular: A case report. J Trauma 1971;11:528-531.

Steinbauer M, Harris A, Leiderer R, et al: Impact of dextran on microvascular disturbances and tissue injury following ischemia/reperfusion in striated muscle. Shock 1998;9:345-351.

Stelzner V, Horatz K: Correction of gunshot wounds of extrapericardial ascending aorta. Thoraxchirurgie 1963;10:632.

Stemmer E, Oliver C, Carey J, Connolly JE: Fatal complications of tracheotomy. Am J Surg 1976;131:288-290.

Stewart F: Arteriovenous aneurysm treated by angiography (angiorrhaphy). Abb Surg 1913;57:247-254.

Stich R: Ueber gefaess und organ transplantationen mittelst gefaessnaht. Ergeon Chir Orth 1910;1:1.

Stiles Q, Cohlmia G, Smith J, et al: Management of injuries of the thoracic and abdominal aorta. Am J Surg 1985;150:132-140.

Stinnett D, Graham JM, Edwards W: Fibromuscular dysplasia and thrombosed aneurysm of the popliteal artery in a child. J Vasc Surg 1987;5:769-772.

Stipa S, Vollmar J: Arterial Trauma. Rome, Italy, Ares-Serono Symposia, 1986.

Stokes J, McAfee C: Increasing limb survival in vascular injury with fracture. J Trauma 1965;5:162.

Stollone R, Ecker R, Samson P: Management of major acute thoracic vascular injuries. Am J Surg 1974;128:249-254.

Stone H, Oxford W, Austin JT: Penetrating wounds of the abdominal aorta. South Med J 1973;66:1351-1355.

Stone H, Fabian TC, Turkleson M: Wounds of the portal venous system. World J Surg 1982;6:335-341.

Stone K, Walshaw R, Sugiyama G, et al: Polytetrafluoroethylene versus autogenous vein grafts for vascular reconstruction in contaminated wounds. Am J Surg 1984;147:692-695.

Stone W: Observations on the treatment of wounded arteries, with cases. New Orleans Med Surg J 1857;2:168.

Stoney R, Roe B, Redington J: Rupture of the thoracic aorta due to closed chest trauma. Arch Surg 1964;89:840-847.

Storey C, Nardi G, Sewell W: Traumatic aneurysms of the thoracic aorta: Report of two cases, one successfully treated by resection and graft replacement with the aid of a shunt. Ann Surg 1956;144:69-78.

Stothert JJ, McBride L, Tidik S, et al: Multiple aortic tears treated by primary suture repair. J Trauma 1987;27:955-956.

Strandness DE Jr: Collateral Circulation in Clinical Surgery. Philadelphia, WB Saunders, 1969.

Strandness DE Jr, Bell JW: Peripheral vascular disease: Diagnosis and objective evaluation using a mercury strain gauge. Ann Surg 1965;161(suppl 1):3-35.

Strassmann G: Traumatic rupture of the aorta. Am Heart J 1947;33:508-515.

Straus R: Pulmonary embolism caused by a lead bullet following a gunshot wound of the abdomen. Arch Pathol 1942;33:63-68.

Stringer W, Kelly DJ: Traumatic dissection of the extracranial internal carotid artery. Neurosurgery 1980;6:123-130.

Strodel W, Eckhauser F, Lemmer J: Presentation and perioperative management of arterioportal fistulas. Arch Surg 1987;122:563.

Stromberg B: Symptomatic lead toxicity secondary to retained shotgun pellets: Case report. J Trauma 1990;30:356-357.

Stubbs D, Dorner D, Johnson R: Thrombosis of the iliofemoral artery during revision of a total hip replacement: A case report. J Bone Joint Surg [Am] 1986;68:454-455.

Sturm J, Strate R, Mowlem A, et al: Blunt trauma to the subclavian artery. Surg Gynec Obstet 1974;138:915-918.

Sturm J, Perry JJ, Cass AS: Renal artery and vein injury following blunt trauma. Ann Surg 1975;182:696.

Sturm J, Marsh D, Bodily KC: Ruptured thoracic aorta: Evolving radiological concepts. Surgery 1979;85:363-367.

Sturm J, Bodily KC, Rothenberger D, Perry JF: Arterial injuries of the extremities following blunt trauma. J Trauma 1980;20:933-936.

Sturm J, Cicero J: The clinical diagnosis of ruptured subclavian artery following blunt thoracic trauma. Ann Emerg Med 1983;12:17-19.

Sturm J, Perry JF Jr, Olson F, Cicero J: Significance of symptoms and signs in patients with traumatic aortic rupture. Ann Emerg Med 1984;13:876-878.

Sturm J, Billiar TR, Dorsey J, et al: Risk factors for survival following treatment of traumatic aortic rupture. Ann Thorac Surg 1985;39:418-421.

Sturm J, Perry JJ: Brachial plexus injuries form blunt thoracic trauma: A harbinger of vascular and thoracic injury. Ann Emerg Med 1987;16:404-406.

Sturm J, Billiar TR, Luxenberg M, Perry JF: Risk factors for the development of renal failure following the surgical treatment of traumatic aortic rupture. Ann Thorac Surg 1987;43:425-427.

Sturm J, McGee M, Luxenberg M: An analysis of risk factors for death at the scene following traumatic aortic rupture. J Trauma 1988;28:1578-1580.

Suarez C, Bernstein DM, Goldberger J, et al: The role of nuclear scanning in the evaluation of arterial injuries. Am Surg 1983;49:209-210.

Sugg S, Gerndt S, Hamilton B, et al: Pseudoaneurysms of the intraparenchymal splenic artery after blunt abdominal trauma: A complication of non-operative therapy and its management. J Trauma 1995;39:593-595.

Sugg W, Rea W, Ecker R: Penetrating wounds of the heart: An analysis of 459 cases. J Thorac Cardiovasc Surg 1986;56:531-545.

Sullivan M: Rupture of the brachial artery from posterior discoloration of the elbow treated by vein graft. Br J Surg 1971;58:470-471.

Sullivan M, Smalley R, Banowsky LH: Renal artery occlusion secondary to blunt abdominal trauma. J Trauma 1972;12:509-515.

Sullivan W, Thorton F, Baker LH, et al: Early influence of popliteal vein repair in the treatment of popliteal vessel injuries. Am J Surg 1971;122:528-531.

Summerall C, Lee WJ, Boone JA: Intracardiac shunts after penetrating wounds of the heart. N Engl J Med 1965;272:240-242.

Sumpio G, Gusberg R: Aortic thrombosis with paraplegia: An unusual consequence of blunt abdominal trauma. J Vasc Surg 1987;6:412-414.

Sutorius D, Schreiber J, Helmsworth J: Traumatic disruption of the thoracic aorta. J Trauma 1973;13:583-590.

Svane H, Ottosen T: Traumatic vascular lesions. J Cardiovasc Surg 1963;4:303-305.

Svensson L, Antunes MDJ, Kinsley R: Traumatic rupture of the thoracic aorta: A report of 14 cases and a review of the literature. S Afr Med J 1985;67:853-857.

Swan KG, Hobson RW II, Reynolds D, et al: Venous surgery in the lower extremities. In Swan KG, Hobson R, Reynolds D, et al (eds): St Louis, Warren H Green Publishers, 1975.

Sweetman W: Subclavian steal syndrome following trauma: Case report. Am Surg 1965;31:463-466.

Swetnam J, Hardin WD, Kerstein MD: Successful management of trifurcation injuries. Am Surg 1986;52:585-587.

Symbas P, Vlasis-Hale S, Picone A: Missiles in the heart. Ann Thorac Surg 1989;48:192-194.

Symbas P, Pourhamidi A, Levin J: Traumatic rupture of the aortic arch between the left common carotid and left subclavian arteries and avulsion of the left subclavian artery. Ann Surg 1969;170:152-156.

Symbas P, Sehdeva J, Abbott OA, et al: Penetrating wounds of the thoracic aorta and great arteries. South Med J 1970;63:853-857.

Symbas P, Sehdeva J: Penetrating wounds of the thoracic aorta. Ann Surg 1970;171:441-450.

Symbas P, Tyras D, Ware R, Hatcher CJ: Rupture of the aorta. Ann Thorac Surg 1973;15:405-410.

Symbas P, Tyras D, Ware R, Diroio D: Traumatic rupture of the aorta. Ann Surg 1973;178:6-12.

Symbas P, Kourias E, Tyras D, Hatcher CJ: Penetrating wounds of great vessels. Ann Surg 1974;179:757-762.

Symbas P, Harlaftis N, Waldo W: Penetrating cardiac wounds: A comparison of different therapeutic methods. Ann Surg 1976;183:377-381.

Symbas P, Harlaftis N: Bullet emboli in the pulmonary and systemic arteries. Am Surg 1977;185:318-320.

Symes J, Eadie D, Maclean A: Traumatic aorto-caval fistula associated with horse-shoe kidney. J Trauma 1974;14:402-408.

Symonds F, Garnes A, Porter V, Crikelair G: Pitfalls in the management of penetrating injuries of the forearm. J Trauma 1971;11:47-52.

Synder C, Eyer S: Blunt chest trauma with transection of the azygos vein: Case report. J Trauma 1989;29:889-890.

Synder S, Wheeler J, Gregory R, et al: Freshly harvested cadaveric venous homo-grafts as arterial conduits in infected fields. Surgery 1987;101:283-291.

Syracuse D, Seaver PR Jr, Amato JJ: Aortic gunshot injury and paraplegia: Pre-operative definition with arteriography and computerized axial tomography. J Trauma 1985;25:271-273.

Szentpetery S, Lower R: Changing concepts in the treatment of penetrating cardiac injuries. J Trauma 1977;17:457-461.

Szentpetery S: Management of aortic cannulation site blowouts. Ann Thorac Surg 1992;54:582-583.

Szilagyi D: Discussion on "Choice of vascular graft material for patients." In Wesolowski S, Dennis C (eds): Fundamentals of Vascular Grafting. New York, McGraw-Hill, 1963, pp 397-419.

Szilagyi D: Spinal cord damage in surgery of the abdominal aorta. Surgery 1978;83:38-56.

Szuchmacher P, Freed J: Immediate revascularization of the popliteal artery and vein: Report of a case. J Trauma 1978;18:142-144.

Tailor A, Granger D: Role of adhesion molecules in vascular regulation and damage. Curr Hyperten Rep 2000;2:78-83.

Takeuchi M, Maruyama K, Nakamura M, et al: Posttraumatic inferior vena caval thrombosis: Case report and review of the literature. J Trauma 1995;39:605-608.

Tamim W, Arbid EJ, Andrews LS, Arous EJ: Percutaneous induced thrombosis of iatrogenic femoral pseudoaneurysms following catheterization. Ann Vasc Surg 2000;14:254-259.

Tarlow S, Achterman CA, Hayhurst J, Ovadia D: Acute compartment syndrome in the thigh complicating fracture of the femur: A report of three cases. J Bone Joint Surg 1986;68:1439-1443.

Tassi A, Davies A: Pericardial tamponade due to penetrating fragment wounds of the heart. Am J Surg 1969;118:535-538.

Tawes RJ, Etheredge S, Webb R, et al: Popliteal artery injury complicating arthroscopic meniscectomy. Am J Surg 1988;156:136-138.

Taylor B, Rhee R, Muluk S: Thrombin injection versus compression of femoral artery pseudoaneurysms. J Vasc Surg 1999;30:1052-1059.

Taylor LJ, Troutman R, Feliciano P, et al: Late complications after femoral artery catheterization in children less than five years of age. J Vasc Surg 1990;11:297-306.

Taylor TKF, Wardill JC: Successful primary repair of rupture of the popliteal artery in association with compound dislocation of the knee-joint. Br Surg 1964;51:163-166.

Tector A, Reuben C, Hoffman J, et al: Coronary artery wounds treated with saphenous vein bypass grafts. JAMA 1973;225:282-284.

Tector A, Worman L, Romer J, et al: Unusual injury to the aortic arch: A case report. J Thorac Cardiovasc Surg 1974;67:547-552.

Tegner Y, Bergdahl L, Ekestrom S: Traumatic disruption of the thoracic aorta. Acta Chir Scand 1984;150:635-638.

Tepas J, Alexander RH, Snyder J: Real time ultrasonography as a diagnostic screen in experimental arterial injury. J Trauma 1985;25:720.

Thal E, Perry MO, Crighton J: Traumatic abdominal aortic occlusion. South Med J 1971;64:653-656.

Thal E, Snyder WH III, Hays R, Perry MO: Management of carotid artery injuries. Surgery 1974;76:955-962.

Theodorides T, de Keizer G: Injuries of the axillary artery caused by fractures of the neck of the humerus. Injury 1976;8:120-123.

Theunis P, Coenen L, Brouwers J: Traumatic injuries to the porta hepatis. Injury 1989;20:152.

Thevenet A, DuCailiar C: Chronic traumatic aneurysms of the thoracic aorta. World J Surg 1989;13:112-116.

Thio R: False Aneurysm of the ulnar artery after surgery employing a tourniquet. Am J Surg 1972;123:604-605.

Thio R, Stanton P, Logan W: Simultaneous avulsion of the innominate and left intrathoracic subclavian arteries. J Thorac Cardiovasc Surg 1973;66:96-98.

Thomas A, Goodman P, Roon A: Role of angiography in cervicothoracic trauma. J Thorac Cardiovasc Surg 1978;76:633-638.

Thomas CJ, Carter J, Lowder S: Pericardial tamponade from central venous catheters. Arch Surg 1969;98:217-218.

Thomas D, Wilson R, Wieneck R: Vascular Injury about the knee: Improved outcome. Ann Surg 1989;55:370-377.

Thomas T: Management of cardiac and intrathoracic great vessel injuries. Surg Gynecol Obstet 1967;125:997-1002.

Thomford N, Curtiss P, Marable S: Injuries of the iliac and femoral arteries associated with blunt skeletal trauma. J Trauma 1969;9:126-134.

Thomford N, Pace W, Meckstroth C: Traumatic rupture of the thoracic artery. Am Surg 1969;35:244-249.

Thorlacius H, Vollmar B, Westermann S, et al: Effects of local cooling on microvascular hemodynamics and leukocyte adhesion in the striated muscle of hamsters. J Trauma 1998;45:715-719.

Tilney N, McLamb J: Leg trauma with posterior tibial artery tear. J Trauma 1967;7:807.

Timberlake G, O'Connell RC, Kerstein MD: Venous Injuries, to repair or ligate, the dilemma. J Vasc Surg 1986;4:533-538.

Timberlake G, Adinolfi MF, McSwain N Jr: Problem: Rupture of the thoracic aorta. Emerg Med 1987;19:45-49.

Timberlake G, Kerstein MD, McSwain N Jr: Penetrating thoracic aortic injuries: Rare but potentially salvageable sequelae of urban warfare. South Med J 1989;82:970-972.

Timberlake G, Kerstein MD: Venous injury: To repair or litigate, the dilemma revisited. Am Surgeon 1995;61:139-145.

Tipton W, D'Ambrosia R: Vascular Impairment as a result of fracture-dislocation of the ankle. J Trauma 1975;15:524-527.

Tisnado J, Tsai F, Als A, Roach J: A new radiographic sign of acute traumatic rupture of the thoracic aorta: Displacement of the nasogastric tube to the right. Radiology 1977;125:603-608.

Todd G, Bregman D, Voorhees A, Reemtsma K: Vascular Complications associated with percutaneous intra-aortic balloon pumping. ArchSurg 1983;118:963-964.

Toguri A, Liu T, Bayliss C: Traumatic bilateral renal artery thrombosis. J Urol 1974;112:430.

Toivio I, Karlsson B: Treatment of ischemia of extremity caused by a shotgun blast. Ann Med Milit Fenn 1975;4:159.

Tomatis L, Doornobs F, Beard JA: Circumferential intimal tear of the aorta with complete occlusion due to blunt trauma. J Trauma 1968;8:1096-1101.

Tomiak M, Rosenblum J, Messersmith R, Zarins C: Use of CT for diagnosis of traumatic rupture of the thoracic aorta. Ann Vasc Surg 1993;7:130-139.

Toursarkissian B, Allen BT, Petrinec D: Spontaneous closure of selected iatrogenic pseudoaneurysms and arteriovenous fistulae. J Vasc Surg 1997;25:803-809.

Towne JB, Delbert D, Smith J: Thrombosis of the internal carotid artery following blunt cervical trauma. Arch Surg 1972;104:565-568.

Townsend R, Colella J, Diamond D: Traumatic rupture of the aorta: Critical decisions for trauma surgeons. J Trauma 1990;30:1169-1174.

Traber D: Nitric oxide synthase and tissue injury. Shock 2000;14:243-244.

Trask A, Richards F, Schwartzbach C, Kurtzke R: Massive orthopedic, vascular, and soft tissue wounds from military type assault weapons: A case report. J Trauma 1995;30:1169-1174.

Travers B, Cooper A: On wounds and ligature of veins. Surgical Essays (Lond) 1818;1:243.

Treiman G, Yellin AE, Weaver FA, et al: Examination of a patient with a knee dislocation: The case for selective angiography. Arch Surg 1992;127:1056-1063.

Treiman R, Doty D, Gaspar MR: Acute vascular trauma: A fifteen year study. Am Surg 1966;111:469-473.

Trent M, Parsonnet V, Shoenfeld R: A balloon expandable-intravascular stent for obliterating aortic dissection. J Vasc Surg 1990;11:707-717.

Tribble C, Crosby I: Traumatic rupture of the thoracic aorta. South Med J 1988;81:963-968.

Trimble C: Arterial bullet embolism following thoracic gunshot wounds. Ann Surg 1968;168:911-916.

Trinkle JK, Marcos J, Grover FL, Cuello L: Management of the wounded heart. Ann Thorac Surg 1974;38:181-182.

Trinkle JK, Toon R, Franz J, et al: Affairs of the wounded heart: Penetrating cardiac wounds. J Trauma 1979;19:467-472.

Trinkle JK: Penetrating heart wounds: Difficulty in evaluating clinical series (editorial). Ann Thorac Surg 1984;38:181-182.

Trueblood H, Wuerflein R, Angell WW: Blunt trauma rupture of the heart. Ann Surg 1973;177:66-69.

Trunkey DD, Blaisdell FW: Abdominal vascular injuries. West J Med 1975;123:321-324.

Trunkey DD: Trauma: Accidental and intentional injuries account for more years of life loss in the U.S. than cancer and heart disease. Among the prescribed remedies are improved prevention efforts, speedier surgery and further research. Sci Am 1983;249:28-35.

Tse D, Slabaugh P, Carlson P: Injury to the axillary artery by a closed fracture of the clavicle. J Bone Joint Surg 1980;62:1372-1373.

Tuffier M: Contemporary French surgery. Br J Surg 1915;3:100-112.

Turner G: Gunshot wounds of the heart. War Medicine, a Symposium. In Pingh WS (ed): Podolsky Edward, 1942.

Turney SZ, Attar S, Ayella R, et al: Traumatic rupture of the aorta: A five-year experience. J Thorac Cardiovasc Surg 1976;72:727-734.

Turney SZ, Attar S, Ayella R, et al: Is arteriography necessary in the management of vascular trauma of the extremities? Surgery 1978;84:557-562.

Turney SZ, Rodriguez A, Attar S: Repair of traumatic thoracic aortic rupture: Risk factors of paraplegia. J Cardiovasc Surg 1990;31:107.

Turpin I, State D, Schwartz A: Injuries to the inferior vena cava and their management. Am J Surg 1977;134:25-34.

Tuzeo S, Saad S, Hastings O, Swan KG: Management of brachial artery injuries. Surg Gynec Obstet 1978;146:21-24.

Tyburski JG, Wilson RF, Dente C, et al: Factors affecting mortality rates in patients with abdominal vascular injuries. J Trauma 2001;50:1020-1026.

Uhlmann D, Uhlmann S, Spiegel H: Endothelin/nitric oxide balance influences hepatic ischemia-reperfusion injury. J Cardiovasc Pharmacol 2000;36:S212-S214.

Ulflacker R, Saadi J: Transcatheter embolization of superior mesenteric arteriovenous fistula. AJR Am J Roentgenol 1982;139:1212.

Ulvestad L: Repair of laceration of superior mesenteric artery acquired by nonpenetrating injury to the abdomen. Ann Surg 1954;140:752-754.

Utley J, Singer M, Roe B, et al: Definitive management of innominate artery hemorrhage complicating tracheostomy. JAMA 1972;220:577-579.

Valle A: War injuries of heart and mediastinum. Arch Surg 1955;70:398-404.

Van De Wal H, Draaisma J, Vincent J, Goris R: Rupture of the supradiaphragmatic inferior vena cava by blunt decelerating trauma: Case report. J Trauma 1990;30:111-113.

Van Gilder J, Coxe W: Shotgun Pellet embolus of the middle cerebral artery. Neurosurgery 1970;32:711-714.

van Leeuwen J, Broos P, Rommens P, Nevelsteen A: Combined blunt rupture of the diaphragm and the thoracic artery. Injury 1990;21:117-119.

Van Niekerk J, Heijstraten F, Goris R, et al: Spinal cord injury following surgery for acute traumatic rupture of the thoracic aorta. Thorac Cardiovasc Surg 1986;34:30-34.

Van Way C: Intrathoracic and intravascular migratory foreign bodies. Surg Clin North Am 1989;69:125-133.

Varner J, Oliver R: Superior mesenteric arteriovenous fistula. Ann Surg 1969;170:862.

Vasko J, Raess D, Williams TE Jr: Non-penetrating trauma to the thoracic aorta. Surgery 1977;82:400-406.

Vaughan G, Mattox KL, Feliciano DV, et al: Surgical experience with expanded polytetrafluorethylene (PTFE) as a replacement graft for traumatized vessels. J Trauma 1979;19:403-408.

Vauthey J, Maddern G, Balsiger D, et al: Superselective embolization of superior gluteal artery pseudoaneurysms following intramuscular injection: Case report. J Trauma 1991;31:1174.

Veith F, Gupta S, Daly V: Technique for occluding the supraceliac aorta through the abdomen. Surg Gynec Obstet 1980;151:426-428.

Veith F, Ascer E, Gupta S, Wengerter K: Lateral approach to the popliteal artery. J Vasc Surg 1987;6:119.

Verdant A, Mercier C, Page A, et al: Major mediastinal vascular injuries. Can J Surg 1983;26:38-42.

Verdant A, Cossette R, Dontigny L, et al: Acute and chronic traumatic aneurysms of the descending thoracic aorta: A 10-year experience with a single method of aortic shunting. J Trauma 1985;25:601-607.

Verdant A: Major mediastinal vessel injury: An underestimated lesion. Can J Surg 1987;30:402-404.

Verdant A: Traumatic rupture of the thoracic aorta. Ann Thorac Surg 1990;49:686-687.

Veterans Administration Cooperative Study Group 141: Comparative evaluation of prosthetic, reversed, and in situ vein bypass grafts in distal popliteal and tibioperoneal revascularization. Arch Surg 1988;123:434-438.

Vignon P, Gueret P, Vedrinne J, et al: Role to transesophageal echocardiography in the diagnosis and management of traumatic aortic disruption. Circulation 1995;92:2959-2968.

Vij D, Simoni E, Smith R: Resuscitative thoracotomy for patients with traumatic injury. Surgery 1983;94:554-561.

Vincent K, Blair WF: A false aneurysm of the ulnar artery after a forearm compartment syndrome. Orthopedics 1984;7:1834-1836.

Visser P, Hermreck A, Pierce G, et al: Prognosis of nerve injuries incurred during acute trauma to peripheral arteries. Am J Surg 1980;140:596-599.

Vitale G, Richardson JD, George SM Jr, Miller F: Fasciotomy for severe, blunt, and penetrating trauma of the extremity. Surg Gynecol Obstet 1988;166:397-401.

Vitelli C, Scalea T, Phillips T, et al: A technique for controlling injuries of the iliac vein in the patient with trauma. Surg Gynecol Obstet 1988;166:551-552.

Vollmar J, Krumhaar D: Surgical experience with 200 traumatic arteriovenous fistulae. In Hiertonn T, Rybeck B (eds): Traumatic Arterial Lesions. Stockholm, Försvarets Forskningsanstalt, 1968.

Vollmar J: Surgical experience with 197 traumatic arterial lesions (1953-66). In Hiertonn T, Rybeck B (eds): Traumatic Arterial Lesions. Stockholm, Försvarets Forskningsanstalt, 1968.

Vollmar J: Knochenbruch und Gefässverletzung. Langenbecks Arch Chir 2001;339:473-477.

von Horoch C: Die Gefässnaht. Allg Wien Med Ztg 1888;33:263-279.

von Oppell U, Beningfield SJ, Odel J, Reichart B: Cardiac rupture caused by blunt trauma as well as false angiographic aortic rupture: A case report. S Afr Med J 1988;74:519-520.

von Oppell U, Dunne T, DeGroot M, Zilla P: Traumatic aortic rupture: Twenty year metaanalysis of mortality and risk of paraplegia. Ann Thorac Surg 1994;58:585-593.

Von Zoege-Manteuffel: Demonstration eines Präparates von aneurysma arteriosovenosum ossificans der art femoralis profunda. Verhandl Deutsch Gesellsch Chir 1895;24:167-170.

Vorwerk D, Günther R, Wendt G: Chronic aortoiliac dissection treated by self-expanding stent placement. Cardiovasc Intervent Radiol 1995;18:43.

Vosloo S, Reichart B: Inflow occlusion in the surgical management of a penetrating aortic arch injury: Case report. J Trauma 1990;30:514-515.

Waddell J, Lenczer E: Arterial injury associated with skeletal trauma. Injury 1974;6:28-32.

Waddell W, Vogelfanger I, Prudhomme P, et al: Venous valve transplantation. Arch Surg 1964;88:5-15.

Wagner W, Calkins E, Weaver FA: Blunt popliteal artery trauma: 100 consecutive cases injuries. J Vasc Surg 1988;7:736-748.

Wagner W, Calkins E, Weaver FA, et al: Blunt popliteal artery trauma: One hundred consecutive injures. J Vasc Surg 1988;5:736-743.

Wagner W, Yellin AE, Weaver FA, et al: Acute treatment of penetrating popliteal artery trauma: The importance of soft tissue injury. Ann Vasc Surg 1994;8:557-565.

Waibel P, Ludin H: Unusual sources for peripheral arterial embolization: A case report. Arch Surg 1966;92:105-106.

Waigand J, Uhlich F, Gross C: Percutaneous treatment of pseudoaneurysms and arteriovenous fistulas after invasive vascular procedures. Catheter Cardiovasc Interv 1999;47:157-164.

Walden R, Lynn M, Golan M, Garniek A: Plastic bullet arterial embolization following gunshot injury to the heart: Case report and review of the literature. J Cardiovasc Surg 1990;31:482-485.

Walker A, Walker R: Traumatic thrombosis of the aorta. Br Med J 1961;5238:1514.

Walker M, Poindexter J, Stovall I: Principles of management of shotgun wounds. Surg Gynecol Obstet 1990;170:97-106.

Walker P, Dake M, Mitchell R, Miller D: The use of endovascular techniques for the treatment of complications of aortic dissection. J Vasc Surg 1993;18:1042-1051.

Walker T, Geller S, Brewster DC: Transcatheter occlusion of a profunda femoral artery pseudoaneurysm using thrombin. AJR Am J Roentgenol 1987;149:185-186.

Walker W, Pate J: Medical management of acute traumatic rupture of the aorta. Ann Thorac Surg 1990;50:965-967.

Walker W, Cooley DA, Duncan J, et al: The management of aortoduodenal fistula by in situ replacement of the infected abdominal aortic graft. Ann Surg 1987;205:727-732.

Wall MJ Jr, Pape PE, Martin RR, et al: Immediate versus delayed fluid resuscitation for hypotensive patients with penetrating torso injuries. N Engl J Med 1994;331:1105-1109.

Wall MJ Jr, Granchi T, Liscum K, Mattox KL: Penetrating thoracic vascular injuries. Surg Clin North Am 1996;76:749-761.

Wallenhaupt S, Huspeth A, Mills S, et al: Current treatment of traumatic aortic disruptions. Am Surg 1989;55:316-320.

Waller B, Girod D, Dillion J: Transverse aortic wall in infants after balloon angioplasty for aortic valve stenosis: Relation of aortic wall damage to diameter of inflated angioplasty balloon and aortic lumen in seven necropsy cases. J Am Coll Cardio 1984;4:1235-1241.

Walls J, Curtis J, Boley T: Sarns centrifugal pump for repair of thoracic aortic injury: Case report. J Trauma 1989;29:1283-1285.

Walls J, Boley TM, Curtis J, Schmaltz R: Experience with four surgical techniques to repair traumatic aortic pseudoaneurysm. J Thorac Cardiovasc Surg 1993;106:283-287.

Walsh J, Meyer JP, Rosenbloom M: Production and treatment of mechanically induced arterial vasospasm in a rabbit model. Surg Fo 1987;38:313-314.

Wand J, Zuckerman J: Delayed rupture of false aneurysm following a femoral fracture. J Bone Joint Surg 1989;71B:700.

Wang N, Sparks S, Bailey LL: Staged repair using omentum for posttraumatic aortoesophageal fistula. Ann Thorac Surg 1994;58:557-559.

Wang P, Singh G, Rana M, et al: Preheparinization improves organ function after hemorrhage and resuscitation. Am J Physiol 1990;259:R645-R650.

Wang P, Ba ZF, Chaudry IH: Endothelial cell dysfunction occurs after hemorrhage in nonheparinized but not in preheparinized models. J Surg Res 1993;54:499-506.

Wang P, Tait S, Ba ZF, Chaudry IH: ATP-MgCl2 administration normalizes macrophage cAMP and beta-adrenergic receptors after Hhemorrhage and resuscitation. J Physiol 1994;267:G52-G58.

Wang P, Ba ZF, Chaudry IH: Chemically modified heparin improves hepatocellular function, cardiac output, and microcirculation after trauma: Hemorrhage and resuscitation. Surgery 1994;116:169-175.

Wang P, Ba ZF, Chaudry IH: Nitric oxide. To block or enhance its production during sepsis? Arch Surg 1994;129:1137-1142.

Wang P, Ba ZF, Chaudry IH: ATP-MgCl2 restores depressed endothelial cell function after hemorrhagic shock and resuscitation. Am J Physiol 1995;268:H1390-H1396.

Wang P, Ba ZF, Chaudry IH: Endothelium-dependent relaxation is depressed at the macro- and microcirculatory levels during sepsis. Am J Physiol 1995;269:R988-R994.

Wang P, Ba ZF, Stepp K, Chaudry IH: Pentoxifylline attenuates the depressed endothelial cell function and vascular muscle contractility following trauma and hemorrhagic shock. J Trauma 1995;39:121-126.

Wang P, Ba ZF, Reich S, et al: Effects of nonanticoagulant heparin on cardiovascular and hepatocellular function after hemorrhagic shock. Am J Physiol 1996;270:H1294-H1302.

Wang P, Ba ZF, Cioffi W, et al: Salutary effects of ATP-MgCl₂ on the depressed endothelium-dependent relaxation during hyperdynamic sepsis. Crit Care Med 1999;27:959-964.

Ward P, Suzuki A: Gunshot wound of the heart with peripheral embolization. J Thorac Cardiovasc Surg 1974;68:440.

Warren R: Report to the Surgeon General. Washington, DC, Department of the Army, 1952.

Warren R, Akins CW, Conn A, et al: Acute traumatic disruption of the thoracic aorta: Emergency department management. Ann Emerg Med 1992;21:391-396.

Warrian R, Shoenut J, Iannicello C, et al: Seatbelt injury to the abdominal aorta. J Trauma 1988;28:1505-1507.

Wascher R, Gwinn B: Air rifle pellet injury to the heart with retrograde caval migration. J Trauma 1995;38:379-381.

Watson W, Silverstone S: Ligature of the common carotid artery in cancer of head and neck. Ann Surg 1939;109:1-27.

Waxman K, Soliman M, Braunstein P, et al: Diagnosis of traumatic cardiac contusion. Arch Surg 1986;121:689-692.

Waxman K: Shock: Ischemia, reperfusion, and inflammation. New Horiz 1996;4:153-160.

Weaver FA, Rosenthal R, Waterhouse G, Adkins RB: Combined skeletal and vascular injuries of the lower extremities. Am Surg 1984;50:189-197.

Weaver FA, Yellin AE, Wagner W, et al: The role of arterial reconstruction in penetrating carotid injuries. Arch Surg 1988;123:1106-1111.

Weaver FA, Suda R, Stiles G, Yellin AE: Injuries to the ascending aorta, aortic arch and great vessels. Surg Gynecol Obstet 1989;169:27-31.

Weaver FA, Yellin AE, Bauer MAP, et al: Is arterial proximity a valid indication for arteriography in penetrating extremity trauma? A perspective analysis. Arch Surg 1990;125:1256-1260.

Weber T, Dent T, Lindenaur S: Viable vein graft preservation. J Surg Res 1975;18:247-255.

Wei J, Chang C, Chang Y: Traumatic sinus of Valsalva fistula. Ann Thorac Surg 1991;52:852-854.

Weiland A, Robinson H, Futrell J: External stabilization of a replanted upper extremity: Case report. J Trauma 1976;16:239-241.

Weimann S, San Nicolo M, Sandbichler P, et al: Civilian popliteal artery trauma. J Cardiovasc Surg 1987;28:145-151.

Weinstein M, Golding A: Temporary external shunt bypass in the traumatically amputated upper extremity. J Trauma 1975;15:912-915.

Weisberg D, Goetz R: Necrosis of arterial wall following application of methyl-2-cyanoacrylate. Surg Gynecol Obstet 1964;119:1248.

Weiser M, Gibbs S, Valeri C, et al: Anti-selectin therapy modifies skeletal muscle ischemia and reperfusion injury. Shock 1996;5:402-407.

Weiss J, Bernadine HB, Hutchins G, Mason S: Two-dimensional echocardiography recognition of myocardial injury in man: Comparison with postmortem studies. Circulation 1981;63:401-408.

Welborn MJ, Sas J: Acute abdominal aortic occlusion due to nonpenetrating trauma. Am J Surg 1969;118:112-116.

Welling R, Kakkasseril J, Cranley J: Complete dislocations of the knee with popliteal vascular injury. J Trauma 1981;21:450-453.

Welling R, Kremchek T, Rath R, et al: Blunt arterial injuries associated with multiple trauma. Ann Vasc Surg 1989;3:345-350.

Werne C, Sagraves S, Costa C: Mitral and tricuspid valve rupture from blunt trauma sustained during a motor vehicle collision. J Trauma 1989;29:113-115.

Wernly J, Campbell C, Replogle R: Traumatic avulsion of the innominate and left carotid arteries. J Thorac Cardiovasc Surg 1982;84:392-397.

Wexler L, Silverman J: Traumatic rupture of the innominate artery: A seat belt injury. N Engl J Med 1970;282:1186-1187.

Whelan TJ, Baugh JH: Non-Atherosclerotic Arterial Lesions and Their Management: Current Problems in Surgery. Chicago, Year Book Medical Publishers, 1967.

White GH, White RA, Kopchok G, Wilson SE: Angioscopic thromboembolectomy: Preliminary observations with a recent technique. J Vasc Surg 1988;7:318-325.

White GH, White RA, Kopchok G: Endoscopic intravascular surgery removes intraluminal flaps, dissections and thrombus. J Vasc Surg 1990;11:280-299.

White J: Shark attack in Natal. Injury 1975;6:187-197.

White J, Talbert J, Haller JA Jr: Peripheral arterial injury in infants and children. Ann Surg 1968;167:757-766.

Whitehouse W, Coran A, Stanley JC: Pediatric vascular trauma. Arch Surg 1976;111:1269-1275.

Whitesides T, Haney T, Morimoto K: Tissue pressure measurement as a determinant for the need for fasciotomy. Clin Orthop 1975;113:43-51.

Whitman G, McCroskey B, Moore EE, et al: Traumatic popliteal and trifurcation vascular injuries: Determinants of functional limb salvage. Am J Surg 1987;154:681-684.

Wholey M, Bocher J: Angiography in musculoskeletal trauma. Surg Gynecol Obstet 1967;125:730-736.

Wholey M, Bocher J: Angiographic features of aortic and peripheral arterial trauma. Arch Surg 1968;97:68-74.

Whye D, Barish R, Alquist T, et al: Echocardiographic diagnosis of acute pericardial affusion in penetrating chest trauma. Am J Emerg Med 1988;6:21-23.

Wiechert R, Hewitt RL: Injuries to the vena cava: Report of 35 cases. J Trauma 1970;10:649-657.

Wiedeman J, Mills J, Robison JG: Special problems after iatrogenic vascular injuries. Surg Gynecol Obstet 1988;166:323-326.

Wiencek R, Wilson R: Abdominal venous injuries. J Trauma 1986;26:771-778.

Wiencek R, Wilson R: Injuries to the abdominal vascular system: How much does aggressive resuscitation and prelaparotomy really help. Surgery 1987;102:731-736.

Wiener I, Flye M: Traumatic false aneurysm of the vertebral artery. J Trauma 1984;24:346-349.

Wigle R, Morgan J: Spontaneous healing of a traumatic thoracic aortic tear: Case report. J Trauma 1991;31:280-283.

Wildegans H: Verletzungen der aorta. Deutsch Med Wchnschr 1926;52:1810-1812.

Williams C, Brenowitz JB: Sequential aortic and inferior caval clamping for control of suprarenal vena caval injuries: Case report. J Trauma 1977;17:164-167.

Williams C, Robinson D: Traumatic abdominal aorta-inferior vena cava fistula with immediate repair. Ann Surg 1961;154:998-1000.

Williams D: Stab wound of the heart and pericardium-recovery-patient alive three years afterward. Medical Record 1897;51:437-439.

Williams D: Embolization of a bullet to the posterior tibial artery following a gunshot wound of the thorax. J Trauma 1964;4:258-265.

Williams D, Brothers T, Messina L: Relief of mesenteric ischemia in type III aortic dissection with percutaneous fenestration of aortic septum. Radiology 1990;171:450-452.

Williams G: Peripheral vascular trauma: Report of 90 cases. Am J Surg 1968;116:725-730.

Williams G, Crumpler J, Campbell G: Effect of sympathectomy on the severely traumatized artery. Arch Surg 1970;101:704-707.

Williams J, Silver D, Laws H: Successful management of heart rupture from blunt trauma. J Trauma 1981;21:534-537.

Williams J, Graff J, Uku JM, Steinig J: Aortic injury in vehicular trauma. Ann Thorac Surg 1994;57:726-730.

Williams J, Sherman R: Penetrating wounds of the neck: Surgical management. J Trauma 1973;13:435-442.

Williams T, Knopp R, Ellyson J: Compartment syndrome after anti-shock trouser use without lower extremity trauma. J Trauma 1982;22:595-597.

Wilson C: Aortic bypass graft in a child. Am J Surg 1974;128:797-798.

Wilson J: Fracture of the pelvis complicated by ischemia of the lower limb. J Bone Joint Surg 1952;34-B:68-69.

Wilson L: Dispersion of bullet energy in relation to wound effects. Milit Surg 1921;49:241-251.

Wilson R, Bassett JS: Penetrating wounds of the pericardium or its contents. JAMA 1966;195:513-518.

Wilson R, Arbulu A, Basset JS: Acute mediastinal widening following blunt chest trauma: Critical decisions. Arch Surg 1972;104:551-558.

Wilson R, Wiencek R, Balog M: Predicting and preventing infection after abdominal vascular injuries. J Trauma 1989;29:1371-1375.

Wilson R, Wiencek R, Balog M: Factors affecting mortality rate with iliac vein injuries. J Trauma 1990;30:320-323.

Wilson SE, Veith F, Hobson RW II, Williams R: Noninvasive Diagnosis of Venous Obstruction and Insuficency. New York, McGraw-Hill, 1987.

Wilson S, Au FC: In extreme use of a Foley catheter in a cardiac stab wound. J Trauma 1986;26:400-402.

Wind G, Finley R, Rich NM: Three-dimensional computer graphic modeling of ballistic injuries. J Trauma 1988;28:S16-S20.

Wiser E, Cheek R, Britt L: Gunshot wounds of the suprarenal abdominal aorta. Am Surg 1976;42:430-435.

Witte C, Smith C: Single anastomosis vein bypass for subclavian vein obstruction. Arch Surg 1966;93:664-666.

Wixon C, Philpott J, Bogey WM, Powell C: Duplex-directed thrombin injection as a method to treat femoral artery pseudoaneurysms. J Am Coll Surg 1998;187:464-466.

Wolf R, Berry RE: Transaxillary intra-aortic balloon tamponade in trauma. J Vasc Surg 1986;4:95-97.

Wolf Y, Reyna T, Schropp K, Harmel R: Arterial trauma of the upper extremity in children. J Trauma 1990;30:903-905.

Wolfel G, Moore EE, Cogbill TH: Severe thoracic and abdominal injuries associated with lap-harness seatbelts. J Trauma 1984;24:166-167.

Wood J, Fabian TC, Mangiante E: Penetrating neck injuries: recommendations for selective management. J Trauma 1989;29:602-605.

Wood M, Nykamp P: Traumatic arteriovenous fistula of the superior mesenteric vessels. J Trauma 1980;20:378.

Woodhall B, Nulsen F: Peripheral nerve wounds. In Bowers WF (ed): Surgery of Trauma. Philadelphia, JB Lippincott Co, 1953.

Woodhurst W, Robertson W, Thompson G: Carotid injury due to intraoral trauma: Case report and review of the literature. Neurosurgery 1980;6:559-563.

Woodring J, Fried A, Hatfield D, et al: Fractures of first and second ribs: Predictive value for arterial and bronchial injury. AJR Am J Roentgenol 1982;138:211-215.

Woodruff C: The cases of the explosive effect of modern small caliber bullets. N Y J Med 1898;67:593.

Woodson G, Kendrick B: Laryngeal paralysis as the presenting sign of aortic trauma. Arch Otol Head Neck Surg 1989;115:1100-1102.

Woolsey R: Aortic laceration after anterior spinal fusion. Surg Neurol 1986;25:267-268.

Wright CB, Swan KG: Hemodynamics of venous occlusion in the canine hindlimb. Surgery 1973;73:141-146.

Wright CB, Swan KG: Hemodynamics of venous repair in the canine hind limb. J Thorac Cardiovasc Surg 1973;65:195-199.

Wright CB, Hobson R: Hemodynamic effects of femoral occlusion in the subhuman primate. Surgery 1974;75:453-460.

Wright CB, Hobson RW II, Swan KG, Rich NM: Extremity venous ligation: Clinical and hemodynamic correlation. Am Surg 1975;41:203-208.

Wright CB, Hobson RW II: Prediction of intestinal viability using Doppler ultrasound techniques. Am J Surg 1975;129:642-645.

Wright CB, Hobson RW II, Giordano J, et al: Acute femoral venous occlusion: Management by segmental venous replacement. J Cardiovasc Surg 1977;18:523-529.

Wright CB, Hiratzka L, Hobson RW II, et al: Management of vena caval injuries: The Vietnam Vascular Registry review. J Cardiovasc Surg 1981;22:203-212.

Wright R, Edwards W: Manifestations and management of acute arterial injuries. J Trauma 1973;463-468.

Wyatt D, Kellum CD, Joob A, Daniel T: Isolated injury of the proximal vertebral artery associated with blunt chest trauma. J Vasc Surg 1986;4:196-198.

Yajko R, Trimble C: Arterial bullet embolism following abdominal gunshot wounds. J Trauma 1974;14:200-211.

Yamada S, Kindt G, Youmans J: Carotid artery occlusion due to nonpenetrating trauma. J Trauma 1967;7:333-342.

Yamada T, Sato H, Seki M, et al: Successful salvage of aortoesophageal fistula caused by a fish bone. Ann Thorac Surg 1996;61:1843-1845.

Yamaguchi Y, Matsumura F, Liang J, et al: Neutrophil elastase and oxygen radicals enhance monocyte chemoattractant protein-expression after ischemia/reperfusion in rat liver. Transplantation 1999;68:1459-1468.

Yao JST, Vanecko RM, Printen K, Shoemaker WC: Penetrating wounds of the heart: A review of 80 cases. Ann Surg 1968;168:67-78.

Yao J, Suri R, Patt N, et al: An unusual subclavian artery injury. J Trauma 1970;10:176-180.

Yarbrough DR III, Grooms G, Flint L: Repair of two traumatic aneurysms of the supraceliac abdominal aorta in a single patient. Surgery 1972;72:371-377.

Yaw P, Van Beek A, Glover JL: Successful repair of a gunshot wound to the first part of the superior mesenteric artery. J Trauma 1974;14:885.

Yeager RA, Hobson RW II, Lynch TG, et al: Popliteal and infrapopliteal arterial injuries: Differential management and amputation rates. Am Surg 1984;50:155-158.

Yee L, Olcott E, Knudson M, Lim RC Jr: Extraluminal, transluminal, and observational treatment for vertebral artery injuries. J Trauma 1995;39:480-486.

Yellin A, Golan M, Klein E: Penetrating thoracic wounds caused by plastic bullets. Thorac Cardiovasc Surg 1992;2:381.

Yellin AE, Shore E: Surgical management of arterial occlusion following percutaneous femoral angiography. Surgery 1973;73:772-777.

Yellin AE, Lundell C, Finck E: Diagnosis and control of post-traumatic pelvic hemorrhage. Arch Surg 1983;118:1378-1388.

Yelon J, Scalea T: Venous injuries of the lower extremities and pelvis: Repair versus ligation. J Trauma 1992;33:532-538.

Yelon J, Barrett L, Evans J: Distal innominate artery transection and cervical spine injury. J Trauma 1995;39:590-592.

Yeo M, Domanskis E, Bartlett RH, Gazzaniga A: Penetrating injuries of the abdominal aorta. Arch Surg 1974;108:839-844.

Yoder R, Merck D: Innocuous appearing stab wounds to the neck: Is exploration always indicated? South Med J 1969;62:113-114.

Yoshioka H, Seibel R, Pillai K, Luchette F: Shotgun wounds and pellet emboli: Case reports and review of the literature. J Trauma 1995;39:596-601.

Yosowitz P, Hobson RW II, Rich NM: Iliac vein laceration caused by blunt trauma to the pelvis. Am J Surg 1972;124:91-93.

Youkey J, Clagett GP, Rich NM, et al: Vascular trauma secondary to diagnostic and therapeutic procedures: 1974 through 1982. Am J Surg 1983;146:788-791.

Young J, Stallone R, Iverson L, et al: Surgical management of traumatic disruption of the descending aorta. West J Med 1989;150:662-664.

Young P: Following microdiskectomy: Laceration of the abdominal aorta and vena cava. IMJ 1988;174:93-94.

Zabin A: Cholecystectomy complicated by hemorrhage from the inferior vena cava. N Y J Med 1950;50:1500.

Zakharia AT: Cardiovascular and thoracic battle injuries in the Lebanon war. J Thorac Cardiovasc Surg 1985;89:723.

Zakharia A: Thoracic battle injuries in the Lebanon war: Review of the early operative approach in 1,992 patients. Ann Thorac Surg 1985;3:209-213.

Zehnder M: Delayed posttraumatic rupture of the aorta in a young healthy individual after closed injury: Mechanical-etiological considerations. Angiology 1956;7:252.

Zehntner MK, Petropoulos P, Burch HB: Arterial injuries associated with fractures of the extremities. Proc of the First Mediterranean Congress of Angiology 1988;223-226.

Zeiger M, Clark DE, Morton JR: Reappraisal of surgical treatment of traumatic transection of the thoracic aorta. J Cardiovasc Surg 1990;31:607-610.

Zelenock G, Kazmers A, Whitehouse W: Extracranial internal carotid artery dissections. Arch Surg 1982;117:425-432.

Zelenock G, Kazmers A, Graham L, et al: Nonpenetrating subclavian artery injuries. Arch Surg 1985;120:685-692.

Zellweger R, Ayala A, Zhu X, et al: A novel nonanticoagulant heparin improves splenocyte and peritoneal macrophage immune function after trauma: Hemorrhage and resuscitation. J Surg Res 1995;59:211-218.

Zhou M, Wang P, Chaudry IH: Endothelial nitric oxide synthase is downregulated during hyperdynamic sepsis. Biochim Biophys Acta 1997;1335:182-190.

Zilkha A: Traumatic occlusion of the internal carotid artery. Radiology 1970;97:543-548.

Ziperman H: Acute arterial injuries in the Korean War: A statistical study. Ann Surg 1954;139:1-8.

Zuckerman J, Flugstad D, Teitz C, King H: Axillary artery injury as a complication of proximal humeral fractures. Clin Orthop 1984;189:234-237.

Zweifach S, Hargens A, Evans K, et al: Skeletal muscle necrosis in pressurized compartments associated with hemorrhagic hypotension. J Trauma 1980;20:941-947.

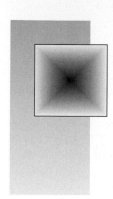

INDEX